HANDBOOK of
Institutional
Pharmacy
Practice

4TH EDITION

Thomas R. Brown, MS, Pharm.D., FASHP
Professor Emeritus
School of Pharmacy
University of Mississippi
Oxford, Mississippi

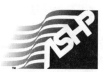

American Society of Health-System Pharmacists®
Bethesda, Maryland

Any correspondence regarding this publication should be sent to the publisher, American Society of Health-System Pharmacists®, 7272 Wisconsin Avenue, Bethesda, MD 20814, attn: Special Publishing. Produced in conjunction with the ASHP Publications Production Center.

The information presented herein reflects the opinions of the authors and contributors. It should not be interpreted as an official policy of ASHP or as an endorsement of any product.

Drug information and its applications are constantly evolving because of ongoing research and clinical experience and are often subject to professional judgment and interpretation by the practitioner and to the uniqueness of a clinical situation.

The authors, contributors, and ASHP have made every effort to ensure the accuracy and completeness of the information presented in this book. However, the reader is advised that the publisher, authors, contributors, and reviewers cannot be responsible for the continued currency or accuracy of the information, for any errors or omissions, and/or for any consequences arising from the use of the information in the clinical setting.

The reader is cautioned that ASHP makes no representation, guarantee, or warranty, express or implied, that the use of the information contained in this book will prevent problems with insurers and will bear no responsibility or liability for the results or consequences of its use.

Director of Acquisitions: Cynthia Conner
Acquisitions Editor: Hal Pollard
Senior Editorial Project Manager: Dana A. Battaglia
Project Editor: Kristin C. Eckles
Cover and page design: DeVall Advertising

ASHP is the 30,000-member national professional association representing pharmacists who practice in hospitals and health systems. ASHP members practice across the continuum of care, including acute care, long-term care, home care, and ambulatory care. ASHP believes the mission of pharmacists is to help people make the best use of medicines. For more information about ASHP or ASHP products, call ASHP Customer Service at 301-657-4383 or browse our website at www.ashp.org.

ASHP® is a service mark of the American Society of Health-System Pharmacists, Inc.; registered in the U.S. Patent and Trademark Office.

ISBN: 1-58528-114-x

Dedication

To Bonnie
"It's been great!"

Table of Contents

Foreword

America's health care services system has changed dramatically over the course of the past 40 years. A plethora of entitlements funded through federal and state funding formulas, expansion of health benefits through employers, program-specific coverage for diseases such as AIDS and end-stage kidney disease, and the list continues. Simultaneously, several scientific revolutions have occurred to bring improvements in preventive, trauma, acute, restorative, and behavioral care. Utilization of the services embedded in the health care services system rose right along with the expenditures necessary to finance the providers and organizations that rendered the care. In response to increased utilization and costs, we witnessed the formation of Health Maintenance Organizations, managed care, hospital mergers, and a variety of other "experiments" to keep these variables in check.

Pharmacists, pharmacies, and pharmaceuticals were important pieces of the ever-changing landscape created by the revolutions. These integral components of the infrastructure of our health care services system went through revolutionary periods of their own, most often as a result of the changes occurring in the macrosystem. The preparatory education of pharmacists was dramatically changed, mail order pharmacies appeared, innovative chemical and biological agents were discovered, and a host of other changes appeared. Change became the constant to which pharmacists in all practice settings had to adapt. And the revolution continues.

Pharmacy practice in hospitals and health systems has witnessed profound and dynamic changes over these past decades. Moving away from large-scale and bulk manufacturing and taking responsibility and accountability for drug therapy regimens represents just one such area of change. Presently, embracing automated systems for handling the logistics issues in the hospital or health system is coupled with a strong emphasis on quality and safety in care services. Pharmacists in hospitals and health systems are being privileged in a number of institutions to carry out largely autonomous care functions such as managing antithrombotic clinics and following up with organ transplant patients. And the development of the electronic medical record, managing large databases of integrated data, and information and electronic application of point-of-care verification systems are the present applications and evolutions being seen in a number of institutions and pharmacy practice sites as a result of the "electronic revolution."

Since its first introduction in 1979, the *Handbook of Institutional Pharmacy Practice* has guided students and practitioners alike in understanding and preparing for practice in the institutional environment. This new and revised version continues in the same tradition while also capturing the issues and areas of hospital and health-system practice that have changed substantially over the course of the last several decades. New topics that reflect current and forecasted directions are also captured in this volume.

Some have said that the 21st century may be the century of pharmacy and pharmacists because, indeed, pharmacists in hospitals and health systems have appeared on the ever-widening radar screen. JCAHO Standards and the National Patient Safety Goals call upon pharmacists to be at the point of prospective decision making regarding drug therapy. The National Quality Forum underscores that a best practice in the care of patients includes having a pharmacist on the patient care team. Numerous studies and literature citations point to the cost benefit and safety enhancements associated with collaborative patient care that engages a pharmacist. Editor Tom Brown and the array of authors used in the preparation of the chapters in the current edition address these trends, opportunities, and challenges.

Reading this 4th edition in conjunction with staying current with the *American Journal of Health-System Pharmacy* and the *ASHP Best Practices for Hospital and Health-System Pharmacy* will provide a solid base of literature that is descriptive and proscriptive for pharmacists' services in hospitals and health systems. This text will also serve to be a useful resource for those occasional issues and questions that arise during the course of practice and discussion with pharmacy colleagues and other health professionals. It will be a "go to" reference.

Tom Brown and his nationally renowned colleagues have selected the right topics, have written about them in an authoritative fashion, and have constructed a well-integrated overview of the various elements of pharmacy practice in the complex tapestry of our health care system. The reader is encouraged to take it in with pause and reflection, knowing that the current content serves as the starter yeast for the next batch of change, challenge, and frontier.

Henri R. Manasse, Jr., Ph.D., Sc.D.
Executive Vice President and Chief Executive Officer

July 7, 2005

Preface

It hardly seems possible that 26 years have passed since the initial edition of the *Handbook of Institutional Pharmacy Practice* was published. Dr. Mickey Smith and I began considering the first effort about 3 years prior to publication, thus we approach 30 years since the initial idea was conceived. The first edition was based upon a statement of competencies required of hospital pharmacists, which had been adopted and published by the American Society of Health-System Pharmacists (ASHP). Although this statement of competencies no longer exists as a published entity, its effects and other such statements and positions fostered by ASHP in *Best Practices for Health-System Pharmacy* have profoundly affected the contents of this edition and the practice of pharmacy over time. ASHP has for many decades guided the practice of pharmacy through the development and publication of standards as useful tools for practice.

This edition, like its predecessors, is "designed for both student and practitioner." In retrospect, there are significant changes that have occurred between the publication of the first and fourth editions. Certainly, technological advances in computer utilization and automation have had a tremendous impact on many, if not most, of the elements of pharmacy practice. Home care, managed care, hospice and palliative care along with ambulatory care and long-term care have undergone significant changes; federal law and regulations as well as accreditation standards have dictated many of these changes. There has been considerably more emphasis on medication safety in all institutional settings and formal methods to ensure this safety are noticeably changed. Practice settings have become a much more formalized setting for pharmacy education as well, which has likely improved both.

It is my sincere wish that this book "be equal to the task of providing the student with a thorough grounding in institutional pharmacy and providing the practitioner with a ready reference to use in addressing any problem in practice." If I have learned anything as an educator, practitioner, and editor it certainly includes the inability of a single individual to do justice to the ever changing profession that is pharmacy in one publication. To research, even with guidance from experts, every aspect of the profession and enlist the services of worthy expert authors is more than a daunting task, it is a highly unlikely occurrence.

The reader of this text is urged to go beyond the material as well as the topics covered in this book to ensure their adequacy for practice-specific issues, "Read it, study it, and by all means go beyond it." The Editor wholeheartedly endorses the utility of *Best Practices for Health-System Pharmacy* as the gold standard for practice-related issues.

I have been asked many times by students, practitioners, and young educators in pharmacy, what areas do I need to focus on in pursuing my career, should it be the cardiovascular drugs, those to treat diabetes, asthma, just where should I invest much of my time in skill development for practice? My response is uniform that it is a given that you must be proficient in the aforementioned areas and many others. I strongly urge each individual to develop their communication skills. Without the ability to write and speak effectively, our knowledge and ability to aid in patient care will be silenced.

Thomas R. Brown, Editor

Acknowledgments

A publication of this magnitude cannot be accomplished by one individual; anyone who attempts to make such an investment of time and effort should know that before they begin. Although the editorial work is challenging, the authors of each chapter are ultimately responsible for the success of a reference text. Therefore, I owe a large debt of gratitude to those who contributed their expertise to the wide variety of topics which are included in this text. There is no question that pharmacy is blessed with many talented individuals who contribute by sharing their expertise through its literature and thus assure the viability of a dynamic profession.

At the outset of this edition, an editorial board was established who offered considerable assistance in the development of the book particularly in the development of topic areas, organization of those areas, and recommending authors for specific topics. These individuals were very important in the initial development and I am deeply grateful to each of them for their assistance. They are Paul Abramowitz, Wayne Conrad, Harold Godwin, Cliff Hynniman, John Murphy, Phil Schneider, and Bill Smith.

Without the assistance of ASHP and their staff it is doubtful that the book would have been completed. Cynthia Conner first contacted me early in 2004 and encouraged me to begin work on this edition with the belief that it could be published in time for the Midyear Clinical Meeting in 2005; I had serious doubts and quietly I think she did as well. With her encouragement and gentle prodding the book began to come together and eventually we both believed it was possible to complete by late 2005. As work continued into the serious editing phase, Dana Battaglia became the pivotal ASHP figure in getting over the difficult hurdles. Our almost daily e-mails kept the chapters moving through the process; she has been a joy to work with and a very positive influence on this work. I am extremely grateful to Cynthia, Dana, Kristin Eckles, and others at ASHP who diligently worked to achieve our mutual goals.

For over 35 years, I have had the pleasure of participating in academic endeavors as a faculty member of the University of Mississippi School of Pharmacy. I have learned a great deal from the students I have taught and my colleagues have been extraordinarily important to my professional development. I will ever be indebted to "Ole Miss."

Personally, I am grateful each day for my family. My wife, Bonnie, is always encouraging and our sons, Dennis and Jeff, pharmacist and physician, have made us both very proud. My sincere thanks to my family for the support I have received over many years and I continue to be blessed each day. On July 4, 1939, Lou Gehrig, the great NY Yankee slugger, said that he considered himself the "luckiest man on the face of the earth." On a smaller scale, I know how he felt.

Thomas R. Brown, Editor

Contributors

Kenneth N. Barker, Ph.D., R.Ph.
Director
Center for Pharmacy Operations and Designs
Sterling Professor
Harrison School of Pharmacy
Auburn University
Auburn University, Alabama

Christina Martin Barnett, Pharm.D.
Associate Director of Academic Affairs
Professional Compounding Centers of America (PCCA)
Houston, Texas

Gus Bassani, Pharm.D.
Manager
Product Development
Professional Compounding Centers of American (PCCA)
Houston, Texas

Peter A. Bauer, Pharm.D.
Geriatric Pharmacy Practice Resident
Department of Veterans Affairs Medical Center
Idaho State University College of Pharmacy
Boise, Idaho

Ilisa B.G. Bernstein, Pharm.D., JD
Senior Advisor for Regulatory Policy
Office of the Commissioner/Office of Policy
U.S. Food and Drug Administration
Rockville, Maryland

Cynthia Brennan, Pharm.D., MHA
Assistant Director
Ambulatory Pharmacy
Harborview Medical Center Pharmacy
Clinical Professor
University of Washington School of Pharmacy
Seattle, Washington

E. Clyde Buchanan, MS, FASHP
Pharmacy Consultant
Retired Director of Pharmacy
Visiting Clinical Professor
Mercer University Southern School of Pharmacy
Atlanta, Georgia

Robert A. Buerki, Ph.D., R.Ph.
Professor
Division of Pharmacy Practice and Administration
The Ohio State University College of Pharmacy
Columbus, Ohio

Paul W. Bush, Pharm.D., MBA, FASHP
Director
Pharmacy Services
MUSC Medical Center
Clinical Associate Dean & Associate Professor
South Carolina College of Pharmacy–MUSC Campus
Charleston, South Carolina

Jannet M. Carmichael, Pharm.D., FCCP, BCPS
VISN 21 PBM Manager
VA Sierra Pacific Network
Reno, Nevada

Barry L. Carter, Pharm.D., FCCP, FAHA, BCPS
Professor
Division of Clinical and Administrative Pharmacy
College of Pharmacy and Department of Family Medicine
Roy J. and Lucille A Carver College of Medicine
University of Iowa
Iowa City, Iowa

Bruce W. Chaffee, Pharm.D.
Clinical Pharmacist and Clinical Associate Professor
Department and College of Pharmacy
The University of Michigan Health System
Ann Arbor, Michigan

Kathy A. Chase, Pharm.D.
National Project Manager
Pharmacy Consulting
Cardinal Health
Prairie Village, Kansas

Daniel J. Cobaugh, Pharm.D., FAACT, DABAT
Director of Research
ASHP Research and Education Foundation
Bethesda, Maryland

Charles P. Coe, BS Pharm., R.Ph.
President
Eagle Rx Health-System Pharmacy Services
Spring, Texas

Wayne F. Conrad, BS, Pharm.D., FASHP
Professor and Chair
Division of Pharmacy Practice
University of Cincinnati College of Pharmacy
Cincinnati, Ohio

Rowell Daniels, Pharm.D., MS
Clinical Assistant Professor
UNC School of Pharmacy
Associate Director
Department of Pharmacy
UNC Hospitals and Clinics
Chapel Hill, North Carolina

George J. Dydek, Pharm.D., BCPS, FASHP
Director
Department of Pharmacy
Madigan Army Medical Center
Tacoma, Washington

Fred M. Eckel, M.Sc., FAAAS, FASHP
Professor of Pharmacy
University of North Carolina at Chapel Hill
Executive Director
North Carolina Association of Pharmacists
Chapel Hill, North Carolina

Stephen F. Eckel, Pharm.D., BCPS
Assistant Director of Pharmacy
University of North Carolina Hospitals
Chapel Hill, North Carolina

Elizabeth A. Flynn, Ph.D., R.Ph.
Associate Research Professor
Center for Pharmacy Operations and Designs
Auburn University
Auburn, Alabama

Karl F. Gumpper, R.Ph., BCNSP, BCPS, FASHP
Director of Pharmacy
Pharmacy Practice Residency Director
Children's National Medical Center
Washington, DC

Rusty Hailey, Pharm.D., D.Ph., MBA
Chief Pharmacy Officer and Senior Vice President
Pharmacy Services
Coventry Health Care, Inc.
Executive Vice President
Coventry Prescription Management Services, Inc.
Franklin, Tennessee

Bruce G. Hancock, R.Ph., MS
Director
Pharm.D. Experiential Programs
College of Pharmacy & Health Sciences
Butler University
Indianapolis, Indiana

Michael D. Hogue, Pharm.D.
Assistant Professor of Pharmacy Practice
Samford University
McWhorter School of Pharmacy
Birmingham, Alabama

Stephen K. Huffines, Pharm.D.
Associate Director
Pharmacy
Vanderbilt University Medical Center
Nashville, Tennessee

William N. Jones, MS
Pharmacy Program Manager for Clinical Services
Southern Arizona VA Health Care System
Tucson, Arizona
Associate Clinical Professor of Pharmacy Practice
  and Science
The College of Pharmacy
The University of Arizona
Tucson, Arizona

Sandra G. Jue, Pharm.D., FASHP
Clinical Pharmacy Teaching Coordinator
Veterans Affairs Medical Center
Boise, Idaho
Clinical Professor of Pharmacy Practice
Idaho State University
College of Pharmacy
Pocatello, Idaho

Laurence A. Kennedy, Ph.D.
Associate Professor of Pharmacy Administration
College of Pharmacy & Health Sciences
Butler University
College of Pharmacy and Health Science
Indianapolis, Indiana

James R. Knight, D.Ph., MS, FASHP
Director of Pharmaceutical Services
Vanderbilt University Medical Center
Nashville, Tennessee

Contributors, continued

David A. Kvancz, MS, R.Ph., FASHP
Chief Pharmacy Officer
The Cleveland Clinic Foundation
Department of Pharmacy
The Cleveland Clinic
Cleveland, Ohio

William Letendre, MS, R.Ph., MBA
Vice President
Pharmacy Management Department
Professional Compounding Centers of America (PCCA)
Houston, Texas

Scott M. Mark, Pharm.D., MS, M.Ed., FACHE, FASHP,
  FABC
Director of Pharmacy
Director, Pharmacy Management Residency Program
University of Pittsburgh Medical Center
Assistant Professor
University of Pittsburgh School of Pharmacy
Pittsburgh, Pennsylvania

Barb J. Mason-Kennedy, Pharm.D., FASHP
Professor and Vice Chair
College of Pharmacy
Idaho State University
Ambulatory Care Pharmacist
Home Health Care Consultant
Boise VA Medical Center
Boise, Idaho

Scott R. McCreadie, Pharm.D., MBA
Strategic Projects Coordinator and Clinical Assistant Professor
Department and College of Pharmacy
The University of Michigan Health System
Ann Arbor, Michigan

Thomas J. McGinnis, R.Ph.
Director of Pharmacy Affairs
U.S. Food and Drug Administration
Rockville, Maryland

Mary Lynn McPherson, Pharm.D., BCPS, CDE
Professor
University of Maryland School of Pharmacy
Baltimore, Maryland

Michelle C. Mercado, Pharm.D.
Clinical Specialist
Medication Safety and Quality Assurance
Department of Pharmacy
Children's National Medical Center
Washington, DC

Jessica L. Milchak, Pharm.D, BCPS
Pharmacy Practice Specialist
Division of Clinical and Administrative Pharmacy
College of Pharmacy
University of Iowa
Iowa City, Iowa

William A. Miller, M.Sc., Pharm.D., FCCP, FASHP
Professor
Division of Clinical and Administrative Pharmacy
College of Pharmacy
University of Iowa
Iowa City, Iowa

Jerrod Milton, R.Ph.
Chief Pharmacist
Director, Campus Transition & Occupancy
The Children's Hospital
Denver, Colorado

Mary R. Monk-Tutor, Ph.D., MS, R.Ph., FASHP
Director of Academic Programs
Associate Professor of Pharmacy Administration
Department of Pharmaceutical, Social, and Administrative
  Sciences
McWhorter School of Pharmacy
Samford University
Birmingham, Alabama

John E. Murphy, Pharm.D., FASHP, FCCP
Professor, Department Head and Associate Dean
The University of Arizona College of Pharmacy
Tucson, Arizona

Robert Navarro, Pharm.D.
Executive Advisory Group
Campbell Alliance
Raleigh, North Carolina

Francis B. Palumbo, Ph.D., JD
Executive Director & Professor
University of Maryland School of Pharmacy
Center on Drugs & Public Policy
Baltimore, Maryland

Renee Remmert Prescott, Pharm.D.
Director of Online Education
Continuing Education Administrator
Professional Compounding Centers of America (PCCA)
Houston, Texas

Carriann E. Richey, BS, Pharm.D.
Assistant Professor of Pharmacy Practice
Director of Postgraduate Education
Butler University College of Pharmacy & Health Sciences
Indianapolis, Indiana

S. Trent Rosenbloom, MD, MPH
Assistant Professor
Department of Biomedical Informatics
Assistant Professor, School of Nursing
Internal Medicine and Pediatrics
Vanderbilt University Medical Center
Nashville, Tennessee

Steve Rough, MS, R.Ph.
Director of Pharmacy
University of Wisconsin Hospital and Clinics
Madison, Wisconsin

Philip J. Schneider, MS, FASHP
Clinical Professor
Director of the Latiolais Leadership Program
Division of Pharmacy Practice and Administration
College of Pharmacy
The Ohio State University
Columbus, Ohio

Cindy C. Selzer, Pharm.D., BCPS
Clinical Pharmacist
Indiana University Hospital
Assistant Professor of Pharmacy Practice
Butler University College of Pharmacy and Health Sciences
Indianapolis, Indiana

Mickey C. Smith, Ph. D.
Barnard Distinguished Professor of Pharmacy Administration,
    Management, and Marketing, Emeritus
School of Pharmacy
University of Mississippi
Oxford, Mississippi

Suellyn J. Sorensen, Pharm.D., BCPS
Clinical Pharmacist, Infectious Diseases
Clinical Pharmacy Manager
Indiana University Hospital
Indianapolis, Indiana

James G. Stevenson, Pharm.D., FASHP
Director of Pharmacy Services
University of Michigan Hospitals and Health Centers
Professor and Associate Dean for Clinical Sciences
University of Michigan College of Pharmacy
Ann Arbor, Michigan

C. Richard Talley
Editor, *AJHP*
Assistant Vice President of Pharmacy Publishing
Publications and Drug Information Systems Office
American Society of Health-System Pharmacists
Bethesda, Maryland

Jack Temple, Pharm.D.
Administrative Resident
Clinical Instructor
University of Wisconsin Hospital and Clinics
Madison, Wisconsin

Kasey K. Thompson, Pharm.D.
Director, Practice Standards and Quality Division
Director, Patient Safety
American Society of Health-System Pharmacists
Bethesda, Maryland

David J. Tomich, Pharm.D., FASHP
Clinical Coordinator
Department of Pharmacy
Madigan Army Medical Center
Tacoma, Washington

John P. Uselton, BS, R.Ph.
Vice President, Operations Improvement
The Pharmacy Management Business of Cardinal Health
Houston, Texas

Louis D. Vottero, MS
Professor Emeritus, Pharmacy
Ohio Northern University College of Pharmacy
Ada, Ohio

Contributors, continued

Andrew L. Wilson, Pharm.D., FASHP
Chief, Department of Pharmacy
National Institutes of Health Clinical Center
Bethesda, Maryland

Karol G. Wollenburg, R.Ph., MS
Vice President and Apothecary-in-Chief
New York-Presbyterian Hospital
New York, New York

William A. Zellmer, MPH
Deputy Executive Vice President
American Society of Health-System Pharmacists
Bethesda, Maryland

Chapter 1

Health Systems: An Overview

Bruce G. Hancock, Laurence A. Kennedy, Carriann E. Richey

Introduction

Hot topics of discussion regarding health care today include the costs of care, the uninsured, rural access to care, and the role of technology. Reviewing the history and current structure of our health care system affords us the opportunity to put today's health care challenges in perspective and prepare for future advances. First, we recognize that our system is primarily market driven, that is without government regulation and price or salary controls. Second, we consider that physician salaries and prescription drug costs are amongst the highest in the world. Administration of the complex system bears its own significant costs. For those individuals with private insurance, premiums are 21% of the national median household income.[1] Some may argue that our health care system is not a system at all. According to a recent RAND Corporation study, Americans received only 50–60% of the recommended care.[2]

Based on current ranking by the World Health Organization, the U.S. fails to top the list.[3] Reasons for this include a shorter life expectancy at birth, higher infant mortality, no universal coverage and a less well-developed health care system. We spend more per capita on health care than other industrialized countries, and health care expenditures are the highest share of gross domestic product (15%).[4] And yet we do not produce the best results as measured by the health status of our population. We don't have the most technologically intensive system nor the most hospital admissions or services used per capita.

In the article, "Health Care in the United States—Is it the Best in the World?," the author discusses how other health care systems control the supply and specialty mix of health care professions.[3] Notably practice areas in the U.S. with more specialty providers have improved health outcomes; however, this improvement is not proportional either to the number of specialists or their cost. In all countries surveyed, a need was demonstrated for systems originally designed for acute care and infection control to now manage long-term chronic disease. It was this author's opinion that no

country has created an effective system for this type of care. The reasons included poor coordination of care, poor communication between health care practitioners and patients, management of errors, and polypharmacy. In countries with national health care systems, the supply of physicians, technologies and facilities are barriers to access, whereas in the United States the cost of care and lack of coverage are the major barriers. Hospitals and providers must constantly balance the latest technology, clinical practice, medical knowledge, and research.

The U.S. health care system may be best categorized as a set of subsystems. These subsystems serve different segments of the population and may be completely inclusive or may overlap with others. Depending on the population, the subsystem may be funded publicly or privately and these patients may or may not use the same facilities. This chapter will look vertically through each subsystem and evaluate how care is accessed, delivered, utilized, and reimbursed. For each section key terminology will be introduced along with application to the current structure.

Definitions

Access—Access to health care refers to being able to get the care you need from a suitable source in a timely manner. Access is a function of two main factors, existence of adequate numbers of appropriate facilities and providers in your area, and the ability to obtain care. In the United States this means that you must be able to pay for care through your own resources, be covered by health insurance, be covered by a government program such as Medicaid or Medicare, or be able to obtain care as a veteran. Those without funding may be able to obtain care at a public hospital that is funded through tax dollars to provide care for the indigent. The wait for such care is usually long and the care lacks the amenities that other patients may receive. According to the Census Bureau, about 45 million (14%) Americans do not have health insurance coverage from any of the sources named above. About 11% of children (8.4 million) are uninsured. Access is a complicated topic varying as a function of geographic location, race, and rates of uncompensated care offered by providers.

Diagnostic Related Groups (DRG)—Refers to the classification of hospital case types according to the resources that will be necessary to treat a patient with a given diagnosis. The use of DRGs allows third party payers a convenient method of deciding what treatment, length of stay, and consequently the human resources a patient with a given diagnosis will require. Based on that information they can decide the amount that is reasonable to pay providers for treatment of the case. For example, the third party determines the cost of treating the typical uncomplicated broken leg. They will then pay the health care provider what the insurance company deems is an appropriate amount. A compound fracture that requires greater expenditure of resources due to a lengthy hospital stay would fall into a separate diagnostic related group and the reimbursement payment would be greater. If complications (comorbidities) develop during the treatment of a routine illness (e.g., an infection develops) the patient's care enters a new DRG classification and providers are paid accordingly. Because hospitals lose money when they provide more care than a given DRG will pay, the incentive is for hospitals to provide efficient care and discharge patients as soon as is reasonably possible.

Distribution—Refers to the distribution of hospitals, physicians, and ancillary health care in proportion to the area population. During recent decades the government has encouraged equitable distribution of these resources through financial incentives to students to practice in a given geographic area of need upon graduation. The government has also offered capitation funds to schools encouraging the education of a greater number of students. Additionally, as health insurance organizations changed from fee for service to prospective reimbursement, the lucrative hospital market became competitive and many hospitals were forced to close their doors. This phenomenon forced a more equitable distribution of acute care facilities. The distribution of the type of health care facilities in an area may also be significant.

Delivery—The methods, mechanisms, and conditions under which care is provided to patients.

E-Prescribing—Refers to the use of electronic media to improve efficiency, efficacy, and safety of patient care. Prescriptions are entered by physicians electronically. This results in a legible order that is less likely to be misread. The physician has a choice of wired and wireless devices to use, including pocket PC, smartphone, palm devices, and web-based browser. System suppliers such as RxNT also supply software that provides a comprehensive drug database, patient medication history, patient drug and food allergy screen, drug interaction screen, formulary reference, and frequently prescribed drug and directions list. Automated care and reminders, work flow management, and other features are also available.

Health Care Facilities—Refers to the assortment of facilities that provide care for patients:

1. *Acute care* hospitals provide care for serious illnesses that require the continuous and ongoing attention of physicians, nurses, pharmacists, and ancillary health care providers. Emergency care, surgery, intensive care, and routine care are provided here. Hospital pharmacists monitor care, provide expertise to other professionals, and provide medications for use.

2. *Long-term care* facilities may be used to provide care to patients after discharge from the acute care hospital. In this case the patient does not need the diagnostic tests or level of care required in the hospital; however, nursing care is available to support the patient through short or lengthy periods of recuperation. The number of nursing homes and level of care provided have increased significantly as a result of third party requirements for rapid discharge of patients from hospitals.

3. *Immediate care* centers provide the type of care a patient would receive at the physician's office but have extended hours of operation and do not require an appointment.

Health Literacy—"The capacity of an individual to obtain, interpret and understand basic health information and services in ways that are health-enhancing."[5] Some patients are illiterate, uneducated, or unfamiliar with basic concepts of anatomy, medicine, and medication; reluctant to ask questions of the health care provider for fear of looking ignorant; or are simply intellectually impaired. When interacting with our patients it is important to ascertain their level of understanding and give special attention to those that are most in need.

Interdisciplinary—Refers to health care provided with more than one or several disciplines contributing to the care of a patient. This can include physicians of differing specialties, pharmacists, nurses, physical therapists, nutrition experts, and others. Each discipline contributes their expertise to the development of the overall diagnostic and treatment plan for a given patient.

Managed Care—Refers to medical care that is managed by the payer (third party) with the purpose of holding down unnecessary costs. This approach provides good quality of care at minimal cost. The intent is that health care dollars go further, thus enabling the same dollars to provide care to more people or simply reducing the total health care bill for that insured group.

Multidisciplinary—Refers to health care providers working independently to provide patient care.

National Health Care—Denotes a system of health care in which the government provides care for all of its citizens. Care is paid from tax revenue. Many nations employ such systems, the United States does not. Ideally the system would provide excellent and timely care for all citizens when needed. In reality there are typically long waits for care and, on occasion, denial of certain categories of care for specific classes of persons (e.g., the elderly). Wealthy citizens often opt to pay for faster and perhaps better quality care by going outside of the system.

Price—In general terms, "the amount of money needed to purchase something" in today's complicated health care market, pricing cannot follow the simple pricing rules of typical goods and services.[6] Additionally, the health care market itself has changed dramatically over the last three decades and continues to evolve. Under the fee for service system, a physician, pharmacist, or hospital was free to set prices and bill insurance companies for services provided. The incentive was to provide as much care (prescriptions, lab tests, radiology studies, etc.) to a given patient as reasonable because you would be paid a reasonable price for whatever services you provided. There was also an incentive to purchase and possess the latest in technology as this was a measure of the quality of care in the eyes of public and providers alike. Patients felt they were well-cared for. Under the various third party schemes of more recent times, the payers set the price and the provider either accepts the terms of the particular plan or does not do business with that third party. In pharmacy, prices are set so low that many chain retail pharmacies consider the prescription area itself to be a loss leader. In other words, an area of the business that produces little if any revenue but serves as a method of bringing customers into the business so that they will make other purchases.

Reimbursement—Strictly speaking, refers to paying back for services rendered. For our purpose it refers to the method that a third party uses to pay a provider for delivery of care and the amount of payment provided.

1. *Reimbursement plans* include fee for service systems under which the provider simply bills the third party for service and is paid whatever amount is billed.

2. *Managed care organizations (MCOs)* such as Health Maintenance Organizations (HMOs). In this type of organization a provider is typically paid a fixed amount per month to provide all of the care that a patient needs. If the patient needs more care than the "average patient" used as a reference, the provider may lose money caring for that patient. Other patients, however will require less care than the average; on those patients the provider makes money. Reimbursement rates here must be carefully set through actuarial study to assure that the provider receives a fair income but that the HMO does not pay excessive amounts. The incentive to a provider is to provide as little care as possible that is consistent with good patient care and to keep patients healthy so that they will need less care. Another type of MCO is the preferred provider organization (PPO). Here, providers agree to provide care to a PPO's patients at discounted prices. In other words, a procedure that would ordinarily result in a $100 charge will be provided for a charge of $75. As a result, the PPO and, consequently, the employer and patient save money. The provider receives the benefit of having an adequate number of patients to care for. Patients may experience the disadvantage of not being able to utilize the physician that they would most prefer because that physician has not elected to be a provider associated with that PPO plan.

3. *Cost plus*, also known as *retrospective reimbursement* refers to reimbursement by a third party for all allowable costs resulting from the care of a patient; additionally a reasonable amount above cost is paid. Under this system there is no incentive to reduce costs or operate efficiently.

4. *Prospective reimbursement* refers to reimbursement plans where fixed reimbursement amounts are set in advance by the third party payer. These are based on such criteria as diagnostic related groups as defined above. The incentive for providers is to minimize cost while meeting the standards of good patient care.

Utilization—Refers to the use of health care services and/or goods. The term includes both appropriate and inappropriate use of facilities, personnel, and health care goods. Inappropriate use of health care facilities and personnel would include seeing a physician when not necessary or utilization of an emergency department for nonemergent care. Managed care organizations are very concerned with inappropriate use of care because of the resulting waste of resources. Most MCOs will exclude certain types of inappropriate care from coverage. Coverage for the misuse of emergency department facilities is a typical example of care that might be excluded if not essential based on the patient's symptoms and diagnosis.

Utilization Review—Referred to as monitoring the appropriateness of usage or delivery of health care services. Multidisciplinary utilization review boards are established by third parties, by hospitals, and by state governments to oversee various aspects of health care consumption including acute care length of stay, treatments ordered, and medication (drug utilization review board). Utilization management is intended to provide adequate care yet keep cost of care minimal. Prospective reviews determine the appropriateness of care before care is delivered to the patient. Concurrent utilization review may be used to monitor a specific patient to assure an appropriate but not excessive length of stay. Retrospective reviews may focus on a specific patient's care to review for possible over billing or may evaluate a class of patients to determine treatment strategies resulting in greater cost containment for future use.

Background

Historical Overview of the U.S. Health Care System and Evolution of Care Services

The first health care provided in the colonial U.S. was provided by family, friends, and those in the community with some knowledge of *healing*. Care was provided in the home, no hospitals and few physicians existed.[7]

At a later date, during the 1600s, almshouses and poorhouses existed in Europe. These institutions provided food and domicile to the poor, orphans, unemployed, elderly, and mentally handicapped. Some of these persons were ill and some were not. They also served to quarantine citizens with contagious disease. "Medical care, if provided at all, was of secondary importance. In essence, the earliest U.S. hospitals were the infirmaries of poorhouses."[7]

Voluntary hospitals funded by charitable people or local governments were not established until the late 1700s and early 1800s.[7] These hospitals provided the best institutional care available at the time, but still they treated relatively few patients.[7] This changed during the late 1800s and early 1900s with new technologies and a better understand of cleanliness and hygien.[7]

Health Care from the Civil War to the Early 1900s

Wars usually bring about advancements in health care. The Civil War was no exception. Hospitals now became the places of healing. Henceforth, whatever technology was available was to be found in the hospital. The advent of anesthetics and cleanliness meant that successful surgery became a reality. After the Civil War, medical education became increasingly formalized and defined. The American Medical Association (AMA) was founded in 1847. But in spite of these changes, undoubtedly owing to the shortage of formally trained physicians, anyone could still practice medicine.[8] In keeping with new capabilities in medicine and a growing need to be able to afford them, in 1850 the first bodily injury insurance plan was offered in the U.S. In 1866 the first health insurance policies were offered.[9]

Between 1900 and 1910, membership in the AMA rose from 8,000 to 70,000 physicians, making the AMA a powerful, professional, and political force in the U.S.[8] Because of the remote and dangerous work involved in these occupations, railroads and logging companies lead the way in the provision of care by offering health care to their employees.

- *The 1910s*—In 1910 the Western Clinic in Tacoma, Washington, offered a prepaid health plan, (a forerunner of the HMO concept).[9] U.S. hospitals have become modern, clean, scientific institutions, utilizing antiseptics and anesthetics.[8] During this period, The Flexner Report was published, defining the model for medical education used to this day. Because of the uniformity in medical education there is a greater unity and consequently political power in the medical profession.[8]

- *The 1920s*—General Motors signs a contract with Metropolitan Life to insure 180,000 workers.[8]

- *The 1930s*—In 1933, hospitals created Blue Cross, the first structured pooled financing mechanism. These plans are limited to coverage of hospital services only.[8,9] Physicians then offer Blue Shield which covers payments to physicians. Some employers begin to provide health benefits to their workers.[8] "A few employers rely on and some even create group practices (e.g., Kaiser, Ross-Loos), which are the early health maintenance organizations (HMOs)."[8]

- *The 1940s*—Wage and price controls enacted during World War II lead employers to offer health benefits to employees as a recruitment tool. These benefits did not fall under the control of wage freezes. This more than any other event led to the widespread and commonly accepted provision of health insurance by employers in the U.S.

- *The 1950s*—During the 1950s, significant advances in medical technology and surgical procedures and medication led to the beginning of spiraling health care costs. In 1950, the nation spent 4.5% of the Gross National Product (GNP) on health care.[8]

- *The 1960s*—The amount of health insurance offered by employers continued to grow as employees came to expect it as part of a benefits package. What differs is the fact that the economy is not as strong and health care prices are rising. The cost of providing insurance begins to be a burden for employers. From 1965 to 1970, Congress enacts two programs to provide health care coverage to citizens. The first is Medicare (for those over 65). The second is the joint federal and state-funded Medicaid programs (for the economically disadvantaged).[8,9] By late 1969, a substantial majority of Americans are covered by some form of public or private coverage. Government policymakers are becoming aware that actual Medicare and Medicaid spending is exceeding the original projections by a fair margin."[8,9] The nation spent 5.3% of GNP (gross national product currently called gross domestic product) on health care in 1969.[9]

- *The 1970s*—"By the end of the decade, 80% of the population is covered by third-party public and private insurance. Forty-two percent of those individuals are covered by federal government programs (i.e., Medicare, Medicaid, and CHAMPUS)."[8] Health care insurers come up with numerous new plans in an attempt to keep cost down but retain the quality of care.

- *The 1980s*—Due to efforts of third party providers, the length of stay of patients or "hospital bed days" begins to drop. In addition, mental health patients are now rarely institutionalized, and much patient care is now offered on an outpatient rather than inpatient basis. Long-term care facilities begin to care for large numbers of patients that do not need continued hospital stays.[8] In the past, some or all of the bills for indigent patients were paid by cost shifting. Vigilant managed care providers no longer allow the "fat" previously allowed in billing that paid for those without coverage.[8]

- *The 1990s*—In spite of efforts to hold down costs, the national health care expenditure reaches 12.2% of GNP.[9] The rate of rise is double the rate of inflation.[8] Employers make a concerted effort to get out of the health care insurance issue by discontinuing insurance benefits, or by covering employees but not families, or by decreasing coverage while increasing copays and deductibles. As a result, 43% of the uninsured in 1998 were in families in which at least one person worked full-time all year. Three-quarters of uninsured workers are never offered insurance by their employer. Those earning low wages are less likely to be offered insurance by their employer according to the Census Bureau's Current Population Survey.

- *The 2000s*—The number and percentage of Americans who are uninsured increased in 2001 and 2002, after falling the previous 2 years.[10] From 2000 to 2002, the number of nonelderly people who were uninsured increased from 39.4 million to 43.3 million, or from 16.1% of the nonelderly population to 17.3%.[11,12]

Attempts at National Health Care

Through the decades many groups have presented arguments for a National Health Care System. The Government has discussed and made some attempts to establish some meaningful aspects of a National Health Care System. An overview of events is best described by the historic timeline presented below:

- *The 1900s*—Not surprisingly, when compared to the older nations of Europe, America is far behind these nations in assuring access to health care for citizens.[13]

- *The 1910s*—In an attempt to protect laborers, the American Association for Labor Legislation organized a conference to discuss "social insurance."[13] Reform seems to be moving forward but opposing voices, such as physicians, stall the progress. In 1917, the First World War diverts attention away from domestic matters.[13]

- *The 1930s*—During the Great Depression, the nation's attention once again begins to turn to domestic matters, and the Social Security Act is passed but does not contain provisions for the still controversial health care insurance.[13]

- *The 1940s*—"President Roosevelt asks Congress for an 'economic bill of rights,' including the right to adequate medical care."[13] President Truman proposes a National Health Insurance Plan that would cover all citizens. This plan is defeated by special interest groups such as the AMA and Americans fearful of the new perceived threat of communism.[13]

- *The 1950s*—"Many legislative proposals are made for different approaches to hospital insurance, but none succeed."[13]

- *The 1960s*—President Lyndon Johnson, as part of his plan for the Great Society proposes Medicare and Medicaid. When these laws providing only partial coverage become law, supporters of National Health Insurance for all begin to feel that the public, feeling that something meaningful had been done, will loose interest in the issue.[13]

- *The 1970s*—President Nixon's plan for national health insurance is rejected by both liberals and labor unions alike. Health care costs continue to rise due to a combination of social and technological reasons. The health care system is seen as being "in crisis."[13]

- *The 1980s*—In an effort to control costs, President Reagan institutes Diagnostic Related Groups (DRG) for Medicare payment. Private insurance, seeing the cost saving of this mechanism, is quick to adopt the system for widespread use.[13]

- *The 1990s*—With health care costs rising at double the rate of inflation, insurance companies employ managed care to hold down costs. No health care bills are passed by congress. "By the end of the decade there are 44 million Americans, 16% of the nation, with no health insurance at all."[13]

- *The 2000s*—With the cost of health care continuing to rise and the base of young taxpayers shrinking in proportion to those qualifying for Medicare, it is becoming more difficult to fund a national health care system. No meaningful solutions have yet been offered by the Government.[13]

Health Care Statistics

- *Number of Practicing Pharmacists and Projected Need*—According to the Bureau of Labor Statistics (BLS), in 2002 there were 230,000 pharmacists working in the field. Sixty-two percent worked in community pharmacies, and 22% worked in hospital pharmacies. The remainder "works in clinics, mail-order pharmacies, pharmaceutical wholesale, home health agencies, or the Federal Government."[14] BLS projections indicate the demand for pharmacists is expected to exceed supply through 2012. This is due to changes in demographics resulting in a growing number of elderly persons in our society. Even though the number of students enrolled in pharmacy schools has recently increased, the shortage of practitioners is expected to remain through at least 2012.[14]

- *Number of Prescriptions Issued per Year*—The number of prescriptions written continues to increase yearly. The main reasons for the increases are an increasing elderly population and many new medications entering the market. The number of prescriptions written has increased from 2 billion in 1993 to 3.4 billion in 2003. This represents an increase of 70% even although the population itself has increased only 13%. The number of prescriptions per capita per year increased from 7.8 to 11.8 during a given year. Obviously, a specific patient may only take a given prescription for a few days and have periods during the year where they take none at all. Other patients may take several prescriptions throughout the year.[15,16]

- *Number of Physicians*—There are about 745,000 physicians in the United States at this time. For many years the AMA stated that the number of physicians and number being trained were adequate. In recent times, there have been increasing numbers of predictions that we face a growing shortage of physicians. Recent predictions estimate a shortfall of as many as 85,000 to 200,000 physicians by the year 2020.[17] Recommendations are that 3,000 to 27,000 additional physicians be trained yearly.[17,18] Currently, the number of applications to medical schools is down from 42,806 in 1993 to 34,785 in 2003.[17] But the most significant problem seems not to be the number of physicians but the mix and distribution.[18,19] "In every other developed country, 50% to 70% of the physicians are generalists. In the United States, however, the proportion of generalists (family physicians general internists, and general pediatricians) has declined from 42% in 1965 to less than 30% today."[19] It is easy to see the dynamics behind this situation. Physicians may choose their specialty over general practice for a variety of reasons, but one is the striking difference in earnings between a family practice, pediatrics, or internal medicine physicians (~$152,000) and an anesthesiologist, general surgeon, or OBGYN physician ($234,000–$307,000). These differences in earning also drive up the cost of health care if indeed a general practitioner could have provided the same care for less.[20] In addition, as has always been the case, physicians prefer to live in urban and suburban settings rather than rural settings and their earnings are substantially higher there as well. As a result there are significant shortages of primary care physicians in rural areas, especially in Public Health Region IV. Region IV is composed of states with vast rural regions: AL, FL, GA, KY, MS, NC, SC, and TN.[21]

Public Perceptions of the Health Care System

An authoritative document assessing the status and perceptions of Americans living, using and experiencing our health care system presents some sobering facts of consequence for citizens, politicians, and health care provider's alike.[22] This study found that life under the U.S. health care system presents few problems for those in the upper income classes. They are able to obtain and pay for the very best in physicians, medications, equipment, and facilities that our country offers. About 20% of Americans think the system works pretty well. For those in lower income brackets life can be a

very different experience leading to serious heath and financial problems. These problems often affect the middle income class as well. In fact, the research shows that even the upper income classes are worried that the troubles experienced by others may extend to them as well.[22]

Access to Health Care

Distribution of Health Care Personnel

Since the mid-1990s, the first reports of pharmacist shortages were recognized. It has been widely reported in the popular media that the shortage of pharmacists and other selected health care professionals continues. Surveys by both the National Association of Chain Drug Stores (NACDS) and the American Society of Health-System Pharmacists (ASHP) have focused attention on specific areas of need.[23] The surveys indicate a number of factors have contributed to the shortage of pharmacists. These include the following:

- Increased utilization of health care facilities
- Increased prescription volumes
- Decreased ability to increase the supply of pharmacists
- Regional shifts of pharmacists
- Increased percentage of female pharmacists

There does appear to be data to support the fact that filling positions in community pharmacy settings is less difficult than institutional settings. Current trends indicate that more states improved their shortage status, but the overall system still shows signs of inadequate supply.

The greatest concern related to shortage is in the institutional practice setting. A May, 2003 survey of hospital pharmacy directors by ASHP showed a 5–6% vacancy rate.[24] A similar survey in 2004, reported a vacancy rate average of 5%, a downward trend from 8.9% in 2000. Smaller hospitals have the greatest challenge in securing pharmacists. Particularly hard-hit are institutions with fewer than 100 beds, which report higher vacancy and staff turnover rates when compared to larger institutions. In facilities with 1 to 99 beds, the turnover rate was 12.5%, compared with 5.4% in facilities with 400 or more beds. The fact that small hospitals make up approximately 44% of all hospitals nationwide compounds the situation.[25] It stands to reason that rural areas will be more affected by these shortages.

A variety of solutions have been proposed to improve the shortage situations as it directly relates to institutional practice:

- Establish more competitive salary and benefit packages as compared to community practice settings
- Create innovative approaches to grants for loans for students interested in institutional practice
- Increase admissions to pharmacy schools
- Increase number of pharmacy schools
- Broaden recruitment strategies
- Provide job-sharing/shift-sharing

Based on current surveys, results would indicate that in most areas of the United States the shortage situation is improving as of 2005.[24]

Distribution of Facilities

Rural access to health care presents a unique blend of challenges as compared to urban areas. As previously noted, the shortage of pharmacists is more pronounced in smaller, rural institutions. With respect to specific patient demographics for the rural setting, the following contribute to problems in accessing health care[26]:

- Less educated
- More disabled
- More elderly
- More chronic disease states
- More frequently uninsured
- Decreased access to health care facilities and to providers
- Higher incidence of Medicare and Medicaid reliance
- Lack of public transportation

One recent solution to these challenges is the use of technology in the form of telepharmacy to reach areas with limited access to medications and pharmacists. A variety of approaches have been utilized including video, telephonic, computer links, and automated dispensing systems to provide better access to health care. These approaches have also focused on decreasing the costs of care and improving the quality of care.[27]

Urban areas are not without their own issues related to the provision of health care. Where access and transportation may be improved in the urban setting, the number of uninsured in urban areas is staggering.

With approximately 70% of the United States population in urban areas, the current national total of over 40 million uninsured indicates that close to 30 million people are uninsured in urban areas.[28]

Many reasons are used to explain and predict the growing number of uninsured throughout the country. Although a variety of safety-net processes are in place, the numbers continue to increase at an alarming rate.[29,30] The increase has been attributed to the following:

- Unemployment
- Underinsured
- Decreasing employer benefits
- People not aware of benefits available to them
- Unhealthy lifestyles
- State budgets cannot provide continued level of support

As discussed previously, access to health care is a significant issue in both rural and urban areas. This is compounded by the fact that the uninsured are three times more likely to not fill a prescription as those with insurance. A situation leading to serious health care consequences might result. In many cases, this results in emergency department visits as the initial point of health care. This may result in hospitalization and longer lengths of stay that further challenge the health care system.

A variety of programs have been implemented to provide service to the uninsured in both rural and urban settings, ranging from volunteer services to sophisticated community health centers that provide high quality ambulatory care.[31] The majority of these sites offer some type of patient assistance programs to provide better access to medications and services. In planning a program such as this, it truly requires a multidisciplinary approach to determine what needs the patient population has and who will best provide the needed services.[29–31]

Medication access plays an integral part in the planning process for providing services to the underserved. Pharmacists have the opportunity to provide a wide variety of services to assist in the planning and implementation of these processes. Medication access for seniors may be somewhat improved with the Medicare Modernization Act (MMA), but it is still anticipated that a number of people will still not have adequate prescription coverage.[32] Some of the current options used to improve medication access:

- Drug samples
- Drug discount cards
- Bulk donations
- Manufacturer assistance programs
- Contracted pharmacy services
- Federal programs
- Sliding scale payment systems

Numerous examples exist demonstrating how organizations have improved access to medications by utilizing the items listed.[33] With improved access, sites have been able to show significant improvements in health care costs based on shifting services to the ambulatory setting from the institutional setting.

Beyond the provision of better medication access, pharmacists have also been involved in patient education, formulary and protocol development, policy and procedure preparation, and disease management strategies. Pharmacists involved in these types of programs are given an excellent opportunity to collaborate with other health care professionals and together, improve patient care.[33,34]

Delivery of Health Care

Managed Care

The rising costs of health care are not only a concern for patients, but also for providers of health care and the organizations that provide health care insurance to patients. Over the last 30 years an attempt to control costs, while maintaining quality, has made inroads into the provision of health care to over 30% of the population of the United States.[35] The approach is commonly known as managed care, which is a planned and coordinated approach to providing health care in the most cost-effective manner with a significant emphasis on preventive care. As these programs have evolved over the last several decades, a variety of options are available to patients and employers. Payment for these services is most often prepaid to a provider for services on a per-member, per-month basis. In the majority of cases a primary care physician is the "gatekeeper" to specialized services for patients. Referrals from the primary care physician are required for a number of these services.

Over the years debate has raged over the effectiveness or ineffectiveness of the managed care approach to provision of health care. From the negative perspective, the most commonly reported concerns are[36]:

- Rising costs
- Problems with access to specialized services
- Lack of preferred access to specific health care facilities
- Confusion about what is provided and by whom

As reported in a recent survey, it was shown that the level of dissatisfaction may not be as significant as thought from earlier reports. This particular survey indicated that the primary concern voiced by patients was related to out-of-pocket costs for prescription medications.[37] Although earlier surveys indicated a number of problems existed with current systems, it is apparent that enrollments are increasing and in fact, in some areas of the country enrollments in managed care programs may be as high as 50% of the population.[35,38]

Regardless of the latest survey results, the focus of any managed care organization is to support the delivery of evidence-based, affordable, and accessible health care. A major focus of this process is the management of pharmacy benefits. Nationwide this has allowed pharmacists to become actively involved in both operational and clinical components of the managed care system.[39] The role of the pharmacist in these organizations is an excellent example of interdisciplinary involvement in a health care system. A variety of involvement opportunities exist for pharmacists involved in managed care organizations. As a rule, the following activities are typical:

- Development of formularies or select drug lists
- Drug utilization evaluations (DUE)
- Education of health care providers about pharmacotherapy
- Compliance
- Promotion of step therapy regimens
- Therapeutic interventions (i.e., polypharmacy)
- Provide feedback to prescribers on trends of care
- Disease state management

As managed care organizations continue to evolve and new challenges such as specialty drugs, biotech products, new delivery systems and changes in federal insurance plans affect health care delivery, the pharmacist is well-suited to provide expertise in assisting in this change process.

Quality of Care/Interdisciplinary Teams

Quality of care is a term that is repeated frequently in discussions regarding provision of health care. This concept has been a major contributor to the movement from multidisciplinary to interdisciplinary approach to care. Simply stated it is the standard of care provided in all patient-directed services. A number of parameters may be used to assess the quality of care, including: length of stay, adverse medication reactions, and conversion from intravenous to oral therapy. Traditionally, care was provided in a multidisciplinary manner. Multidisciplinary refers to everyone working independently to provide patient care. As health care delivery systems became more efficient and cost-focused, more interest was shown in an interdisciplinary approach to care.[40] Interdisciplinary refers to the fact that health care professionals are working together to coordinate and optimize patient care.

Over the last several decades, a number of factors related to quality have had a tremendous impact on health care systems. With the development of DRGs, Medicare implemented a plan to make institutional delivery of health care more effective and efficient. Some of the desired results of this system included the following:

- Decreased length of stay
- Higher acuity of patients in the hospital
- Less financial support for certain aspects of care
- More emphasis on ambulatory care
- Developing interest in preventive medicine

All of these factors created a high degree of competition among providers and caused many institutions to find ways to improve processes, consolidate functions, or face some form of decline of services.

As institutions dealt with this change, it became clear that quality was the focal point for success both financially and in patient outcomes. Quality was defined as "the degree to which health services for individuals or populations increase the likelihood of desired health outcomes and are consistent with current professional knowledge." This set in motion a variety of approaches to improve patient care.[37] With any approach to improving quality of care, the following goals are critical:

- Provide continuity of care
- Decrease fragmentation of services
- Guide family and patient through the process
- Optimize cost effectiveness, utilizing well-documented approaches to care
- Increase patient, family, and employee satisfaction

Continuous quality improvement (CQI) initiatives became commonplace and were quickly adopted in all institutional settings. Organizations determined methods to improve provision of services and achieve positive patient outcome. Concepts such as *patient-focused care* were implemented which resulted in more emphasis on decentralized services, cross-training of providers, and redesign of health care delivery systems that promoted simplification of work.[41] This concept also promoted the interdisciplinary approach to care that has been previously discussed. An excellent example of the role pharmacists can play in this model is the provision of services to geriatric patient populations. Inappropriate prescribing is common in the geriatric population and pharmacists have been able to document their contribution to improvement in patient outcomes specific to this type of patient.[42]

A further evolution of patient-focused care was the development of critical pathways that concentrated resources to improve patient outcomes. Critical pathways were many times designed for specific DRGs that were associated with high costs, complications, and increased lengths of stay. The process focused on optimizing steps and interventions by health care providers with the primary goals of minimizing delays and resources and improving the quality of care. Pharmacists have been able to play an integral part in these processes by providing assessments of medication orders by screening for drug allergies and monitoring specific medications as well as educating patients. They also assess drug dosing based on renal function, participate in the selection of appropriate medications and ultimately provide feedback on appropriateness of medication use once a plan is initiated.[43]

The shortage of pharmacists in institutional settings has the potential to have direct negative effects on the quality of patient care. The incidence of medical errors in one report noted that 44,000 to 98,000 deaths per year occurred due to medical errors, with the largest component being medication errors.[44] The increasing complexity of medical therapies and the acuity of patients in institutions have made the interdisciplinary role of the pharmacist more critical.

Utilization of Health Care

Patient Populations

Trends in U.S. population changes have enormous ramifications for the health care system and the cost of providing care. In 1900, when the life expectancy was 47 years of age, a patient was likely to die relatively quickly of an acute illness. At that time the technology available for treatment was minimal and inexpensive. Table 1-1 below shows the changes in life span expectancy that has occurred and is projected in the U.S. With each passing year, new and expensive technology becomes available. As genetics based therapies become common, it is reasonable to expect radical shifts in health care costs. The therapies themselves will be expensive but may cure or prevent conditions that would have cost far more to treat by conventional means. When considering the problems generated by an older population, it is important to consider that there are scientists working on life span expansion technology that have bet $500 million that there will

Table 1-1

Historic and Projected Lifespan for Average U.S. Citizens by Year of Birth[a,b]

Year of Birth	Average Lifespan	
(Total U.S. Population, Average of Both Sexes)		
2100	90	(projected)
2050	83.5	(projected)
2025	80.6	(projected)
2002	77.3	
2000	77	
1990	75.4	
1980	73.7	
1970	70.8	
1960	69.7	
1950	68.2	
1940	62.0	
1930	59.7	
1920	54.1	
1910	50.0	
1900	47.3	

[a] Projections: U.S. Census Bureau Methodology and Assumptions for the Population Projections of the United States. Population Division Working Paper No. 38 Ref. 19. Population Projections Branch Population Division; January 2000.

[b] Historic Data: U.S. Census Bureau. National Vital Statistics Reports. November 10, 2004 (Vol 53, No. 6).:Table 12, Reference 20.

be someone alive at the age of 150 years by January 1, 2150.[45] Considering the rate at which genetic technology is progressing, this may be a reality before that time.

With advancing age each organ system is subject, on the average, to a greater likelihood of problems. By examining just one common physical condition that arises in old age, atrial fibrillation, we can illustrate the significant increase in health care costs that is almost certain with the average elderly person. Atrial fibrillation is a simple irregular heartbeat that can lead to stroke. "About 80,000 strokes occur in America each year that can be attributed to atrial fibrillation (AF)."[46] An inexpensive blood thinning agent, warfarin, lowers the risk of stroke in AF patients, but less than half of patients that should take it do take it. Either their physician does not prescribe it, they cannot afford it, are afraid to take a blood thinner, or lack the health literacy to understand the importance of taking it. The use of warfarin to prevent stroke would "save an estimated $1.45 million each year per 100,000 people aged 65 and older, of who about 6,000 would have AF."[46] This illustration demonstrates the cost of one chronic condition. Other studies have looked at the number of chronic physical illnesses by age. One of these also looked across six social classes (highly professional to unskilled manual).[47] When this study compared age 15–34 to 65 years and over, they found a range from 1.8 times as much chronic disease in skill manual laborers to 11 times more for lower professional workers. The average across all groups was 4.6 times more disease for the older age group.

Health Literacy

Health Literacy is defined as "the capacity of an individual to obtain, interpret, and understand basic health information and services in ways that are health-enhancing."[5] While statistics regarding the exact rate of problems in health literacy differ by study, it is clear that medical directives are difficult enough to understand and follow even for the fully literate. Those who are impaired by reason of poor reading ability or lack of education and experience in health care issues are at greater risk of making mistakes or not following the instructions of health care professionals. Studies find that 20% of Americans read at or below the 5th grade level, and the average citizen reads at the 8th or 9th grade level. This means that any written instructions as well as our verbal instructions must be appropriately geared for the patient's level of understanding.[48] While anyone may experience health literacy problems, as pharmacists we can be prepared to give the greatest educational effort to those in high-risk groups. These include a disproportionate number of minorities. It is important to make special efforts to educate and train the elderly, as 66% of adults over age 60 have health literacy problems, and they are the most likely to have multiple chronic illnesses and be prescribed multiple medication therapy.[49] Not only are health literacy problems a serious health risk and, consequently, a financial risk for the patient, but they cost the nation tens of billions of dollars each year. This money could be used by the individual patient to pay for needed care and by the nation to preserve precious health resources and provide a greater range and depth of care for all.[50] There are countless references and guides available from many publishers and organizations to assist pharmacists regarding proper counseling in light of health literacy issues.

Chronic Disease Management (CDM)

There are a multitude of definitions for chronic disease found in good health care texts and online. Most indicate that a chronic disease is one lasting greater than 30 days duration, cannot be cured but may be controlled or treated. Illnesses such as asthma, diabetes, hypertension, and arthritis are included in the chronic disease category. For the pharmacists, CDM involves getting to know the patient, their level of medical literacy, their illness and coexisting illnesses, lifestyle (e.g., smoking), and determining a baseline for the patient.[50] One study illustrated precisely what a pharmacist might do and accomplish to care for diabetic patients.[51] The approach of the pharmacist included "(1) Identifying patients at risk for Type II diabetes due to known risk factors, (2) conducting blood glucose screening of patients with risk factors, (3) offering point-of-dispensing services including reminders for proper preventive care and glucose testing, (4) disease state management, and (5) providing patient education."[51] The improvements in patient health and quality of life are perhaps best indicated by clinical and financial indicators. "Within the first eight months, the average A1c was at or below 7% and has been sustained for five years."[51]

Employer total mean medical costs decreased by $1,622 per patient to $3,356 per patient per year compared with baseline. Days of sick time decreased every year for one employer, with estimated increases in productivity estimated to be $18,000 annually. The number of patients having influenza vaccinations went from 40% to 75% by the sixth visit. On the first visit only 28% had current foot exams; by the sixth visit 80% had current foot exams. On the first visit only 34% had current eye exams; by the sixth visit 80% had current eye exams. On the first visit 73% had current blood pressure readings; by the sixth visit 92% had current readings. And finally, on the first visit only 49% had lipid profiles, by the sixth visit 94% had them.[51] It is clear that these markers translate into fewer sick days and greater productivity. What are unmeasured are the long-term effects of less long-term disability, amputation, and blindness. This is a successful illustration of excellent chronic disease management by the pharmacist in only one disease state. The quality of life and financial savings would be multiplied many times if pharmacists were as involved with the management of all chronic disease states.

Price and Reimbursement of Health Care

The area of price and reimbursement varies within each subsection of our health care structure. You have already received an introduction to public health payment mechanisms and the managed care system and detailed information will be provided in subsequent chapters. Various cost control mechanisms have been introduced in the last 30 years.

Four basic models for financing health care are out-of-pocket payment, individual private insurance, employment or association based group private insurance, and government financing.

TV shows placed in the Old West or on the prairie portray the original out-of-pocket payment system in the U.S. Physicians were paid in goods and services when cash was not available. Because health care expenditures are unpredictable, necessary, and require the guidance of a health care practitioner, it is difficult for the average American to prepare for these costs. Individuals without government support or private insurance may still pay out-of-pocket for any or part of the health care services. Charitable and religious organizations continue to provide circumstantial assistance to those in need through shelter, clinics, and direct support.

With private insurance, individuals pay a regular fee to receive assistance with significant medical bills. These types of insurance plans can insure single individuals and families—individual plans or groups of individuals—group plans. Health risk is accessed by an underwriter who is trained in risk factor analysis and actuarial science. Because other individuals health risk is not available to offset the cost of the plan nor is an employer contributing to the costs, these plans are more costly than employer based plans. Currently, less than 10% of the U.S. population utilizes individual health insurance plans. Group health insurance shares the risk across individuals. Group plans which are offered through employment are employer based plans. Therefore, those who are healthy are able to offset the insurance cost for those who are not. Another insurance option for individuals who are unemployed or self-employed may seek insurance through an association group. These groups based on profession, hobbies, or location may offer these individuals a cheaper alternative.

During World War II wage and price controls prevented wage increases but allowed the growth of benefits. This, combined with a competition for a limited labor source health insurance, became an employer benefit. Unions furthered the existence of group health benefits, and the role of the employer or union as negotiators for the best plan at the best cost. Traditionally employers pay the majority of the premiums for employer-based health insurance; however, with an increase in health care costs employee contributions are on the rise.

Government financial assistance for health care services is primarily supplied by two mechanisms: Medicare and Medicaid. Both programs began in 1965—Medicare specifically for the elderly is primarily funded through federal and social security taxes, and Medicaid specifically for the poor is primarily administered by the states responsibility funded by both state and federal taxes. Medicare has been divided into Part A and Part B: hospital and outpatient services, respectively.[52]

Becoming aware that a fee-for-service payment system supported overuse and nonessential behavior within the system cost containment mechanisms were developed. One method still used today, particularly for inpatient services, is diagnosis-related groups (DRGs). Medicare established hundreds of DRGs. This method of reimbursement linked a diagnosis with a standard reimbursement rate, and this rate included the anticipated length of stay, costs of procedures, etc. Hospitals could make a profit by keeping the actual cost of services under the reimbursement rate. For patients whose actual costs of services are greater than the reimbursement rate, the hospital loses money. DRGs are one example of how cost containment can compromise the care delivered to patients.[52]

The current reimbursement cycle within our system supports that our health care remains market driven. Current medical research suggests that preventive medicine might decrease health care expenditures on chronic disease which continues to plague our system as life expectancy increases. Health economists might suggest that insurance should begin to support preventive medication services in addition to the treatment options currently available. Challenges to the practicality of this change under the current system would require a market shift toward preventive behavior. In addition, with the rapid turnover of insurance companies by employers seeking the best rates, little incentive exists today to support such behavior. The cost of insurance would likely rise to cover new benefits while supporting those who previously had no access or incentive for preventive care. The rise of insurance costs ultimately limits the number of insured and increases the reliance on public health programs in turn increasing the cost of government subsides. As the battle with cost continues, insurers will continue to seek methods for cost containment and limitations of benefits.

Other Cost Containment Mechanisms

Prescription drug expenditures in the United States continue to rise. In 2003, total spending reached a total of over $216 billion. It is estimated that in 2005, there will be a 10–12% increase in drug expense in the outpatient settings, a 12–15% increase in clinics, and 6–9% in hospitals.[53] The challenges of an ever-increasing pattern of expenditures on drugs provides an excellent opportunity for pharmacists to provide their expertise in the management of drug-related expenditures.

Although a number of factors will affect the level of drug expenditures, a primary focus for pharmacists is through formulary management strategies. As health care has evolved over the years, new treatments have created controversy over which ones may be the best. A critical decision-making step to determine the most effective therapy is the concept of evidence-based medicine.[54] This concept promotes the critical review of pertinent studies to determine best practice models that focus on both quality and positive patient outcomes.

With the concept of evidence-based medicine as a guiding principle for the formulary process, pharmacists have been able to play an integral role in the determination of quality approaches to care. The drug formulary system is "an ongoing process in which a healthcare organization through its physicians, pharmacists, nurses and other health care professionals establish policies on the use of drug products and therapies that were the most medically appropriate and cost-effective to best serve the health interests of a given patient population."[55] A variety of approaches have been utilized to develop drug formularies, including the following concepts:

- Generic substitution
- Therapeutic alternatives
- Category review
- Therapeutic substitution
- Therapeutic interchange

Each of these approaches is based on careful review of a variety of data points and is not just limited to cost of therapy.

When making recommendations in the drug formulary process, one should use the following approach as a template for decision-making[56–58]:

- Base decisions on sound scientific evidence and practice standards by utilizing peer-reviewed literature. Studies that are well-designed, statistically sound, and that focus on outcomes are preferred.
- Consider patient compliance and ease of administration
- Review risk versus benefit ratios with a focus on adverse events and potential interactions
- Include costs on monitoring or administration costs associated with a drug in the review process
- Compare the drug being reviewed to currently available products on formulary and determine if the new drug does establish a therapeutic niche
- Review financial incentives as a final item once therapeutic efficacy has been determined

In this process it is also important to determine the potential usage patterns of an agent if it is going to be added to the formulary and to estimate what impact that will have on the drug budget and patient outcomes.[59]

In most health care systems, the group that coordinates the drug formulary system is the Pharmacy and Therapeutics (P&T) Committee. The P&T Committee is most often comprised of physicians, pharmacists, administrators, and nurses. Physician members may include a variety of practice backgrounds from family medicine to specialty practice, with subject matter experts available for consultation. The primary function of the pharmacist member is to provide thorough reviews of items on the agenda and present recommendations to the committee. The P&T Committee will develop, monitor, and revise the formulary on an ongoing basis. Given the dramatic increases in new drug development, the P&T Committee faces the daunting task of keeping current with an ever-changing, dynamic process. The process also faces the challenges of continued marketing by manufacturers, which further emphasizes the need for critical review of the literature and perhaps counter-detailing critical issues with physicians.

The P&T Committee may have slightly different functions given the specific environment (i.e., hospital, managed care group, state Medicaid). As a rule, the following functions are generic to their administrative responsibilities:

- Drug selection and formulary maintenance
- Drug Use Evaluations (DUE)
- Periodic review and analysis or appropriateness of use
- Compiling data into educational programs
- Adverse medication reaction and medication error reporting
- Develop trending data models
- Develop strategies to correct
- Develop protocols to effectively utilize formulary drugs
- Establish procedures for nonformulary drugs

It is important to realize the educational component of the formulary process. Numerous approaches such as newsletters, comparison charts, in-services, and counter-detailing have been used to update practitioners on decisions made by the committee.[56–59]

Pharmacist Reimbursement

Over the years, pharmacists have developed numerous strategies to be compensated for cognitive services. Most of these attempts were in situations where pharmacists were working in collaboration with a recognized health care provider who could bill for services. As the role of pharmacists has changed to one of a greater focus on nondistributive, clinical activities, there has been an increased interest in seeking reimbursement for patient-focused activities.[60] Reports have consistently shown the positive impacts that pharmacists can have in the provision of health care, with specific emphasis on decreasing costs related to the overall care of a patient.[61,62] This confirmation of contribution to health care delivery has led to the initiation of discussions regarding pharmacists having specific Current Procedural Terminology (CPT) codes covering medication therapy management services.[63] Trial programs in several states have also allowed pharmacists to be reimbursed for cognitive services to state Medicaid recipients. Perhaps one of the best examples of documentation of impacts resulting in recognition of is the Asheville project that provided sound data showing the positive interventions made by pharmacists in diabetes management.[64]

Medicare Modernization Act/Medicaid

All of these examples have set the stage for the more recent changes at the federal level of health care insurance. The concept of Medicare was enacted by Congress in 1965 and has evolved over the last 40 years to provide health insurance to primarily people over 65 years of age. For the most part this insurance did not include prescription benefits. Medicare recipients had to depend on out-of-pocket payments, their own additional insurance, state Medicaid, or patient assistance programs to obtain their medications. In 2003, the latest iteration of Medicare was signed into law. This update is known as the *Medicare Modernization Act of 2003 (MMA)*.[65] Numerous attempts were made during both the 1980s and 1990s to revamp the system, but this was the first success at change. The significance of MMA is that it provides prescription coverage for the first time to eligible individuals through Medicare Part D.

One of the opportunities for pharmacists with the new legislation is the possibility of an expanded role in the delivery of health care to those covered individuals. Specifically this relates to the inclusion of medication therapy management services to recipients with certain types of chronic disease states who are taking multiple medications. In the current wording of MMA, this could include a variety of health care professionals, but for the first time pharmacists have been recognized as providers of direct patient care at a national level.[66,67]

The path forward for MMA is still confusing and many details need to be further refined over time. The following are key steps with MMA as it has rolled out:

- Access to Medicare Drug Discount Cards, June 2004 to December 2005—savings were estimated at 10–15% on drug costs with online comparisons available

- Beginning January 2006, beneficiaries will have

a choice of original Medicare with a Medicare Prescription Drug Plan or Medicare Advantage Plan through a health maintenance organization that covers Medicare benefits and drugs. Recipients will have between November 15 and December 31, 2005 to sign up for Prescription Drug Plan.

The process also involves dual eligible recipients that have both Medicare and Medicaid if low-income subsidies are met based on federal poverty level status. Through this process, pharmacists will play a vital role in helping patients understand the options available, perhaps assist in the application for Part D and enroll patients in prescription drug plans. Pharmacists will be in a unique position to provide guidance in these early stages of the program's roll out. They will also have the potential to provide medication therapy management in the year's ahead.[67]

Legislative and Regulatory Changes:

Technology Advancement

Technology trends seek to advance medicine itself while redesigning access, delivery, utilization, and reimbursement of care. Internet pharmacies, telemedicine, and electronic prescribing improve access to health care. Individuals in rural settings can be seen by specialists miles away. Automation in pharmacies and the use of electronic records improves the care delivered to the patient. Pharmacists can better access patient health records and limit dispensing errors. Technology that translates instructions into multiple languages assists patients in utilizing their medications correctly. Development of an electronic insurance card similar to a credit card would improve communication and management of health care expenditures.

Hints on How to Monitor Legislative and Regulatory Changes

Pharmacists must be involved in the status and future of the current health care system. National associations utilize lobbyists who track legislation and communicate the interest of pharmacists to legislators at a state and local level. Accessing your state government website or state association will allow pharmacists to locate local legislation related to the practice of pharmacy in their state. Federal legislation can also be tracked directly by utilizing the library of congress website, *www.thomas.loc.gov*. Finally, by attending state board of pharmacy meetings or reviewing minutes, pharmacists can learn about regulations developed from new legislation. These rules are primarily developed by subcommittees and must be made available for public review and comment prior to adoption.

Summary

Future Opportunities for Pharmacists in the Changing Environment

With the knowledge of the history of the health care system, recognition of the attempts at national health care, acknowledgement of the deficiencies in our health care system, and challenges for improvement, pharmacists must decide what their role will be.

To improve access to health care, pharmacists must consider the shortage of pharmacists particularly in the rural setting and small hospitals. Pharmacists should improve their knowledge of public assistance mechanisms and options for uninsured patients. Finally technology in the pharmacy may improve options in all pharmacy settings.

Delivery of health care includes efforts toward pharmaceutical care including use of evidence-based medicine.[68] Pharmacists will continue to serve as a part of interdisciplinary teams functioning in roles such as formulary management, provider education, disease management, quality improvement, etc. Understanding the cost savings techniques of managed care and working with payer companies may provide additional support to patients not currently offered by any profession.

Pharmacists who continue to practice skills related to health literacy will likely see improved utilization of pharmacy and health care services by their patients. Pharmacists will adjust their workflow so that patient counseling and communication becomes a priority. Education and experience with chronic disease management will improve service to customers beyond acute care and prescription filling.

Legislative support for pharmacist reimbursement supports the roles for pharmacists mentioned above. Pharmacists must increase their knowledge on reimbursement strategies and consider business opportunities for practice advancement. Maintaining legislative support will require lobbying support as well as documented health care improvement by pharmacists. At the local, state, regional, and federal level, pharmacists have the opportunity to improve current health care deficiencies, bridging the gaps in the current health care system.

References

1. Frist W. Health care in the 21st century. *N Engl J Med.* 2005;352:267–72.

2. McGlynn EA, Asch SM, Adams J, et al. The quality of health care delivered to adults in the United States. *N Engl J Med.* 2003;348(26):2635–45.

3. Carpenter C. Health care in the United States—Is it the best in the world? *Journal of Financial Service Professionals.* 2005;59(2):29–31.

4. Reinhardt UE, Hussey PS, Anderson GF. U.S. Health spending in an international context. *Health Aff.* 2004;23:10–25.

5. Joint Committee on National Health Education Standards. 1995. Available at: www.nhsinherts.nhs.uk/hp/glossary.htm.

6. www.cogsci.princeton.edu/cgi-bin/webwn.

7. Fincham J, Wertheimer A. *Pharmacy and the U.S. Health Care System.* 2nd ed. New York: The Pharmaceutical Products Press; 1984:241–2.

8. Law and medicine: health care law prof. Mayo U.S. health care timeline. Available at: http://faculty.smu.edu/tmayo/health%20care%20timeline.htm.

9. Health insurance history. Available at: http://www.ehealthhelp.com/images/InsuranceHistory.gif.

10. Researchers disagree about how the CPS estimates of the uninsured should be interpreted. Like many health care analysts, CBO believes that those estimates provide a close approximation of the number of people who are uninsured at a specific point in time. See Congressional Budget Office, How Many People Lack Health Insurance and for How Long?

11. Fronstin P. *Sources of Health Insurance Coverage and Characteristics of the Uninsured: Analysis of the March 2003 Current Population Survey. Issue Brief No. 264.* Washington, DC: Employee Benefit Research Institute; December 2003.

12. CBO Testimony. Statement of Douglas Holtz-Eakin (Director of Health Care Spending and the Uninsured) before the Committee on Health, Education, Labor, and Pensions. United States Senate; January 28, 2004. Available at: http://www.cbo.gov/showdoc.cfm?index=4989&sequence=0.

13. PBS. Healthcare crisis: healthcare timeline. Available at: http://www.pbs.org/healthcarecrisis/history.htm.

14. U.S. Department of Labor Bureau of Labor Statistics occupational outlook handbook. Available at: http:/stats.bls.gov/ocoocos079.htm.

15. Kaiser Family Foundation. Prescription drug trends. October 2004. Available at: www.kff.org/rxdrugs/loader.cfm?url=/commonspot/security/getfile.cfm&PageID=48305.

16. Number of prescriptions grow faster than population. *Managed Care Magazine.* December 2004. MediMedia, USA. Available at: http://www.managedcaremag.com/archives/0412/0412.snapshot.html.

17. USA Today examines national physician shortage. *USA Today*. March 4, 2005. Available at: http://www.medical newstoday.com/medicalnews.php?newsid=20679.

18. American Academy of Family Physicians. Workforce study says marketplace should determine specialty distribution. August 13, 2004.

19. Schroeder SA, Sandy LG. Specialty distribution of physicians—the invisible driver of health care costs. *N Engl J Med*. 1993 Apr 1;328(13):961–3.

20. U.S. Department of Labor, Bureau of Labor Statistics. Occupational outlook handbook: physicians and surgeons, 2003. Available at: http://stats.bls.gov/oco/ocos 074 .htm.

21. Federal Office of Rural Health Policy. Facts about… rural physicians. Health Resource and Services Administration, U.S. Department of Health and Human Services. Available at: http://www.shepscenter.unc.edu/ research_programs/rural_programs/phy.html.

22. NPR/Kaiser/Harvard Kennedy School Poll on Health Care. America faces problems, but don't want radical change. Available at: http://www.npr.org/news/specials/ helathcare poll/index.html. June 5, 2002.

23. Facts at a Glance: the pharmacist shortage. Available at: http://www.afpenet.org/news_facts_at_a_glance. Accessed April 5, 2005.

24. Knapp KK, Quist RM, Walton SM, et al. Update on the pharmacist shortage: national and state data through 2003. *Am J Health-Syst Pharm*. 2005:62:492–9.

25. Vecchione A. ASHP survey shows pharmacy leadership crisis looming. Available at: http://www.drugtopics.com. Accessed March 31, 2005. (From November 22, 2004.)

26. Office of Technology Assessment. *Health Care in Rural America*. Washington, DC: U.S. Congress; 1990.

27. Stubbings T, Miller C, Humphries TL, et al. Telepharmacy in a health maintenance organization. *Am J Health-Syst Pharm*. 2005;62:406–10.

28. Sarrafizadeh M, Waite NM, Hobson EH, et al. Pharmacist-facilitated enrollment in medication assistance programs in a private ambulatory care clinic. *Am J Health-Syst Pharm*. 2004;61:1816–20.

29. Duke KS, Raube K, Lipton HL. Patient-assistance programs: assessment of and use by safety-net clinics. *Am J Health-Syst Pharm*. 2005:62:726–31.

30. Adams D, Wilson AL. Structuring an indigent care pharmacy benefit program. *Am J Health-Syst Pharm*. 2002;59:1669–75.

31. Dent LA, Stratton TP, Cochran GA. Establishing an onsite pharmacy in a community health center to help indigent patients access medications and to improve care. *J Am Pharm Assoc*. 2002;42:497–507.

32. Meyer BM, Cantwell KM. The Medicare Prescription Drug, Improvement, and Modernization Act of 2003: implications for health-system pharmacy. *Am J Health-Syst Pharm*. 2004;61:1042–51.

33. Strain JD, Jorgenson JA, Martin S. Development and implementation of a pharmacy directed community health education and screening program. *Hosp Pharm*. 2005;40:54–60.

34. Knapp KK, Blalock SJ, Black BL. ASHP survey of ambulatory care responsibilities of pharmacists in managed care and integrated health systems—2001. *Am J Health-Syst Pharm*. 2001;58:2151–66.

35. Aventis Pharmaceuticals. *Managed Care Digest Series®*. Bridgewater, NJ: Aventis Pharmaceuticals; 2002.

36. American Journal of Health-System Pharmacists (ASHP). Hospitals, physicians gain clout against managed care. *Am J Health-Syst Pharm*. 2001;58(9):756–7.

37. Motheral BR, Heinle SM. Predictors of satisfaction of health plan members with prescription drug benefits. *Am J Health-Syst Pharm*. 2004;61:1007–14.

38. Berk ML, Schur CI, Yegian R. Public perceptions of cost containment strategies: mixed signals for managed care. *Data Watch Magazine*. Available at: http://www.healthaffairs,org. Accessed February 17, 2005.

39. Curtis FR, Fry RN, Avey SG. Framework for pharmacy services quality improvement—a bridge to cross the quality chasm. *J Manage Care Pharm*. 2004;10: 60–78.

40. Bodenheimer T. The American health care system: the movement for improved quality in health care. In: Lee PR, Estes CL, eds. *The Nation's Health*. 7th ed. Sudsbury, MA: Jones and Bartlett Publishers; 2003:445–52.

41. Vogel DP. Patient-focused care. *Am J Health-Syst Pharm*. 1993;50:2321–9.

42. Lam S, Ruby CM. Impact of an interdisciplinary team and drug therapy outcomes in a geriatric clinic. *Am J Health-Syst Pharm*. 2005;62:626–9.

43. American Society of Health-System Pharmacists (ASHP). ASHP guidelines on the pharmacist's role in the development, implementation, and assessment of critical pathways. *Am J Health-Syst Pharm*. 2004;61 939–45.

44. Bond CA, Raehl CJ, Franke T. Clinical pharmacy services, hospital pharmacy staffing, and medication errors in the United States hospitals. *Pharmacotherapy*. 2002; 22:134–47.

45. Klein B. ImmInst.org. Human lifespan—is there a limit? Average and maximum lifespan. Available at: http://www.imminst.org/forum/index.php?act=ST&f=67 &t=680&s=. January 7, 2003.

46. Agency for Healthcare Research and Quality. Health care costs: fact sheet. AHRQ Publication No. 02-P033. Available at: http://www.ahrq.gov/news/costsfact.htm. September 2002.

47. www.ucc.ie/medstud/downloads/med5/Table2_Chronic_ Physical_Illnesses_by_Age_and_Social_Class.doc.

48. Doak CC, Doak LG, Root JH. The literacy problem. In: *Teaching Patients With Low Literacy Skills*. 2nd ed. Philadelphia: J.B. Lippincott Co.; 1996:1–9.

49. Center for Health Care Strategies, Inc. Who suffers from poor health literacy? Fact sheet. Available at: http://www.chcs.org/resource/hl.html.1997.

50. Weiss BD, ed. *20 Common Problems in Primary Care*. New York: McGraw Hill; 1999:468–81.

51. Garrett DG, Martin LA. The Asheville Project: participants' perceptions of factors contributing to the success of a patient self-management diabetes program. *J Am Pharm Assoc.* 2003;43(2):185–90.

52. Williams SJ, Torrens PR, eds. *Introduction to Health Services.* Albany, NY: Delmar Publishers Inc.; 1993.

53. Hoffman JM, Shah ND, Vermeulen LC, et al. Projecting future drug expenditures—2005. *Am J Health-Syst Pharm.* 2005;62:149–67.

54. Young D. Policymakers, experts review evidence-based medicine. *Am J Health-Syst Pharm.* 2005;62 (4):342–3.

55. Wang Z, Salmon JW, Walton SM. Cost-effectiveness analysis and the formulary decision making process. *J Manag Care Pharm.* 2004;10:48–59.

56. American Society of Hospital Pharmacists (ASHP). ASHP technical assistance bulletin on the evaluation of drugs for formularies. *Am J Hosp Pharm.* 1988;45:386–7.

57. American Society of Hospital Pharmacists (ASHP). ASHP guidelines on formulary system management. *Am J Hosp Pharm.* 1992;49:648–52.

58. American Society of Hospital Pharmacists (ASHP). ASHP technical assistance bulletin on drug formularies. *Am J Hosp Pharm.* 1991;48:791–3.

59. American Society of Hospital Pharmacists (ASHP). ASHP technical assistance bulletin on assessing cost-containment strategies for pharmacists in organized health care settings. *Am J Hosp Pharm.* 1992;49:155–60.

60. American Society of Hospital Pharmacists (ASHP). ASHP statement on third-party compensation for clinical services by pharmacists. *Am J Hosp Pharm.* 1985;42:1580–1.

61. Johnson JA, Bootman JL. Drug-related morbidity and mortality: a cost-of-illness model. *Arch Intern Med.* 1995;155(18):1949–56.

62. Kohn LT. *To Err is Human: Building a Safer Health System.* Washington, DC: National Academy Press, Institute of Medicine; 1999.

63. Thompson CA. Billing codes for pharmacy clinical services advance. *Am J Health-Syst Pharm.* 2005;62(1):20–1.

64. Cranor DW, Bunting BA, Christensen DB. The Asheville Project: long-term clinical and economic outcomes of a community diabetes care program. *J Am Pharm Assoc.* 2003;43(2):173–84.

65. Department of Health and Human Services, Centers for Medicare and Medicaid Services. Medicare program: Medicare prescription drug benefit—2004. *Fed Register.* 2004;69:46632–46863.

66. American Society of Health-System Pharmacists (ASHP). Summary of the executive sessions on medication therapy management programs. *Am J Health-Syst Pharm.* 2005;62:585–92.

67. Young D. Imperfect Medicare has positive implications for pharmacists. *Am J Health-Syst Pharm.* 2004;61(2): 126–8.

68. Fincham JE, Wentheimer AL, eds. *Pharmacy and the U.S. Health Care System.* 2nd ed. Binghamton, NY: The Haworth Press, Inc.; 1998.

Chapter 2

Overview of the History of Hospital Pharmacy in the United States

William A. Zellmer

Introduction

Hospitals today offer immense opportunities for pharmacists who want to practice in an environment that draws on the full range of their professional education and training. It was not always so.

This chapter tells the story of how hospital pharmacy developed in this country, analyzes the forces that shaped the hospital pharmacy movement, and draws lessons from the changes in this area of pharmacy practice. The historical facets discussed here are highly selective, reflecting the author's judgment about the most important points to cover within the limits of one chapter.

Hospital Pharmacy's Nascence[a,1–4]

Hospital pharmacy practice in the United States did not begin to develop into a significant movement until the 1920s. Although there were important milestones before that era (including the pioneering hospital pharmacy practices of Charles Rice [1841–1901][5]—see Figure 2-1—and Martin Wilbert [1865–1916]), many factors kept hospital pharmacy at the fringes of the broader development of pharmacy practice and pharmacy education.[6] When the Pennsylvania Hospital (the first hospital in Colonial America) was established in 1752 and Jonathan Roberts was appointed as its apothecary, medicine and pharmacy were commonly practiced together, with drug preparation often the responsibility of a medical apprentice.[7] In 1800, with a population of 5 million, the nation had only two hospitals. Even by 1873, with a population of 43 million, the United States had only 178 hospitals with fewer than 50,000 beds.[2] Hospitals, which were "places of

dreaded impurity and exiled human wreckage," and doctors had little to do with each other.[8] Hospitals played a small role in health care, and pharmacists played a very small role in hospitals.

In the early 1800s, drug therapy consisted of strong cathartics, emetics, and diaphoretics. From the 1830s to the 1870s, clean air and good food rather than medicines were the treatments emphasized in hospitals. In

Figure 2-1

Hospital Pharmacy Department, Bellevue Hospital, New York City, Late 1800s[a]

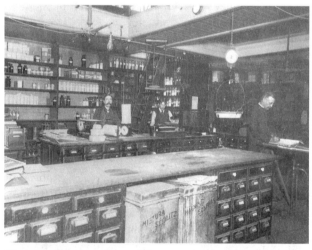

[a] The bulk medicine area, where medicines were packaged for use on the wards, at Bellevue Hospital, New York City, in the late 1800s. Standing on the right is Charles Rice, the eminent chief pharmacist at Bellevue, who headed three revisions of the United States Pharmacopeia.

Source: *AJHP.*

---

[a] Well-documented accounts of the development of hospital pharmacy practice in the United States were published by the American Society of Health-System Pharmacists (ASHP) in conjunction with anniversaries of its 1942 founding. Particularly noteworthy are the "decennial issue" of the *Bulletin on the American Society of Hospital Pharmacists* and articles that marked ASHP's 50th anniversary.[1–3] Readers who have an interest in more detail are encouraged to seek out those references and others.[4] This section of the chapter is based closely on Reference 2.

the mid-1800s, the medical elite avoided drug use or used newer alkaloidal drugs such as morphine, strychnine, and quinine. An organized pharmacy service was not seen as necessary in hospitals, except in the largest facilities. The situation changed somewhat during the Civil War when hospital directors sought out pharmacists for their experience in extemporaneous manufacturing and in purchasing medical goods.[2]

In the 1870s and 1880s, responding to the influx of immigrants, the number of hospitals in cities doubled. Most immigrants in this period were Roman Catholic, and they built Catholic hospitals. This was significant for two reasons—Catholic hospitals charged patients a small fee (which allowed services to be improved) and they were willing to train, or obtain training for, nuns in pharmacy. This era of hospital expansion coincided with reforms in nursing, development of germ theories, and the rise of scientific medicine and surgery. The general adoption of aseptic surgery in the 1890s made the hospital the center of medical care. Advances in surgery led to growth of community hospitals, most of which were small and relied on community pharmacies to supply medicines.[2]

By the early twentieth century, hospitals had developed to the point of having more division of labor, more specialization in medical practice, a greater need for professional pharmaceutical services for handling complex therapies, and recognition that it was more economical to fill inpatient orders in-house. Hospital pharmacists retained the traditional role of compounding, which fostered a sense of camaraderie among them and an impetus to improve product quality and standardization. The advent of the hospital formulary concept persuaded many hospital leaders about the value of professional pharmaceutical services. An important reason for hiring a hospital pharmacist in the 1920s was Prohibition—alcohol was commonly prescribed, and a pharmacist was needed for both inventory control and to manufacture alcohol-containing preparations, which were expensive to obtain commercially.[2]

By the 1930s, pharmacy-related issues in hospitals had coalesced to the point that the American Hospital Association (AHA) created a Committee of Pharmacy to analyze the problems and make recommendations. The 1937 report of that committee was considered so seminal by hospital pharmacy leaders that even a decade later they saw value in republishing it.[9] The aim of the committee was to develop minimum standards for hospital pharmacy departments and to prepare a manual of pharmacy operations. The committee

characterized pharmacy practices in hospitals as "chaotic" and commented, "Few departments in hospital performance have been given less attention by and large than the hospital pharmacy." In the committee's view, "…any hospital larger than one hundred beds warrants the employment of a registered pharmacist…. Unregistered or incompetent service should not be countenanced, not only because of legal complications but to insure absolute safety to the patient."[9] The proliferation of unapproved and proprietary drug products in hospitals was the target of extensive criticism by the committee.

A Fifty-Year Perspective

There is much that can be learned by comparing contemporary hospital pharmacy with practice of 50 years ago. Fifty years is a comprehensible period of time for most people and, in hospital pharmacy's case, the past half century was a period of astonishing advancement.

The data sources for making such a comparison are remarkably good. A major study of hospital pharmacy was conducted between 1957 and 1960—the Audit of Pharmaceutical Services in Hospitals—under the direction of Donald E. Francke and supported by a federal grant (see Figure 2-2). The results were published in a book, *Mirror to Hospital Pharmacy*, which remains a reference of monumental importance.[10] In more recent times, ASHP has conducted an annual survey of hospital pharmacy, yielding contemporary data for comparison with the figures of an earlier era.

Four major themes emerge from an examination of changes over this period:

1. Hospitals have recognized universally that pharmacists must be in charge of drug product acquisition, distribution, and control.

2. Hospital pharmacy departments have assumed a major role in patient safety.

3. Hospital pharmacy departments have assumed a major role in promoting rational drug therapy.

4. Hospital pharmacy departments have come to see their mission as fostering optimal patient outcomes from medication use.

It is important to keep in mind what was happening over this period in the United States as a whole. Since 1950, the U.S. population has grown 86%. Expenditures for health care services have grown from about 5% of gross domestic product to 14%. This growth has fostered an endless stream of public and private initia-

Figure 2-2
Authors of the *Mirror to Hospital Pharmacy*[a]

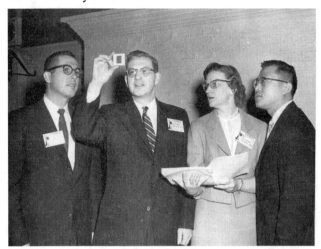

[a] The authors of the *Mirror to Hospital Pharmacy* examining a slide containing data from the results of the Federal *Audit of Pharmaceutical Services in Hospitals* that was conducted in 1957. From left, Clifton J. Latiolais, Donald E. Francke, Gloria Niemeyer Francke, and Norman F. H. Ho. The results were published by ASHP in the book, *Mirror to Hospital Pharmacy*, in 1964.

Source: ASHP Archives.

tives to curtail health care spending. Average daily hospital census, on a per-population basis, has declined by 24% during this period as a result of public and private initiatives to reduce hospital use. Nonfederal, short-term general hospitals in 1950 numbered 5,031 and rose to a zenith of 5,979 in 1975; in 2003 the number stood at 4,918, nearly 18% fewer than the peak of three decades before. On a per-capita basis, the number of inpatient hospital beds has declined 65% since 1950. Since 1965 (the first year AHA reported these data), hospital outpatient visits have increased more than fourfold.[11]

Drug Product Acquisition, Distribution, and Control

Fifty to sixty years ago, pharmaceutical services were of marginal importance to hospitals. The 1949 hospital standards of the American College of Surgeons had only three questions related to pharmacy in its point-rating system, and responses to those questions con-

tributed only 10% to the overall rating. Pharmacy was perceived as a complementary service department, not as an essential service.[12]

Fewer than half the hospital beds in the nation (47%) in the late 1950s were located in facilities that had the services of a full-time pharmacist.[10] Fewer than four out of 10 hospitals (39%) had the services of a pharmacist. Hospital size was an important determinant of the availability of a pharmacist. All larger short-term institutions—those with 300 beds or more—employed a full-time pharmacist. This performance declined sharply with decreasing hospital size:

200–299 beds	96%
100–199 beds	72%
50–99 beds	18%
under 50 beds	3.5%

Today, the vast majority of hospitals in the United States have the services of one or more pharmacists. Important exceptions are small rural hospitals that still rely on the services of local community pharmacists. About 7% of the nation's hospitals have fewer than 25 beds; it is not known how many of them employ a pharmacist.

In 1957, the total number of hospital pharmacists was 4,850 full time and about 1,000 part-time.[10] Today, there are about 50,000 full-time equivalent pharmacists providing inpatient services in nonfederal short-term hospitals.[b,13] (Hospitals employ an equal number of pharmacy technicians.) About one-fourth of all actively practicing pharmacists in the U.S. today are in hospitals.

Today's hospitals employ approximately twelve full-time equivalent pharmacists per 100 occupied beds.[13] The comparable figure for 1957 was approximately 0.4 FTE pharmacists per 100 occupied beds. In other words, pharmacist staffing in hospitals is 30-fold more intensive today. During the same interval, the intensity of hospital staffing as a whole increased approximately sevenfold.[c]

Reflective of more intensified pharmacist staffing, 30% of hospitals today offer 24-hour inpatient pharmacy services. In the largest hospitals (400 beds), 95% of pharmacy departments are open around the clock.[13]

In the middle of the 20th century, nurses and community pharmacists had significant responsibility for

[b] Throughout this chapter, pharmacy data from recent ASHP surveys refer to U.S. nonfederal short-term hospitals.
[c] Calculated based on data in Reference 11.

hospital drug product acquisition, distribution, and control. The *Mirror to Hospital Pharmacy* estimated that 4,000 nurses were engaged in pharmacy work. Here are specific data collected in 1957 showing who handled drugs for the 2,200 hospitals that did not have a full-time pharmacist:

Nonpharmacist personnel (generally nurses)	45%
Nonpharmacist personnel plus community pharmacist	45%
Supervision by local community pharmacist	9%

Table 2-1 shows the services hospital pharmacists were providing in 1957–1960. Two types of services—bulk compounding and sterile solution manufacturing—were a major element of the hospital pharmacists' professional identity in the 1950s (Figure 2-3). Hospital pharmacy leaders of the day cited the following factors in explaining the heavy involvement in manufacturing:

- The unsuitability of many commercially available dosage forms for hospital use
- The close relationship between physicians and pharmacists in hospitals
- The opportunity to serve a need of physicians and patients
- The opportunity to offer a professional service and build interprofessional relations[10]

Today, bulk compounding or manufacturing is no longer a significant activity in U.S. hospital pharmacies. In sharp contrast to 50 years ago, hospital pharmacists now prefer to purchase commercial products whenever they are available, in the interests of appropriate deployment of the workforce and of using products of standard commercial quality. Changes in the laws and regulations that govern drug product manufacturing and distribution, the development of a well-regulated generic pharmaceutical industry, and a shift in the perceived mission of pharmacy practice were among the factors that led to the relegation of manufacturing to hospital pharmacy's past.

In summary, from mid-twentieth century to today, hospital pharmacy in the United States moved from an optional service to an essential service. It used to be that the administrator, the physicians, and the nurses in many institutions, especially smaller facilities, believed that they could function adequately with a drug room controlled by nurses. Today it is beyond question by

Table 2-1
Percentage of U.S. Hospitals Providing (or Desiring to Provide) Specific Pharmacist Services, 1957–1960[a,10]

Service	Provide	Would Like to Provide
Supply drugs to nursing units	97	1
Inpatient prescriptions	95	1
Prescription compounding	94	1
Interdepartmental drug needs	91	1
Drug information	84	9
Outpatient prescriptions	64	6
Formulary system	53	25
Bulk compounding program	41	12
Teaching program	28	23
Product development/research	13	23
Sterile solution manufacturing	11	15

[a] Hospitals with a chief pharmacist.

anyone in the hospital field that medications need to be controlled by a pharmacy department that is run by qualified pharmacists. Moreover, as pharmacists have become firmly established in hospitals, they have been recognized for their expertise beyond drug acquisition, distribution, and control functions, which has led to greatly intensified pharmacy staffing. The growing opportunities in hospitals have attracted more practitioners to the field, which has made hospital practice a major sector of the profession.

Patient Safety

The clarion call to professionalism in hospital pharmacy in recent times has been the patient safety imperative. Hospital pharmacists have made immense progress in this arena. Initially, that progress was tied to greater accuracy in dispensing and administration of medications, but it has evolved to also focus on improving prescribing and monitoring the results of therapy. But it all started with a desire to improve drug product distribution for inpatients.

In 1957, there were two ways in which drug products were distributed to hospital inpatients: as ward

Figure 2-3

Sterile Solution Laboratory, Cardinal Glennon Memorial Hospital for Children, St. Louis, Missouri, circa 1950s[a]

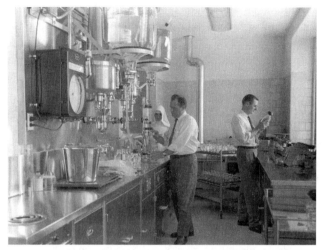

[a] Production of distilled water and the manufacture of large-volume sterile solutions were major pharmacy activities in medium and large hospitals in the 1950s and 1960s.

Source: ASHP Archives.

stock or as individual prescriptions. If the patient was charged for the medication, individual prescriptions were generally used. Otherwise, it was most common for stock containers of medications to be available to the nurse for administration to the patient as needed.[10]

The authors of the *Mirror to Hospital Pharmacy* highlighted a critical limitation of medication systems of that era:

> "From the viewpoint of patient safety, one of the major advances in dispensing procedures would be the interpretation by the pharmacist of the physician's original ... order for the patient. In many hospitals, the pharmacist never sees the physician's original order. In cases where the physician does write an original prescription, he does so only for a limited number of drugs, the other drugs being stock items on the nursing units. In many cases the pharmacist receives only an order transcribed by a nurse or even more commonly by a lay person such as a ward clerk. As a result, errors made by the prescribing physician and errors made in transcribing his orders

often go undetected, while the patient receives the wrong drug, the wrong dosage form, or wrong amount of the drug, or is given the drug by injection when oral administration was intended, and vice versa."[14]

Concerns about medication errors and about overall efficiencies and best use of hospital personnel led to the development of improved drug distribution systems.[15] Two major studies were done in the early 1960s on unit dose drug distribution. At the University of Arkansas Medical Center, a centralized system was developed, and at the University of Iowa, a decentralized system was studied (see Figure 2-4).[16,17] Both projects documented important benefits to unit dose drug distribution, including greater nursing efficiency, better use of the pharmacist's talents, cost savings, and improved patient safety.

The key elements of unit dose drug distribution, as the system has evolved from the original studies, are as follows:

1. The pharmacist receives the physician's original order or a direct copy of the order.

Figure 2-4

Pioneers in Unit Dose Drug Distribution—William Heller (circa 1965) and William Tester (circa 1965)[a]

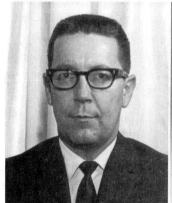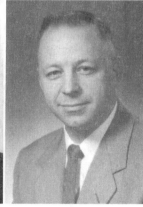

[a] The pharmacy departments led by these two prominent hospital pharmacists— William M. Heller (left), University of Arkansas Medical Center, and William W. Tester (right), University of Iowa Hospital—conducted important studies on unit dose drug distribution in the 1960s. This method of drug distribution was devised in response to the results of medication error studies.

Source: ASHP Archives.

2. A pharmacist reviews the medication order before the first dose is dispensed.

3. Medications are contained in single-unit packaging.

4. Medications are dispensed in as ready-to-administer form as possible.

5. Not more than a 24-hour supply of doses is delivered or available at the patient-care area at any time.

6. A patient medication profile is concurrently maintained for each patient.[18]

These precepts for state-of-the-art drug distribution are met widely in U.S. hospitals today. For example, in a 2002 survey, in 79% of hospitals, pharmacists reviewed and approved all medication orders before the drug was administered to patients. The figure for the largest hospitals (≥400 beds) was 92%.[19]

There has been much debate in hospital pharmacy over the years about the virtues of centralized versus decentralized drug distribution. With a decentralized system, pharmacists come in contact more regularly with physicians, nurses, and patients, which is consistent with contemporary views about how the profession should be practiced. Among all hospitals, 20% use a decentralized system; the figure is 41% for the largest hospitals.[19] Many hospitals indicate that they would like to move toward decentralized pharmacy services in the future (see Table 2-2).

U.S. hospitals have shown a remarkable rate of adoption of point-of-use automated storage and distribution devices, which are now used to some extent in 58% of facilities. Point-of-use dispensing is now the primary method of dose delivery in about one-fourth of U.S. hospitals.[19]

Pharmacy-based IV admixture services have been widely adopted by U.S. hospitals. Development of such services, as a professional imperative, was a topic of intense interest in the 1960s.[20] For short-term hospitals as a whole, ASHP estimates that about 80% of IV admixtures are now prepared by the pharmacy department.[19]

ASHP's 2002 survey showed that most hospitals regularly engage in a number of programs designed to increase the safety of injectable medications, including educational programs on IV administration equipment (82%), administration and precautions associated with high-risk therapies (71%), and administration of IV push medications (62%); promulgating lists of approved IV push medications (57%); and affixing supplemental labels for IV push medications (53%).[19]

There is immense interest in U.S. hospitals in applying computer technology to improve the safety of medication prescribing, dispensing, and administration. Computer-generated medication administration records are used in 64% of all hospitals and in 75% of the largest hospitals.[19] The foregoing data notwithstanding, the cost of such technology is having a decided moderating effect on the rate of adoption. For example, in 2002, only about 2% of hospitals used computer-readable coding technology to improve accuracy of medication administration, and, in 2004, only about 3% of hospitals used a computerized prescriber order entry system that was linked to a decision support system.[13,19]

Because of the concerns of groups such as the Institute of Medicine and various federal agencies, improving patient safety is now a major national priority.[21] When that general interest in patient safety embraces medication-use safety, hospital pharmacists have cheered and felt "it's about time!" Further breakthrough advances in medication-use safety will depend on a fundamental reengineering of the entire medication-use process, a shift toward a true team culture in providing care, and wider application of computer technology.[22] As new technologies or new patterns of health professional behavior evolve, history suggests that hospital pharmacists will be at the leading edge of those advances.

Table 2-2
Hospitals with Decentralized Drug Product Distribution[19]

	Year 2002	Future Desire
All hospitals	20%	44%
Largest hospitals (≥400 beds)	41%	56%

Promoting Rational Drug Use

In U.S. hospitals, the concept of a pharmacy and therapeutics (P&T) committee, as a formal mechanism for the pharmacy department and the medical staff to communicate on drug-use issues, was first promulgated in 1936 by Edward Spease (dean of the School of Pharmacy at Western Reserve University) (Figure 2-5) and Robert Porter (chief pharmacist at the University's

Figure 2-5

Advocate of the Pharmacy and Therapeutics Committee—Edward Spease (1883–1957), circa 1952[a]

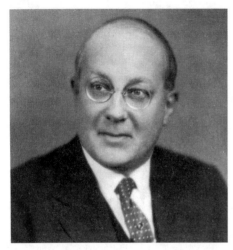

[a] Edward Spease established one of the first college courses in hospital pharmacy and developed the Minimum Standards for Hospital Pharmacies for the American College of Surgeons in 1936. At the time, Spease was dean and professor at Cleveland's Western Reserve University School of Pharmacy.

Source: ASHP Archives.

hospitals).[23] Subsequently, the American Hospital Association and the American Society of Hospital Pharmacists jointly developed guidance on the P&T committee and on the operation of a hospital formulary system. The formulary system is a method whereby the medical staff of a hospital, working through the P&T committee, evaluates, appraises, and selects from among the drug products available those that are considered most useful in patient care. The formulary system is also the framework in which a hospital's medication-use policies are established and implemented.

A major imperative for the advocates of the formulary system in the mid-1900s was to manage the proliferation of drug products. The number of new market entries for just one year, 1951, were as follows:

New drug products, 332
New drug entities, 35
Duplications of drug entities, 74
Combination products, 221[24]

In 1957, slightly more than half of all hospitals operated under the formulary system.[10] Today, essentially all hospitals do so.[13]

In 1957, 58% of hospitals had an active P&T committee, and a similar percentage of hospitals had a formulary or approved drug list. However, about one fourth of the P&T committees were inactive.[10] Today, nearly all hospitals in the U.S. have an active P&T committee that meets an average of seven times a year.[13]

In the late 1950s, the functions of P&T committees focused on very basic activities such as delegating to the chief pharmacist responsibility for preparing product specifications and selecting sources of supply (66% of committees) and approving drugs by nonproprietary name (50%).[10] In most hospitals today, the P&T committee has authorized pharmacists to track and assess adverse drug events (ADEs), conduct retrospective drug-use evaluations, and identify and monitor patients on high-risk therapies.[13]

In summary, concepts first advanced in the 1930s regarding a formal communications linkage between the hospital pharmacy department and the medical staff with respect to drug-use policy have taken hold firmly. Hospital pharmacists are heavily engaged in helping the medical staff establish drug-use policies, in implementing those policies, in monitoring compliance with those policies, and in taking corrective action. The invention of the pharmacy and therapeutics committee and the hospital formulary system has facilitated the deep involvement of pharmacists in promoting rational drug use in hospitals.

Fostering Optimal Patient Outcomes

U.S. hospital pharmacists have evolved markedly in their self-concept over the past 50 years. As recently as 20 years ago, the traditional pharmacist mission prevailed, a mission that was captured in the words, *right drug, right patient, right time,* connoting a drug-product-handling function. *Right drug* in this context meant whatever the physician ordered. Today's philosophy about the mission of pharmacists focuses on achieving optimal outcomes from medication use. The overarching question for the hospital pharmacist is whether the right drug is being used in the first place. A popular phrase used to summarize this philosophy is, "The mission of pharmacists is to help people make the best use of medicines." These words reflect a profound paradigm shift with respect to the primary purpose of pharmacy practice.[25,26]

In the 1950s, hospital pharmacy's Spartan staffing levels did not leave much time for work beyond the basics of acquiring, storing, compounding, and distributing medications. Nevertheless, chief pharmacists of the time were called upon frequently by physicians and nurses to answer drug information questions related to dosage, dosage forms, and pharmacology. Somewhat less frequently, pharmacists were asked for advice on adverse drug reactions and clinical comparisons of products. In analyzing pharmacist consultations, the authors of the *Mirror to Hospital Pharmacy* suggested that both weakness in the pharmacist's scientific knowledge and lack of time contributed to limited progress in this realm.

The transformation of the hospital pharmacy department from a product orientation to a clinical orientation was stimulated by active consensus-building efforts by hospital pharmacy leaders. One important example of such efforts was the ASHP Head conference.[25]

Hilton Head refers to a consensus-seeking invitational conference conducted in 1985 in Hilton Head, South Carolina, officially designated as an invitational conference on Directions for Clinical Practice in Pharmacy (see Figure 2-6). The purpose of the meeting was to assess the progress of hospital pharmacy departments in implementing clinical pharmacy. What emerged from the event was the idea that clinical pharmacy should not be thought of as something separate from pharmacy practice as a whole. Rather, hospital pharmacies should function as clinical departments with a mission of fostering the appropriate use of medicines. This was a very important idea because most hospital pharmacists thought in terms of adding discrete clinical services (such as pharmacokinetic monitoring) rather than conceptualizing the totality of the department's work as a clinical enterprise.

Working through its affiliated state societies, ASHP supported repetitions of the conference on a regional basis. ASHP leaders spoke at meetings around the country about the ideas of Hilton Head, and the *American Journal of Hospital Pharmacy* published numerous papers on the subject.

As a result, many individual pharmacy departments began to hold retreats of their staffs to reassess the fundamental mission of their work. It was common for departments to adopt mission statements that, for the first time, framed their work not in terms of drug distribution but in terms of achieving optimal patient outcomes from the use of medicines.

The most important indirect indicators of hospital pharmacist clinical activity in the current era are

Figure 2-6
Hilton Head Conference, 1985[a]

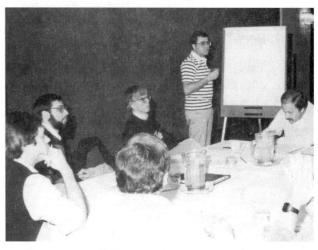

[a] A workshop session at ASHP's Hilton Head conference in 1985. This invitational consensus-seeking program was designed to assess the progress of hospital pharmacy departments in implementing clinical pharmacy; as a result of the discussions, many hospital pharmacy departments began to conceptualize their mission in terms of fostering appropriate use of medicines. Standing at the flip chart at one of the break-out sessions is Henri R. Manasse, Jr., at the time dean of the School of Pharmacy, University of Illinois at Chicago

Source: ASHP Archives.

shown in Table 2-3. There is a growing body of scientific evidence, published in both the medical and pharmacy literature, about the positive outcomes achieved through pharmacist involvement in direct patient care.[27–30]

In summary, U.S. hospital pharmacists today are engaged in extensive clinical activity, which is a major change from practice of 50 years ago. We are not yet at the point where a majority of hospital patients who are on medication therapy receive the benefit of clinical oversight by the pharmacist, but progress in this direction continues to be made.

Recap of Major Themes

Thus we have a picture of the major thrust of changes in hospital pharmacy over the past 50 years. The four major themes have been, first, the universal recognition by hospitals that pharmacists must be in charge of drug product acquisition, distribution, and control; second, hospital pharmacy departments have assumed a major role in patient safety; third, pharmacy departments have assumed a major role in promoting rational drug therapy; and, finally, pharmacy departments

Table 2-3
Indicators of Contemporary Hospital Pharmacist Clinical Activity

	All Hospitals	Largest Hospitals (≥400 beds)
Hospitals with decentralized pharmacists (1999 data)[a]	29%	82%
Percentage of decentralized pharmacists time spent on clinical activities (1999)	59%	-
Pharmacists have authority to initiate medication orders (2001)	52%	62%
Pharmacists attend rounds (2004)	35%	79%
Pharmacists provide drug information consultations (2004)	90%	-
Pharmacists monitor prescriber compliance with medication-use policies (2004)	81%	92%

[a] All data are from ASHP national surveys of the year shown.

have defined their mission in terms of optimal patient outcomes from medication use. Taken together, these changes signify that pharmacy practice in U.S. hospitals over the past 50 years has become more intensive in its professional staffing, more directly focused on patient care, and more directly influential on the quality and outcome of patient care. In short, hospital pharmacy has been transformed from a marginal, optional activity into a vital profession contributing immensely to the health and well being of patients and to the stability of the institutions that employ them.

Explaining the Transformation

A combination of indirect and direct factors helps explain this transformation in hospital pharmacy. Indirect factors are those forces external to hospital pharmacy that fostered development of the field. These factors include the following:

- Shift of national resources into health care, especially hospital care (stimulated immensely by implementation of Medicare in 1965 and expansion of other health insurance coverage).
- Expanded clinical research and drug product development.

- Greater complexity and cost of drug therapy accompanied by sophisticated pharmaceutical product marketing.
- Growing interest in improving the quality of health care services.

More important for this chapter's discussion are the internal factors within hospital pharmacy that precipitated the changes discussed above. In this category, five points merit discussion:

1. Visionary leadership
2. Professional associations
3. Pharmacy education
4. Postgraduate residency education and training
5. Practice standards

Visionary Leadership

One cannot read the early literature of hospital pharmacy in the U.S. without being impressed by the clear articulation of an exciting, uplifting vision by that era's practice leaders. These views were being expressed at a time when pharmacy was a marginal profession in the U.S.; when most pharmacists were engaged primarily in retail, mercantile activities; when hospital pharmacy had little visibility and respect; and when hospital pharmacy was a refuge for pharmacists who preferred minimal interactions with the public. Out of this environment emerged a number of hospital pharmacists, many of them at university teaching hospitals, who expressed an inspiring vision about the development of hospital pharmacy and about the role of hospital pharmacy in elevating the status of pharmacy as a whole.

These were leaders such as Arthur Purdum, Edward Spease, Harvey A. K. Whitney, and Donald E. Francke (to mention only a few) who were familiar with the history of pharmacy and had a sense of pharmacy's unfulfilled potential. Many of them had seen European pharmacy firsthand and decried the immense gap in professional status and scope of practice between the two continents.

A sense of the deep feelings of these leaders may be gained from the following comment by Edward Spease, a retired pharmacy dean speaking in 1952 about his initial exploration of hospital pharmacy 40 years earlier:

"I expected to see true professional pharmacy in hospitals and was much disappointed that it did not exist there. The more I observed and heard about the growing tendency towards commercial-

ism in drugstores, the more I felt that if professional pharmacy was to exist, let alone grow to an ideal state, it would have to be in the hospital where the health professions were trained....
Good pharmacy is as important in hospitals away from teaching centers as it is in the teaching and research hospital. It can be developed to a high degree of perfection there, too, *if the pharmacist can get the picture in his mind.*" (Emphasis added.)[31]

"...if the pharmacist can get the picture in his mind." Those are key words that reflect that early hospital pharmacy leaders were trying to create a new model for pharmacy practice in hospitals and not allow this practice setting to become an extension of the type of practice that prevailed in community pharmacies. These leaders were change agents with a missionary zeal, and they were blessed with the ability to infect others with their passion.

It is noteworthy that the *Mirror to Hospital Pharmacy* framed the entire Audit project in the context of professional advancement. The report laid out the essential characteristics of a profession and articulated goals for hospital pharmacy that would bring pharmacy as a whole into better alignment with those characteristics.

Professional Associations

The national organization of hospital pharmacists— the American Society of Health-System Pharmacists (ASHP)—has had a profound effect on the advancement of the field. The visionary hospital pharmacists of the early 1900s focused much of their energies on the creation of an organizational structure for hospital pharmacy. One landmark event was the creation of the Hospital Pharmacy Association of Southern California in 1925. On a national level, organizational efforts were funneled through the American Pharmaceutical Association (APhA), the oldest national pharmacist organization in the country. For years, hospital pharmacists participated in various committee activities of APhA focused on their particular interest. Then, in 1936, a formal APhA subsection on hospital pharmacy was created. This modest achievement evolved to the creation of ASHP in 1942 as an independent organization affiliated with APhA[32] (see Figure 2-7).

There are two essential things that ASHP has done for the advancement of hospital pharmacy. One is to serve as a vehicle for the nurturing, expression, and actualization of the professional ideals and aspirations of hospital pharmacists. In its early years, ASHP conducted a series of educational institutes that were very influential in enhancing knowledge and skills and in building esprit de corps among hospital pharmacists.[33] Also noteworthy, especially as the organization has grown in size and diversity, is ASHP's efforts to develop consensus about the direction of practice.[25,26]

The second essential act of ASHP has been its creations of resources to assist practitioners in fostering the development of hospital pharmacy practice. One example is the *AHFS Drug Information* reference book (and, in recent times, electronic versions for central information systems, desktop computers, and handheld devices), which is the most widely used independent source of drug information in U.S. hospitals. Another example is the *American Journal of Health-*

Figure 2-7

A Leading Force in the Creation of ASHP—Harvey A. K. Whitney (1894–1957) circa, 1940[a]

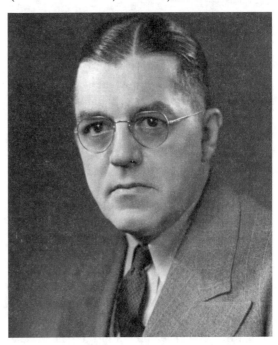

[a] Harvey A. K. Whitney took the lead in organizing hospital pharmacists in the United States. He was chief pharmacist at the University of Michigan Hospitals when he became ASHP's first chairman (president) in 1942. Whitney was also a pioneer in developing postgraduate training in hospital pharmacy.

Source: ASHP Archives.

System Pharmacy. These two publications, and other ASHP activities such as the Midyear Clinical Meeting, have produced a source of funds beyond membership dues that ASHP has used to develop a broad array of services that help members advance practice.

The original objectives of ASHP were as follows:

- Establish minimum standards of pharmaceutical service in hospitals

- Ensure an adequate supply of qualified hospital pharmacists by providing standardized hospital pharmacy training for four-year pharmacy graduates

- Arrange for interchange of information among hospital pharmacists

- Aid the medical profession in the economic and rational use of medicines

The core strengths of ASHP today are as follows:

- Practice standards and professional policy

- Advocacy (government affairs and public relations)

- Residency and technician training accreditation

- Drug information

- Practitioner education

- Publications and communications

One of the reasons for ASHP's success has been its clarity about objectives and its concentrated focus on a limited number of goals. It is a testament to the wisdom of ASHP's early leaders that the goals expressed in 1942 still serve to guide the organization, although different words are used today to express the same ideas, and some other points have been added. The organization continues as a powerful force in the ongoing efforts to align pharmacists with the needs that patients, health professionals, and administrators in hospitals have related to the appropriate use of medicines.

Pharmacy Education

There are three important points about the role of pharmacy education in transforming hospital pharmacy. First, as pharmacy education as a whole has been upgraded over the years, hospital pharmacy has benefited by gaining practitioners who are better educated and better prepared to meet the demands in hospital practice. Second, hospital pharmacy leaders have put considerable pressure on pharmacy educators to up-grade the pharmacy curriculum, to make it more consistent with the needs in hospital practice. This is significant because practice demands have always been far more intense in hospitals than in community pharmacy, so pressure to meet the demands in hospitals served to elevate education for all pharmacists. Also, beginning in the 1970s, corresponding with increased emphasis on clinical pharmacy in the curriculum, hospital pharmacies played a much larger role in pharmacy education as clerkship rotation sites for pharmacy students. Third, in the early days of clinical education, faculty members from schools of pharmacy began establishing practice sites in hospitals, which often had a large impact on the nature of the hospital's pharmacy service.

Table 2-4 shows how the minimum requirements for pharmacy education have evolved over the years. It took a very long time for pharmacy in the U.S. to settle on the Pharm.D. as the sole degree for pharmacy practice. Many bitter fights—between educators, between practitioners, among educators and practitioners, and among educators and the retail employers of pharmacists—occurred over this issue. Now that the matter is settled, everyone seems to be moving on with the intention of making the best application of the pharmacist's excellent education.

Over the past 20 years, pharmacy education in the U.S. has been transformed completely from teaching primarily about the science of drug products to teaching primarily about the science of drug therapy. Trans-

Table 2-4

Evolution of Minimum Requirements for Pharmacist Education in the United States

Year	Minimum Requirement (Length of Curriculum and Degree Awarded)
1907	2 years (Graduate in Pharmacy)
1925	3 years (Graduate in Pharmacy or Pharmaceutical Chemist)
1932	4 years (B.S. or B.S. in Pharmacy)
1960	5 years (B.S. or B.S. in Pharmacy)[a]
2004	6 years (Pharm.D.)

[a] Transition period; some schools offered only the B.S. or the Pharm.D. degree; many schools offered both degrees, with the Pharm.D. considered an advanced degree.

formation of hospital pharmacy practice from a product orientation to a patient orientation could not have occurred without this change in education.

Postgraduate Residency Education and Training

Stemming from its early concerns about the inadequacy of pharmacy education for hospital practice, ASHP leaders advocated internships in hospitals and worked for years to establish standards for such training. This led to the concept of residency training in hospital pharmacy and a related ASHP accreditation program.[33-35]

Early hospital pharmacy leaders noted the following imperatives for hospital pharmacy residency training[36]:

- Hospitals were expanding, thereby creating a growing unmet need for pharmacists who had been educated and trained in hospital pharmacy.

- Pharmaceutical education was out of touch with the needs in hospital pharmacy.

- The internship training required by state boards for licensure was not adequate preparation for a career in hospital pharmacy practice.

- Hospital pharmacists required specialized training in manufacturing, sterile solutions, and pharmacy department administration.

- Organized effort was needed to achieve improvements in hospital pharmacy internships or residencies.

There are well over 10,000 pharmacists in practice who have completed accredited residency training. These individuals have been trained as change agents and practice leaders. Early in their careers, they came to understand the complexity of hospital pharmacy, including inpatient operations, outpatient services, drug product technology and quality, and medication-use policy. Residency training is the height of mentorship in professionalism in American pharmacy. Dreams are fostered in residency training—dreams of the profession becoming an ever more vital force in health care; dreams of patients improving their health status more readily because pharmacists are there to help them.

Practice Standards

Numerous legal and quasi-legal requirements affect hospital pharmacy practice. On the legal end of the spectrum are various federal laws governing drug products and state practice acts governing how the pharmacist behaves and how pharmacies are operated. At the opposite end of the spectrum are voluntary practice standards promulgated by organizations such as ASHP.

A practice standard is an authoritative advisory document, issued by an expert body, that offers advice on the minimum requirements or optimal method for addressing an important issue or problem. A practice standard does not generally have the force of law. Methods used to foster compliance with practice standards include education and peer pressure. ASHP's practice standards have been very important in elevating hospital pharmacy in the United States.

The origins of hospital pharmacy practice standards go back to 1936 when the American College of Surgeons adopted the *Minimum Standard for Pharmacies in Hospitals*. This document was semidormant for a number of years, but it served as a rallying point for hospital pharmacists and revision and promulgation of the Standard became a priority for ASHP.[37]

The revision pursued by ASHP in the 1940s specified the following minimum requirements:

- An organized pharmacy department under the direction of a professionally competent, legally qualified pharmacist

- Pharmacist authority to develop administrative policies for the department

- Development of professional policies for the department with the approval of the pharmacy and therapeutics committee

- Ample number of qualified personnel in the department

- Adequate facilities

- Expanded scope of pharmacist's responsibilities:
  - Maintain a drug information service
  - Nurse and physician teaching
  - File periodic progress reports with administrator

- P&T committee must establish a formulary

From this modest beginning, ASHP has developed more than 60 practice standards that deal with most aspects of hospital pharmacy operations and several major controversies in therapeutics.[38]

ASHP practice standards have been used effectively over the years as a lever for raising the quality of hospital pharmacy services. The standards have been used in the following ways:

- Requirements for pharmacy practice sites that conduct accredited residency programs

- Guidance to practitioners who desire to voluntarily comply with national standards

- Guidance to the Joint Commission on Accreditation of Healthcare Organizations in developing standards for pharmacy and the medication-use process

- Tools for pharmacy directors who are seeking administrative approval for practice changes

- Guidance to regulatory bodies and courts of law

- Guidance to curriculum committees of schools of pharmacy

Summary of Internal Factors

In summary, five internal factors have played a large role in transforming U.S. hospital pharmacy over the past 50 years: (1) visionary leadership, (2) a strong professional society, (3) reforms in pharmacy education, (4) residency training, and (5) practice standards. The common element among these forces has been dissatisfaction with the status quo and burning desire to bring hospital pharmacy in better alignment with the needs of patients and the needs of physicians, nurses, other health professionals, and administrators in hospitals.

Summary

From the author's perspective, clouded to be sure by participation in the hospital pharmacy movement for many years, four tentative lessons may be drawn from the history of U.S. hospital pharmacy:

1. Fundamental change of complex endeavors requires leadership and time. Hospital pharmacists are sometimes frustrated by the slow pace of change. Wider study of history might help practitioners dissolve that discouragement.

2. It is important to engage as many practitioners as possible in assessing hospital pharmacy's problems and identifying solutions, so that a large number of individuals identify with the final plan and are committed to pursuing it.

3. It is critical to recognize and capitalize on changes in the environment that may make conditions more favorable to the advancement of hospital pharmacy. This requires curiosity about the world at large.

4. It is important to regularly and honestly assess progress and embark on a new approach if the existing plan for constructive change is not working or has run its course. This requires open-mindedness and a good sense of timing.

Today's challenges in hospital pharmacy are no more daunting than those that faced hospital pharmacy's leaders and innovators in the past. Fortunately, hospital pharmacy is imbued with a culture of taking stock, setting goals, making and executing plans, measuring results, and refining plans. If hospital pharmacy sticks to this time-tested formula, it will continue to be a beacon for the profession as a whole.

References

1. Niemeyer G, Berman A, Francke DE. Ten years of the American Society of Hospital Pharmacists, 1942–1952. *Bull Am Soc Hosp Pharm.* 1952;9:279–421.

2. Higby G. American hospital pharmacy from the colonial period to the 1930s. *Am J Hosp Pharm.* 1994;51: 2817–23.

3. Harris RR, McConnell WE. The American Society of Hospital Pharmacists: a history. *Am J Hosp Pharm.* 1993;50(suppl 2):S3–S45.

4. Berman A. Historical currents in American hospital pharmacy. *Drug Intell Clin Pharm.* 1972;6:441–7.

5. Wolfe HG. Charles Rice (1841–1901), an immigrant in pharmacy. *Am J Pharm Educ.* 1950;14:285–305.

6. Burkholder DF. Martin Inventius Wilbert (1865–1916): hospital pharmacist, historian, and scientist. *Am J Hosp Pharm.* 1968;25:330–43.

7. Williams WH. Pharmacists at America's first hospital, 1752–1841. *Am J Hosp Pharm.* 1976;33:804–7.

8. Starr P. The reconstitution of the hospital. In: Starr P. *The Social Transformation of American Medicine.* New York: Basic Books; 1982:145–79.

9. Hayhow EC, Amberg G, Dooley MS, et al. Report of committee on pharmacy, American Hospital Association, 1937. *Bull Am Soc Hosp Pharm.* 1948;5:89–96.

10. Francke DE, Latiolais CJ, Francke GN, et al. *Mirror to Hospital Pharmacy—A Report of the Audit of Pharmaceutical Services in Hospitals.* Washington: American Society of Hospital Pharmacists; 1964.

11. *AHA Hospital Statistics, 2005.* Chicago: Health Forum; 2005.

12. Purdum WA. Minimum standards and the future. *Bull Am Soc Hosp Pharm.* 1951;8:114–7.

13. Pedersen CA, Schneider PJ, Scheckelhoff DJ. ASHP national survey of pharmacy practice in hospital settings: prescribing and transcribing—2004. *Am J Health-Syst Pharm.* 2005;62:378–90.

14. Francke DE, Latiolais CJ, Francke GN, op. cit. p 115.

15. Barker KN, McConnell WE. The problems of detecting medication errors in hospitals. *Am J Hosp Pharm.* 1962;19:361–9.

16. Barker KN, Heller WM. The development of a centralized unit dose dispensing system, part one: description of the UAMC experimental system. *Am J Hosp Pharm.* 1963;20:568–79.

17. Black HJ, Tester WW. Decentralized pharmacy operations utilizing the unit dose concept. *Am J Hosp Pharm.* 1964;21:344–50.

18. ASHP technical assistance bulletin on hospital drug distribution and control. *Am J Hosp Pharm.* 1980;37:1097–103.

19. Pedersen CA, Schneider PJ, Scheckelhoff DJ. ASHP national survey of pharmacy practice in hospital settings: dispensing and administration—2002. *Am J Health-Syst Pharm.* 2003;60:52–68.

20. Holysko Sr, MN, Ravin RL. A pharmacy centralized intravenous additive service. *Am J Hosp Pharm.* 1965;22:266–71.

21. Committee on Quality of Health Care in America (Institute of Medicine). *Crossing the Quality Chasm—A New Health System for the 21st Century.* Washington: National Academy Press; 2001.

22. Re-engineering the medication-use system—proceedings of a national interdisciplinary conference conducted by the Joint Commission of Pharmacy Practitioners. *Am J Health-Syst Pharm.* 2000;57:537–601.

23. Francke DE, Latiolais CJ, Francke GN, op. cit. p 139.

24. Francke DE. Hospital pharmacy looks to the future. In: Harvey A. K. *Whitney Award Lectures (1950–2003).* Bethesda, MD: ASHP Research and Education Foundation; 2004:19–25.

25. Directions for clinical practice in pharmacy—proceedings of an invitational conference conducted by the ASHP Research and Education Foundation and the February 10–13, 1985, Hilton Head Island, South Carolina. *Am J Hosp Pharm.* 1985;42:1287–342.

26. Implementing pharmaceutical care. Proceedings of an invitational conference conducted by the American Society of Hospital Pharmacists and the ASHP Research and Education Foundation. *Am J Hosp Pharm.* 1993;50:1585–656.

27. Leape LL, Cullen DJ, Clapp MD, et al. Pharmacist participation on physician rounds and adverse drug events in the intensive care unit. *JAMA.* 1999;282:267–70.

28. Kucukarslan SN, Peters M, Mlynarek M, et al. Pharmacists on rounding teams reduce preventable adverse drug events in hospital general medicine units. *Arch Intern Med.* 2003;163:2014–8.

29. Boyko WL, Yurkowski PJ, Ivey MF, et al. Pharmacist influence on economic and morbidity outcomes in a tertiary care teaching hospital. *Am J Health-Syst Pharm.* 1997;54:1591–5.

30. Bjornson DC, Hiner WO, Potyk RP, et al. Effect of pharmacists on health care outcomes in hospitalized patients. *Am J Hosp Pharm.* 1993;1875–84.

31. Spease E. Background to progress. *Bull Am Soc Hosp Pharm.* 1953;10:362–4.

32. Niemeyer G. Founding and growth. *Bull Am Soc Hosp Pharm.* 1952;9:299–338.

33. Niemeyer G. Education and training. *Bull Am Soc Hosp Pharm.* 1952;9:363–75.

34. Francke DE. Contributions of residency training to institutional pharmacy practice. *Am J Hosp Pharm.* 1967; 24:193–203.

35. ASHP residency and accreditation information. Available at: http://www.ashp.org/rtp/index.cfm?cfid=4992632&CFToken=35717293. Accessed February 1, 2005.

36. Francke DE, Latiolais CJ, Francke GN, op. cit. p 157–67.

37. Niemeyer G. Establishment of minimum standard. *Bull Am Soc Hosp Pharm.* 1952;9:339–46.

38. ASHP policy positions, statements, and guidelines. Available at: http://www.ashp.org/bestpractices/index.cfm?cfid=4992632&CFToken=35717293. Accessed February 1, 2005.

Chapter 3

The Pharmacy Staff

William A. Miller

Introduction

The number one resource of the pharmacy department is the pharmacy staff. For this reason, it is critical that the pharmacy staff be carefully selected, effectively managed, and provided benefits and an environment conducive for staff retention. The modern hospital pharmacy department offers a wide range of pharmaceutical services requiring a diverse pharmacy staff. In addition to the provision of patient care services by pharmacists and pharmacy technicians, the pharmacy department must be well-managed and operated as a business unit of the organization.

Over the last 40 years, the well-developed hospital pharmacy department has transitioned from a department primarily focused on drug preparation and dispensing to a department primarily focused on the provision of patient care services. The terms *clinical pharmacy* and *pharmaceutical care* are now widely used to characterize the transition of pharmacy from a profession primarily focused on drug preparation and dispensing to a profession primarily focused on the use of drug knowledge to provide safe and effective patient drug therapy.[1] To contrast the present focus of hospital pharmacy services to the past, pharmacy service descriptions for today's hospital pharmacy departments include the provision of pharmaceutical care and clinical pharmacy services as well as other services, which focus primarily on the distribution, compounding, and control of drug use. As pharmacists become essential members of interdisciplinary teams caring for patients, pharmacists are being viewed as patient care providers along with physicians, nurses, and other health professionals involved in direct patient care. In the future, pharmacists are likely to focus more exclusively on the provision of pharmaceutical care to patients. Thus, it is clear that the character of the professional pharmacy staff will continue to evolve as pharmacy evolves as a clinical profession. It is also likely that critical thinking, problem solving, and patient care skills of the future hospital pharmacist will need to be more advanced than today as medical care advances and the role of pharmacists evolve.

This chapter will address factors affecting present and future needs for pharmacy staff: the type, mix, and numbers of pharmacy staff needed by pharmacy departments to deliver hospital pharmacy services today and in the future; personnel management and leadership; management staff relations; and effective strategies to recruit, hire, develop, review, and retain staff in today's hospital environment.

Factors Affecting Present and Future Needs for Pharmacy Staff

The staff needed by a department of pharmacy is driven by the mission and scope and depth of services provided by the department. Today the mission of the pharmacy department in most hospitals emphasizes improving patient care outcomes and patient safety through the provision of patient care, clinical, and drug distribution services. Pharmacy departments in academic or academically affiliated settings are more likely to emphasize teaching and research in addition to service as a part of their mission. The *ASHP Guidelines: Minimum Standard for Pharmacies in Hospitals* describes a minimum level of practice that all hospital pharmacy departments should consistently provide.[2] These guidelines state that pharmacy departments should have a written mission statement, short and long-term goals, and a scope of services consistent with the hospital's mission and patient care services. When possible, 24 pharmaceutical services should be maintained in all hospitals. Pharmacy services should typically include the following:

- Pharmacy administrative services
- Medication-use policy development and drug information services
- Drug distribution and control services
- Drug preparation and compounding services
- Clinical pharmacy or patient care services to inpatients and outpatients served by the hospital
- Investigational drug services when warranted

ASHP has developed numerous positions, statements, and guidelines to help hospital pharmacists establish best practices for pharmacy and medication use systems in hospitals and health care systems. These guidelines are annually published as *Best Practices for Hospital and Health-System Pharmacy*.[3] In addition, ASHP has developed a *Best Practice Self Assessment Tool* (available at www.ashp.org) for use by pharmacy directors and managers to assess compliance of their department to nationally recognized hospital pharmacy best practices. Best practices are derived from the opinions of expert panels, ASHP councils and task forces, opinion leaders, and original research. Pharmacy directors and managers who complete a pharmacy self-assessment using this tool are able to identify and measure major and minor practice gaps as compared to ASHP practice guidelines. Pharmacy managers can use the results of the self-assessment to develop a prioritized quality improvement plan to address the practice gaps identified through the self-assessment. Managers can periodically rescore their practices as a part of their departmental performance improvement plan to track and demonstrate practice improvements over time. Performance improvements plans, resulting from self-assessments by pharmacy managers, will undoubtedly call for additional staff, information technology, and other resources needed to more closely approximate best practices.

ASHP conducts national pharmacy surveys to assess the state of pharmacy services in hospitals. Drug distribution and control, drug preparation and compounding, and administrative pharmacy services are provided to support patient care in all hospitals. The degree of involvement of pharmacists in patient drug therapy monitoring varies significantly among hospitals. Some hospitals primarily provide targeted drug monitoring while others have decentralized pharmacy services with pharmacists more actively engaged in drug therapy monitoring and patient care.[4] The last survey examining drug dispensing and administration indicates that the majorities of hospitals use a centralized inpatient drug distribution system (80%), but 44% of hospitals indicated that they planned to further decentralize the drug distribution system. Decentralization of the drug distribution system occurs more frequently in large hospitals (e.g., greater than 300 beds) than small (e.g., less than 100) and medium-sized (e.g., 200 beds) hospitals. Concurrent with decentralization of the drug distribution system, pharmacy departments in medium and large hospitals are deploying decentralized phar-

macists to provide drug distribution support and clinical services on various patient care units.[5] Data from these surveys show a gradual but consistent movement to greater involvement of pharmacists in drug therapy monitoring, patient education, physician consultation, physician education through the provision of drug information, and involvement of pharmacists in medication-use policy development.[6] Inpatient clinical services are most often more comprehensive than outpatient clinical services. In some hospitals, pharmacists are given prescriptive authority to manage specific drug therapy and/or provide disease state management of inpatients and outpatients. A greater number of pharmacists are being placed in clinics to provide physician consultation and disease state management services. These services are growing particularly in hospitals with large ambulatory clinics that treat indigent patients that use the hospital's clinics for primary care.

As pharmacists are expected by hospital administrators, other health providers, and accrediting bodies to be more directly involved in patient care, it is anticipated that a greater number of hospitals of all sizes will decentralize pharmacists to enable them to review and monitor drug therapy and provide drug information to physicians, nurses, and other providers as a member of interdisciplinary patient care teams. It is also anticipated that a greater number of pharmacists will be a part of interdisciplinary ambulatory care teams in hospitals with large ambulatory patient populations.

Bond has studied patient care and cost outcomes in hospitals with varying degrees of clinical pharmacy services and has found that hospitals that have more comprehensive clinical pharmacy services have improved patient care and cost outcomes.[7] He has suggested that evidenced-based core clinical pharmacy services should be present in all hospitals. The core services he suggests are drug information, adverse drug reaction management, drug protocol management, medical rounds, and admission drug histories. Today in most hospitals, physicians do not currently round with patient care teams. However, a greater number of hospitals are employing hospitalists who work full-time in the hospital taking care of patients for admitting physicians. In these hospitals, pharmacists often develop collaborative relationships with hospitalists and round with them to monitor and improve the pharmaceutical care of their patients. Bond has projected that implementing these four core clinical services in 2020 for 100% of inpatients in the United States would require

14,508 additional pharmacists, which would lead to increased pharmacy staffing in most hospitals. He believes this model is feasible given overall pharmacy manpower projections over this time period.[8,9]

The presence of pharmacists in patient care units to allow direct interaction with physicians, nurses, and other health care providers appears to be the most important factor in achieving good patient outcomes. As JCAHO and ASHP best practice requirements for hospitals evolve to require the presence of pharmacists in patient care areas, the type, mix, and number of staff needed to deliver pharmacy services in various types of hospitals will change.

Additional factors affecting the type and mix of pharmacy staff needed today and in the foreseeable future are the emphasis on improving patient safety and medication-use systems in hospitals. In the last decade the safety of the medication-use system in hospitals has come under scrutiny and has led to efforts by the government and JCAHO to take steps to further improve medication safety in hospitals. JCAHO introduced national patient safety goals and new medication management standards for hospitals in 2004.[10,11] These new medication management standards require the pharmacy department to provide greater oversight and control for all drugs used throughout hospitals. These standards have also established greater expectations for hospitals to have pharmacists prospectively review medication orders before drug dispensing and administration occurs to help ensure efficacious and safe drug therapy. Many of the national patient safety goals established by JCAHO involve medication safety. Pharmacy is expected to play a major role along with physicians and other involved providers in the establishment of safe medication-use systems throughout the hospital. Pharmacy is expected to present evidence based recommendations for consideration of the Pharmacy and Therapeutics Committee or other policy making committees of the hospital to help ensure safe prescribing, dispensing, administration, and monitoring of drug therapy. Pharmacist review of drug orders for appropriateness is becoming the most cognitively complex responsibility of pharmacists. Required review of all nonemergent drug prescriptions or orders by pharmacists prior to dispensing and administration is becoming the standard of care expected by JCAHO surveyors. These changes in the expectations for pharmacy services will dramatically affect the type and number of pharmacists needed by pharmacy departments in the future.

Hospitals are moving to establish electronic medical records, computerized physician order entry systems, and bar-coding of drug doses to allow confirmation of the right drug, dose, and time against a computerized medication profile prior to administration of the drug by nurses or other care givers. Order-entry systems are being programmed to check drug orders against other computerized patient information and standards of care used by the hospital to optimize drug selection, dosing, and administration. These changes will require the pharmacy department to employ more staff with information technology and automation qualifications.

Long range forecasts of pharmacy manpower needs and demand are based upon the assumption that pharmacists will predominantly function as providers of patient care and pharmacy technicians will utilize information technology and automation to largely assume responsibility for the drug distribution function of the profession of pharmacy. As a component of strategic planning, pharmacy directors must annually assess the use of pharmacy technicians, information technologies, and automation as methods to decrease the time spent by pharmacists in distributive work and increase the time they spend providing patient care services. Obviously new technologies and automation have to be included into financial and human resource planning for the pharmacy department and implemented when the technologies are mature and economically feasible.[12,13]

Collectively, these changes will require pharmacists to be more involved in the provision of clinical pharmacy services on patient care units and/or teams and greater involvement of pharmacists will be needed to establish the medication-use policies and systems used by hospitals now and in the future. These changes will also require expanded use of pharmacy technicians and staff with information technology and automation backgrounds. It is clear that the pharmacy staff of the future will be more diverse as pharmacy practice becomes more patient care focused and information technology and automation are used to improve the efficiency and safety of the medication use process.

Other chapters of this textbook describe the current and the projected future state for various pharmacy services. As briefly described in this chapter, the services provided by a pharmacy department reflect its mission and influence the type, mix, and number of professional and technical staff needed by a department today and in the future.

Type, Mix, and Number of Pharmacy Staff Needed by Pharmacy Departments

The provision of pharmacy services requires a diverse staff including a director of pharmacy and other pharmacy manager positions as needed, pharmacists, technicians, business, clerical, secretarial, and information technology support personnel. Each staff category must have an appropriate job description that describes the duties and responsibilities for each position. There may be more than one position for each category of pharmacy staff. For example, today pharmacists are employed by hospitals as staff pharmacists, clinical pharmacists, and clinical pharmacy specialists. The key duties and responsibilities for each type of pharmacist position differ. The job description for a staff pharmacist is more likely to emphasize drug preparation and dispensing than the job description for a clinical pharmacist or clinical pharmacy specialist. The credentials required for candidates for each position may also differ. For example, clinical pharmacy specialists are often required to have completed postgraduate residency training as a qualification for pharmacy practice positions in patient specific or specialized areas of practice (e.g., critical care, oncology, pediatrics, psychopharmacy, and geriatrics) while staff pharmacist positions require at a minimum a degree in pharmacy with previous hospital work experience being a desirable credential. Although board certification as a pharmacy specialist is not routinely required for clinical pharmacist or clinical specialist positions today, it is a desirable credential and in the future more pharmacy employers will require board certification.

The number, type, and mix of pharmacy positions varies dependent upon the mission, size, and types of patients treated by the hospital; the expectations of hospital leadership for pharmacy services; the mission and scope and depth of pharmacy services provided by the department; and the model for the delivery of pharmacy services used by the pharmacy department.

Larger hospitals often have a broader mission and scope and depth of pharmacy services and, thus, have a larger and more diversified pharmacy staff. Larger hospitals are more likely to have a greater number of intensive care beds and offer emergency trauma services and specialized medical and surgical services. A patient care acuity index is used as a gauge for the complexity of patient care provided by a hospital. Hospitals with high patient care acuity indexes are more likely to require decentralized, clinical pharmacy services and 24 pharmacy services leading to increased pharmacy staffing levels.

Hospital leaders including the hospital's chief executive office, chief nursing office, chief financial officer, and medical leaders may have limited expectations for pharmacy primarily focused on pharmacy's role in drug dispensing and control. For this reason it is still, unfortunately, not uncommon for some pharmacy department's mission to be primarily focused on drug distribution services, which, in turn, limits the diversity and number of staff needed by the pharmacy department.

Some pharmacy managers prefer using an integrated staff model for the delivery of pharmaceutical care with pharmacists providing both distributive and clinical services. This model often requires pharmacists to rotate between central and decentralized pharmacy areas. Pharmacists working under this model must have both good distributive and clinical pharmacy service skills. Other managers use a coordinated service delivery model, with some pharmacists assigned to central pharmacy service areas primarily to provide drug distribution related services, while other pharmacists are decentralized and assigned to particular patient populations or patient care units primarily to provide clinical pharmacy services. There are many variations and combinations of decentralized and centralized staffing models. There are no research papers in the pharmacy literature that clearly demonstrate the advantages of one model over another on overall patient care and economic outcomes. Numerous papers have demonstrated the value of the clinical pharmacy services on patient outcomes and cost avoidance.[14,15] Future pharmacy staffing models should primarily focus on achieving best patient and economic outcomes. Research is needed to establish optimum staffing models for various types of hospitals and health care systems.

To illustrate the difference in staffing requirements, two different types of hospital pharmacy departments are contrasted as case examples for staffing. A pharmacy mission and scope of pharmacy services statement for a 500-bed acute care hospital in a large metropolitan area is shown in Appendix 3-1. The pharmacy department in this hospital is affiliated with a college of pharmacy for teaching purposes. Job responsibilities for staff pharmacists, clinical pharmacists, or patient care unit pharmacists and clinical pharmacy specialists employed by this hospital are shown in Appendices 3-2 through 3-4. The hospital offers emergency and trauma services through an emergency department and has cardiovascular, neurological, medical, and surgical intensive care units with a combined total of 95 beds. The hospital offers oncology services including bone marrow transplantation as well as renal, liver, and heart transplants. The pharmacy department provides 24-hour services 7 days a week. The director of pharmacy for this department is primarily involved in planning, decision making, financial management, building relations with key administrative physician and nursing leaders, representing pharmacy within the institution on key committees, and overseeing the work of pharmacy mangers responsible for the day-to-day operations of the department. Based upon the mission and scope of services, the pharmacy department employs 126 staff. The distribution and numbers of staff needed to provide these services are listed in Appendix 3-5. A pharmacy mission and scope of pharmacy services for a 75-bed general community hospital in a rural community with a population of 18,000 is shown in Appendix 3-6. Sample lists of the job responsibilities for a staff pharmacist employed by this hospital are shown in Appendix 3-7. This hospital offers general medical and surgical units and has an obstetrics and gynecology unit. The hospital has one combined medical and surgical intensive care unit of 9 beds. Patients needing emergency, trauma and specialized services not provided by the hospital are referred to larger, acute care hospitals in a nearby large metropolitan area. The pharmacy department is staffed from 7 a.m. to 9 p.m. 5 days a week and is open from 8 a.m. to 12 noon on weekends. A pharmacist is on call to handle emergency pharmacy needs, but nurses have access to a drug cabinet for drugs needed after the pharmacy is closed. The rural community hospital's pharmacy mission is limited primarily to drug distribution, compounding, and drug control. The director of pharmacy in this setting serves as the pharmacy administrator, as a supervisor, and also participates in routine staffing of the department. Pharmacists dispense, compound, and review routine drug orders. They also serve as a source of drug information for physicians and nurses. They occasionally leave the pharmacy to review orders or solve drug-related problems for specific patients. Based upon the mission and scope of services, the pharmacy department employs 9 staff. The distribution and numbers of staff needed to provide these services are listed in Appendix 3-8. These two different hospital examples illustrate the differences in the number, type, and mix of pharmacy staff needed to provide pharmacy services.

Pharmacy Job Descriptions

Job descriptions are used to define employee responsibilities and accountabilities, establish performance expectations, write performance evaluations, and as a recruitment tool. Position descriptions should contain detailed information on the knowledge, skills, abilities, and experiences that acceptable candidates should possess. ASHP has developed the following suggested guidelines for information to be included in job descriptions[14]:

- Position title
- Duties, essential job functions, and responsibilities of the position
- Education, training, experience, and licensure required
- Knowledge, skills, and abilities required to perform assigned duties
- Reporting relationships
- Pay grade and salary range
- Education and training required to maintain competence
- Other specifications of the position that may be required to meet legal requirements

Key responsibilities for different types of pharmacist positions have been previously provided in Appendices 3-2, 3-3, 3-4, and 3-7. Readers may review these responsibilities as well as job descriptions from other hospitals and the pharmacy literature to craft pharmacist positions suitable to the needs of various pharmacy departments. Job descriptions should be reviewed annually and changed as the model for pharmacy services evolves in a pharmacy department and as additional expectations are established for pharmacy departments by hospital administration. For example, as previously noted patient safety is being emphasized by JCAHO and all hospitals are implementing quality improvement projects to improve the safety of their medication-use system. Job descriptions for pharmacists are being changed in hospitals to reflect this new emphasis area. Due to the trends towards decentralization of pharmacists, previously noted in many hospitals, pharmacist job descriptions are slowly evolving to require pharmacists to spend a greater percent of their effort providing patient care services.

To achieve high retention and low staff turnover rates, pharmacy managers must also create and or modify existing job descriptions to meet the needs of pharmacists and other staff for work they can enjoy and that fully utilize their knowledge and skills. Pharmacists and nonpharmacists come to work with different needs and work expectations. Today's pharmacy graduates are educated and trained by colleges of pharmacy to be providers of pharmaceutical care. Faculties instill in students the notion that their primary professional goal should be to become a provider of pharmaceutical care. One of the tenets of pharmaceutical care is that pharmacists are responsible and accountable for optimizing drug therapy for their patients. Many new graduates and pharmacists in practice desire positions that will allow them to focus on the provision of patient care services. Hospital pharmacy jobs advertised as decentralized pharmacist positions with an emphasis on the provision of clinical pharmacy services are very attractive. However, sometimes advertised jobs, upon closer inspection, may not be very attractive to pharmacist candidates. For example, if upon closer examination of a decentralized pharmacist job advertisement, a candidate discovers that the job requires the pharmacist to provide daily pharmaceutical care to over 150 patients, the candidate may conclude that the job is not a good match for them because he or she will be unable to effectively provide pharmaceutical care beyond reviewing prescription orders and monitoring laboratory and other test results for potential drug-related problems. Pharmacists who are working in decentralized pharmacist positions, with heavy patient loads like this advertised position, may likewise become frustrated and look for another decentralized pharmacist position that would require them to take care of fewer patients. This example illustrates the importance of the development of job descriptions matched to the needs of the pharmacy department while also meeting the needs of pharmacists for satisfying work.

Staffing Levels and Work and Productivity Measurement

Pharmacy departments and the profession as a whole have not developed good metrics to measure the work performed and productivity of pharmacy departments. The most common measure of work performed by pharmacy departments continues to be based on the number of prescriptions dispensed as inpatient doses or outpatient prescriptions. Consulting groups, based at large accounting companies, pool data from various hospital clients and develop pharmacy staffing ratios primarily based on doses dispensed. Hospitals use external consultants to help them reduce costs and

pharmacy staffing is often targeted as a potential cost reduction strategy for hospital administrators to consider.

Work measurement systems that rely solely on drug dispensing ratios for calculating pharmacy staffing levels do not take into account services other than drug dispensing aimed at improving patient care outcomes. Hospitals with extensive drug information and clinical pharmacy services appear to be over staffed using work measurement models that are primarily based on drug dispensing. ASHP has advocated the implementation of pharmacy productivity monitoring systems that analyze productivity changes in terms of their impact on patient outcomes. ASHP and other pharmacy organizations continue to communicate with health-system leaders and administrators and consulting firms on the value of clinical pharmacy services provided by pharmacists and on the use of accurate data to assess pharmacy productivity and staffing levels.

Some hospitals have developed internal work measurement systems to document work output and productivity and use these data for justifying the number of full-time equivalents employed by the department. Many hospital pharmacy departments collect clinical pharmacy intervention data to document the efforts of pharmacists to improve patient care outcomes through effective, safe, and cost-effective use of drugs. Drug information requests, recommendations, and interventions made by pharmacists subsequent to drug therapy monitoring are tracked using hospital specific or commercially available software. Cost avoidance savings are projected based on the recommendations or interventions made by pharmacists. The significance of pharmacotherapy recommendations made by pharmacists is also often tracked by pharmacy departments to show the impact of clinical services on improving the quality and safety of patient care.

Numerous studies have been performed to document the value and economic benefits of clinical pharmacy services.[15,16] These studies along with hospital specific intervention data can be used by pharmacy directors to support the need for clinical pharmacy services and additional staff. In spite of the lack of good work and productivity systems that measure clinical as well as distributive pharmacy services (as hospital administrators and medical and nursing leadership within hospitals perceive or recognize the value of clinical services and decentralized pharmacy services), pharmacy staffing increases have been approved. Better productivity and work measurement systems are needed and will most likely evolve to help hospitals monitor pharmacy work, productivity, and the impact of pharmacy services on patient care outcomes.

Human Resource Planning

As a component of strategic planning and pharmacy human resource planning and management, today's pharmacy directors and other managers must regularly plan, adjust, and review the type, mix, and number of pharmacy personnel needed to deliver pharmacy services provided by the department. Human resource planning often starts with the creation of a vision for the future state of the pharmacy department. ASHP national surveys on the status of pharmacy services ask questions about the future plans for the pharmacy. As previously noted, decentralization of pharmacists is a priority for many hospital pharmacy directors. Achieving decentralization starts as a vision. To achieve this vision, the director must convince hospital administration, nursing, and key medical leaders of the advantages of decentralization. Pharmacists who are comfortable in their role as centralized pharmacists may also need to be convinced and brought along with the advantages of decentralization. It is important for the director and management team to involve staff in human resource planning and to keep them aware of the time frame for significant staffing changes. For example, if the department is currently centralized without any decentralized pharmacy services, the staff should be involved in planning the role for decentralized pharmacists and be aware of the time frame for decentralization to begin before interested stakeholders outside pharmacy including physicians and nurses are made aware of the implementation plan.

Leadership and Management of Pharmacy Staff

Management and *leadership* are terms that are often used interchangeably by pharmacy staff. Managers are automatically viewed by the staff as being leaders, but managerial science suggests that not all managers are also leaders. Management is often described as getting things done through others. In contrast leadership is described as getting people or employees to share the leader's view of the mission, vision, beliefs, and values of the organization in order to achieve organizational goals. A mix of management and leadership is going on concurrently in the typical pharmacy department. Pharmacy directors and other managers use a variety of management and leadership styles to lead and manage the pharmacy staff and advance the pharmacy department. Managers must balance their leadership and management responsibilities. Some pharmacy directors spend more of their time on supervision and management and do not take advantage of the opportunities to create change and achieve goals through leadership. Many clinical pharmacists and clinical specialists have a negative attitude about management because they see it as controlling, rigid, conservative, uncreative, and bureaucratic. To fully involve pharmacists as direct, patient care providers, there is a need for more effective leadership and less management.

Leadership

Pointers has defined leadership as the process through which an individual attempts to intentionally influence another individual or group to accomplish a goal.[17] Numerous papers and books on leadership have described leadership theories, leadership qualities, and leadership processes. Holdford described leadership as a process because it is a series of actions exerted by individuals to accomplish goals.[18] Leaders exert influence to achieve their values and goals. Individuals who do not influence others are not leaders. Leaders use power available to them to influence staff perceptions and behavior. Holdford describes various types of power available to leaders including formal, reward, punishment, expert, charismatic, and information power.[18] Each of these types of power can be used by pharmacy managers to create influence to change staff perceptions and behavior. There are various theories about what makes an effective leader. Holdford reviews these theories.[18] The trait theory says that the traits of leaders are developed at birth or early in life. The behavioral theory says that leaders develop the behaviors and abilities expected of leaders over time. The situational theory states that good leaders adapt to the situation at hand and use the right combination of behaviors to achieve desired outcomes. Bennis defined the basic or essential ingredients for leadership as consisting of a guiding vision, integrity, passion, curiosity, and daring.[19] Leaders have a clear idea or guiding vision for what they want to achieve and persist in spite of failures. Leaders have a passion for their profession and life. Leaders demonstrate integrity characterized by self-knowledge, candor, and maturity. Because of their integrity leaders are trusted. Leaders are curious and explore new ways of doing things and adventure. Leaders are daring and are willing to accept failure in their pursuit of excellence.

Zilz and other pharmacy leaders described core components of leadership needed for high- performance pharmacy practice: core self, vision, relationships, learning, and mentoring.[20]

Bennis distinguishes managers and leaders as follows[19]:

- The manager administers; the leader innovates.

- The manager is a copy; the leader is an original.

- The manager imitates; the leader originates.

- The manager focuses on systems and structure; the leader focuses on people.

- The manager relies on control; the leader inspires trust.

- The manager has a short-range view; the leader has a long-range perspective.

- The manager focuses on the bottom line; the leader has an eye on the horizon.

- The manager accepts the status quo; the leader challenges it.

- The manager is the classic good soldier; the leader is his or her own person.

- The manager does things right; the leader does the right thing.

Pharmacy leaders and managers want staff to buy into their vision for pharmacy services and want to accomplish goals through the staff. Leaders and managers have to generate trust to get staff to buy in and support the vision and goals of the pharmacy department. Bennis identified four ingredients that generate and sustain trust between leaders and/or managers and staff.[19] Leaders demonstrate constancy, "stay the course," and avoid surprising staff. Leaders demonstrate congruity. There is no difference in the theories they espouse and the life they practice. Leaders demonstrate reliability and are there when it counts and support staff in the moments that matter. Leaders demonstrate integrity by honoring their commitments and promises.

Management

In 1960, McGregor, an early management theorist, described two different types of workers requiring two different management styles, which he labeled as *Theory X* and *Theory Y*. Theory X is based upon the assumption that humans inherently dislike working and will try to avoid it if they can. Because people dislike work they have to be coerced or controlled by management and threatened so they work hard enough. McGregor described Theory X employees as being lazy, less than intelligent, resistant to change, and requiring close supervision and direction. Theory X management is representative of an autocratic, authoritative, or hard management style.[21] In a work environment characterized by Theory X employees, McGregor postulated that managers need to be autocratic and unilaterally assume responsibility for all planning and decision making. This management style is conducive to large-scale, efficient operations as seen in mass production and other manufacturing facilities. Theory Y employees are described by McGregor as being people who view work as natural as play and rest and who expend the same amount of physical and mental effort in their works as in their private lives. Provided people are motivated; they will be self-directing to the aims of the organization. For these employees, job satisfaction is the key to engaging them and ensuring their commitment. Theory Y employees accept and seek responsibility and are imaginative and creative. Their ingenuity can be used to solve work problems. Theory Y management is representative of a participative or soft management style and is thought to be conducive to the management of professionals, knowledge workers, and managers. In 1981, Ouchi described a variant of Theory X and Y, which he labeled *Theory Z*.[22] He combined American and Japanese management practices at that time together. Theory Z assumes that people are innately self-motivated to not only do their work, but also to be loyal toward the company or organization and to want to make the organization succeed. Theory Z managers have a great deal of trust that their workers can make sound decisions. They act more as a coach to workers and let workers make most work-related decisions. Japanese management practices tend to rotate workers so they become generalists and are very knowledgeable about the company or organization. Theory X workers are often more specialized and are less knowledgeable about the company or organization. Theory Z requires mutual trust between workers and managers. Workers trust managers because they believe management will take care of them and their family and will let them make most of the work decisions. Workers resolve conflicts while managers play more of an arbitrator role in managing conflict and decision making. Theory Z is closer to Theory Y than X. Workers in a Theory Y organization may participate in decision making, but workers are not delegated as much decision-making powers as in a Theory Z organization. There are many interpretations and variants on these basic management styles that have described by other authors. Rather than labeling managers as a Theory X, Y, Z or any other type of manager, it is more practical to think of managers as using a mix of autocratic, democratic, and permissive management styles. A variety of autocratic, democratic, and permissive styles has been described by grouping managers into one of the following four management styles[23]:

- *Directive Democrat*—This type of manager makes decisions using a participative manner but closely supervises subordinates.

- *Directive Autocrat*—This type of manager makes decisions unilaterally and also closely supervises subordinates. This type of manager is often referred to as a *micromanager*.

- *Permissive Democrat*—This type of manager makes decisions using a participative manner and gives subordinates latitude in carrying out their work.

- *Permissive Autocrat*—This type of manager makes decisions unilaterally but gives subordinates latitude in carrying out his or her work.

There are textbooks, papers, and short articles describing a whole host of popular management styles and techniques. A quick search of management websites found numerous descriptions of various management styles. Following is a list of techniques or styles found on the web.[24] Some of these styles have been around for a long time with entire books written to describe how to use the style as a manager.

- *Management by Coaching and Development (MBCD)*—This type of manager sees himself or herself primarily as an employee trainer and heavily invests in staff development.

- *Management by Consensus (MBC)*—This type of manager constructs methods to allow individual employees to provide input into decision making and makes decisions as often as possible based upon consensus.

- *Management by Exception (MBE)*—This type of manager delegates as much responsibility and activity as possible to those below them, stepping in only when absolutely necessary to make decisions or manage situations.

- *Management by Objectives (MBO)*—The organization sets overall objectives and then this type of manager works with employees to set objectives aimed to achieve the organization's objectives.

- *Management by Performance (MBP)*—This type of manager seeks quality levels of performance through motivation and employee relations. Employees with high performance are rewarded.

- *Management by Styles (MBS)*—This type of manager adjusts his or her style to meet situational needs.

- *Management by Walking Around (MBWA)*—This type of manager walks around the organization, getting a feel for people and operations, and stopping to listen and talk. Information gathered by the manager is then used in decision making.

Although most managers have a predominant management style, there is a range of styles between the manager who is totally autocratic, to the manger who engages staff in decision making, to the manager who uses laissez-faire or "hands-off" style and delegate's decision making and autonomy in completing work to staff. Most managers vary their management style based on the situation at hand with different styles being appropriate given varying circumstances. No one management style is considered right or wrong although individual workers or employees prefer one style to another based on their own needs and outlooks on work.

These and other descriptions of management styles can be useful to both pharmacy managers and pharmacy staff. Managers can review management styles and decide which one or more of the styles are descriptive of their behavior as a manger. They can reflect on their style and decide to modify or change it. For example, if a manager's primary style is autocratic, he or she may work hard to use a more participative style in planning and decision making and to allow individual staff as well as staff groups or teams to make more decisions about how work will be done and completed. An effective way for managers to change their management style is to discuss their management style with staff, obtain feedback, and then, as deemed desirable, work to change their management habits. This takes courage since the manager may not want to openly discuss particular aspects of his or her management style that may not be well-liked by staff.

Managers may decide that part of the reason they act in an autocratic mode with staff is because their boss or manager is autocratic and is focused on quickly obtaining results. Thus, it is easier for the manager to be autocratic and to get work done quickly. In this instance, an autocratic style may or may not yield the best results, but the manager is focused on meeting expectations of his or her boss. It may be necessary for managers who are trying to change their management style to discuss this with their boss, particularly if the desired change in style is different that the style used by their boss.

Staff members unconsciously analyze the management style of their manager. However, if they consciously think about the management style of their manager, they may be able to better manage their relationship with their boss. For example, if your boss is primarily autocratic or a Type X manager, he or she is likely to be very results-oriented so it would make sense to focus your discussions with your manager around results in terms of what you can deliver and when. You also may want to make suggestions to improve workflow or processes in the context of improved results since this type of manager is often very results-oriented.

Pharmacists may follow the directions of an autocratic pharmacy manager out of respect for the manager's knowledge and success or out of a fear of retribution if not compliant with the wishes of the manager. Pharmacy technicians and other nonpharmacists working in pharmacy departments are more likely to follow the directions of an autocratic pharmacy manager, but many technicians also want to be involved with planning and decision making and also do not need close supervision to carry out their responsibilities.

If staff respect and trust the autocratic manager to make good decisions, overall staff morale can be acceptable. If staff do not respect and trust the autocratic manager to make decisions, staff morale will suffer. Democratic and permissive managers permit subordinates to participate in decision making and also give staff a considerable degree of autonomy in completing routine work activities. Staff that need to work in an environment that fosters self-esteem and self-actualization are happier working with more democratic or permissive managers that allow them to participate in decision making and complete work without a lot of supervision. Pharmacists and nonpharmacist staff positions are often readily available so dissatisfied or unhappy staff may leave a pharmacy department if the management environment is not matched to their needs.

Understanding leaders and managers is not as simple as reading any of the papers or books referenced for this chapter section. Leaders and managers should read and learn more about leadership and management to develop a greater awareness of their personal leadership and management skills and work to improve their skills over time. Leaders and managers can benefit from openly discussing their leadership and management style with staff to obtain feedback and better understand staff perceptions and viewpoints on the direction and management of the department.

Management-Staff Relations

Beliefs, Values, Needs, and Motivation of Pharmacy Staff

Managing people is the primary function of all organizational activities. For pharmacy leaders and managers to achieve their goals they must have cooperation from staff. Dwyer suggests that all behavior is designed, albeit subconsciously much of the time, to serve the values or beliefs of the person who engages in the behavior.[25] Managers should never expect staff or anyone to engage in a behavior that serves their values unless they give the staff member adequate reason to do so. To influence the behavior of pharmacy staff and to gain approval and support for goals of the department, the pharmacy leader, manager, and/or supervisor needs to tap into the values, beliefs, and perceptions of pharmacy staff. Common values and beliefs that managers need to consider when working with staff are listed in Appendix 3-9. A common technique used by managers is to identify the stakeholders that might be affected by a decision made by the manager. A stakeholder is any individual who may be directly or indirectly affected by a decision or change going on in an organization. Depending upon the change under consideration, pharmacists, technicians, clerks, and other pharmacy staff may be stakeholders that the pharmacy manager should consider. By considering how each stakeholder feels about an important decision that may affect them, the manager is more likely to make decisions that will be well-received as well as developing effective solutions to a problem or goal of the organization. Managers should consider the values and perceptions of stakeholders in making major decisions. Relationships are built through mutual respect and trust, both personal and professional trust. Perceptions often have a powerful influence on how staff will react to a goal or decision of a pharmacy manager. Staff values and perceptions also shape or influence their behavior.

People have routine ways of behaving and reacting to various situations that are developed as they progress from being a child, to a teenager, to an adult. Dwyer describes these routine ways of behaving and reacting by people as internal programs.[25] These internal programs or ways of reacting are developed primarily through repetition and become engrained. People consistently react to situations that feed on their values, beliefs, and perceptions. Dwyer suggests that people need to install new programs in their minds, which become new habits to change their behavior. For example, managers who usually communicate unclearly need to install a new program in their mind that reminds them each time they communicate that they need to do so in a way that is clear. Managers must give staff adequate reason to change their internal program or way of reacting into new habits. Managers must reinforce the need for staff to change their internal programs or habits by giving staff cues to remind them of the new program until they are reprogrammed. For example, if you want staff members to improve their communication with patients, physicians, nurses, and other customers, you need to remind them of this goal, collect and distribute customer satisfaction data to show them progress, and get them to perceive the value of this desired change in performance to improve their communication behavior. As a manager, what you want a staff member to do is often irrelevant in his or her decision. What is critical is the staff member's perception of the relationship between what you want he or she to do and the staff member's values. This is the personal or subjective state that controls behavior. Dwyer describes a positive five-part model to influence human behavior.[25] To illustrate this model, let's assume that a pharmacy manager wants centralized pharmacists who have primarily been performing tasks related to drug dispensing to become decentralized pharmacists providing clinical and patient care services. The first condition the manager must consider before approaching the pharmacists—and having them move from central to decentralized positions—is whether they are capable of performing in the new roles. The manager must be competent and confident that they can move into the new roles. If the manager approaches the pharmacists and they do not feel capable, it is unlikely the manager can persuade them to accept the change without forcing them. If the manager expects them to question their capability, he or she can indicate that they will receive staff development training to prepare them in becoming decentralized

pharmacists. The second condition is for the manager to present the proposed change in a manner that will allow involved staff pharmacists to perceive value satisfaction. The involved pharmacists may perceive value satisfaction because their new role may be perceived as a sign of recognition or appreciation of their value to the department, an achievement, or an increase in status. The third factor is the perception by the involved pharmacists of the probability of value satisfaction from the role change. This will be linked to their trust of the pharmacy manager. If they trust the manager they are more likely to believe the probability of value satisfaction will occur. The fourth condition is that the pharmacists involved must not perceive the cost of the change as being significant. For example, if the change is perceived to potentially affect friendships with other pharmacists or family relationships because of increased job or work expectations, the pharmacists may perceive the cost of the move to be too great. The fifth condition relates to the involved pharmacists perception of the risk of making the change. For example, they may fear failure or embarrassment if they are not able to effectively function in the new role. Managers can consider these conditions in making major changes that will affect pharmacists and other staff members. An example of a major role change for pharmacy technicians might include compounding of TPN and chemotherapy admixtures in addition to routine admixtures.

Managers should recognize that staff members have different work needs as well as values and beliefs that may affect their work habits. These differences in work needs may be the result of different family, cultural, and educational backgrounds or may be generational in nature. Maslow described a hierarchy of employee needs from basic survival needs to complex needs reinforcing the value of the individual.[26] His hierarchy of needs includes biological, safety, socialization, self-esteem, and self-actualization needs. Some pharmacy employees view work primarily as a source of income to support themselves and their families. For others work is only fulfilling if it satisfies their need for self-esteem and accomplishments.

Pharmacy managers cannot possibly take time to critically evaluate every decision they make. However, if they get to know their staff, they will intuitively know how staff groups and individual staff are likely to react to a change under consideration. However, if a major change is under consideration (e.g., change in job responsibilities, change in work flow design, change in salary and benefits) the pharmacy manager may more likely be able to implement the change with maximum stakeholder buy in if stakeholders' values, perceptions, and needs have been considered.

David McClelland developed an achievement-based motivational theory and models and promoted improvements in employee assessment methods using competency-based assessments and tests. He described three types of motivational needs: the need for achievement, the need for authority and power, and the need for affiliation.[27] Individuals needing achievement are motivated and therefore seek achievement, attainment of challenging goals, and job advancement. These individuals have a strong need for feedback so as to achieve and progress, as well as a need for a sense of accomplishment. Individuals needing power and authority want to be influential, effective, and to make an impact in their work environment. Individuals needing affiliation have a need for friendly relationships and are motivated toward interaction with other people. These individuals need to be liked and held in popular regard and are often effective team players.

According to McClelland most people possess and exhibit a combination of these characteristics.[27] Some people exhibit a strong bias to a particular motivational need, and this motivational need affects their behavior and style as managers or workers.

McClelland suggested that strong, affiliated, and motivated people undermine a manager's objectivity because of their need to be liked, and that this affects a manager's decision-making capability.[27] Strong, power-seeking, and motivated people have a determined work ethic and commitment to an organization and while they are attracted to leadership positions, they may not possess the required flexibility and people-centered skills to be effective leaders. McClelland believes that strong, achievement-oriented, and motivated people make the best leaders, although they may have a tendency to demand too much of their staff, believing that all staff are highly achievement focused and results driven, which, of course, most people are not.

Pharmacy managers should also consider the motivations of their employees and select employees with motivations matched to the particular task. For example, staff members who need affiliation are good individuals to plan social events for the department. Managers may appoint staff members as team leaders or as chair-of-task forces or standing committees because these individuals will want to achieve the task at hand.

Communications

Communication is the basic foundation for effective personnel management. Communication within a pharmacy department must be both upward and downward based upon the organizational structure for the department. Professional and technical staffs need to be able to communicate upward to pharmacy managers to obtain information, provide recommendations, and express their opinions on workplace issues that may affect their work. Pharmacy managers need to communicate downward to staff so they have all of the information to successfully perform the responsibilities, duties, and activities associated with their work. Managers should provide staff members with enough of the big picture concerning a particular issue or topic so they understand the need for them to perform certain duties or activities. Good communication by directors and pharmacy mangers will make staff members feel a sense of belonging and will stimulate them to more actively participate in departmental activities that will enhance the likelihood of achieving departmental goals.

The precise mechanisms used to transmit information up and down in an organization vary depending on the size of the staff, the degree of staff empowerment as reflected by the key job responsibilities of each staff position, ease of access to staff for direct communication, and the leadership and management styles of the pharmacy director and other managers.

Pharmacy managers must employ good written, verbal, and nonverbal communication to effectively manage pharmacy staff. Verbal communication serves as a fundamental means by which leaders and managers are able to build trust with staff and get buy in to the established goals of the pharmacy department. Verbal communication between managers and staff is important when changes affecting staff are being considered or implemented. For example, if a pharmacy manager feels that work hours for pharmacists and technicians need to be changed to better distribute pharmacy workload, this potential change might be best first presented for discussion and feedback from involved staff before being finalized and written as a new policy and procedure. Written communication is necessary to convey important operational information in a consistent and retrievable manner for future reference. For example, revisions in pharmacy policies and procedures, formulary additions, drug shortages, and other routine and usually noncontroversial communications should be distributed in a written format.

Written memorandums can be distributed as hard copy or posted onto an intranet website for the pharmacy department for easy access and review by pharmacy staff. Once staff are aware a change is under consideration that will affect them, managers may use email and written communication to distribute preliminary information or pending changes for staff feedback.

Managers should be aware of the verbal and nonverbal messages they are sending and avoid giving unclear or mixed messages. For example, pharmacy managers who say they have an open-door policy but then tells employees to please make an appointment to see them is sending a mixed message. Managers should recognize that nonverbal signals can be misinterpreted and give the opposite of their verbal message and be negative to staff relationships. Staff can detect a manager's lack of sincerity from nonverbal facial expressions. Managers should assume that staff will interpret their verbal or written messages differently and should encourage and answer questions through emails, staff meetings, or personal encounters to make sure messages are clear and understood by all.

When interacting with pharmacy staff, managers should avoid keeping subordinates or staff members waiting to see them for an appointment; avoid interrupting staff members' sentences before they have a chance to complete their own thoughts; use appropriate eye contact when talking with staff; avoid brow beating employees to get them to do what the manager wants; avoid yawning when talking to staff; and avoid failing to respond to staff suggestions. Managers should try to eliminate barriers between them and staff when they are talking with staff in their office. The manager should come out from behind the desk and should avoid excessive office space and overly pretentious furnishings, which may send a message to staff that the manager is more important and cannot relate to staff views or concerns. Managers should also respect people's personal space to avoid them feeling intimidated.

Periodic staff meetings are a common means to communicate important information to staff and to provide clarification of messages that have been formally sent out between staff meetings. If the pharmacy department has a large staff, meetings with all staff may be held on a bi-monthly or quarterly basis to review and discuss issues, policies, or changes affecting all staff. Meetings of the entire pharmacy staff allow for transmission of identical information to all and make all feel that they are a part of the organiza-

tion. Smaller staff meetings may be held for work teams for larger pharmacy departments. These meetings may be formally held in a reserved conference room or may be held more informally in a work team area (e.g., a pharmacy satellite) to minimize disruption of pharmacy services. Smaller staff meetings for staff working as a team in an area of the pharmacy (e.g., central pharmacy, pharmacy satellites, decentralized pharmacists) foster teamwork and allow the meeting agenda to primarily focus on unique problems and issues.

Practical Management Guidelines for Effective Management-Staff Relations

Management and leadership theory suggest there are some fundamental approaches that benefit and make people effective managers and lead to good management-staff relations. These fundamentals for good pharmacy managers include the following:

- Managers should view staff as the primary asset for achieving departmental goals. If the pharmacy manager keeps this perspective in mind he or she will more likely engage staff in planning, decision making, and will more likely employ a more democratic or permissive management style. Employees sense when a manager views them as an important asset and react favorably.

- Managers should put themselves in the position of the employees they are supervising and ask themselves the question of how they want to be treated and supervised. Managers should employ this strategy when making major organizational changes that will affect employees. People skills apply to all facets of life, and managers should use the same people skills at work that they would use with their family, friends, etc.

- Managers should recognize that loyalty comes out of mutual respect, is built upon honesty, and is a willing commitment and not an obligation, which is frequently linked to staff feeling subservient and out of necessity following the directives of a supervisor.

- Managers should assign reasonable responsibilities, accountabilities, and deadlines so staff members know their expectations. Work should be broken into smaller projects to avoid overwhelming staff.

- Managers should be consistent in their supervisory approach without being rigid. Managers should make sure that rules and regulations applying to any one person/position apply to everyone in comparable positions.

- Mangers should not hide mistakes they make but should publicly acknowledge mistakes to demonstrate that they are human like everyone else.

Emotional intelligence has been defined as the intelligent use of emotions. Leaders and managers use emotional intelligence to help guide their behavior and thinking in ways that enhance results. Leaders and managers with good emotional intelligence are able to accurately perceive, appraise, and express emotion. They are able to regulate their emotions and use emotional intelligence to better understand other people and enhance their relationships and social skills. These skills are important for pharmacy leaders and managers to employ in building staff relationships.[28]

Pharmacy Staff Development

To achieve job satisfaction and staff retention, managers should provide or provide access to various types of staff development programs to help staff develop and maintain the skills needed for their respective jobs. Staff development should be a component of the annual review and performance improvement plan for each staff member.

Human resource departments of hospitals often offer staff development programs such as computer training, handling stress, communications, performance improvement, and other skills common to most employees. In addition, many pharmacy departments offer seminars, case discussion, and journal clubs as ways to help staff maintain and develop new knowledge and skills. Groups of pharmacists at hospitals with extensive clinical services may form study groups to prepare for pharmacotherapy or other pharmacy specialty board certification. Pharmacy departments may also pay for pharmacists to complete traineeships such as those offered by ASHP and self-study programs such as the *Pharmacotherapy Self Assessment Program* offered by ACCP (available at www.accp.org). Pharmacy departments may also provide training and support the costs for pharmacy technicians to become certified through the Pharmacy Technician Certification Board that is housed at the American Pharmacists Association (www.aphanet.org).

Pharmacy Staff Reviews

Most hospitals require annual performance reviews of all staff. Performance improvement plans are developed by a supervisor or manager for each staff member following policies and procedures and using forms required by the hospital. These summative evaluations focus on the performance of the staff member and usually include the identification of some personal goals for development over the next 1-year period. Staff should not be surprised by the findings of the annual summative evaluation. Good managers and supervisors provide periodic and informal formative feedback to both praise and recognize good work and to help the employee identify areas for improvement as well as specific strategies the employee can take to improve performance. It is important for managers to provide praise as well as specific constructive, performance-related feedback when appropriate to increase morale, motivation, and productivity. Staff members who feel unappreciated will not give anything extra to the organization. The more informal and unthreatening the feedback is, the more likely a staff member will listen to it and take steps to improve his or her performance. Managers should take care to never criticize an employee in front of other employees or the managers will risk losing respect from those that observe them criticizing someone else. When it is necessary to provide a staff member with constructive criticism, it should be targeted at improvement on a specific task or duty and should not be an attack on the individual staff member.

As the majority of pharmacists in hospitals become involved in providing clinical and patient care services, it will be necessary for pharmacy mangers to develop more effective methods in evaluating clinical competence and skills of pharmacists. ACCP has developed a template for the evaluation of a clinical pharmacist for this purpose.[29]

JCAHO requires assessment and documentation of staff competence related to various roles of pharmacists and other providers in patient care. In some hospitals pharmacists are credentialed through the medical staff, allowing them to provide medication therapy management for various patient populations (e.g., lipid, diabetes, and hypertension). As the job expectations change for pharmacists, technicians, and other pharmacy workers, managers have the responsibility of identifying methods for each member to achieve the skill levels required. Training of pharmacists and other staff members may occur through in-house mentoring programs, shadowing and training of pharmacists by other pharmacists (with the desired skill level for a particular task or function), attending workshops or programs outside the hospital to obtain training, or self-directed study and development.

Recruitment, Hiring, and Retention of Pharmacy Staff

Pharmacy managers use many methods to recruit pharmacy staff. They advertise positions in newsletters, professional journals, newspapers, and online recruitment sites offered by pharmacy organizations. They also use personnel placement services that are available at national or regional organizational meetings to connect employers with graduating pharmacy students and pharmacists in practice looking for a position. Executive search firms are also frequently used to recruit pharmacy directors and other managers through various channels. Depending upon the type of pharmacist desired (e.g., pharmacist, clinical pharmacist, clinical specialist) and the scarcity of pharmacists in the area, a hospital may recruit locally, regionally, or on a national basis. Human resource or personnel departments for hospitals have to follow federal guidelines as an equal opportunity employer. These guidelines require employers' hiring practices to not discriminate based on age, race, color, sexual orientation, and other diversity factors. The rules for recruitment have become complex, and pharmacy managers have to comply with the rules and procedures established by their hospital. Applicants for a pharmacist position will consider many factors in deciding whether to apply for a position including the job description, location of the hospital and cost of living for the area, salary and fringe benefits, opportunities for professional growth and development, and the hospital's and pharmacy department's reputation. Most pharmacy managers collect applicant information including a letter of interest, application form, reference letters, and curriculum vitae and then screen applicants and select the candidates that are the best match for interviews. Screening may be completed by a pharmacy manager or several managers, or there may be a formal search committee for the position in which the committee will screen candidates. Applicants are then contacted for an initial discussion of the position by a pharmacy manager or search committee chair. An initial interview may take place over the phone or an on-site interview may be

setup as the initial interview. Interviews may be done by individuals or a group of interviewers such as a search committee. Interviews may be short (a few hours) or may be longer than a day depending on the type of position being recruited. Interviews may be formally structured with predetermined questions that all candidates are asked or loosely and informally organized. Candidates may be asked to formally present a seminar to demonstrate their knowledge in the field of practice (e.g., oncology, critical care) and communication skills. After all of the interviews are completed, the manager recruiting for the position or the search committee will compare candidates and make a decision on which candidate is best matched for the position. Before or after the candidate is made an offer, applicants may be screened to make sure they are licensed pharmacists, do not have a criminal record, and are not abusing drugs. The top candidate is then contacted and made an offer. Candidates will be given adequate time to consider the offer and may wish to obtain additional information or to negotiate concerning the job description, hours of work, salary, or concerns about other aspects of the job. Usually the offer is made verbally with a final offer made in writing after any negotiation is concluded.

Staff turnover is costly and may have a negative impact on staff morale because remaining workers will have to cover staff vacancies. As previously noted staff members have different work needs, which may change over time and which may be affected by changes within the hospital or pharmacy department (e.g., changes in organizational structure, work environment, work expectations, salary, and fringe benefits).

A recent national survey of pharmacists' attitudes toward work life revealed that over 68% of pharmacists in community and hospital settings experienced job stress, role overload, and role ambiguity, and 48% experienced work-home conflict. Many hospitals are experiencing difficult financial times when patient care acuity is increasing. This causes pharmacy managers and staff to do more work with fewer resources. Staff pharmacists and other staff can tolerate periods of stress, but over time unless the role stress is lessened, the personal physical and mental health of staff may suffer. High-stress positions may also lead to increased staff turnover.[30]

ASHP guidelines for retention of pharmacy personnel list the following factors among others that may affect staff retention:

- Job satisfaction
- Pay and benefits
- Performance management through employee assessment and appraisals
- Recognition and awards
- Promotion opportunities
- Job design
- Peer relations
- Staff development opportunities
- Management style
- Physical working conditions
- Staff scheduling

These factors reflect the leadership and management styles, needs of individuals, and work motivators that have been previously described. Readers are referred to the *ASHP Guidelines on the Recruitment, Selection, and Retention of Pharmacy Personnel* for a more in-depth discussion of each of these retention factors.[14]

Summary

The pharmacy staff is the most important asset of a pharmacy department. Pharmacy leaders and managers primarily achieve departmental goals through the work performed by the pharmacy staff. If leaders and managers are vigilant of this basic management principle, engage staff in decision making, and obtain feedback from staff about the work environment, the pharmacy department will benefit because the leaders and managers have created an environment that respects the value and optimizes the use of all staff to achieve departmental goals. Good communication between pharmacy managers and staff is essential in creating a positive work environment. Staffs will more likely value, enjoy, and be motivated to achieve their full potential when they feel they are important to the success of the department.

There are many types of leadership and management styles that leaders and managers can use to influence staff behaviors. Pharmacists, by virtue of their training, are professionals and most desire to have input in decision making and prefer working independently or as a part of work teams to complete the duties and responsibilities of their position. Pharmacy leaders and managers are more likely to obtain staff support and motivation when they use a participative rather than an autocratic management style.

There are many factors that affect the type, mix, and number of pharmacy staff needed for progressive pharmacy departments. It is clear that in the future pharmacists will spend the majority of their time providing clinical and patient care services. As the mission and responsibilities of pharmacy as a profession evolve, pharmacy directors must adjust staffing plans and models by changing job descriptions and responsibilities for pharmacists and other staff, changing the mix and numbers of staff, and adjusting the work environment to optimize staff retention.

The life of a leader and manager is not always easy or fun. The rewards of leaders and managers are to achieve their personal and departmental goals and to proudly watch and help staff develop.

References

1. Hepler CD. Clinical pharmacy, pharmaceutical care, and the quality of drug therapy. *Pharmacotherapy.* 2004;24(11):1491–8.

2. American Society of Health-System Pharmacists (ASHP). ASHP guidelines: minimum standard for pharmacies in hospitals. *Am J Health-Syst Pharm.* 1995;52: 2711–7.

3. American Society of Health-System Pharmacists (ASHP). *Best Practices for Hospital and Health-System Pharmacy.* Bethesda, Maryland: American Society of Health-System Pharmacists; 2005.

4. Pedersen CA, Schneider PJ, Santell JP, et al. ASHP national survey of pharmacy practice in acute care settings: monitoring, patient education, and wellness-2000. *Am J Health Syst Pharm.* 2000;57:2171–87.

5. Pedersen CA, Schneider PJ, Scheckelhoff DJ. ASHP national survey of pharmacy practice and settings: dispensing and administration-2002. *Am J Health Syst Pharm.* 2003;60:52–68.

6. Pedersen CA, Schneider PJ, Scheckelhoff DJ. ASHP national survey of pharmacy practice in hospital settings: prescribing and transcribing-2004. *Am J Health Syst Pharm.* 2005;62:378–90.

7. Bond CA, Raehl CL, Franke T. Clinical pharmacy services, pharmacy staffing, and drugs costs in United States hospitals. *Pharmacotherapy.* 2000;20:609–21.

8. Bond CA, Raehl CL, Patry R. Evidence-based core clinical pharmacy services in United States hospitals in 20020: services and staffing. *Pharmacotherapy.* 2004;24(4):427–40.

9. Bond CA, Raehl C, Patry R. The feasibility of implementing an evidence-based core set of clinical pharmacy services in 2020: manpower, marketplace factors, and pharmacy leadership. *Pharmacotherapy.* 2004;24(4):441–52.

10. Joint Commission on Accreditation of Healthcare Organizations (JCAHO). *A Guide to JCAHO's Medication Standards.* Oakbrook Terrace, IL: Joint Commission on Accreditation of Healthcare Organizations; 2004.

11. Joint Commission on Accreditation of Healthcare Organizations (JACHO. *National Patient Safety Goals for 2005 and 2004.* Oakbrook Terrace, IL: Joint Commission on Accreditation of Healthcare Organizations; 2005. Available at: http://www.jcaho.org/accredited+organizations/patient+safety/index.htm. Accessed March 8, 2005.

12. Knapp DA. Professionally determined need for pharmacy services in 2020. *Am J Pharm Educ.* 2002;66:421–9.

13. Law AV, Ray MD, Knapp KM, et al. Unmet needs in the medication use process: perceptions of physicians, pharmacists, and patients. *J Am Pharm Assoc.* 2003;43:394–402.

14. American Society of Health-System Pharmacists (ASHP). ASHP guidelines on the recruitment, selection, and retention of pharmacy personnel. *Am J Health Syst Pharm.* 2003;60:587–93.

15. Schumock GT, Butler MG, Vermeulen LC, et al. Evidence of the economic benefit of clinical pharmacy services: 1996–2000. *Pharmacotherapy.* 2003;23(1):113–32.

16. Hatoum HT, Catizone C, Hutchinson RA, et al. An eleven-year review of the pharmacy literature: documentation of the value and acceptance of clinical pharmacy. *Drug Intell Clin Pharm.* 1986;20:33–41.

17. Pointers DD, Sanchez JP. Leadership a framework for thinking and acting. In: Shortell SM, Kaluzny AD, eds. *Health Care Management: Organizational Design and Behavior.* 3rd ed. Albany, NY: Delmar; 1994:85–112.

18. Holdford DA. Leadership theories and their lessons for pharmacists. *Am J Health Syst Pharm.* 2003;60:1780–6.

19. Bennis W. *On Becoming a Leader.* Reading, MA: Addison-Wesley Publishing Company; 1989.

20. Zilz DA, Woodward BW, Thielke TS, et al. Leadership skills for a high-performance pharmacy practice. *Am J Health Syst Pharm.* 2004;61:2562–74.

21. McGregor D. *The Human Side of Enterprise.* New York: McGraw-Hill; 1961.

22. Ouchi, W. *Theory Z.* Reading, MA: Addison-Wesley Publishing Company; 1981.

23. Anonymous. Management styles. Available at: http://www.rpi.edu/dept/advising/esl/free_enterprise/business_structures/management_styles.htm. Accessed March 8, 2005.

24. The Institute for Management Excellence. Management styles. Available at: http://www.itstime.com/index.html. Accessed March 8, 2005

25. Dwyer CE. Managing people. In: Roven S, Ginsberg L, eds. *Managing Hospitals.* San Francisco, CA: Jossey-Bass Publishers; 1991.

26. Maslow AH. A theory of human motivation. *Psychol Rev.* 1943;50(4):29–47.

27. McCelland DC. *Human Motivation.* Cambridge, UK: Cambridge University Press; 1987.

28. Weisinger H. *Emotional Intelligence at Work.* San Francisco, CA: Jossey-Bass Publishers; 1998.

29. American College of Clinical Pharmacy. Template for the evaluation of a clinical pharmacist. *Pharmacotherapy.* 1993;13(6):661–7.

30. Mott DA, Doucette WR, Gaither CA, et al. *J Am Pharm Assoc.* 2004;44(3):326–36.

Appendix 3-1
Mission
Department of Pharmaceutical Services
Large Community Hospital with Comprehensive Pharmacy Services

The mission of the Department of Pharmaceutical Services is to help ensure safe and appropriate clinical outcomes for the use of drugs in patients treated in the medical center. All services provided by the department are aimed at improving patient drug therapy or preventing drug related problems.

Functions Provided by the Department of Pharmaceutical Services

From a functional viewpoint the professional, administrative, technical, clerical, and other staffs employed by the department are committed to

- assuming responsibility for the prospective review of all routine drug orders for appropriateness and safety;
- providing an effective drug distribution system, which assures that all drugs required in the care and treatment of patients are provided where needed;
- maintaining an electronic medication profile and medication administration record (indicating what drugs are prescribed, what drugs were dispensed, what drugs were administered, and other pertinent drug-related information such as patient weight, drug sensitivity, and allergies, etc.) on all patients;
- packaging, formulating, and preparing all drugs required for patient care;
- extemporaneously providing drug information to physicians, nurses, and other care providers, and answering in-depth questions requiring extensive drug literature searches, analysis, and recommendations;
- monitoring all significant drug therapy with regard to efficacy, safety, and cost effectiveness;
- playing a leading role in the development of medication-use policy by the Pharmacy and Therapeutics Committee and other patient care committees;
- actively participating in emergency care by providing and preparing, when necessary, all drug needs and providing drug information;

- providing information to physicians and other care providers by interviewing the patient and obtaining a drug history of prescription, herbal remedies, and over-the-counter medications and identifying drugs the patient brings to the hospital;
- providing radiopharmaceuticals needed for inpatient and outpatient treatment;
- playing a lead role in efforts of the hospital to continuously improve the safety of the medication-use system;
- developing pharmacy quality assurance and quality improvement programs to help ensure the quality of pharmaceutical services and the quality and cost-effectiveness of drug therapy;
- developing pharmacy information systems to support the medication-use system and track drug therapy outcomes; and,
- providing a system to help ensure the correct and safe distribution and administration of investigational drugs.

Pharmaceutical Services

The following distinct pharmaceutical services have been established to provide these functions:

- Inpatient drug distribution service
- Outpatient drug distribution service
- Intravenous admixture service
- Drug information service
- Patient care unit pharmacy service
- Medical team specialized clinical pharmacy service
- Nuclear pharmacy service
- Clinical pharmacy consult service
- Pharmacy packaging and manufacturing service
- Administrative service

Appendix 3-2
Large Community Hospital with Comprehensive Pharmacy Services
Staff Pharmacist Responsibilities

Prescription Review (50% Effort)

1. Review fax copies of prescription orders and enter into the pharmacy computer system. Orders to be reviewed for right drug, dose, schedule, and potential interactions.

Provide Oversight of Pharmacy Technicians (15% Effort)

1. Supervise pharmacy technicians involved in the unit-dose drug distribution system in the central pharmacy. Check unit-dose carts and first doses prepared for dispensing by technicians.

2. Supervise pharmacy technicians involved in the centralized, intravenous admixture service. Check intravenous admixtures prepared by technicians.

Coordinate Care with Patient Care Unit Pharmacists and Clinical Specialists (10% Effort)

1. Work with patient care unit pharmacists and clinical specialists to resolve drug-related problems detected through prescription order review.

2. Work with patient care unit pharmacists and clinical specialists to dispense stat and now medications in a timely manner.

Education (10% Effort)

1. Answer drug information questions from physicians, nurses, and other providers.

2. Participate in pharmacy staff development programs and staff meetings.

3. Participate in the provision of in-service education to physicians, nurses, and other health professionals.

Preparation of Medications for Dispensing (10% Effort)

1. Prepare stat and now medication doses and routine doses for oral or intravenous admixtures when necessary.

Other Duties (5% Effort)

1. Perform other duties as directed by the pharmacy manager.

Appendix 3-3
Large Community Hospital with Comprehensive Pharmacy Services Responsibilities for Patient Care Unit Pharmacists

Direct Clinical Activities (50% Effort)

1. Provide initial review and evaluation of physician's orders for proper disposition of the order; therapeutic appropriateness, proper dosing in regard to patient's age, weight, and renal function; drug interactions; allergic reactions; route and rate of administration; and therapeutic redundancy.

2. Clarify physician's orders, when necessary, through direct and timely contact with the prescriber or designated practitioner. This includes promoting adherence to the formulary.

3. Respond to CPR (Mayday) emergencies on assigned units and provide coverage to other pharmacists involved in these emergencies.

4. Provide general and patient specific drug information as required to other health care professionals or patients. This service may take the form of in-services, drug literature searches, development or teaching aids such as compatibility charts and medication cards, and formal presentations.

5. Effectively communicate and coordinate activities with pharmacy clinicians and residents, outpatient pharmacists and technicians, physicians, nurses, and other health care professionals with regard to patient drug therapy and departmental policies and procedures. This includes collaboration on drug studies and trials within a specific area of practice.

6. Actively participate in drug usage evaluations as assigned.

7. Identify through direct patient contact or chart review and forward any adverse drug reactions and forward to the Drug Information Center.

8. Implement all drug use policy and formulary decisions of the Pharmacy and Therapeutics Committee.

9. Provide initial work-up and routine monitoring of patients being administered drugs identified in the department's monitored drug program and provide formal documentation of these activities.

10. Evaluate antibiotic regimen for appropriateness of therapy and renew order as indicated.

11. Facilitate and assure adherence to pharmacy-related issues in investigational drug protocols including confirmation of consent form, timely dispensing and administration of medications, identification, and reporting any adverse drug reactions.

12. Actively participate in multidisciplinary programs that are focused on the improvement of patient care (food-drug interactions, patient medication education, etc.).

Distribution Support Services (40% Effort)

1. Enter physician's orders or supervise technician order entry into the patient record in the pharmacy computer system, and document allergies, diagnoses, weights, and ages.

2. Complete daily review of patient medication administration records and charts to ensure the following:

   - Accuracy of MAR and medication cart

   - Reconciliation of medication administration times and other discrepancies

   - Resolution of compatibility issues and drug interactions

   - Appropriateness of PRN dispensing levels

   - Appropriate scheduling of medications to optimize their therapeutic effect

Educational and Training Activities (5% Effort)

1. Assist in the training of new employees, supportive personnel, residents, and students. Act as a preceptor for Bachelor of Science pharmacy students as well as a mentor for pharmacy residents functioning in the patient care unit pharmacist roll.

2. Attend and participate in national/local professional organizations as well as hospital and departmental in-service or continuing education programs.

Other Activities (5% Effort)

1. Perform quality control measures and quality assurance studies as directed. This includes monthly inspections of patient care areas for outdated drugs, overstock, and proper storage.

2. Actively participate in the development of departmental policy and procedures as well as departmental committees and work groups.

3. Demonstrate commitment to the profession of pharmacy through active advancement of pharmacy practice within the department and on a state and national level.

4. Perform other position-related duties as assigned by the immediate supervisor.

5. Facilitate daily renewal of parenteral nutrition and identify patients in which therapy is to be discontinued.

6. Review the cause of missing doses and assure delivery of replacement doses.

7. Dispense first doses of new physician's orders for emergent (stat) medications.

8. Provide daily reconciliation of unit medication carts with pharmacy computer-generated cart fill list.

9. Perform inventory control duties for assigned satellite on a daily basis.

Appendix 3-4

Large Community Hospital with Comprehensive Pharmacy Services Responsibilities for Clinical Specialists

Provision of Clinical Pharmacy Services (60% Effort)

1. Participates as an integral member of the patient care team by assisting physicians with therapeutic decisions such as drug and drug product selection, therapeutic drug monitoring, and drug dosing. Participates in the planning and development of patient treatment under the direction of the physician team leader and appropriately documents pharmacy services in the patient's medical record.

2. Investigates therapeutic alternatives and recommends or initiates the management of patient-related problems based on interpretation of relevant medical literature and clinical experience. Communicates, orally and/or in writing, the results of these investigations to health care practitioners, peers, patients, the public, and health care managers in a manner appropriate to the training, skill, and needs of that individual.

3. Reviews patient records and orders regarding drug therapy and recommends and initiates changes as appropriate with regard to age, weight, organ function (e.g., renal, hepatic, etc.). Assists in the management, monitoring, and modification of drug therapy in patients with acute and chronic diseases.

4. Evaluates patients by means of interview and, if appropriate, physical assessment to determine past medical history, previous medication use, present medical condition, and response to therapy.

5. Interprets laboratory and other patient-specific data to aid in the development of treatment plans and monitors response to therapy in order to achieve desired outcomes.

6. Interprets and applies pharmacokinetic drug data in order to achieve efficacious, safe, and economical pharmacotherapeutic regimens, thus ensuring optimal patient care.

7. Solves therapeutic queries posed by physicians and other health care providers.

8. Identifies potential and existing drug-related problems such as complications resulting from drug therapy, ineffective therapy, allergic, and other adverse drug reactions and recommends or initiates the necessary treatment alternatives to minimize or negate them.

9. Utilizes available state-of-the-art knowledge and technology to assess, improve, and monitor drug therapy regimens.

10. Establishes procedures for detecting significant drug-drug, drug-laboratory, and drug-food interactions and develops the necessary means to minimize adverse patient consequences, which might result from such interactions.

11. Assesses and participates in the management of patients with drug overdose and patients exposed to poisons.

12. Performs basic cardiac life support and assesses and participates in drug therapy management during medical emergencies, when appropriate.

13. Assures the appropriateness of discharge planning and medications when necessary. Works with other health professionals and outside health organizations to ensure continuance of medical care and advises patients in proper drug usage.

14. Counsels patients and/or care giver as to the proper administration potential adverse reactions, storage of their medications, etc.

15. Works with the Indigent Care Coordinator and other financial support personnel to help acquire medications.

Systems of Care: Clinical specialists Work as Part of Interdisciplinary Teams to Improve Clinical Processes and Systems of Care (10% Effort)

1. In conjunction with other team members, develops, manages, and assists in the implementation of critical pathways, treatment algorithms, treatment guidelines, and protocols.

2. Works with other health care providers and relevant committees to establish policy or implement process improvements that improve drug therapy outcomes (efficacy, safety, cost effectiveness) and overall quality of patient care.

3. Identifies therapeutic categories or individual therapeutic agents warranting medication use evaluations. In conjunction with drug information staff, physicians, and other health professionals conducts medication use evaluations for selected agents.

Documentation of Pharmaceutical Care (5% Effort)

1. Evaluates and documents the impact of clinical pharmacy services upon patient care outcomes (clinical outcomes, quality of life outcomes, costs outcomes).

2. Participates as members of interdisciplinary teams to decide on allocation of resources (staffing, technology, supplies, etc.) to provide quality and cost effective patient care.

3. Participates in departmental documentation programs such as clinical documentation, process improvement, monitored drug program, etc.

Distributive Pharmacy Services (2% Effort)

1. Coordinates the timely, accurate preparation, delivery, and administration of medications to patients in conjunction with other pharmacy and nursing team members.

2. Prepares and dispenses medications when necessary to provide patient focused care in a timely manner.

Drug Information and Scholarly Activities (5% Effort)

1. Retrieves, analyzes, evaluates, and interprets the scientific literature as a means of providing patient- and population-specific drug information to health care professionals and patients.

2. Participates in hospital medical and pharmacy departmental conferences and attends meetings to learn more about pharmacotherapy.

3. Participates in the generation of new knowledge relevant to the practice of pharmacotherapy, clinical pharmacy, and medicine, such as clinical research projects and case reports.

4. Prepares and presents formulary reviews of drugs or drug therapy classes for use by the Pharmacy and Therapeutics Committee.

5. Serves as a Pharmacy and Therapeutics Liaison to obtain information and formulate recommendations on formulary issues pertinent to practice areas.

Staff Development, Education and Training Activities (15% Effort)

1. Provides in-service education to physician's nurses and other health care professionals.

2. Serves as a preceptor for Pharm.D. students, residents, and staff.

Other Activities (3% Effort)

1. Administrative activities including committee work

2. Performs other related and nonrelated job duties as assigned by his or her immediate supervisor.

Appendix 3-5
Pharmacy Staff
Large Community Hospital with Comprehensive Pharmacy Services

Director of Pharmacy	1	Technicians Inpatient	40
Pharmacy Managers	4	Technicians Outpatient	6
Team Coordinators	4	Information Technology Specialists	3
Staff Pharmacists Inpatient	15	Automation Technicians	2
Staff Pharmacists Outpatient	8	Accounting Staff	3
Patient Care Unit Pharmacists	24	Administrative Assistants	2
Clinical Specialists	8	**Total**	**126**
Residents	6		

Appendix 3-6
Mission Statement
Department of Pharmacy
Small Community Hospital

To provide all drugs needed in the care of patients in a safe and efficient manner and provide drug information to physicians, nurses, and other providers to improve drug therapy.

The department provides the following services:

- Inpatient unit dose drug distribution service
- Intravenous admixture service
- Drug information
- Pharmacy administration

Appendix 3-7
Small Community Hospital
Staff Pharmacist Responsibilities

Prescription Review (40% Effort)

1. Review fax copies of prescription orders and enter into the pharmacy computer system. Orders to be reviewed for right drug, dose, schedule, and potential interactions.

Preparation of Medications for Dispensing (30% Effort)

1. Prepare stat and now medication doses and routine doses for oral or intravenous admixtures when necessary.

Provide Oversight of Pharmacy Technicians (15% Effort)

1. Supervise pharmacy technicians involved in the unit-dose drug distribution system in the central pharmacy. Check unit-dose carts and first doses prepared for dispensing by technicians.

2. Supervise pharmacy technicians involved in the centralized intravenous admixture service. Check intravenous admixtures prepared by technicians.

Education (10% Effort)

1. Answer drug information questions from physicians, nurses, and other providers.

2. Participate in staff development programs and staff meetings.

3. Participate in the provision of in-service education to nurses.

Other Duties (5% Effort)

1. Perform other duties as directed by the pharmacy manager.

Appendix 3-8
Pharmacy Staff
Small Community Hospital

Director of Pharmacy	1
Staff Pharmacists	3
Pharmacy Technicians	4
Pharmacy Clerk	1
Total	**9**

Appendix 3-9
Values

Acceptance

Affiliation

Authority

Autonomy

Concern for the welfare of others

Control

Duty or obligation

Empowerment

Ethics

Fun

Morality

Power

Professional expertise

Professionalism

Recognition

Respect

Rights

Responsibility and authority

Self-esteem

Success

Chapter 4

Ambulatory Care

Jessica L. Milchak, Barry L. Carter

Introduction

In recent decades, our health care system has undergone major changes. Restrictions on reimbursement have resulted in shortening of hospital stays and a greater emphasis on outpatient care as a cost-effective alternative.[1,2] In addition, an enlarged focus on health care promotion and disease prevention has led to greater provision of nonacute care services by acute care institutions. As a result of these changes, ambulatory care has emerged as a new paradigm for the delivery of health care services, resulting in increasing opportunities for pharmacists. The purposes of this chapter are to describe common ambulatory care settings in which pharmacy is involved, review the impact of ambulatory care services, and outline standards of practice in these settings.

Background

Dramatic expansions in pharmacy practice have occurred in recent years, due in part to changes in the structure of health care institutions and changes in mechanisms of reimbursement for pharmacy services. Efforts to control costs during the 1980s triggered major restructurings of medical care, including reduced hospital stays and increased outpatient surgeries and procedures. Major incentives for alternative health care delivery systems were created, resulting in a proliferation of ambulatory care centers, home health care services, and outpatient care.[1] Another outcome of cost-containment efforts was the growth of preferred provider organizations, health maintenance organizations, and primary-care networks.[1] Through these organizations and networks, hospitals became able to provide more diverse services. Ambulatory centers were located within the hospital, adjacent to the hospital, or in freestanding buildings on hospital grounds. Hospital-affiliated satellite clinics also became common, providing automatic referral sources to the hospital. Pharmacy practice has evolved to meet the needs of these restructured health care settings.

Recent legislation, at both the federal and state levels, has provided unprecedented opportunities for pharmacists to play a significant role in improving medication use and receive reimbursement for patient care services. At the federal level, Congress enacted the Medicare Prescription Drug Improvement and Modernization Act (MMA) of 2003, a landmark piece of legislation with many important implications for the pharmacy profession.[2] The MMA requires Medicare drug plan sponsors to move forward with several quality assurance measures, including drug utilization management and medication therapy management programs. This legislation marks the first time that pharmacists will be eligible to receive reimbursement from Medicare for providing related patient care services.[2] However, the pharmacy community will need to continue educating drug program sponsors in order to ensure that pharmacists assume and maintain critical roles in the advancement and implementation of these programs.

State Medicaid programs currently in place authorize payment for pharmacist services. For example, the Iowa pharmaceutical case management (PCM) program was implemented in 2000 with funds appropriated by the state's legislature as part of an amendment to the state Medicaid plan.[3,4] This program utilizes eligible pharmacist-physician teams in the ambulatory and community setting to identify, prevent, and resolve drug therapy problems. The pharmacist assesses the patient and makes written recommendations to the physician regarding goal-directed drug treatment, patient education, and monitoring. Eligible pharmacists are reimbursed for the provision of these services to patients with one of 12 select disease states who are treated with four or more nontopical medications. Reimbursement through these types of medication therapy management programs represents an important step forward for pharmacy practice.

Definitions and Philosophy

Ambulatory care encompasses those health-related services that, by definition, are provided to patients who walk to seek their care and who, therefore, are not confined to a bed in an institutional setting.[5] The term *ambulatory care* covers a wide range of service areas including outpatient pharmacies, emergency departments, primary care clinics, ambulatory care centers, and family medicine groups; this chapter focuses on these types of ambulatory settings. Home health care, residential homes and nursing home facilities, other examples of ambulatory care health systems or care settings, are covered elsewhere in this handbook.

Family medicine is a subspecialty primary care practice. Central to its philosophy is the provision of total care to patients of all ages and their families regardless of their state of health.[7] This highly personalized type of care rests upon practitioners' willingness to accept responsibility for the management of long-term comprehensive care, including disease prevention as well as disease management.[7] Family medicine also considers the patient's family members and the contribution of family and social dynamics to the expression of disease.

Primary care, the subset of ambulatory care that provides patients with an initial point of contact with the medical system, has unique features and a specific philosophy. Primary care practitioners serve patients who present with a wide variety of illnesses or multiple disease states, many of which are rarely managed by inpatient or tertiary care. The primary care physician commonly assumes a coordinating role for a patient's overall health care needs, facilitating access to and integration of inpatient, long-term, subspecialty, mental health, and social services.[6] Even when a patient is referred for secondary or tertiary care, the primary care physician continues to provide chronic and preventative care and coordinate overall care. As a result, continuity of care is enhanced. The three most common primary care specialties are general pediatrics, general internal medicine, and family medicine.

Primary care physicians frequently practice, either conceptually or physically, with an interdisciplinary team. As leader of the team, the primary care physician consults with social workers, dieticians, behavioral counselors, and clinical pharmacists. Patient care, teaching and research activities are provided by the team members at a level and scope that correspond to their level of expertise.

Functions and Standards of Practice

The types of pharmaceutical services offered will differ from one setting to another. A good general description of the functions that are typically performed in the ambulatory setting was found in the previous learning objectives and standards for the American Society of Hospital Pharmacists (ASHP) accredited training in primary care. These standards are listed in Table 4-1.[8]

Prior to providing clinical services, it is important that the pharmacist establish a scope of practice. This scope of practice serves as a guideline or protocol for the practicing pharmacist and describes their functions in the clinic as a member of the health care team. It may also be used to ensure quality or evaluate performance.[6] A collaborative drug therapy management (CDTM) agreement may exist as part of this scope of practice, which allows pharmacists to engage in specific activities including initiating, adjusting, or evaluating drug therapy, performing physical assessment, counseling and educating patients, and administering drug therapy. Elements of the CDTM may require advanced training and/or certification such as completion of a residency or board certification, authority to document activities in the medical record, accountability, and provisions to allow for compensation for drug therapy management services.

Pharmacists should attempt to provide a high quality service consistent with the definition of pharmaceutical care. This involves personalized care aimed at achieving outcomes that can improve the patient's quality of life. These outcomes have been defined as (1) cure of a disease; (2) elimination or reduction of symptoms; (3) arrest or slowing of the disease process; or (4) prevention of disease or symptoms.[9] It is also important that pharmacists attempt to measure the impact of their intervention by evaluating these patient outcomes in some way. This assessment can provide a meaningful measure of the quality of care delivered.

The clinical and legal implications of the pharmacist-patient relationship are important for the pharmacist practicing in the ambulatory care setting to understand.[6] In establishing a relationship with a patient, a pharmacist assumes a "duty to care" and is responsible for practicing professionally, ethically, and skillfully. This relationship continues as long as pharmaceutical attention is required, and a patient must receive appropriate notice if a pharmacist desires to end the relationship. It is important that pharmacists carefully document any care-related activities in the patients' medical record.

In addition to their clinical duties, many ambulatory care pharmacists spend a considerable amount of time conducting research and publishing scholarly

Table 4-1
Functions Performed in Ambulatory Settings

- Conduct a patient interview and interpret the result of the interview

- List and explain the monitoring parameters and therapeutic endpoints for the safe and efficacious use of each drug used in a patient

- Prospectively monitor drug therapy for potential drug-drug, drug-laboratory test, drug-diet, drug-disease, and drug-condition interactions and recommend modifications in drug therapy, when appropriate to minimize such interactions

- Use interviews, physical assessment skills, and interpretation of laboratory test results to monitor therapy for adverse and therapeutic effects

- Take a medication history, assess the patient's attitude toward compliance, and evaluate the influence of these factors on therapeutic response; initiate strategies to correct noncompliant behavior

- Effectively counsel patients on drug use

- Serve on a health care team providing primary or consultative care

- Prospectively formulate individualized drug regimens based on the purpose of the medication(s), concurrent disease(s) and drug therapies, pharmacokinetic parameters of the drug(s), and the patient's clinical condition

- Competently devise individualized drug regimens and recommend adjustments based on therapeutic response

- Describe the clinical manifestations of potential toxicities associated with a patient's medication, assess the significance of the toxicity, and recommend an appropriate course of action

- Develop and conduct or assist in a collaborative clinical research project

- Evaluate drug studies in the literature in terms of research design, validity of results, and clinical applicability

- Communicate effectively with patients, physicians, nurses, other health professionals, and peers

- Manage a patient's drug therapy by
  - designing a drug therapy treatment plan, and advising prescribers on its implementation
  - using established therapeutic protocols
  - independently prescribing or adjusting drug therapy in instances where supportive legislation exists

- Develop criteria for safe and effective drug use and coordinate drug use review and patient care audits

- Identify factors to measure the quality of care provided by the pharmacy service which could be used in the development of a departmental quality assurance program

- Explain the organization and operation of the outpatient pharmacy department; this could include physical accommodations, reference sources, computer applications, professional and supportive personnel, budgeting, relationships with other health care departments, assumed or designated responsibilities, and documentation of services

- Use personal computers to assist in the conduct of professional activities; these uses may include word processing, data base management, statistical analysis, graphics, and communication software

---

work. Most of these practitioners have responsibilities for teaching pharmacy students, residents and fellows, medical students, and residents.

Ambulatory Care Settings

Pharmacists provide ambulatory care services in a variety of settings, including free standing pharmacies and clinics, hospital outpatient departments and clinics, long-term-care or assisted living centers, home health care settings, and mail-order services.[10] (Table 4-2) Ambulatory care services can be offered either separate from or in conjunction with more traditional pharmaceutical services that are associated with distribution functions. Two distinct practices for the clinical pharmacist providing primary care have been described, one in which the pharmacist is independently respon-

sible for providing care and one in which the pharmacist participates in collaborative patient management as a member of an interdisciplinary team.[6] The intent of this chapter is to discuss the provision of comprehensive pharmacy services offered independently of distribution services in outpatient pharmacy settings or group practices.

Pharmacy Services in Primary Care Clinics

Pharmacists involved in primary care generally are members of a multidisciplinary team comprised of a broad representation of caregivers in a general medicine or specialty clinic. In this model, the pharmacist works collaboratively with members of the team during each scheduled clinic time to optimize drug therapy for the patient. Practice privileges vary among collabo-

Table 4-2

Selected Examples of Ambulatory Pharmacist Practice Settings

Outpatient Pharmacy Services

    Community pharmacy

    Hospital outpatient pharmacy

    Emergency room

    Private group practice

General Medicine (Primary Care) Clinics

    Pharmacy clinics

    Family medicine clinics

Specialty Medicine Clinics

    Anticoagulation

    Diabetes

    Hypertension

    Hyperlipidemia

    Infectious disease

    Oncology

    Psychiatry

    Pulmonology

    Rheumatology

Pediatrics

    General pediatrics

    Asthma or allergy

Home Health Care

Managed Care Organizations

---

rative primary care settings, depending on the extent of authority and responsibility given to the pharmacist.[11] Pharmacists frequently assist with designing therapeutic regimens, identifying untreated conditions and designing long-term follow-up and monitoring plans. Pharmacists can establish relationships with patients and provide them with education and medication counseling services to enhance compliance, therapeutic monitoring of drug-therapy and refills. They commonly provide drug information, education, and consultation to physicians. Primary care pharmacists also can run pharmacist-managed specialty clinics in which the pharmacist offers direct patient care services. Pharmacist-managed specialty clinics are prevalent in academic health centers and Veterans Affairs Medical Centers (VAMCs) and have been utilized effectively for a variety of chronic disease states.[12–22] Pharmacist services can be designed to complement and supple-

ment the care provided by the physician and can be influenced by the specific needs of the patient population, physician, or setting. The extent of integration of pharmacy services in the primary care clinic and opportunities for pharmacist-managed specialty clinics depend largely on the degrees of support from the senior management and the medical staff, and on the type of pharmacy leadership that exists.[23]

Pharmacists' experiences in early pharmacist-managed clinics were integral to extending their roles beyond distribution and increasing their provision of patient-oriented pharmaceutical services.[24–27] As a result, pharmacist-managed clinics, in which pharmacists manage care for a wide range of patients with multiple disease states, are increasingly found in the primary care setting.[13]

Pharmacy clinics, or *pharmacotherapy clinics,* are innovative pharmacist-managed primary care clinics that rely on pharmacists as an integral part of the health care team that have been implemented by many academic centers and VAMCs in an attempt to enhance primary health care accessibility, timeliness and continuity of care.[28–29] Clinical pharmacists work both alone and collaboratively with a specific primary care team to provide comprehensive pharmaceutical services. These services may include counseling patients on new prescriptions, helping providers with specific medication-related problems, identifying untreated conditions, therapeutic duplication, drug-related problems, processing narcotic prescriptions, seeing walk-in patients with medication issues, determining strategies to optimize medication adherence, providing drug information, assessing nonformulary prescriptions, evaluating and completing drug therapy plans for home and nursing home care, and teaching pharmacy students and residents.[28,30] Patients can be referred to the pharmacy clinic by any team member for drug therapy management. Pharmacists may utilize protocols or clinical drug use criteria and practice under CDTM to see individual patients during scheduled appointments. These types of agreements at the VAMCs allow pharmacists to autonomously initiate, modify, continue, and monitor a patient's drug therapy. Common conditions managed in the pharmacy clinic include hypertension, heart failure, dyslipidemia, diabetes, pain management, chronic obstructive pulmonary disease, smoking cessation, H. pylori infection, and cases of polypharmacy. In this type of setting, physicians have demonstrated high rates of acceptance of pharmacists' recommendations and scheduled visit care plans.[30–31]

Pharmacist-managed clinics in the primary care setting have demonstrated a variety of improved clinical outcomes for patients. Anticoagulation clinics have been particularly successful, and the number of such clinics where pharmacists are providing direct patient care is increasing. According to a national survey, between 1995 and 1998 the number of U.S. hospitals with pharmacists offering direct care in ambulatory anticoagulation clinics doubled to 14%.[32] In these clinics, the physician typically maintains responsibility for the overall care of the patient and is available for consultation if the patient requires immediate medical attention. The pharmacist obtains a detailed patient history, orders pertinent laboratories, makes long-term dosage adjustments and provides detailed patient education.[33–34] The pharmacist may also measure a patient's INR using a point-of-care device. A cost-benefit evaluation demonstrated that the pharmacist-managed anticoagulation clinic decreased complications and hospitalizations, resulting in marked cost reduction.[35]

Pharmacists are also active in many subspecialty clinics within the primary care setting, where they have demonstrated significant improvements in a variety of outcomes. Cioffi et al. demonstrated a significant reduction in HbA1c, total cholesterol, triglycerides, blood pressure, and microalbuminuria in Type II diabetic patients in a pharmacist-managed diabetic clinic.[19] Coast-Senior and colleagues showed an improvement in glycemic control in diabetic patients managed in a VAMC setting.[15] In a randomized controlled study of African-American patients in an urban setting, Jaber et al. showed improved glycemic control in the pharmacy intervention group compared to patients receiving usual care from physicians.[36] Pauley and colleagues determined that the number of emergency department visits for acute exacerbations of asthma was reduced as a result of participation in a pharmacist-managed comprehensive educational asthma clinic.[37] Pharmacist interventions have also been shown to enhance blood pressure control and lipid control in primary care patient populations.[14,17,38–42]

In recent years, the number of pharmacists providing direct patient care services in oncology has increased significantly.[32] The needs of the typical patient undergoing chemotherapy are complex and can include antiemetic prophylaxis, nutritional support, mucositis prophylaxis and therapy, and pain management.[43] With their expertise in drug therapy, the pharmacist can have a significant impact on a patient's quality of life. Pharmacists play an integral role on multidisciplinary teams in providing supportive care and limiting therapy-associated toxicities. Pharmacists are commonly utilized to monitor therapeutic drug levels, provide drug information, nutritional support, and pain management in the ambulatory setting.

Numerous studies have demonstrated the value of clinical pharmacists in the management of patients with a variety of chronic diseases.[30,34,37,42,44–46] Clinical pharmacy services have also been well-described in general pediatric clinics and pediatric allergy clinics. These services have resulted in disease control that is at least as good as physicians for conventionally managed patients.

Pharmacy Services in Family Medicine Clinics

Clinical pharmacy services in family medicine have been well-established for nearly 30 years.[47–55] One of the earliest examples was developed by the Cedar Rapids Family Practice Residency and the University of Iowa College of Pharmacy in the rural town of Mechanicsville, IA.[56–57] This practice employed a physician, a nurse, a pharmacist, and a receptionist. No written prescriptions were provided to the patients. Instead, the pharmacist filled all prescriptions from the medical record and made many of the treatment decisions including dose titration and initiation. Several other programs have incorporated this model into private practice groups. The Area Health Education Centers in North Carolina and other states commonly incorporate a family physician-clinical pharmacist model into their programs.[49,52,58] Approximately 25% of all family medicine residency programs (FMRP) approved by the Accreditation Council for Graduate Medical Education (ACGME) and the American Osteopathic Association (AOA) have clinical pharmacist involvement.[59] Clinical pharmacist involvement may vary depending on the program's location. For example, the affiliated network of eight family medicine residency training programs in Iowa has a clinical pharmacy faculty member in all eight programs. Typically, the clinical pharmacist in these programs holds a doctor of pharmacy degree, has completed a residency, and spends a high percentage of their time dedicated to the residency program.[59]

There are sometimes major differences between pharmacy practice in the primary care clinic and in the family medicine clinic. Pharmacists in FMRPs perform a variety of educational and clinical functions, scholarly activities, and administrative duties. In these settings, the clinical pharmacist may be less likely to serve as an independent primary care provider, since the majority of patients are seen by medical residents completing their training. Instead, a major component of the clinical pharmacists' services is education of both health care professionals and patients. The clinical pharmacist is actively involved in teaching medical residents, faculty, and medical and pharmacy students through formal lectures, small-group discussions, evidence-based precepting, and participation in daily teaching rounds.[47–48] During more than 2,000 precepting encounters with a clinical pharmacist, medical residents rated the pharmacist as a highly useful, available, and effective teacher.[60] It is not uncommon for pharmacy faculty to be recognized for their outstanding contributions to the FMRPs through teaching awards from medical residents. Exposing medical residents to clinical pharmacists during training might foster long-term collaborative relationships. A nationwide survey of family medicine medical residents concluded that clinical pharmacists had a positive impact on residents' attitudes toward multidisciplinary team care and clinical pharmacy services.[61] Clinical pharmacists in the family medicine setting also have favorable effects on patient attitudes regarding their care. Helling et al. demonstrated that perceptions of overall medical care were significantly higher in patients who encountered a clinical pharmacist than those who did not encounter a clinical pharmacist during their visit to a family practice office.[62]

Although the majority of a clinical pharmacist's time in an FMRP is typically devoted to teaching and patient care, their involvement in scholarly activities and administrative functions is increasing. Pharmacists are active in collaborative clinical research with clinic faculty members and residents and may also participate in investigative drug trials.[59] Their participation in administrative duties such as committee work, promotion and tenure evaluation, resident recruitment, pharmaceutical representative meetings, medication sample management, and indigent drug program management is not uncommon.[63]

Clinical pharmacy services have been shown to increase the appropriateness of physician prescribing in family medicine settings. Brown and colleagues used a blinded physician/pharmacist review panel to assess family medicine physician consultations with the clinical pharmacist.[64] Physicians implemented 96% of the pharmacist recommendations. Furthermore, the prescribing physicians rated 92% of the pharmacists'

recommendations as moderately to very useful. None of the recommendations were rated as not at all useful or were deemed to be inappropriate. Similar results were demonstrated by Haxby et al. when they evaluated pharmacist recommendations using physician questionnaires.[65] In this study, physicians reported implementing 96% of the pharmacist recommendations and rated 97% of the recommendations as very useful or mostly useful. In addition, 77% of physician respondents felt that the recommendations greatly improved or somewhat improved the clinical status of their patients.

Carter et al. used a blinded physician/pharmacist peer review panel to compare the appropriateness of prescribing at four family medicine model offices in the Iowa-affiliated network, two with active clinical pharmacy services and two without such services.[66] The panel judged that significantly more prescriptions were "most appropriate" or "acceptable" in the offices with clinical pharmacists. Furthermore, the prescriptions that resulted from direct consultation with a clinical pharmacist were given significantly higher ratings for drug choice, dose, and benefit to the patients when compared to prescriptions that did not result from consultation, even though the consulted cases were judged to be significantly more difficult. Other studies have found that prescribing improved with an educational intervention by a clinical pharmacist.[67–68] In addition, clinical pharmacy services have been shown to be cost effective in the family medicine setting.[69–71]

CDTM agreements are less common in FMRP than in primary care clinics. A major reason for this is that medical residents in these training programs see many patients as part of their education that a pharmacist may otherwise follow in a primary care setting. However, this is not to say that pharmacists do not have an independent role in the family medicine setting. Family medicine pharmacists can be active in a variety of direct patient care activities, including disease state management activities. In many family medicine programs, the physician will delegate certain drug- related responsibilities to the pharmacist. At a particular visit, a given patient might be seen by both the physician and the pharmacist. The physician performs diagnostic functions, while the pharmacist provides recommendations for selection of drugs and dosages, write prescriptions, educates patients, or creates a plan for long-term monitoring. Dosage adjustments, adverse reactions, and refills can then be managed by the pharmacist through either subsequent office visits or telephone follow-up.

The pharmacist can also, at the physician's request, provide formal consultation services for conditions such as smoking cessation, asthma, diabetes, hypertension, or hyperlipidemia.

Several studies have demonstrated the high quality of care provided in pharmacist-managed anticoagulation clinics in the family medicine setting. Wilt et al. conducted a retrospective chart review to determine if pharmacist-managed anticoagulation service improved the outcomes of patients receiving warfarin compared to patients managed by a physician.[72] Patients in the physician-managed group had a significantly greater number of major hemorrhagic events, defined as gross hematuria, major hematoma, and upper gastrointestinal bleeds. The number of unplanned clinic visits, emergency room visits, and hospital admissions was also significantly higher for patients in the physician-managed group, and care was significantly more costly. The authors concluded that pharmacists had a positive impact on the quality and cost of patient care.

Ernst and colleagues evaluated patient outcomes in an anticoagulation case management service over a 4-year period in a rural private office.[73] Patients were referred to the service by their primary physician and managed by the pharmacist based on a written protocol. Compared to values obtained prior to enrollment, the investigators found a significant increase in the number of after-enrollment therapeutic INRs for patients managed by the pharmacist (37.6% versus 57.8%, p<0.001). Supratherapeutic INRs were infrequent, occurring in only 1% of patients. Both provider and patient satisfaction with the clinical services were very high. All physicians surveyed agreed or strongly agreed that the service added value to patient care, improved continuity of care, and provided a greater margin of patient safety.

Jameson and colleagues evaluated the effects of a pharmacotherapy consult service in a randomized study of family medicine patients at high risk for medication-related problems.[74] Patients in the intervention group received a 45–60-minute consultation focused on simplifying the medication regimen, improving the effectiveness of the regimen, and decreasing adverse effects. The pharmacist recommended changes to the patient's physician in order to decrease drug-related problems with therapy and provided education to the patient regarding any resultant changes in drug-therapy. The intervention resulted in a significant decrease in the number of drugs, number of daily doses, and the 6-month cost of therapy.

Pharmacy Services in Outpatient Community Pharmacies

Credentialed with Pharm.D. degrees and educated in the concept of pharmaceutical care, many community pharmacists are eager to take advantage of opportunities to expand their traditional roles and responsibilities.[9] Innovative practice models are widespread in this setting.[22] Pharmacy in the community is evolving from a product-centered to a patient-centered practice. For many patients, the community pharmacist represents the most trusted and accessible health care practitioner. An increasing number of community pharmacists are taking advantage of their unique position to implement disease state management services. Many community pharmacies are located within the same building as a primary care or specialty clinical practice, facilitating the provision of clinical pharmacy services to patients of those clinics. The community pharmacist is an important component of ambulatory pharmacy practice.

Numerous research studies have examined the effects of clinical pharmacy services in community settings. The effects of pharmacist disease state management services in the community setting were measured in a classic study by McKenney et al. in 1973, in which a clinical pharmacist worked independently in a community pharmacy setting but maintained close communication with physicians in a model neighborhood comprehensive health program in Detroit.[75] A cohort of hypertensive patients was divided into a control group and an intervention group. The intervention group received comprehensive individualized education and monitoring by the pharmacist when they received prescriptions and the pharmacist interacted frequently with physicians in order to modify antihypertensive therapy. In addition, the pharmacist visited the physician's office in order to review medical records and make drug-therapy recommendations. Patients in the control group received usual care from their physician and access to commercial hypertension literature. Patient compliance, knowledge of hypertension, and blood pressure control were significantly improved in the intervention group compared to the control group as a result of the intervention. After the intervention was discontinued, compliance and blood pressure control deteriorated.

The effects of pharmaceutical care on blood pressure control were evaluated by Carter et al. in a controlled single-blind parallel group study in a community pharmacy located within a rural medical clinic.[76] Patients in the intervention group were scheduled to see the pharmacist for monthly follow-up appointments, while control group patients were seen at baseline and 6 months. Systolic blood pressures in the intervention group were significantly improved after 6 months of follow-up compared to baseline, (p<0.001). There was no change in mean blood pressures in the control group. The appropriateness of blood pressure regimen was significantly improved in the intervention group based on blinded peer review panel ratings. Patients in both groups indicated that they were very satisfied with pharmacy services; however, responses from the intervention group indicated they more strongly agreed that services were valuable, high in quality, and improved their understanding.

Bluml and colleagues conducted a large observational study in 26 community-based ambulatory care pharmacies to improve persistence and compliance with lipid lowering therapies, improve lipid levels, and increase communication among patients, physicians, and pharmacists.[77] A point-of-care cholesterol testing device was used to obtain a fasting lipid profile. Patients were seen by the pharmacist every month for the first 3 months and quarterly thereafter and were actively involved in their treatment plan and goals. Pharmacists intervened with physicians throughout the study in order to optimize drug therapy. A high percentage, 62.5%, of patients achieved the National Cholesterol Education Program's recommended goals of therapy. Physicians accepted and implemented 76.6% of the pharmacist recommendations. This project demonstrated a successful model for community pharmacist collaboration with patients and physicians to provide an advanced level of care.

Another large study was conducted in 54 community pharmacies in Canada targeting patients with high cardiovascular risk.[78] The primary endpoint of the study was the measurement of a complete fasting cholesterol panel by the physician or a prescription for a new lipid lowering therapy or an increase in the current therapy. Patients in the pharmacy intervention group had their cholesterol checked using a point-of-care device and were educated on cardiac risk factors by the pharmacist. Follow-up visits in person or by telephone occurred at 2, 4, 8, 12, and 16 weeks in the intervention group. The control group received usual care with minimal follow-up. In the intervention group, pharmacists communicated the lipid results, the patients' risk factors and medications and their therapeutic recommenda-

tions to the patients' primary care physicians via facsimile. Patients in the control group received general information on cardiovascular risk factors from the pharmacist and a telephone call at 8 and 16 weeks. Significantly more patients in the intervention group achieved the primary endpoint compared to the control group (57% vs. 31%, p<0.001). This study was stopped early due to the significant benefit incurred in the intervention group. A separate economic analysis of the project determined that costs associated with providing the program were minimal from both a government and pharmacy manager perspective.[79] The results of this study speak to the value of the clinical pharmacist in providing pharmaceutical care.

One of the longest studies conducted in the community setting is the Asheville Project, which was conducted in 12 community pharmacies in Asheville, NC to evaluate the clinical, economic, and humanistic short- and long-term outcomes of pharmaceutical care services for patients with diabetes.[80] The intervention consisted of pharmacists meeting with patients to offer pharmaceutical care services including diabetes and lipid education, glucose monitor instruction, adherence strategies, and goal monitoring. Physical assessment of patients' feet, skin, blood pressure, and weight was also performed by the pharmacists. Short-term outcomes were assessed after 7 to 9 months of follow-up. At this time period, the number of patients with A1c values less than 7% increased significantly compared to baseline, with 37% of patients having a decrease in their A1c of at least 1%.[81] There was also a significant improvement in patient satisfaction with pharmacy services. To assess long-term outcomes, data from participating patients with up to 5 years of follow-up were analyzed. Compared to baseline, hemoglobin A1c levels at every follow-up were improved. Patients indicated improved adherence to American Diabetes Association recommended diabetes care including foot exam, A1c measurement, ACE-inhibitor use, and self-test of blood glucose. Improvements in LDL and HDL levels also were seen. Overall, the total direct medial costs paid per patient per year, including costs from physician visits, hospitalizations, emergency room visits, laboratory tests, and prescriptions, decreased every year compared to baseline. This study demonstrated the sustainability of community-based pharmaceutical care interventions.

Early outcomes of the PCM program in Iowa were described by Carter et al.[3] The study evaluated an intensity score representing the scope of services provided by pharmacists in 117 community pharmacies to 2,931 eligible patients. An individual patient score was derived by assigning points for each aspect of the pharmaceutical care process, including meeting with the patient, providing a written work-up of the patient, sending drug-therapy recommendations to the physician, and receiving a physician response. Each pharmacy received a score derived by summing the individual patient scores. Higher pharmacy intensity scores indicated a higher level of services provided and/or a greater number of patients served. Total scores were calculated quarterly for each pharmacy. Pharmacists, on average, met with 33.3% of patients, evaluated 26.9% of patients, provided recommendations for 17.6% of patients, and received physician replies for 11.5% of patients. In the first quarter, 19 (17.4%) pharmacies were ranked as "high intensity," while in quarters two to four, only one to three (1.4–3.9%) of the 117 pharmacies were highly ranked. Pharmacists indicated they were unable to provide PCM services to a high percentage of eligible patients. A survey found that the most commonly cited reasons for not providing PCM services were difficulties with pharmacy start-up of services, inadequate staffing, and inability to gain access to patients. The study concluded that despite start-up difficulties, the large number of pharmaceutical care services provided must be considered a success.

A second study of Iowa's PCM program evaluated the outcomes of medication safety and health care utilization.[4] Measures of safety included a Medication Appropriateness Index (MAI) score for all patients and the use of "high risk" medications for those patients age 65 and older. The MAI score was constructed for each patient using pharmacist SOAP note documentation. This score, which ranges from 0 to 18, is based on 10 domains and includes elements such as the indication, effectiveness, correct dosage and directions, interactions, and cost. At baseline, a high percentage of patients (92.1%) and medications (46.1%) were classified as having at least one medication problem. After 9 months of follow-up, the percentage of medications with problems was decreased in eight out of 10 MAI domains and the percentage of medications with any identified problems was significantly decreased (p<0.001) in the patients who received the PCM service. High-risk medication use was significantly reduced in recipients of PCM >65 years of age compared to baseline and compared to the group of patients who were eligible for PCM but did not receive PCM services. Interestingly, the greatest benefit was seen in

patients of pharmacies that were rated as high intensity, and this benefit was significantly higher than pharmacies rated as low or zero intensity, (p<0.001). There was no difference in health care utilization between eligible patients who received PCM services and those who did not, indicating that the program did not increase costs to Medicaid. Initiating pharmaceutical care activities in the community setting is challenging. The success of programs like the PCM requires long-term commitment and dedication by participants. The authors underscored the importance of supporting efforts to expand the Iowa PCM program by enrolling more pharmacy providers, informing patients of eligibility, increasing provider awareness, and developing a *best practice* model to facilitate pharmacist-physician collaboration in the community setting.[4]

Community pharmacists can play an important role in improving the continuity of care between inpatient and ambulatory settings. Enhancing the continuity of care after hospital discharge by improving information transfer and communication between providers and patients may help reduce adverse drug events (ADE). Kuehl et al. evaluated the effects of pharmacy-to-pharmacy facsimile transmission of medication regimen at admission and discharge on pharmacist interventions.[82] Significantly more interventions were documented in patients for whom information had been supplied compared to those who did not. Other studies indicate that increased communication have reduced medication problems and ADEs.[83–85] In a study evaluating the incidence and severity of adverse events following hospital discharge, Forster and colleagues suggested there should be better assessment and communication of unresolved problems at discharge, better monitoring following discharge, and follow-up telephone contact with a clinical pharmacist within 5 days of discharge.[86] The community pharmacist is well-positioned to play an integral role in provider-to-provider information transfer.

Many successful pharmaceutical care type practices exist in the community setting.[87] The changing roles of community pharmacists and their growing involvement in patient-based services create exciting practice opportunities in this area. Day-to-day accessibility to patients puts the community pharmacist in an ideal position to serve as a drug therapy interventionist and clinical manager. Although many community pharmacists do not practice in a traditional institutional setting, they are an important part of ambulatory care practice and many health systems have incorporated community pharmacies into their system.

Developing an Ambulatory Care Practice

The most important activity in developing an ambulatory practice is appropriate planning. The practice philosophy or team philosophy must be known, understood, and incorporated into the planning phase. For instance, is patient care the only mission of the practice? Is there any role for management of patients by a clinical pharmacist? Do medical residents or medical students have a major role, and how will they impact clinical pharmacy services? Is a significant research program in progress or desired? The answers to these questions will determine the major thrust of any proposed clinical pharmacy service.

If personnel resources are limited, the scope of services might also need to be limited upon initiation of the service. For example, a new practitioner in a group practice could not provide direct patient care services, pharmacokinetic monitoring, physician education, and small group pharmacotherapeutic teaching. Rather, the practitioner could evaluate which of those services best fit the clinic's specific needs and concentrate efforts on developing that service. Once the service becomes established, other services could be added. The pharmacist should carefully consider the overall time commitment for each service and plan appropriately for the potential long-term growth of the service and the resultant impact on their schedule. This is especially important if the pharmacist has other obligations like teaching or scholarship. Direct patient management services such as anticoagulation or services such as refill clinics can be very time-consuming and can grow rapidly, quickly over committing and overwhelming a pharmacist. Careful consideration of the types of services offered and a long-term plan will help the pharmacist successfully maximize the quality and efficiency of their services.

The administrator who plans to hire an ambulatory clinical pharmacist must ensure that the individual is competent and can effectively perform the standards of practice listed in Table 4-1. The pharmacist must have exceptional interpersonal skills and perform effectively as an integral member of an interdisciplinary team. The administrator should strongly consider requiring advanced residency or fellowship training in primary care or family practice and board certification as a pharmacotherapy specialist.

There are numerous possibilities for providing pharmacy services in a developing clinic setting, including the models cited in this chapter. In addition, the ambulatory pharmacy literature can provide valuable ideas for clinical services and examples of successful new practitioners. It is important to remember that each setting or specialty practice will be unique. All clinical pharmacy services or models for delivering those services will not be appropriate for every setting.

One of the most important features of an effective ambulatory care practice is the involvement of the clinical pharmacist in therapeutic decision making. The pharmacist must be available and accessible at the time the patient is seen by the caregiver. In large practices, where it is not possible to interact during each prescribing event, a combination of methods for improving drug therapy might be necessary: prospective chart review before patients present to the clinic; population-based management of electronic databases, physician bench-marking and feedback, academic detailing, and group or one-on-one interactions with the physicians; or retrospective chart review to identify common drug-therapy problems that are correctable through pharmacy intervention. Koecheler and coworkers identified six prognostic indicators that could be used to identify ambulatory patients with high risk of adverse outcomes: (1) five or more medications in the drug regimen; (2) 12 or more medication doses per day; (3) medication regimen changes four or more times during the past 12 months; (4) more than three concurrent disease states present; (5) history of noncompliance; and (6) presence of drugs that require therapeutic drug monitoring.[88] These criteria were automated by the IMPROVE investigators to screen large numbers of patients electronically who might benefit from clinical pharmacy services.[89] Clinical pharmacists in a very busy practice might focus their effort on patients who meet these criteria and prospectively interact with their physicians to assist with decision making and long-term management.

It is clear that successful ambulatory pharmacy services must be comprehensive and continual.[51] Some family medicine, general medicine, or pediatric groups see patients 40 hours per week. If clinical pharmacy services are provided only part of that time, their success and use will be limited. Ideally, pharmacy services should be available to patients and providers 80 to 90% of the time. Providing this degree of service requires a strong commitment from the clinical pharmacist and from the department that employs them. In many circumstances (i.e., when the pharmacist is a faculty member), this level of service is difficult to maintain, and it is important to consider methods of relief. It might be necessary, for example, to have two clinical pharmacists who are able to share the clinical responsibilities.

Lastly, to ensure that the highest quality of care and the most beneficial pharmacy services are continually provided, some method of ongoing evaluation should exist. Pharmacy services can be evaluated through physician surveys of satisfaction or pharmacist use, measures of disease control or patient outcomes, and reviews of drug use. These criteria can be used to benchmark progress or to compare services to other practice sites.

Reimbursement

Many pharmacists are beginning to pursue new avenues for reimbursement for clinical services through collaborative drug therapy monitoring services.[90] Kuo and colleagues described the following 10-step process for establishing this type of service in a family medicine setting: (1) establish a working relationship with physician colleagues; (2) assess the needs of your patients; (3) draft collaborative drug therapy management service (DTMS) protocols and agreements; (4) apply for credentialing status within your health organization; (5) consult the billing office staff at the clinic; (6) design a clinic-encounter form; (7) identify and train support personnel; (8) allocate resources; (9) advertise the DTMS; and (10) evaluate and improve your service.[91]

There are many examples of pharmacists in the community setting who successfully bill for their cognitive services.[81] Other studies have indicated patients willingness to pay for clinical services provided by pharmacists and to accept pharmacists as non traditional providers.[92–94] Widespread reimbursement for cognitive services will require continued efforts by members of the pharmacy profession to raise awareness of the value of these services through documentation of positive economic and clinical outcomes.[95]

Summary

The health care structure continues to shift toward ambulatory care. This movement will provide additional opportunities for numerous types of ambulatory pharmacy services, including pharmaceutical care services, collaborative drug therapy management, and disease state management services. The profession has made progress toward reimbursement for these types of cognitive services through new legislation at the state and federal levels. However, the paradigm shift in health care raises many future challenges for the pharmacy profession. Pharmacists should remain diligent to ensure that new and upcoming legislation values and reimburses pharmacists for clinical services. They should continue to demonstrate high quality service and positive outcomes through clinical research and should embrace high standards to ensure continued positive growth of the profession and the best possible care for the patients they serve.

References

1. Black BL. Competitive alternatives to hospital inpatient care. *Am J Hosp Pharm.* 1985;42(3):545–53.

2. Meyer BM, Cantwell KM. The Medicare Prescription Drug, Improvement, and Modernization Act of 2003: implications for health-system pharmacy. *Am J Health-Syst Pharm.* 2004;61(10):1042–51.

3. Carter BL, Chrischilles EA, Scholz D, et al. Extent of services provided by pharmacists in the Iowa Medicaid Pharmaceutical Case Management program. *J Am Pharm Assoc.* 2003;43(1):24–33.

4. Chrischilles EA, Carter BL, Lund BC, et al. Evaluation of the Iowa Medicaid pharmaceutical case management program. *J Am Pharm Assoc.* 2004;44(3):337–49.

5. Burns LA. Trends and initiatives in hospital ambulatory care. *Am J Hosp Pharm.* 1982;39(5):799–805.

6. Establishing and evaluating clinical pharmacy services in primary care. American College of Clinical Pharmacy. *Pharmacotherapy.* 1994;14(6):743–58.

7. Rakel RE, ed. The family physician. In: *Textbook of Family Practice.* 6th ed. Philadelphia: W. B. Saunders Company; 2002.

8. ASHP supplemental standard and learning objectives for residency training in critical-care pharmacy practice. American Society of Hospital Pharmacists. *Am J Hosp Pharm.* 1990;47(3):609–12.

9. Hepler CD. The future of pharmacy: pharmaceutical care. *Am Pharm.* 1990;NS30(10):23–9.

10. ASHP guideline: minimum standard for pharmaceutical services in ambulatory care. American Society of Health-System Pharmacists. *Am J Health-Syst Pharm.* 1999;56(17):1744–53.

11. ASHP statement on the pharmacist's role in primary care. *Am J Health-Syst Pharm.* 1999;56(16):1665–7.

12. Carter BL. Clinical pharmacy in disease-specific clinics. *Pharmacotherapy.* 2000;20(10 Pt 2):273S–277S.

13. Alsuwaidan S, Malone DC, Billups SJ, et al. Characteristics of ambulatory care clinics and pharmacists in Veterans Affairs medical centers. IMPROVE investigators. Impact of Managed Pharmaceutical Care on Resource Utilization and Outcomes in Veterans Affairs Medical Centers. *Am J Health-Syst Pharm.* 1998;55(1):68–72.

14. Geber J, Parra D, Beckey NP, et al. Optimizing drug therapy in patients with cardiovascular disease: the impact of pharmacist-managed pharmacotherapy clinics in a primary care setting. *Pharmacotherapy.* 2002;22(6):738–47.

15. Coast-Senior EA, Kroner BA, Kelley CL, et al. Management of patients with type 2 diabetes by pharmacists in primary care clinics. *Ann Pharmacother.* 1998;32(6):636–41.

16. Vivian EM. Improving blood pressure control in a pharmacist-managed hypertension clinic. *Pharmacotherapy.* 2002;22(12):1533–40.

17. Cording MA, Engelbrecht-Zadvorny EB, Pettit BJ, et al. Development of a pharmacist-managed lipid clinic. *Ann Pharmacother.* 2002;36(5):892–904.

18. Patchin GM, Wieland KA, Carmichael JM. Six months' experience with a pharmacist-run Helicobacter pylori treatment clinic. *Am J Health-Syst Pharm.* 1996;53(17):2081–2.

19. Cioffi ST, Caron MF, Kalus JS, et al. Glycosylated hemoglobin, cardiovascular, and renal outcomes in a pharmacist-managed clinic. *Ann Pharmacother.* 2004;38(5):771–5.

20. Kennedy DT, Paulson MD, Eddy TD, et al. A smoking-cessation program consisting of extensive counseling, pharmacotherapy, and office spirometry: results of a pilot project in a veteran's administration medical center. *Pharmacotherapy.* 2004;24(10):1400–7.

21. Furmaga EM. Pharmacist management of a hyperlipidemia clinic. *Am J Hosp Pharm.* 1993;50(1):91–5.

22. Carter BL, Helling DK. Ambulatory care pharmacy services: has the agenda changed? *Ann Pharmacother.* 2000;34(6):772–87.

23. Reeder CE, Kozma CM, O'Malley C. ASHP survey of ambulatory care responsibilities of pharmacists in integrated health systems—1997. *Am J Health-Syst Pharm.* 1998;55(1):35–43.

24. McKenney JM, Witherspoon JM, Pierpaoli PG. Initial experiences with a pharmacy clinic in a hospital-based group medical practice. *Am J Hosp Pharm.* 1981;38(8):1154–8.

25. Gardner ME, Trinca CE. The pharmacy clinic: a new approach to ambulatory care. *Am J Hosp Pharm.* 1978;35(4):429–31.

26. Monson R, Bond CA, Schuna A. Role of the clinical pharmacist in improving drug therapy. Clinical pharmacists in outpatient therapy. *Arch Intern Med.* 1981;141(11):1441–4.

27. Sczupak CA, Conrad WF. Relationship between patient-oriented pharmaceutical services and therapeutic outcomes of ambulatory patients with diabetes mellitus. *Am J Hosp Pharm.* 1977;34(11):1238–42.

28. Carmichael JM, Alvarez A, Chaput R, et al. Establishment and outcomes of a model primary care pharmacy service system. *Am J Health-Syst Pharm.* 2004;61(5):472–82.

29. Segarra-Newnham M, Soisson KT. Provision of pharmaceutical care through comprehensive pharmacotherapy clinics. *Hosp Pharm.* 1997;32:845–50.

30. Galt KA. Cost avoidance, acceptance, and outcomes associated with a pharmacotherapy consult clinic in a Veterans Affairs Medical Center. *Pharmacotherapy.* 1998;18(5):1103–11.

31. Hanlon JT, Weinberger M, Samsa GP, et al. A randomized, controlled trial of a clinical pharmacist intervention to improve inappropriate prescribing in elderly outpatients with polypharmacy. *Am J Med.* 1996;100(4):428–37.

32. Raehl CL, Bond CA. 1998 national clinical pharmacy services study. *Pharmacotherapy.* 2000;20(4):436–60.

33. Reinders TP, Steinke WE. Pharmacist management of anticoagulant therapy in ambulant patients. *Am J Hosp Pharm.* 1979;36(5):645–8.

34. Garabedian-Ruffalo SM, Gray DR, Sax MJ, et al. Retrospective evaluation of a pharmacist-managed warfarin anticoagulation clinic. *Am J Hosp Pharm.* 1985;42(2):304–8.

35. Gray DR, Garabedian-Ruffalo SM, Chretien SD. Cost-justification of a clinical pharmacist-managed anticoagulation clinic. *Drug Intell Clin Pharm.* 1985;19(7–8):575–80.

36. Jaber LA, Halapy H, Fernet M, et al. Evaluation of a pharmaceutical care model on diabetes management. *Ann Pharmacother.* 1996;30(3):238–43.

37. Pauley TR, Magee MJ, Cury JD. Pharmacist-managed, physician-directed asthma management program reduces emergency department visits. *Ann Pharmacother.* 1995;29(1):5–9.

38. Morse GD, Douglas JB, Upton JH, et al. Effect of pharmacist intervention on control of resistant hypertension. *Am J Hosp Pharm.* 1986;43(4):905–9.

39. Bogden PE, Abbott RD, Williamson P, et al. Comparing standard care with a physician and pharmacist team approach for uncontrolled hypertension. *J Gen Intern Med.* 1998;13(11):740–5.

40. Cookson T, Rice M, Lacro JP. Blood pressure outcomes in a pharmacist-and-nurse managed hypertension clinic: A team approach. *JMCP.* 1997;3(3):307–12.

41. Erickson SR, Slaughter R, Halapy H. Pharmacists' ability to influence outcomes of hypertension therapy. *Pharmacotherapy.* 1997;17(1):140–7.

42. Okamoto MP, Nakahiro RK. Pharmacoeconomic evaluation of a pharmacist-managed hypertension clinic. *Pharmacotherapy.* 2001;21(11):1337–44.

43. Liekweg A, Westfeld M, Jaehde U. From oncology pharmacy to pharmaceutical care: new contributions to multidisciplinary cancer care. *Support Care Cancer.* 2004;12(2):73–9.

44. Lee AJ, Boro MS, Knapp KK, et al. Clinical and economic outcomes of pharmacist recommendations in a Veterans Affairs medical center. *Am J Health-Syst Pharm.* 2002;59(21):2070–7.

45. Lobas NH, Lepinski PW, Abramowitz PW. Effects of pharmaceutical care on medication cost and quality of patient care in an ambulatory-care clinic. *Am J Hosp Pharm.* 1992;49(7):1681–8.

46. Cowper PA, Weinberger M, Hanlon JT, et al. The cost-effectiveness of a clinical pharmacist intervention among elderly outpatients. *Pharmacotherapy.* 1998;18(2):327–32.

47. Helling DK. Family practice pharmacy service: Part I. *Drug Intell Clin Pharm.* 1981;15(12):971–7.

48. Helling DK. Family practice pharmacy service: part II. *Drug Intell Clin Pharm.* 1982;16(1):35–48.

49. Davis RE, Crigler WH, Martin H, Jr. Pharmacy and family practice: concept, roles and fees. *Drug Intell Clin Pharm.* 1977;11(10):616–21.

50. Johnston TS, Heffron WA. Clinical pharmacy in the family practice residency programs. *J Fam Pract.* 1981;13(1):91–4.

51. Love DW, Hodge NA, Foley WA. The clinical pharmacist in a family practice residency program. *J Fam Pract.* 1980;10(1):67–72.

52. Robertson DL, Groh MJ, Papadopoulos DA. Family pharmacy and family medicine: a viable private practice alliance. *J Fam Pract.* 1980;11(2):273–7.

53. Eichelberger BM. Family practice-clinical pharmacy opportunities in the community setting. *Am J Hosp Pharm.* 1980;37(5):740–2.

54. Maudlin RK. The clinical pharmacist and the family physician. *J Fam Pract.* 1976;3(6):667–8.

55. Moore TD. Pharmacist faculty member in a family medicine residency program. *Am J Hosp Pharm.* 1977;34(9):973–5.

56. Juhl R, Perry P, Norwood G. The family practitioner-clinical pharmacist group practice: A model clinic. *Drug Intell Clin Pharm.* 1974;8:572–5.

57. Perry PJ, Hurley SC. Activities of the clinical pharmacist practicing in the office of a family practitioner. *Drug Intell Clin Pharm.* 1975;9(3):129–33.

58. Robertson DL, Groh MJ. Activities of a clinical pharmacist in a private family practice. *Fam Prac Res J.* 1982;1:188–94.

59. Dickerson LM, Denham AM, Lynch T. The state of clinical pharmacy practice in family practice residency programs. *Fam Med.* 2002;34(9):653–7.

60. Ables AZ, Baughman OL, 3rd. The clinical pharmacist as a preceptor in a family practice residency training program. *Fam Med.* 2002;34(9):658–62.

61. Helling DK, Thies PW, Rakel RE. The effect of clinical pharmacy services on family practice residents' attitudes: a nationwide study. *Drug Intell Clin Pharm.* 1986;20(6):493–6.

62. Helling DK, Hepler CD, Jones ME. Effect of direct clinical pharmaceutical services on patients' perceptions of health care quality. *Am J Hosp Pharm.* 1979;36(3):325–9.

63. Jackson EA. The role of pharmacists in family practice residency programs. *Fam Med.* 2002;34(9):692–3.

64. Brown DJ, Helling DK, Jones ME. Evaluation of clinical pharmacist consultations in a family practice office. *Am J Hosp Pharm.* 1979;36(7):912–5.

65. Haxby DG, Weart CW, Goodman BW, Jr. Family practice physicians' perceptions of the usefulness of drug therapy recommendations from clinical pharmacists. *Am J Hosp Pharm.* 1988;45(4):824–7.

66. Carter BL, Helling DK, Jones ME, et al. Evaluation of family physician prescribing: influence of the clinical pharmacist. *Drug Intell Clin Pharm.* 1984;18(10):817–21.

67. Gehlbach SH, Wilkinson WE, Hammond WE, et al. Improving drug prescribing in a primary care practice. *Med Care.* 1984;22(3):193–201.

68. Ives TJ, Frey JJ, Furr SJ, et al. Effect of an educational intervention on oral cephalosporin use in primary care. *Arch Intern Med.* 1987;147(1):44–7.

69. Chrischilles EA, Helling DK, Rowland CR. Clinical pharmacy services in family practice: cost-benefit analysis. II. Referrals, appointment compliance, and costs. *Drug Intell Clin Pharm.* 1984;18(5):436–41.

70. Chrischilles EA, Helling DK, Rowland CR. Clinical pharmacy services in family practice: cost-benefit analysis. I. Physician time and quality of care. *Drug Intell Clin Pharm.* 1984;18(4):333–41.

71. Nelson AA, Jr., Beno CE, Davis RE. Task and cost analysis of integrated clinical pharmacy services in private family practice centers. *J Fam Pract.* 1983;16(1):111–6.

72. Wilt VM, Gums JG, Ahmed OI, et al. Outcome analysis of a pharmacist-managed anticoagulation service. *Pharmacotherapy.* 1995;15(6):732–9.

73. Ernst ME, Brandt KB. Evaluation of 4 years of clinical pharmacist anticoagulation case management in a rural, private physician office. *J Am Pharm Assoc.* 2003;43(5):630–6.

74. Jameson J, VanNoord G, Vanderwoud K. The impact of a pharmacotherapy consultation on the cost and outcome of medical therapy. *J Fam Pract.* 1995;41(5):469–72.

75. McKenney JM, Slining JM, Henderson HR, et al. The effect of clinical pharmacy services on patients with essential hypertension. *Circulation.* 1973;48(5):1104–11.

76. Carter BL, Barnette DJ, Chrischilles E, et al. Evaluation of hypertensive patients after care provided by community pharmacists in a rural setting. *Pharmacotherapy.* 1997;17(6):1274–85.

77. Bluml BM, McKenney JM, Cziraky MJ. Pharmaceutical care services and results in project ImPACT: hyperlipidemia. *J Am Pharm Assoc.* 2000;40(2):157–65.

78. Tsuyuki RT, Johnson JA, Teo KK, et al. A randomized trial of the effect of community pharmacist intervention on cholesterol risk management: the Study of Cardiovascular Risk Intervention by Pharmacists (SCRIP). *Arch Intern Med.* 2002;162(10):1149–55.

79. Simpson SH, Johnson JA, Tsuyuki RT. Economic impact of community pharmacist intervention in cholesterol risk management: an evaluation of the study of cardiovascular risk intervention by pharmacists. *Pharmacotherapy.* 2001;21(5):627–35.

80. Cranor CW, Bunting BA, Christensen DB. The Asheville Project: long-term clinical and economic outcomes of a community pharmacy diabetes care program. *J Am Pharm Assoc.* 2003;43(2):173–84.

81. Cranor CW, Christensen DB. The Asheville Project: short-term outcomes of a community pharmacy diabetes care program. *J Am Pharm Assoc.* 2003;43(2):149–59.

82. Kuehl AK, Chrischilles EA, Sorofman BA. System for exchanging information among pharmacists in different practice environments. *J Am Pharm Assoc.* 1998;38(3):317–24.

83. Dudas V, Bookwalter T, Kerr KM, et al. The impact of follow-up telephone calls to patients after hospitalization. *Am J Med.* 2001;111(9B):26S–30S.

84. Schnipper JL, Kirwin JL, Cotugno MC, et al. The effect of pharmacist counseling and follow-up on patient outcomes following hospital discharge. *J Gen Intern Med.* 2003;18(Supp 1):137.

85. Cromarty E, Downie G, Wilkinson S, et al. Communication regarding the discharge medications of elderly patients: a controlled trial. *Pharm J.* 1998;260:62–4.

86. Forster AJ, Murff HJ, Peterson JF, et al. The incidence and severity of adverse events affecting patients after discharge from the hospital. *Ann Intern Med.* 2003;138(3):161–7.

87. Rupp MT, McCallian DJ, Sheth KK. Developing and marketing a community pharmacy-based asthma management program. *J Am Pharm Assoc.* 1997;NS37(6):694–9.

88. Koecheler JA, Abramowitz PW, Swim SE, et al. Indicators for the selection of ambulatory patients who warrant pharmacist monitoring. *Am J Hosp Pharm.* 1989;46(4):729–32.

89. Carter BL, Malone DC, Billups SJ, et al. Interpreting the findings of the IMPROVE study. *Am J Health-Syst Pharm.* 2001;58(14):1330–7.

90. Hammond RW, Schwartz AH, Campbell MJ, et al. Collaborative drug therapy management by pharmacists—2003. *Pharmacotherapy.* 2003;23(9):1210–25.

91. Kuo GM, Buckley TE, Fitzsimmons DS, et al. Collaborative drug therapy management services and reimbursement in a family medicine clinic. *Am J Health-Syst Pharm.* 2004;61(4):343–54.

92. Lata PF, Binkley NC, Elliott ME. Acceptability of pharmacy-based bone density measurement by women and primary healthcare providers. *Menopause.* 2002;9(6):449–55.

93. Brown GH, Kirking DM, Ascione FJ. Patient willingness to pay for a community pharmacy based medication reminder system. *Am Pharm.* 1983;NS23(6):69–71.

94. Ernst ME, Bergus GR, Sorofman BA. Patients' acceptance of traditional and nontraditional immunization providers. *J Am Pharm Assoc.* 2001;41(1):53–9.

95. Navarro RP. Reimbursement for cognitive pharmacy services. *Manag Care Interface.* 1998;11(7):57–9.

Chapter 5

Long-Term Care

Barb J. Mason-Kennedy, Sandra G. Jue, Peter A. Bauer

Introduction

In 1996, the Institute of Medicine (IOM) launched an ongoing effort focused on assessing and improving the nation's quality of care. The Institute documented the problems and through various efforts, the health care community is working to solve them. Initiatives have been directed toward health care delivery design, patient and medication safety, electronic information technology implementation, and health care education reform. As a result of these reports and initiatives, many aspects of health care have been affected including long-term care. Although the IOM report was not the first to identify that elderly patients are at risk for medication related problems due to contributing factors such as poor adherence, polypharmacy, inappropriate prescribing, and multiple medical problems, it has assisted in focusing attention on these long- standing problems in the elderly.[1] As a vital member of the health care team, it is the responsibility of the long-term care pharmacist to contribute in addressing these problems through the provision of pharmaceutical care. The purpose of this chapter is to present an overview of long-term care including functions of consultant pharmacists, types of patient populations, levels of care and facilities, and drug distribution pharmacy services in nursing facilities.

Definitions

ADL—Activities of daily living usually done during a normal day, such as getting in and out of bed, dressing, bathing, eating, and using the bathroom.

Center for Medicare and Medicaid Services—Health and Human Services (HHS) federal agency responsible for Medicare and parts of Medicaid.

Clinical Practice Guidelines (CPGs)—Reports written by experts who have studied whether a therapy works and which patients are most likely to be helped by it.

Closed Door Pharmacy—Pharmacy that serves only long-term care facilities.

Community-Based Care—Term used to describe care at a level between a nursing facility and an independent ambulatory patient.

Conditions of Participation—Statutory requirements that facilities are required to comply with, to participate in, and to receive reimbursement from Medicare and Medicaid programs.

Consultant Services—Cognitive or clinical activities

Drug Distribution System—Method of dispensing medications (e.g., modified unit dose [3–30 day supply], unit dose [24–72 hour supply], traditional multidose vial and bottle).

Drug Regimen Review (DRR)—Systematic evaluation of medication therapy viewed within the context of resident-specific data with the goal being optimization of medication therapy, also referred to as Medication Regimen Review (MRR).

Drug Utilization Evaluation or Drug Utilization Review (DUE/DUR)—Structured, ongoing quality assurance process designed to ensure that drugs are used appropriately, safely, and effectively.

Interpretive Guidelines—Provide direction to surveyors of nursing facilities who determine the facility is in compliance with federal regulations.

IOM—Institute of Medicine was chartered by the National Academy of Sciences to enlist distinguished members of health professions in the examination of policy matter pertaining to public health.

Long-Term Care—A variety of services that help people with health or personal needs and activities of daily living over a period of time.

Med Pass Survey—A mechanism to evaluate the outcome of the medication distribution system using direct observation of medication administration.

Medication Administration Record (MAR)—Record carried on the medication cart containing information needed for proper administration of medications, including drug dose, route, frequency of administration and administration times, allergies, and some monitoring requirements.

Nursing Facility—A facility that primarily provides skilled nursing care and related services for the rehabilitation of injured, disabled, or sick persons; or on a regular basis, health-related care services above the level of custodial care.

Nursing Home—A residence that provides a room, meals, and help with ADL and recreation.

Provider Service—Refers to the operation and maintenance of the drug distribution system.

Quality Indicators—Used to identify possible problems that require follow-up and monitor and improve performance.

Prescribing for the Elderly

Elderly persons are often the focus of long-term care consultant pharmacy practice. This population experiences increased medical problems, medication use, and is more likely to have drug-related problems such as adverse drug reactions, drug interactions, and inappropriate and duplicative drug therapy.[2] Healthy People 2010 was established by the United States Department of Health and Human Services in 1997.[3] This initiative has three specific aims that target the elderly population: (1) increase the proportion of primary care providers, pharmacists, and other health care professionals who routinely review all prescription and nonprescription medicines with patients age 65 and older; (2) increase the proportion of adults who are vaccinated against influenza and pneumonia; and (3) reduce hospitalization rates.

The prevalence of inappropriate prescribing is especially high in the nursing home setting.[4,5] It is estimated that approximately $3 billion is spent annually for drug therapy in nursing facilities.[6] For every dollar spent on drugs in nursing facilities, $1.33 is consumed on the treatment of drug-related morbidity and mortality and as many as 70% of medication related problems may be preventable.[7]

Consultant Pharmacy

Consultant pharmacy originated in the provision of pharmacy services to nursing facilities and other long-term care environments over three decades ago. Consultant pharmacists are more than nursing home pharmacists. Consultant pharmacists manage and improve drug therapy of the senior populations and other individuals residing in environments including hospitals,

nursing facilities, subacute care facilities, assisted living facilities, psychiatric hospitals, hospice, and home- and community-based care.

Today, more than 10,000 consultant pharmacists provide a variety of clinical, distributive, and administrative services to more than 1.8 million nursing facility (NF) residents. Pharmacists providing consultation in long-term care do so through a variety of business arrangements. They may be community pharmacy-based and contract with a nursing facility to provide comprehensive pharmacy services. A *closed door* pharmacy refers to a pharmacy that serves only long-term care facilities. Another practice format may be a group of pharmacists specializing in providing comprehensive pharmacy services to a number of nursing facilities either locally or regionally. Some pharmacists may work with the drug distribution system as service providers and others may specialize as consultants. Long-term care corporations are a growing practice format for consultant pharmacists.

Pharmacists' roles in long-term care evolved from chart reviews in back rooms to active recognition for their role in the health care team and administrative and clinical skills directed at appropriate drug use and positive patient care outcomes. Activities are patient focused, such as drug regimen review, and facility focused, such as establishing policies and procedures for medication use. Consultant pharmacists must be clinical practitioners, patient care advocates, educators, regulatory experts, drug information researchers, managers, and entrepreneurs. The consolidation of care, which inherently occurs with nursing home admission, provides the perfect opportunity for review and improvement in drug regimen review. In this environment medication changes may be closely monitored. Pharmacy and medical literature contains many examples of consultant pharmacists' impact on inappropriate medication use in nursing facilities.[8,9,10]

Long-Term Care Patients and Levels of Care

The number of individuals 65 and older could more than double in the next 30 years to approximately 69 million in 2030.[11] More than 8.5 million of this aging population will be 85 and older.[12] In 1994, nearly 17% of the 33 million persons over age 65 received long-term care. While long-term care is not synonymous with nursing home care, the cornerstone of long-term care (LTC) is the nursing facility (NF), also known as nursing home. LTC is interdisciplinary in nature and incorporates services of a wide range of health care providers. Long-term care provides continuity of care and ongoing assessment and follow-up of patient's condition and response to therapy to achieve the highest practical, physical, mental, and psychosocial well-being. Long-term care is a broad topic and is characterized by various care services and settings including medical, social, personal, and supportive and specialized housing for individuals who have lost some capacity to care for themselves. Long-term care services are best described as a continuum that ranges from medical treatment and management of chronic illnesses to assistance with activities of daily living including bathing, dressing, eating, and housekeeping. Common services include adult day care, home care, sheltered housing, residential care facility, assisted living communities, and nursing homes. *Community-based care* is a term used to describe care offered somewhere between the traditional nursing facility environment and the independent ambulatory patient. A focus on institutional care merits further discussion of adult day care, respite care, assisted living communities, intermediate care facilities for persons with mental retardation, psychiatric hospitals, nursing home, and subacute care.[13]

Adult Day Care

Adult day care is best described as a program designed to meet the needs of adults with functional and/or cognitive impairments. Health, social, and other support services are provided in a protective setting during part of the day. Clients of these facilities do not require 24-hour care. Such programs help clients remain in the community while assisting caregivers and families who continue care at home for the individual with a disability. Currently, the law does not require pharmaceutical services in most adult day care settings. Some pharmacists have recognized opportunities in this area of long-term care and provide pharmaceutical care in the form of drug therapy consults.

Respite Care

Respite care describes a program that provides planned, short, intermittent care for a disabled individual for the purpose of providing relief to the regular caregiver. This temporary care can be as short as hours or as long as a limited period of days. Respite care may be delivered in the client's home or at a residential facility or institution. In some settings, pharmacists review patients medication lists during this time and optimize them when appropriate. This can optimize drug therapy management after the respite period.

Assisted Living

Assisted living is best described as an independent living arrangement in which clients receive services such as meal preparation and delivery, assistance with medications and activities of daily living, housekeeping, and transportation. Many facilities have a registered nurse charged with oversight of the limited health services provided. Clients maintain a relatively independent lifestyle and pay a monthly rent for housing and services provided. As with the other forms of non-nursing home care, federal law does not require pharmaceutical care in most assisted living facilities. However, some states are beginning to insist on aspects of pharmaceutical care management. Assisted living facilities offer a new opportunity for the provision of pharmaceutical care. The American Society of Consultant Pharmacists (ASCP) recognized this and issued guidelines for pharmacists seeking to serve clients in this setting.[14] Most elderly persons take multiple drug agents that are prescribed by various prescribers. Such factors can result in various drug therapy problems ranging from drug-drug interactions to monetarily burdensome and cost-ineffective drug regimens. Pharmacists can positively influence this population's drug therapy by solving various drug regimen problems and tailoring cost-effective regimens.

Other Institutionalized Pharmacy Settings

Intermediate care facilities for persons with mental retardation (ICF/MR) and psychiatric hospitals also occupy the landscape of institutional long-term care. An ICF/MR is defined by the Centers for Medicare and Medicaid Services (CMS) as "a facility that provides health-related care above the level of custodial care to mentally retarded individuals" but not at the levels of a skilled nursing facility or hospital. A psychiatric facility is defined by CMS as a facility for "the diagnosis and treatment of a mental illness on a 24-hour basis, by or under the supervision of a physician."[18] CMS has promulgated regulations guiding pharmaceutical care in these settings.

Nursing Home Care

Of all the types of institutionalized long-term care, nursing home care is the most intensive. On average, nursing home clients are frail and require 24-hour supervision. Resident care, organized by the facility includes, the disciplines of nursing, medicine, pharmacy, social work, dietary, and physical therapy.

Subacute Care

Similar to nursing home care in many ways, subacute care offers services distinct from residential nursing home care. This level of care is often used in place of, or after, acute hospitalization. Typically, patients are medically stable, at a level of moderate or low acuity, and require testing and treatments of greater frequency than can be handled in a residential long-term care setting. In subacute care, active or unstable medical conditions or impaired function is evaluated and treated and treatment plans assessed and modified. Some of the treatments provided in subacute care settings have been described as moderately complex requiring significant skill, judgment, or monitoring. The limited time of treatment distinguishes subacute care from residential long-term care. Subacute care is intended to assess and treat specific medical conditions, such as wound care or cardiac monitoring in a limited amount of time. Care of this nature is found in various facilities such as hospitals, rehabilitation hospitals, or nursing homes.[15] Development of the Subacute Care Model has been based largely on economics and the concept that more cost effective care can be provided in this setting. Subacute care requires 24-hour pharmacy services and a pharmaceutical care role similar to the hospital setting.

Consultant Functions

The pharmacy profession and law have defined the role for today's consultant pharmacist. Table 5-1. The requirements stipulated by regulations depend on the institution served by the pharmacist. Thus, one of the major roles of the consultant pharmacist is as a regulatory expert, who has knowledge of laws and regulations of the environment in which they practice. Depending on the setting and location, consultant function may be mandated federally or at the state level. The state regulations vary with each state. Detailed requirements are found in the CMS state operations manual (SOM) pharmacy services section.

Clinical responsibilities are mandated by federal and state regulations. Through their studies, Johnson and Bootman validated the cost-effectiveness of these activities.[16,17] In addition, organizations such as the American Society of Health-System Pharmacists (ASHP) and ASCP developed innovative policy statements and guidelines on the roles of pharmacists in long-term care, found at both organizations' internet websites. These new practices include collaborative

Table 5-1
Roles of Consultant Pharmacists

Drug regimen review

Drug research programs

Pharmacokinetic dosing services

Pain management consults

Intravenous therapy services

Therapeutic drug monitoring

Pharmaceutical care plan

Disease management

Medication utilization evaluation

Policy and procedure

Quality assurance programs

Drug information

In-service education programs

Medication delivery systems

Computer generated forms and reports

Patient safety

Medication error reporting

Adverse drug reaction reports

practice agreements with prescribers, counseling geriatric patients, disease management protocols, software development, laboratory services, nutrition services, pharmaceutical care planning, screening for affective, cognitive, or other psychiatric disorders, monitoring the dosing of the psychoactive drugs, medication use evaluation, clinical research, as well as the oldest function—drug regimen review. Drug information and in-service education of caregivers are also vital services offered by the consultant pharmacist.

Long-term care consultant pharmacy is influenced by changing demographics, the reimbursement environment in which nursing facilities operate, and health care economics. In the past few years, there has been an increase in the use of preadmission screening for nursing homes, expanded role of Medicaid, and introduction of managed care programs. Increasingly, long-term care facilities (LTCF) are taking residents who previously would have been cared for in hospitals. This is evidenced by the growing numbers of subacute centers. A shift to a quality focus began in 2002, when the Center for Medicare and Medicaid Services (CMS) launched a program called the Nursing Homes Quality Initiative. The goal of this was to improve the quality among nursing homes by publicizing survey results.

Since 1991, comprehensive resident assessment has been a federal requirement in all Medicare and Medicaid certified nursing facilities. Every year there is more emphasis on standardized performance measures for judging health care quality, costs, and outcomes. New emphasis on assessment means more expectations of pharmacist consultants.

The Minimum Data Set

In the provision of pharmaceutical care to LTC clients, consultants encounter a data collection tool called the minimum data set. The minimum data set (MDS) 2.0 is a comprehensive assessment instrument required for use on all nursing facility residents for clinical, reimbursement, and licensure survey purposes.[18] It is submitted to Medicaid and Medicare agencies. Resource utilization groups (RUGs) are determined from MDS data which influences reimbursement to nursing facilities. RUGs are based on level of care and the type of services provided to residents. Automated clinical information collected with the MDS assists in patient monitoring and medication regulation. The Minimum Data Set (MDS) is designed to collect data about an individual to use in a comprehensive, outcome oriented care plan for the resident. The Resident Assessment Instrument (RAI) is used to develop outcomes-based care plans that rely on early recognition of problems and risk factors. It is a summary and bridge of the data collected by MDS 2.0 and the care plan. A large component of each Resident Assessment Plan (RAP) requires evaluation of the resident's drug therapy. Certain sections of the MDS 2.0, such as mood and behavior problems, disease diagnosis, and medications can yield a wealth of information for pharmacy applications. MDS 3.0 is being developed with tentative implementation in 2006. The Minimum Data Set for Resident Assessment Instrument (MDRAI) is another acronym utilized.

Psychotropic drug use is one example of information that can be tracked by the MDS, as is the resident's mood, behavior, and function. The staff nurse who abstracts the information from the MDS documents where such information is located in the medical chart. Because the pharmacist's role is to ascertain if psychotropic medications are being used appropriately, she can identify where data may be lacking or insufficient, and bring these matters to the attention of the MDS coordinator.

Drug Regimen Review

Regulation 42 CFR 483.60 (c) requires the medication regimen of each resident be reviewed at least once a month by a licensed pharmacist.[19] This regulation is called the Drug Regimen Review (DRR) or Medication Regimen Review (MRR). The regulation states that the pharmacist must report any irregularities to the attending physician and the director of nursing. Furthermore, these reports must be acted upon. The State Operations Manual (SOM) that guides surveyors in determining whether facilities meet this standard advises that "surveyors check a random sampling of patient charts to determine conformance with frequency of DRR, evidence of monitoring of medications, identification of medication related problems, reporting to medical physician and director of nursing." Additional responsibility requires "medication errors not exceed five percent and that any errors are free of significant errors." It is the "joint responsibility of the pharmacist, prescriber, and nurse to assure that manufacturer's specifications regarding the preparation and administration of the drug or biological be followed." Furthermore, "accepted professional standards and principles which apply to professionals providing services be followed." These "professional standards and principles include various practice regulations in each State and current commonly accepted health standards established by national organizations, boards, and councils."[19]

The requirements for the drug regimen review (DRR) are met by obtaining information gathered by the nursing home through the MDRAI as well as onsite review of the patient's medical and pharmacy records. An example of how information from the MDS RAI can be used to perform DRR is shown on Figure 5-1.

A number of professional organizations have adapted the work of Hepler and Strand, which identified the categories of medication-related problems as the basis of the provision of pharmaceutical care.[20] These categories include (1) untreated medical problems; (2) improper medication selection; (3) too little medication; (4) failure to receive medication for a medical problem; (5) too much medication-overdosage; (6) adverse drug reaction or a condition worsened by a drug; (7) drug interaction; and (8) medication with no indication.

State Operations Manual

As already mentioned, the state operations manual calls special attention to the use of certain drugs evaluated by Beers et al. considered to place a person over age 65 at increased risk of experiencing an adverse drug reaction (ADR).[21] A sample from this list is provided in Table 5-2. It is the responsibility of the consultant pharmacist to call attention to the use of these medications and discourage their use where appropriate so as to decrease the incidence of ADRs. Failure to do so may cause preventable harm to the patient and cause the LTCF to be cited with a deficiency from their respective state health regulatory body.

Use of other medications is also subject to close scrutiny through rules contained in the SOM. Arguably, psychopharmacological drugs including antipsychotics, anxiolytics, and antidepressants attract the most atten-

Figure 5-1
Use MDS 2.0 to Identify At-Risk Elderly

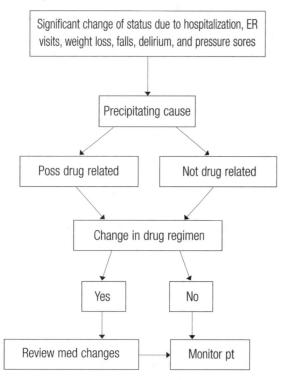

Analyze for trends and suggest programs to prevent hospitalizations (e.g., vaccination for influenza, pneumococci).

Source: Adapted from Losben NL,
http://www.ascp.com/public/pubs/tcp/1197/may/mds.html.

tion. These medications are closely evaluated under the title of "Unnecessary Drugs." F tag 329, a federal regulation addressing unnecessary drugs, states that an "unnecessary drug is any drug when used (1) in excessive dose (including duplicate therapy); (2) for excessive duration; (3) without adequate monitoring; (4) without adequate indications for its use; (5) in the presence of adverse consequences which indicate the dose should be reduced or discontinued; or (6) any combinations of the reasons above."[22] The consultant pharmacist shares a large part of the responsibility in assuring that these medications are being used in a manner that satisfies the aforementioned criteria. Failure to do so on the part of the pharmacist can lead to patient harm, unnecessary drug use, and deficiencies cited by surveyors.[7]

Medication Use Evaluation

Medication Use Evaluation (MUE) is a standard for patient care and quality assurance in long-term care settings. It is used to enhance patient outcomes and contain costs. Individual facility studies of medication use can assess the impact of drug regimen review and education by the consultant pharmacist. Once a baseline usage has been identified, follow-up studies can identify trends and patterns of use. By analyzing trends and patterns of use, MUE can identify appropriate areas for future consultant involvement and subsequent reviews. Utilization data can be most useful when compared with pre- and post-interventions from the same or similar populations. The consultant pharmacist can develop criteria based on current literature and practice standards or adapted from commercial manuals that are peer-reviewed and published periodically.

Throughout the years, MUEs have been performed on individual drugs and drug classes with recent application to disease management systems. Frequently, establishment of medication utilization protocols for specific drug categories evolve as a result of MUE. Cooperation from the medical director of the nursing home, physicians, nurses, and administrators is essential for it to be successful. Challenges to MUE by consultant pharmacists include lack of time, resources, compensation, and formulary.

Pharmacist-Physician Communication

Ongoing communication and a strong relationship between the consultant pharmacist and physician are essential for resident outcomes and to meet federal regulations. Per federal regulations, drug therapy rec-

Table 5-2
Sample of Beer's List Drugs

Drug	Concern	Severity Rating (High or Low)
Propoxyphene (Darvon) and combination products (Darvon with ASA, Darvon-N, and Darvocet-N)	Offers few analgesic advantages over acetaminophen, yet has the adverse effects of other narcotic drugs	Low
Muscle relaxants and antispasmodics: methocarbamol (Robaxin), carisoprodol (Soma), chlorzoxazone (Paraflex), metaxalone (Skelaxin), cyclobenzaprine (Flexeril), and oxybutynin (Ditropan)	Most muscle relaxants and antispasmodic drugs are poorly tolerated by elderly patients since these cause anticholinergic adverse effects, sedation, and weakness; additionally, their effectiveness at doses tolerated by the elderly is questionable	High
Long-acting benzodiazepines: chlordiazepoxide (Librium), chlordiazepoxide-amitriptyline (Limbitrol), clidinium-chlordiazepoxide (Librax), diazepam (Valium), quazepam (Doral), halazepam (Paxipam), and chlorazepate (Tranxene)	These drugs have a long half-life in elderly patients (often several days), producing prolonged sedation and increasing the risk of falls and fractures; short- and intermediate-acting benzodiazepines are preferred if a benzodiazepine is required	High
Digoxin (Lanoxin) (should not exceed >0.125 mg/d except when treating atrial arrhythmias)	Decreased renal clearance may lead to increased risk of toxic effects	Low

Source: Reference 8.

ommendations are to be reported to the resident's physician who is then required to respond to the pharmacist's suggestion. Many variables influence the physician-pharmacist relationship, such as physician perceptions and knowledge of the role of consultant pharmacist, method of communication, and documentation procedures. It is vital that records of consultant pharmacist recommendations be easily retrievable and are based on evidence-based therapeutic guidelines. Professional interaction is usually enhanced if consultant pharmacists respond proactively rather than retroactively. Recommendations should include identification of the concern with specific means to correct the situation and determine how and when outcome results will be measured. Timing of the consultant pharmacist to be there when physicians are at the facility is ideal but not always practical. Pharmacists need to initiate dialog with attending physicians to facilitate long-term care pharmacy consultant functions. While this is not a problem unique to long-term care, one of the frustrations of consultant pharmacists is failure of some physicians to accept pharmacist recommendations. The consultant pharmacists should always remember that the primary responsibility for the care of the patient falls to the prescriber. The SOM requires that the pharmacist notify the nurse and prescriber of medication irregularities. However, the action they take is their own responsibility and may be different from the recommendation of the pharmacist.

Drug Distribution Systems in Long-Term Care

Drug distribution is guided by the same mandates governing drug regimen review. The regulations impose labeling and storage requirements on the facility, but the pharmacist would be immediately responsible for accomplishing these tasks and others (Table 5-3). The service pharmacist is expected to label drugs and biologicals used in the facility in accordance with currently accepted professional principles, including appropriate accessory and cautionary instructions, and expiration dates, when applicable; and in accordance with state and federal laws. The pharmacist must recommend to the facility that it store all drugs and biologicals in locked compartments under proper temperature controls and permit only authorized personnel to have access to the keys. Specifically, guidelines tell surveyors to assure that the lock for the storage of schedule II controlled drugs not be the same key as the key for the lock of non-schedule II drugs.

The standard of care for drug distribution is the unit of use system. Many vendors offer blister, bubble, or bingo cards of 7, 14, or 30 days packaged for a single patient. This system has been shown to reduce errors of omission and commission. Nonetheless, some state Medicaid programs fail to pay for the added costs of packaging, delivery, and inventorying associated with this safer distribution system. The ward stock system has been overshadowed as a cost ineffective method of dispensing medications and should be abandoned.

Among reasons that ward stock and standard prescription vials are ineffective in long-term care are that accountability of doses is virtually nonexistent, medication administration errors are common, and state and federal mandates are not met. Hence, the director of nursing, medical director, administrator, consultant pharmacist, and the service pharmacist must meet to determine a drug distribution system and accept responsibility to teach the nursing staff how to utilize it. The distribution system must maximize efficiency, minimize error, cut waste in staff time, provide for emergency medications, and provide for medications needed on weekends and night times. One of the major remaining challenges is that service pharmacy profiles and nursing home medication administration records fail to record every change that takes place. Over time, these discrepancies can lead to major errors. Communication between the home and the pharmacy is a must. The discrepancies are especially noted with as needed drugs or one-time use drugs.

In other types of long-term care such as assisted living, service pharmacists provide a mixture of systems. Some may provide standard prescription vials. Others may provide 30-day cassettes. State Medicaid programs will not pay for the added cost of filling the cassettes. In addition, in 30-day cassette systems, some state Medicaid programs are revising state pharmacy laws to permit unused doses to be returned to the service pharmacy and requiring pharmacies to credit the Medicaid program for unused drug. The system selected depends on the case mix and the stability of drug regimens for the population served. Some assisted living facilities have nursing staff to administer unit doses; others require the patient to be at a functional level at which they can self-administer from standard prescription vials. Service pharmacists bid on the right to service such facilities.

Emergency and First Dose Drugs

The service pharmacist must design a system for the facility to provide first doses of drugs and emergency drugs in a timely manner. The best approach is to have the executive committee (service and consultant pharmacist, nursing, and medical director) decide on which drugs are emergency drugs that must be provided on-site, because any delay in administration would unduly harm the patient. Often, these medications are provided to the facility in a tamper-evident box. The responsibility for inventory of the contents and replacement of used or expired drugs is jointly held between the facility and the service pharmacist. Additional drugs to provide as first-dose medications, or one-time use medications must also be decided by the committee. The accountability for each dose must be set up by the service pharmacist in order to minimize theft or loss and assure replacement supplies of expired drugs. There is appeal in providing the facility with an extensive inventory so that call-back to the facility at night, weekends, and holidays is minimized. Surveyors pay particular attention to such arrangements because the oversight of the dispensing pharmacist is lost prior to the administration of any doses. Such ward stock also

Table 5-3
Roles of Service Pharmacists

Initial screening of medication orders

Drug packaging and labeling

Drug delivery (routine and emergency)

Medication reordering

Audit system for controlled medications

Emergency medication supply

Monitoring of proper storage of medication

Computer generated-patient medication profile

Medication administration record

Automatic stop orders

Billing statements

exposes the service pharmacist to inventory shrinkage and could result in losses not easily recovered from the facility.

Policy and Procedure Manual

While another chapter discussed the policy and procedure manual, areas specific to the long-term care setting will be discussed here. Essential policy and procedure topics for long-term care facilities include drug supply, destruction of controlled substances, medication administration and monitoring, and consulting services.

Many long-term care facilities do not have in-house pharmacy services and must have pharmaceutical agents supplied by local community pharmacies or pharmaceutical suppliers specializing in long-term care packaging. Policies and procedures pertaining to how drugs are supplied must address timeliness of product delivery, packaging, unused product returns, and emergency/first dose drug supplies.

Policy and procedures must also address the destruction of drug products, especially the destruction of controlled substances. Appropriate documentation and specific witnesses should be discussed in these policies and procedures. State pharmacy rules provide guidance as to specific legal requirements.

A complete long-term care policy and procedure manual also addresses the topic of medication administration and monitoring for therapeutic and toxic effects of medications. Procedures for those individuals authorized to prepare and administer medications to long-term care clients should include steps for preparing and administering medications to clients. Nursing regulations and state departments of health are sources for specific rules. The manual should also address procedures that will aid nursing staff in monitoring for drug effects. Often, manuals will provide guidelines for monitoring effects of certain drugs (e.g., checking pulse rates of patients receiving a beta-blocker).

Policies and procedures relating to consulting services should define how the consultant pharmacist communicates information (based on the drug regimen review) to the nursing and medical staff. Policies should include how levels of information are handled. For instance, a good policy and procedure manual will define how the consultant lodges urgent interventions with other members of the health care team. While this is not an exhaustive list of areas concerning a long-term care pharmacy policy and procedure manual, it highlights areas provided by long-term care.

In-Service Education

Long-term care facilities are mandated to provide education to their staff in the form of short presentations called *in-services*. While in-services address various areas of patient care, long-term care facilities are required to conduct a certain number of in-services on drug therapy every year. Pharmacists often provide these in-services, which treat of a wide variety of topics. Some common topics include diabetes care, pain control, and prevention of medication errors. Some facilities request and include certain in-services as part of a plan to correct deficiencies cited in department of health surveys. Pharmacists present in-services to a broad spectrum of nursing home employees consisting of registered nurses to nursing aides. For these reasons, it is necessary to tailor the content and focus so that all participants can appreciate the education provided.

Committee Responsibility

Pharmacists practicing in long-term care are necessary participants in various committees. Committees in which long-term care pharmacists typically participate include quality assurance, pharmacy services, and infection control. In some cases, these committees may be combined into a larger committee since most of the participants compose the membership of all three committees.

Issues ranging from medication errors to inappropriate drug use may be addressed in this setting. As can be anticipated, these committees address most problems from a policy and procedure standpoint. Other committees also exist in which pharmacists participate. Pharmacists may also take part in care planning, interdisciplinary team, and institutional review board meetings.

Geriatric Education

The clinical role of the pharmacist has been assisted by a significant upgrade in the preparation of pharmacists for their role as consultants. The American Council on Pharmaceutical Education mandated the doctor of pharmacy degree for all schools and colleges of pharmacy beginning in 2000. The curricula of these programs have greatly increased the clinical training of pharmacists. Unfortunately, geriatric training and education in pharmacy curricula are not emphasized. The importance of this was first recognized as far back as the early 1980s. A 1982 survey, by Simonson and Pratt, of 72 accredited schools of pharmacy indicated that 22% of schools had no geriatric coursework, 35% offered courses with some geriatric content, and 43% offered elective courses.[23] A similar survey in 1995, by Kirschenbaum and Rosenberg, showed that only eight programs offered a didactic geriatrics elective and 18 offered a required geriatrics clerkship.[24] As a result, the majority of graduating pharmacists have little training in geriatric pharmacotherapy. This is problematic given the increased need for trained practitioners and consultants in the long-term care setting. The shortage of geriatric-trained health care professionals has even received the attention of the U.S. Senate Special Committee on Aging in 2002.[25]

In an attempt to address these deficiencies, the American Society of Health-System Pharmacists (ASHP) has accredited year-long postdoctoral residency training in geriatric pharmacy practice since 1984. The American College of Clinical Pharmacy also accredits residencies and fellowships in geriatric pharmacy. The American Society of Consultant Pharmacists sponsored the creation of the Commission for Certification in Geriatric Practice in 1997 that administers a standardized national examination on provision of pharmaceutical care to the elderly. Training and resources are now available at websites at these organizations to prepare for these exams.

The Fleetwood Project

To quantify the influence of consultant pharmacist in long-term care, ASCP envisioned and funded a research program called the Fleetwood Project. The Fleetwood Project is a three-phase research initiative designed to demonstrate the impact of consultant pharmacists' services on patient outcomes and health care costs. Phase I was launched in 1995 and was the first pharmacoeconomic study to quantify the cost of medication-related problems in nursing facilities and the value of consultant pharmacists' services.[16] Johnson and Bootman assessed the impact of pharmacist-conducted, federally mandated monthly retrospective review of nursing facility residents' drug regimens in reducing the cost of drug related morbidity and mortality. The cost estimates of drug-related morbidity and mortality with consultant pharmacists services range from a low of $3.3 billion to a high of $6.0 billion versus estimates from $6.7 to $11.5 billion without consultant pharmacist services. The difference represents the drug-related morbidity and mortality costs avoided

with services of consultant pharmacists through retrospective drug regimen reviews.

Phase II of the Fleetwood Project developed a framework for pharmacists to shift their practice focus from the drug regimen to the patient.[26–28] Phase III is measuring the impact of pharmacists' services in improving outcomes and health care costs.[29] Further research is needed on the impact of prospective review by the consultant pharmacist on health care costs of drug related morbidity and mortality.[30]

Long-Term Care Consultant Opportunities

The Centers for Medicare and Medicaid Services (CMS) is in the process of implementing a new Medicare drug benefit. Since approximately 2.5 million Medicare beneficiaries live in long-term care settings, the implementation will have widespread implications for consultant pharmacists. Issues currently being discussed relate to formulary issues, benzodiazepine coverage, access to injectables, and payment for special medication packaging.

The Medicare Prescription Drug, Improvement, and Modernization Act of 2003 has as one of the components a provision for medication therapy management services. Medication-management services is a distinct service or group of services that optimize therapeutic outcomes for individual patients. These services are independent of, but can occur in conjunction with, the provision of a medication product.

Long-term regulations are dynamic and it is important that pharmacists keep themselves up to date with information sources. CMS released proposed changes to the nursing facilities SOM on October 15, 2004. The changes specifically target Pharmacy Services and Unnecessary Drugs sections. These are the first major changes to the SOM since 1999 for these sections. The proposed changes were made by an expert panel, yet the guidelines still focus squarely on unnecessary medications, medication-related problems of Hepler and Strand, and how surveyors should identify them. If these changes are adopted, there will be an increased need for consultant pharmacists to upgrade their skills to use tools such as the MDS RAI to identify patients at risk for drug-related problems. With the growth of the aging population there will also be an increased need for greater numbers of practitioners to become skilled in treating our seniors.

Summary

Topics discussed in this chapter highlight the importance of long-term care consultant pharmacy and the necessity of pharmaceutical care to enhance health care in the elderly. Recent research has clearly identified the contributions of pharmacists in long-term care. Quality initiatives in recent years have also increased the role for consultant pharmacists. Regulations, mandatory pharmaceutical care, and the rewards of interdisciplinary team work make long-term care an ideal career opportunity. To meet this necessity, more pharmacists must be specialty trained in the field of geriatrics. In this specialty area, pharmacists can have a great impact on practice.

Acknowledgments

The authors wish to sincerely acknowledge the never ending, administrative assistant support of Sharlene Hetrick in the preparation of this chapter.

Suggested Readings

Anonymous. 1999 policy statements and guidelines. *Consult Pharm.* 1999;14:1164–80.

Aparasu RR, Mort JR. Inappropriate prescribing for the elderly: Beers criteria-based review. *Ann Pharmcother.* 2000;34:338–46.

Bootman JL, Harrison DL, Cox E. The health care cost of drug-related morbidity and mortality in nursing facilities. *Arch Intern Med.* 1997;157:2089–96.

Clark TR, Gruber J, Sey M. Revisiting drug regimen review, part I: the early history and evolution of DRR. *Consult Pharm.* 2003;18:215–20.

Clark TR, Gruber J, Sey M. Revisiting drug regimen review, part II: art or science. *Consult Pharm.* 2003;18:506–13.

Clark TR, Gruber J, Sey M. Revisiting drug regimen review, part III: a systematic approach. *Consult Pharm.* 2003; 18:656–66.

Dhalla JA, Anderson GM, Mamdani MM, et al. Inappropriate prescribing before and after nursing home admission. *J Am Geriatr Soc.* 2002;50:995–1000.

Gurwitz JH, Field TS, Avorn J, et al. Incidence and preventability of adverse drug events in nursing home. *Am J Med.* 2000;109:87–94.

Hanlon JT, Schmader KE, Boult C, et al. Use of inappropriate prescription drugs by older people. *J Am Geriatr Soc.* 2002;50:26–34.

Keys PA, O'Neil C, Maher R. Geriatric concentration: a new elective sequence in an entry-level doctor of pharmacy program. *Am J Pharm Educ.* 2004;68(1):article:07.

Tett S, Higgins G, Armour C. Impact of pharmacist interventions of medication management by the elderly: a literature review. *Ann Pharmacother.* 1993;27(1):80–6.

References

1. Kohn LT, Corrigan JM, Donaldson MS, eds. Institute of Medicine. *To err is human: building a safer health system.* Washington, DC: Committee on Quality of Health Care in America; 1999.

2. Curtis L, Ostbye T, Serdersky V, et al. Inappropriate prescribing for elderly Americans in a large outpatient population. *Arch Intern Med.* 2004;164:1603–4, 1621–5.

3. Healthy People 2000. Office of Disease Prevention and Health Promotion. U.S. Department of Health and Human Services; 1997. Available at: http://www.health.gov/healthypeople. Accessed November 10, 2004.

4. Beers MH, Ouslander JG, Rollinger I, et al. Explicit criteria for determining inappropriate medication use in nursing home residents. *Arch Intern Med.* 1991;151: 1825–32.

5. Dhalla JA, Anderson GM, Mamdani MM, et al. Appropriate prescribing before and after nursing home admission. *J Am Geriatr Soc.* 2002;50:995–1000.

6. IMS America. IMS Class-of-Trade Analysis: 1995. Plymouth Meeting, PA: IMS American; 1996.

7. Sloane P, Zimmerman S, Brown L, et al. Inappropriate medication prescribing in residential care/assisted living facilities. *J Am Geriatr Soc.* 2002;50:1001–11.

8. Miller S, Warnuck R, Marshall L, et al. Cost savings and reduction of medication-related problems as a result of consultant pharmacy intervention. *Consult Pharm.* 1993;8:1265–72.

9. Laucka PV, Hoffman NB. Decreasing medication use in a nursing home patient care unit. *Am J Hosp Pharm.* 1992;49:96–9.

10. Tett S, Higgins G, Armour C. Impact of pharmacist interventions of medication management by the elderly: a literature review. *Ann Pharmacother.* 1993 21;1:80–9.

11. U.S. Census Bureau. (2000). Demographic data. Available at: http://www.census.gov. Accessed November 10, 2004

12. Desai MM, Zhang P, Hennessy CH. Surveillance for morbidity and mortality among older adults-United States, 1995–1996. *Morbidity and Mortality Weekly Report.* 1999;48(SS-8):1–6.

13. Report of the Special Committee on Aging. United States Senate. *Developments in Aging: 1997 and 1998 Volume 1.* 2000;(Feb 7):154–5, 157.

14. American Society of Consultant Pharmacists. Guidelines for providing consultant and dispensing services to assisted living residents. Available at: http://www.ascp.com/public/pr/guidelines/aliving.html. Accessed October 26, 2004.

15. Levenson, S. The future of subacute care. In: Tumosa N, Moreley JE, eds. *Clinics in Geriatric Medicine: Subacute Care for Seniors.* Philadelphia, PA: W. B. Saunders Company; 2000:683–5.

16. Bootman, JL, Harrison DL, Cox E. The health care cost drug-related morbidity and mortality in nursing facilities. *Arch Intern Med.* 1997;157:2089–96.

17. Johnson JA, Bootman JL. Drug-related morbidity and mortality. A cost-of-illness model. *Arch Intern Med.* 1995;155:1949–56.

18. Centers for Medicare and Medicaid Services. Available at: http://www.cms.hhs.gov/glossary. Accessed October 26, 2004.

19. Centers for Medicare and Medicaid Services. State Operations Manual Appendix PP. Guidance to Surveyors—Long-Term Care Facilities. Rev. 1. May 21, 2004.

20. Hepler CD, Strand LM. Opportunities and responsibilities in pharmaceutical care. *Am J Hosp Pharm.* 1990;47:533–43.

21. Fick DM, Cooper JW, Wade WE, et. al. Updating the Beers criteria for potentially inappropriate medication use in older adults: results of a U.S. consensus panel of experts. *Arch Intern Med.* 2003;163(22)2716–24.

22. Centers for Medicare and Medicaid Services. Appendix P: survey protocol for long-term care facilities. Available at: http://www.hcfa.gov. Accessed November 10, 2004.

23. Simonson W, Pratt CC. Geriatric pharmacy curriculum in U.S. pharmacy schools: a nationwide survey. *Am J Pharm Educ.* 1982;46:249–52.

24. Kirschenbaum HD, Rosenberg JM. Geriatric training programs offered at schools and colleges of pharmacy. *Am J Pharm Educ.* 1995;59:284–6.

25. The Alliance for Aging Research, Medical Never-Never Land. Ten reasons why America is not ready for the coming age boom. Available at: http://www.agingresearch.org. Accessed November 10, 2004.

26. Fouts M, Hanlong JT, Pieper C, et al. Identification of elderly nursing facility residents at high risk for drug-related problems. *Consult Pharm.* 1997;12:2203–11.

27. Harms SL, Garrard J. The Fleetwood Model: an enhanced method of pharmacist consultation. *Consult Pharm.* 1998;13:1350–5.

28. Daschaer M, Brownstein S, Cameron KA, et al. Fleetwood Phase II tests a new model of long-term care pharmacy. *Consult Pharm.* 2000;15:7–19.

29. Harjivan C, Lyles A. Improved medication use in long-term care: building on the consultant pharmacist's drug regimen review. *Am J Manag Care.* 2002;8:318–26.

30. Hanlon JT, Schmader KE, Ruby CM, et al. Suboptimal prescribing in older inpatients and outpatients. *J Am Geriatr Soc.* 2001;49:200–9.

Chapter 6

Evolution of the Management of U.S. Health Care: Managing Costs to Care Management

Robert Navarro, Rusty Hailey

Introduction and Background

The financing and delivery of health care services in the United States has been dramatically transformed over the past 30 years since President Nixon signed the HMO Act in 1973. Managed care existed prior to the 1973, but the HMO Act provided federal funding and encouraged the eventual proliferation of *health maintenance organizations* (HMOs), the initial form of modern managed care. Traditional fee-for-service medicine began its slow death, and the practice of medicine and pharmacy was immutably and profoundly altered forever. Managed care grew because it promised to satisfy two growing societal needs. First, managed care offered to improve the quality of care by encouraging preventive or preemptive care, as well as providing treatment care, and, second, managed care promised to contain a steadily rising and unsustainable health care cost trend. Table 6-1 shows costs by health care delivery segment, percent of total costs, and annual trend rates.

Managed care will be compared to indemnity insurance more fully below, but the essential difference is that managed care offers a prepaid membership with a defined panel of contracted health care providers, compared with an indemnity insurance plan that allows patients to seek care from any community provider, who was then reimbursed on a fee-for-service basis. While managed care began to flourish in many regions in the 1970s, its actual genesis began earlier in the 20th century.[1] The Western Clinic in Tacoma, Washington, began offering health care services for lumber mill employees for a defined monthly premium. A health care cooperative for rural farmers was established in Oklahoma City, Oklahoma, in 1929. Kaiser

Table 6-1
Total Personal Health Care Expenditures by Type of Service (1960–2000)

Type of Service	1960 Amount	Percent	Trend*	1990 Amount	Percent	Trend*	1999 Amount	Percent	Trend*	2000 Amount	Percent
Personal Health Care	$23.4	100.0%	10.0%	$609.4	100.0%	6.0%	$1,062.1	100.0%	6%	$1,130.4	100.0%
Hospital Care	$9.2	39.3%	10.0%	$253.9	41.7%	5.0%	$392.2	36.9%	5%	$412.1	36.5%
Physician/Clinical Services	$5.4	23.1%	10.0%	$157.5	25.8%	6.0%	$270.2	25.4%	6%	$286.4	25.3%
Dental Services	$2.0	8.5%	9.0%	$31.5	5.2%	7.0%	$56.4	5.3%	6%	$60.0	5.3%
Other Professional Care	$0.4	1.7%	12.0%	$18.2	3.0%	8.0%	$36.7	3.5%	6%	$39.0	3.5%
Home Health Care	$0.1	0.4%	16.0%	$12.6	2.1%	10.0%	$32.3	3.0%	<1%	$32.4	2.9%
Prescription Drugs	$2.7	11.5%	10.0%	$40.3	6.6%	12.0%	$103.9	9.8%	17.0%	$121.8	10.8%
Non-Durable Medical Products	$1.6	6.8%	8.0%	$22.5	3.7%	3.0%	$30.4	2.9%	3.0%	$31.2	2.8%
Durable Medical Equipment	$0.7	3.0%	9.0%	$10.6	1.7%	6.0%	$17.6	1.7%	5.0%	$18.5	1.6%
Nursing Home Care	$0.7	3.4%	13.0%	$52.7	8.6%	6.0%	$89.3	8.4%	3.0%	$92.2	8.2%
Other Personal Health Care	$0.6	2.6%	11.0%	$9.60	1.6%	14.0%	$33.7	3.2%	9.0%	$36.7	3.2%

Source: Centers for Medicare & Medicare Services, Office of the Actuary, National Health Statistics Group. Available at: http://www.cms.hhs.gov/review/supp/2001/table4.pdf.

Foundation Health Plans began in 1937 to provide health care for Kaiser construction workers and ship-builders. Similar cooperative *group health plans* developed elsewhere, including Minnesota and Seattle.

Today, health insurance in the United States is commonly offered by employers as an employee benefit and is partially paid by employers. Managed health care benefit plans purchased by private businesses are described as *commercial plans.* Large corporations with adequate financial reserves may qualify to create its own *self-insured plan* that will be developed and customized on its behalf by a health plan for its employees. Self-insured plans are exempt from certain regulations governing commercial health care benefits. Pharmacy benefits are included in over 90% of commercial health plans. All health care in the U.S. is *managed* except the dwindling amount of fee-for-service cash business. Over 90% of all prescription transactions in the U.S. is reimbursed by a private commercial or public (e.g., Medicaid or Medicare) prescription drug program.

Government-sponsored health plans include health and pharmacy benefits for selected populations. Medicaid provides comprehensive care for beneficiaries usually under age 65 and of very low income; Medicare provides health and pharmacy benefits (as of January 1, 2006) for beneficiaries age 65 and over; and the Veterans Administration and Department of Defense plans offer benefits for active and retiree armed forces members and certain government employees. Both private employer groups and government purchasers of health care are known as *payers* because they purchase health care benefits on behalf of their members or beneficiaries. The most broadly sweeping pharmacy benefit changes have recently occurred in Medicare. The Medicare Modernization Act (MMA) signed by President Bush in 2003 provides for an outpatient pharmacy benefit for Medicare members under Part D beginning January 2006. The impact of the MMA on pharmacy benefits for Medicare recipients will be discussed in greater detail elsewhere.

Elements of Managed Care

The essence of managed care is to manage any and all products and services in the health care delivery system. There are two essential aspects of every activity in health care delivery that must be managed: the unit cost of each product or service, and the utilization rate of each product or service. Therefore, managed care attempts to obtain a discount contract from all providers of care, including physicians, dentists, hospitals, long-term care facilities, pharmacies (community, mail service, and specialty pharmacy), chiropractors, and others, as well as from all providers products including pharmaceuticals companies, durable and disposable medical equipment venders, home health care, diagnostic instruments, and any other product used in health care delivery.

While the discounted contracts for all health care products and services control the supply side of resource costs, equally important is controlling the demand for services. Physicians (and other health care professionals with prescriptive authority) are ultimately responsible for ordering the use of health care resources. As a result, health plan participation contracts with physicians require them to use discounted health care resources (e.g., referring patients only to contracted specialists, admitting only hospitals under contract, and prescribing drugs on the formulary). Physicians may have financial incentives or penalties for inefficiently using services or ordering cost-ineffective treatments if not clinically justified.

In addition to physicians, patients (health plan members) are also responsible for causing inefficient use of resources by seeking unnecessary care and requesting unneeded prescriptions and inappropriate use of resources (e.g., visiting the emergency department for trivial illnesses). Therefore, managed care and payers typically require members to share in the plan's financial responsibility by paying part of the health care premium and paying a *user fee* (copayment or coinsurance) when they access health care services. In summary, managed care attempts to share the financial risk with any and all entities that can influence the supply and demand, the cost and utilization, or all health care resources.

Health plans must provide a system that encourages the provision of high quality, cost-effective health care while also controlling health care costs. State courts have held that health plans do not *practice* medicine but provide a financing and delivery system in which physicians practice medicine and remain ultimately responsible for ordering or causing all health care to be provided to eligible health plan members. There is often tension between the health plan that is trying to manage the cost and utilization rate of all health care services and the physician and patient who may request more services or more expensive services that is recommended by the plan. For that reason, all health plans provide an appeal process to review any patient situation in which services are denied and physicians or patients challenge the denial. Therefore, to be successful in the long-term, health plans must develop a benefit design and delivery system structure that rewards physicians to order cost-effective products and services that balance short-term costs and outcomes with longer-term costs and outcomes.

Managed care generally includes the following elements in an attempt to provide cost-effective and high quality health care products:

Defined Inclusion and Exclusion of Benefits

Managed care does not offer unlimited products and services but by contract must specify which benefits are covered and which are excluded. For example, excluded benefits include investigational and experimental medications and procedures. The managed care contract will also specify the monthly premium as well as any copayments or coinsurance requirements. The drug formulary describes drugs eligible for reimbursement as well as prescription limitations (e.g., quantity limits or prior authorization).

Prepaid, Membership Health Care Services

Opposed to paying specifically for and only when health care services are obtained. Members of a managed care system pay a fixed monthly premium regardless if they use services or not. In addition, managed care members often pay a small, fixed copayment or percent coinsurance, which is essentially a user fee, when they actually do utilize covered products and services.

Defined Provider and Vender Network

Managed care organizations contract with specific health care facilities, health providers, and venders to obtain all products and services at discounts for health plan members. Discounted contracts for all products and services are obtained in exchange for the increase in utilization as a result of the health plan encouraging, or requiring, members to use the contracted providers. Some plans will allow access to noncontracted *out-of-network* providers at a higher member copayment or coinsurance cost. To obtain discounted prescription benefits, members must use contracted community and mail service pharmacies for most drugs or contracted specialty pharmacies for certain injectables.

Preventive and Quality Management Services

The original HMO Act of 1973 provided for preventive care. Health plans typically offer preventive health care screening, encourage annual physical exams, and have specific care management or case management programs to manage high cost and high prevalence diseases (e.g., diabetes, obesity, hypertension, dyslipidemia, organ transplants, depression). Drug utilization review, online or telephone drug information, and medication adherence monitoring are common pharmacy benefit quality assurance programs. The National Committee on Quality Assurance (NCQA) accredits achievement of defined health plan quality measures, similar to the JCAHO accreditation of in-patient facilities. Payers often consider the NCQA accreditation status when selecting a health plan.

Types of Managed Care Organizations

In 1973, the term *managed care* signified a health maintenance organization (HMO). This term, allegedly created by Dr. Paul Ellwood, a Minnesota physician and health care advisor to national health care policymakers, promoted the preventive medicine benefits of an HMO with prepaid health care. Early HMOs were typical of a highly controlled staff model or group model plan, such as Kaiser-Permanente Health Plan, which owned medical facilities and employed health care providers. To obtain care, members had to visit the owned medical centers, hospitals, and pharmacies, and were treated by employed physicians. In the late 1970s and early 1980s, a different type of less structured HMO developed. The less controlled network model and independent practice association (IPA) model plans began to flourish. Network model plans and IPAs owned no facilities and employed no physicians but rather contracted with private practice, community-based hospitals, physician groups, and pharmacies to provide services. However, there was a trade-off among model types between the ability to control costs or offer richer benefits. High control such as a staff or group model HMOs (e.g., Kaiser-Permanente Health Plan) were more effective in controlling costs but offered less member freedom of choice of services and community providers. Conversely, less controlled HMOs, such as network and IPA models (e.g., United HealthCare), offered more member freedom of choice, but that choice came at a slightly higher cost.

In an attempt to provide more options to employer groups and members, managed care organizations have developed more plan options, some of which provide even greater freedom of choice. A preferred provider organization (PPO) provides an expanded network of community providers and greater member choice. The point of service (POS) plan combines the benefits of a controlled HMO and a less controlled PPO. In a POS option, members can decide if they would stay within the contracted network (for a lower cost) or go to a noncontracted provider (at a higher cost). We use the term *health plan* or *managed care organization* (MCO) as generic terms to refer to a managed care organization that provides comprehensive inpatient medical, outpatient medical, and prescription drug benefits. At the end of 2003, there were approximately 72 million members in HMOs and 112 million members in PPOs.[2] We use the term *pharmacy benefit managers* (PBMs) to refer to companies that specialize in providing only prescription drugs benefits. Figure 6-1 provides a graphical interpretation of the balance of benefit freedom and cost control.

Figure 6-1

Comparison of Different MCO Types, Level of Control, and Relative Cost

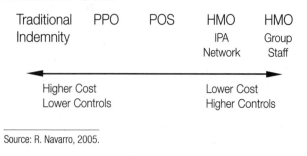

Source: R. Navarro, 2005.

Managed care is neither a singular process nor a static event. Health plan medical and pharmacy benefits, structure, and operations are highly variable based on geographic region, local market competition, state coverage requirements, political considerations, and employer and member demands. And, health plans will evolve over time in response to the same influences and to increase appeal to its customers.

Flow of Money through Managed Care

Managed care is a highly regulated and contracted delivery system. The payers and purchasers of health care (e.g., employer groups, government), heath plan members, providers of care (e.g., physicians pharmacies, hospitals, long-term care facilities), and venders

(e.g., DME companies, home health care agencies) all have a contractual relationship with the health care plans. All of these stakeholders are financially linked or at risk in some way to encourage observance with the cost-containment policies of the health plan.

Purchasers of care (employer groups, government) pay premiums to health plans for health benefits and to PBMs for prescription benefits. Health plans pay hospitals, physicians, and pharmacies a discounted reimbursement for services provided. Pharmacies purchase drugs through wholesalers or directly from pharmaceutical companies. Pharmaceutical companies provide discounts or pay rebates to health plans or PBMs to enhance the cost-effectiveness and formulary position of their products. Patients pay a copayment or coinsurance whenever they access the health care system. In exchange for having access to health plan members, providers and venders under contract agree to provide products and services for a defined discount. Figure 6-2 demonstrates the contractual relationships and flow of money throughout the delivery system.

When examining health plan operations, one must understand how health care providers are reimbursed for their services. Physicians employed by a closed-model plan (e.g., staff or group models) are usually salaried and may receive a bonus linked to plan performance or their own efficiency. Community physicians participating with open-model plan (e.g., IPA or network health models) are generally reimbursed through either a capitation or a discounted fee-for-service arrangement and also may receive a financial incentive for efficient performance. Physicians are usually not at financial risk for the cost of the drugs they prescribe, although there can be geographical and plan-specific variances.

Physician Capitation Reimbursement

Through capitation, a physician (or medical group) receives a fixed monthly fee for providing covered services based upon the number of enrolled members that are assigned to the physician or medical group. The physician or medical group receives the same monthly fee per assigned member regardless of how many times the members may see the physician or how many covered outpatient services the physician provides. Through capitation, the HMO transfers a portion of the financial risk to the physician. Theoretically, this will serve as an incentive to the physician to provide only necessary and cost-effective care. The

Figure 6-2

Flow of Money through a Managed Care Delivery System

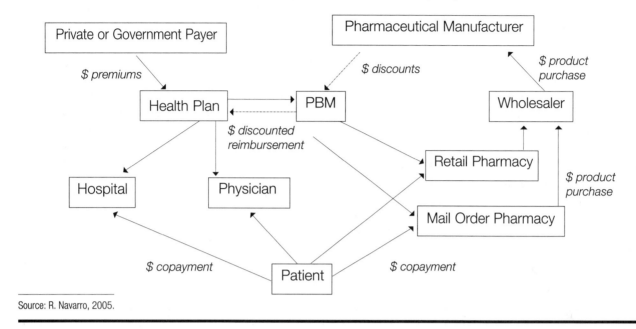

Source: R. Navarro, 2005.

capitated physician is expected to include a full range of services that often include all outpatient visits, preventive care, diagnostic tests, laboratory, and other office-based services. Medical groups that receive a capitation rate that includes drug costs usually create their own formulary, or preferred drug list, in an attempt to manage their drug costs.

Physician Discounted Fee-For-Service (FFS) Reimbursement

Under a discounted FFS reimbursement system, physicians receive payment only when they provide covered services to health plan members. However, their reimbursement is discounted from usual and customary (U&C) payment rates. This provides a mechanism to reduce costs per service. Also, physicians generally receive only a portion of the reimbursement for services rendered (e.g., 80%). The remaining 20% is withheld and maintained in a reserve to be paid out at the end of the year if certain cost and utilization performance objectives are met. High-risk outlier patients (e.g., patients with transplants or AIDS) that may bias the financial performance are eliminated. Inefficient (most costly) physicians may not receive their financial reserve. Physicians that are *average* performers receive their reserve payment. Physicians that are the most

efficient will receive a bonus (essentially the withhold that is not returned to the least efficient physicians).

Hospitals are reimbursed on a per diem, DRG, other fixed-fee basis, or discounted FFS arrangement depending on the service and procedure provided. The cost of inpatient drugs are typically included in the overall hospital fee and are not reimbursed separately (certain expensive drugs may be carved-out and billed separately by mutual agreement). As a result, health plans generally do not have any role or interest in determining inpatient drug formularies. Exceptions include those health plans that own hospitals (e.g., Kaiser-Permanente), where outpatient and inpatient drug purchasing may be coordinated. Hospital reimbursement practices are addressed elsewhere in this book.

Managed Pharmacy Benefits

Outpatient pharmacy benefits are an important component of comprehensive health care benefits offered by managed care organizations and purchased by both commercial and government payers. As of January 2006, Medicare, Medicaid, and over 90% of commercial health plan members will have access to outpatient prescription drug benefits. Arguably, drugs are the most cost-effective form of disease prevention and treatment for many highly prevalent and diseases, including cardiovascular disease, diabetes, migraine headache, asthma, depression, and GERD.

Pharmacists managing prescription drug benefits must provide high quality pharmacy benefits while managing program costs. The quest to manage costs, rather than merely minimize costs, remains the challenge. As pharmacy program costs continue to escalate at an annual trend rate of approximately 20%, it is tempting to merely restrict expensive drugs or increase the patient copayment tier at an equal rate. However, simply focusing on cost-minimization is myopic and ultimately cost-ineffective. Figure 6-3 shows the rate of growth of hospital, physician, and pharmacy costs over the past decade.

Health plan administrators, as well as commercial and government payers, often consider pharmacy benefits only as a cost center, and do not appreciate the value a well managed pharmacy benefit can bring to clinical, economic, and humanistic outcomes. Health

outcomes research in health plans, addressed below, provides the linkage between appropriate use of cost-effective drugs and positive outcomes, and helps administrators and payers shift from cost-minimization to value promotion. To achieve this goal, pharmacy benefit managers attempt to select the most cost-effective drugs for formulary inclusion, implement programs to promote the appropriate use and adherence, and document value by measuring outcomes. These goals are no different than those of hospital pharmacists, but they are more difficult to control as the MCO pharmacy director is often managing prescription benefits for hundreds of thousands of patients with literally every known disease.

Pharmacy Benefit Managers (PBMs)

Many large health plans manage their pharmacy benefit programs through an internal pharmacy department. Even so, the vast majority of health plans also use a

Figure 6-3
Annual Trend Rates for Hospital, Physician, and Pharmacy Costs

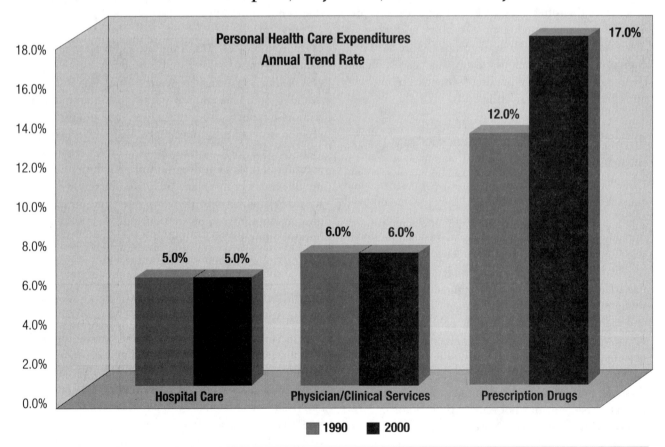

Source: Centers for Medicare & Medicare Services, Office of the Actuary, National Health Statistics Group. Available at: http://www.cms.hhs.gov/review/supp/2001/table4.pdf.

variety of services offered by pharmacy benefit managers, PBMs, which have evolved as experts in pharmacy benefit management. Pharmacy PBMs are specialized companies that provide managed prescription drug benefits to health plans, government plans (e.g., Medicaid, Medicare), or to self-funded employer groups. PBMs do not offer any services a health plan could not develop through an internal pharmacy department. However, PBMs manage millions of lives, and the economies of scale regarding computer services, patient call centers, contracting with pharmacies and with pharmaceutical manufacturers may make PBM services less costly than if an MCO built their own internal PBM.

The amount of PBM services purchased by MCOs, Medicaid plans, and self-insured employers, depends entirely on the needs of the customer. Some of the offered services include the following:

- Pharmacy distribution network (community, mail, and possibly specialty products)

- Drug formulary development and management, including generic substitution program (maximum allowable cost [MAC] list maintenance)

- P&T Committee services including new drug reviews

- Pharmaceutical manufacturer contracting

- Physician and member communication

- Member service help line

- Provider and member website development and maintenance

- Drug utilization review services (prospective, concurrent, and retrospective)

- Clinical pharmacy services (DUR, adherence monitoring, clinical edit development) and disease management programs

- Claims processing and report generation

Some PBMs are captive, or internal PBMs, of a large health care organization. Most PBMs exist as independent companies (e.g., Medco Health Solutions, AdvancePCS/Caremark, Express Scripts, Inc.), although they may be associated with health plans (e.g., Prescription Solutions PBM, a subsidiary of PacifiCare Health Plans, and WellPoint, now a part of Anthem Health Care), or a component of a retail pharmacy chain (e.g., Wallgreens Health Initiatives, CVS PharmaCare). Humana has its own internal PBM that only serves its own commercial members at this time.

However, there has been much consolidation in the PBM market due to mergers, acquisitions, and divestitures. Pharmaceutical companies formerly owned two of the largest PBMs. Merck owned Medco Health Solutions, now an independent company, and SmithKline-Beecham owned DPS, which was borne out of United HealthCare and is now part of Express Scripts, Inc. Table 6-2 provides a list of largest PBMs.

Table 6-2
List of Top PBMs and Membership
Membership of the Largest U.S. Pharmacy Benefit Managers

Caremark/AdvancePCS	105 million
Medco Health Solutions	70 million
Express Scripts, Inc.	53 million
WellPoint	40 million
MedImpact	30 million

Source: R. Navarro, adapted from PBM websites and marketing material, 2005.

Components of a Managed Prescription Drug Benefit Plan

Pharmacists operating health plan pharmacy benefits have borrowed many management strategies from hospital pharmacy programs, including the P&T Committee, the drug formulary, pharmaceutical company contracting, physician education, utilization review, and health outcomes research. However, health plans have had to include additional capabilities, such as development of a community and mail distribution system, member communication and education, and massive computer systems to process millions of claims in a real-time environment.

Certificate of Coverage

Managed care plans do not claim to provide any and all desired health care services. Rather, a payer purchases, and a health plan provides, defined benefits as specified in a state regulated contract (e.g., Certificate of Coverage or other similar name) that is generally renegotiated annually. The contract defines included and excluded benefits, as well as the access rules through which members must obtain benefits. Drugs typically excluded from coverage include the following:

- Experimental or investigational drugs
- Approved drugs when prescribed for unapproved indications (although this is generally unenforceable as community pharmacies generally are not aware of the diagnosis or medication indication; this restriction is usually reserved for expensive drugs or injectables subject to prior authorization, when the drug indication may be verified)
- Drugs used for cosmetic purposes (e.g., Botox for wrinkles) or lifestyle drugs (e.g., PDE-5 inhibitors)
- Brand name drugs for which there are AB-rated generic equivalent that is subject to mandatory generic substitution (e.g., mandatory maximum allowable cost [MAC] program)
- Drug for which there is an identical OTC equivalent, such as ibuprofen 200 mg; insulin is an exception, as it is a nonprescription drug in many states but remains covered by health plans

Health plans use drug formularies to communicate drug coverage as well as member copayment requirements and other restrictions (formularies are discussed below).

Distribution Channels for Outpatient Pharmaceuticals

Managed care organizations must develop a pharmaceutical distribution system that meets member needs for easy access to prescription services as well as containing ingredient and dispensing costs. Closed-model health plans or large employer groups may have in-house, owned pharmacies for member convenience supplemented with community pharmacies, often with mail service. Open-model plans will use a community-based pharmacy including pharmacy chains and independent pharmacies, and often mail service as well. Many pharmacy chains also offer mail service.

Pharmacies participating in the pharmacy provider network agree, by contract, to dispense drugs prescribed by plan physicians to eligible members according to the drug formulary and other benefit design requirements. Pharmacists may participate in many different managed pharmacy programs, and by contract must use the online, real-time point-of-service (POS) computer system to verify coverage information (eligible drug, member, and physician), learn any dispensing limitations or requirements (e.g., quantity limits, step-care protocols), obtain copayment information, and

know the level of reimbursement from the health plan or PBM. Pharmacists received a discounted ingredient cost reimbursement (based on a discount off the AWP) and a dispensing fee. Other payments may exist, such as for a special generic substitution or member clinical consultation.

Specialty Pharmacy Distribution

The increasing use of high cost injectable biotech products that may require special handling has caused the development of many specialty pharmacy distributors (SPDs). Specialty pharmacy services may also be offered by PBMs. SPDs may send injectables directly to a physician office for a patient appointment for drug infusion, or drugs can be mailed directly to a member's home. Volume purchasing by SPDs introduces cost efficiencies into the system that are passed on to payers and members. This system prevents physicians from stocking and storing expensive medications and removes them from the flow of dollars, as the SPD bills the health plan or member directly, and the physician is paid an administration fee by the health plan. The growing availability to biotechnology pharmaceuticals will likely increase the role and importance of SPDs in the future.

Pharmacy and Therapeutics Committee Management

Managed care has borrowed the P&T Committee concept from hospitals as a source for formulary development and drug coverage decisions. In addition to the clinical drug review, the Committee must make recommendations on formulary coverage and copayment tier and other dispensing limitations or restrictions. Managed care P&T Committees typically consist of 10 to 15 physicians and pharmacists and meet quarterly. Clinical pharmacists with the health plan or PBM review available published and manufacturer clinical and economic data, the Academy of Managed Care Pharmacy Format for Formulary Submissions, consider plan-specific expected utilization patterns, other formulary drugs, manufacturer contracts, and present recommendations to the P&T Committee for formulary action. Due to concerns about drug safety and utilization patterns, new drugs are usually not formally reviewed for formulary consideration for at least 3 to 6 months postlaunch. During that time, the drug may be available for reimbursement as a nonformulary or nonpreferred drug, usually on the copayment Tier III.

Clinical data (efficacy/effectiveness and safety) are the primary formulary decision criteria, but net cost ranks quite high as a decision consideration as well. Increasingly, credible health outcomes and economic data are available and considered by managed care P&T Committees, and formulary decisions are based on clinical, economic, and humanistic outcomes rather than solely on pharmacy budget cost minimization. The AMCP Format for Formulary Submissions in particular provides a standardized method for pharmaceutical companies to submit all relevant clinical and economic information on a drug considered for formulary inclusion. The Format for Formulary Submissions supports the informed selection of pharmaceuticals, biologicals, and vaccines by[3]

- standardizing and communicating product and supporting program information requirements

- projecting their impact on both the organization and its enrolled patient population

- making evidence and rationale supporting all choice(s) more clear and valuable by decision makers

Drug Formulary Development and Management

Health plans and PBMs have used drug formularies for the same reasons they are used in hospitals—to promote the most cost-effective pharmaceuticals in the most appropriate manner. The benefit design is enforced through the formulary, which is the basis for the drug and reimbursement information used by the pharmacist to process eligible claims using the POS system. Formulary booklets are mailed to participating physicians and often abridged formulary documents are provided to members, although many plans and PBMs provide pharmacy benefit and formulary information for physicians and members online. Formularies are fundamentally a method of communicating drug coverage and reimbursement policies to physicians and patients.

Some formularies are *open,* signifying most drugs are eligible for reimbursement, although the level of member copayment varies with a drug's formulary position and copayment tier. Other formularies may be *closed,* indicating a select number of drugs are eligible for reimbursement, while others are not covered. Some drugs are *on formulary* but available only if the patient satisfies certain prior authorization (PA) criteria. Drugs

may be subject to a PA based on cost or safety issues, to attempt to control use for labeled indications only or for certain types of patients. The open and closed nature of formularies is cyclical. In the recent past, formularies were more inclusive with most nonformulary products covered on Tier III, but due to rising costs many MCOs are returning to more restrictive formularies and continuing higher and tiered copayments.

Physician and member formulary conformance is enforced using different mechanisms depending on if the formulary is inclusive or exclusive. Closed formularies do not allow for reimbursement of nonformulary products, and pharmacists must contact the prescribing physician to request a change for a formulary product, or the patient must pay cash for a nonformulary product. Open formularies use a tier copayment structure, described below, to encourage physician prescribing and member use of generics or preferred formulary products. Physicians are provided copies of formularies and made aware of formulary changes through mail, newsletters, and email. Some health plans and PBMs employ pharmacists for academic detailing of physicians who continuously disregard the formulary. Many health plans and PBMs provide physicians *formulary conformance report cards* and indicate opportunities for prescribing changes that favor formulary products. Some plans and PBMs offer financial incentives to physicians for high levels of formulary conformance.

Health plans, PBMs, and employer groups often used a tiered formulary structure to apply the member copayment to share costs with utilizing members, and to influence physician prescribing and member acceptance of lower cost drugs when appropriate. There are typically two copayment tier plans, but more plans are adopting three or more copayment tier plans.

Copayment Tier I generically contains generic drugs, and due to the lower generic cost the member copayment is lower to encourage use of generics. *Copayment Tier II* is reserved for preferred or formulary products, and a medium-level copayment amount is assigned. These are generally branded drugs and are more expensive than generics but considered necessary medications. *Copayment Tier III* products are nonformulary or nonpreferred brand drugs, placed on a higher tier due to high cost or because there are cost-effective options on Tier II. Some plans include Tier IV for lifestyle, cosmetic medications, or injectables. The dollar amounts of the various tiers are increasing, as is the delta between tier amounts. Table 6-3 provides examples of a tiered formulary for the HMG Co reductase category.

Critics of high dollar copayments claim the increasing copayment amounts are financial deterrents to members obtaining and remaining on prescribed drugs.

Table 6-3
Example of Statin Formulary Copayment Tiers

Tier I	Tier II	Tier III
Generic	Preferred Formulary Brand	Nonpreferred or Nonformulary Brand
Lovastatin	Lipitor (atorvastatin) Pravachol (pravastatin)	Crestor (rosuvastatin) Leschol (fluvastatin) Zocor (simvastatin)
$12.00	$25.00	$45.00

Source: R. Navarro, 2005.

Research is controversial on the matter and can be criticized by ignoring the numerous other factors that influence drug adherence, such as lack of understanding, forgetfulness, belief that medications are unnecessary, adverse effects, and cultural barriers to medications.

Pharmaceutical Manufacturers Contracts

As hospitals contract for drugs with GPOs and manufacturers, health plans and PBMs similarly negotiated discounts or rebate for selected drugs in exchange for a favorable formulary position. Savings obtained reduce the net price of contracted drugs, and the savings are passed on to customers. Rebates (the favored contract for health plans and PBMs who do not take possession of drugs) generally include an access rebate as well as a performance rebate based on achieving certain market share or volume goals.

Clinical Pharmacy Services

Health plans and PBMs offer an array of clinical pharmacy services, many of which are online and real-time edits provided to the dispensing pharmacist. Others include prospective or retrospective utilization monitoring, adherence intervention, and disease management programs.

Online, real-time point-of-dispensing edits provide commonly used guidance regarding drug interactions, early refill prevention, duplicate medications, age and gender edits, and step-care edits. Health plans and PBMs also provide computerized DUR, screening for drug misuse and abuse, polypharmacy, nonadherence, and other dangerous or inappropriate drug use patterns. Interventions may include patient and or physician communications requesting clarification of the potential dangerous pattern.

Health plans may offer disease-specific management programs to augment health care services provided by plan physicians, which may provide general disease education, diagnostic screening events (e.g., hypertension, diabetes, or dyslipidemia screening), and case management for high-cost and high-risk conditions (e.g., CHF, diabetes, asthma). Pharmaceutical manufacturers may provide some unbranded disease management resources (e.g., physician or patient education) to supplement health plan efforts.

Quality Initiatives

In addition to helping customers manage rapidly rising health care costs, health plans must provide high quality health care delivery services. The National Committee for Quality Assurance (NCQA) is a private, not-for-profit organization dedicated to improving health care quality and provides many mechanisms and reports on quality of care provided by health plans, physicians, disease management providers, and managed behavioral health organizations. NCQA publishes the Health Plan Employer Data and Information Set, or HEDIS measures, which are tools used by health plans to measure performance on important dimensions of care and service. Many employer groups consider NCQA accreditation and HEDIS measure scores to reliably compare the performance of managed health care plans when selecting health plans for their employees.

NCQA 2004 HEDIS measures consist of 60 measures to assess Access/Availability of Care, Satisfaction with the Experience of Care, Health Plan Stability, Use of Services, Health Plan Descriptive Information, and 22 Clinical Effectiveness measures. The Clinical Effectiveness measures that involve the use of pharmaceuticals include the following:

- Childhood and adolescent immunization status
- Appropriate treatment for children with upper respiratory infection

- Osteoporosis management in women who had a fracture

- Beta blocker treatment after a heart attack

- Cholesterol management after acute cardio-vascular event

- Use of appropriate medications for people with asthma

- Antidepressant medication management

- Flu shots for adults

- Management of urinary incontinence in older adults

Assuring the appropriate use of cost-effective pharmaceuticals is an important responsibility for pharmacy directors of managed care organizations. The growing use of HEDIS measures that include drug use help employer groups recognize that pharmacy benefits are not merely a cost center but a source of overall clinical and economic value.

Electronic Prescribing

The rapid expansion of information technology applications in health care presents novel opportunities and challenges for pharmacists. Although electronic prescribing is not widespread and still in a pilot phase, many MCOs are experimenting with electronic data transfer of prescription-related information among trading partners: the health plan, physician, and pharmacy. Electronic prescribing refers to the use of computing devices to enter, modify, review, and output or communicate drug prescriptions.[4] In inpatient care, electronic medication ordering increases prescribing accuracy, dispensing efficiency, and reduces the number of adverse drug events and redundant medications. A number of outpatient pilot projects and initiatives in electronic prescribing are proliferating within managed care organizations to achieve the same goals and are also providing medication history, drug formulary options, drug hypersensitivities, and other clinically relevant data to the prescriber at the point of prescribing.

In the ambulatory environment, recent research shows that adverse events are common and can be serious. The Center for Information Technology Leadership reports that more than 8.8 million adverse drug events occur each year in ambulatory care, of which over 3 million are preventable, many resulting in deaths.[5] In addition to reducing adverse drug effects, electronic prescribing can improve quality, efficiency, and reduce costs through other benefits, including the following[6]:

- Actively promoting appropriate drug usage

- Providing information about formulary options and copay information

- Improving dispensing efficiency and accuracy by providing instant electronic connectivity between the physician, pharmacy, health plans, and PBMs

More than 3 billion prescriptions are written annually.[7] Given this volume, even a small improvement in quality attributable to electronic prescribing would translate into significant health care cost and safety benefits if electronic prescribing is broadly adopted. Studies suggest that the national savings from universal adoption of electronic prescribing systems could be as high as $27 billion, including $4 per member per year savings from preventable adverse drug events and $35–$70 per member per year savings from more appropriate use of medications, for a total savings of $39–$74 per member per year.[8] Electronic prescribing has significant benefits for pharmacists as well. The Institute for Safe Medication Practices estimates that pharmacists spend a significant amount of their time each day clarifying prescription orders and making 150 million phone calls to physicians annually on prescription accuracy-related issues.[9]

PBMs have taken a leadership role in developing and promoting electronic prescribing initiatives. The three largest PBMs—AdvancePCS, Express Scripts, and Medco Health Solutions—sponsored the development of RxHub in 2001 to create a single point of communication of information related to accurate and cost-effective prescription prescribing and dispensing.[10]

Professional Opportunities for Pharmacists in Managed Care

Prescription drugs are the most commonly used health plan benefit and the third largest health care delivery component expenditure, behind inpatient and outpatient physician costs. As a result, cost-efficient pharmacy programs developed and managed by pharmacists are critical to the successful overall operation of a health plan. Many professional opportunities exist for pharmacists within managed care in an overall health plan administration, pharmacy program manager, information technology, provider services, member education, clinical pharmacy services, dispensing activities, and disease management. Specific pharmacy program activities include the following areas of practice:

- *Pharmacy Benefit Management*—Developing and managing the overall pharmacy benefit, health plan business development, staff hiring and development, pharmacy benefit design development, and marketing benefits to prospective customers
- *Pharmaceutical Manufacturer Contracting*—Negotiating and administering discount contracts with drug companies
- *Pharmacy Network Management*—Negotiating contracts with community and mail service pharmacies, and specialty pharmacy distributors
- *Clinical Pharmacy Services*—Developing and executing clinical programs, including utilization review, online clinical edits, adherence interventions, physician and patient education, and disease management programs
- *P&T Committee and Formulary Management*—New drug clinical and economic data review, development of clinical monographs, evaluation of AMCP-compliant formulary guideline submissions from manufacturers, P&T Committee membership, and academic detailing of physicians
- *Health Outcomes Research*—Economic research, pharmacy benefit design impact research, research result publishing, and support of P&T Committee activities related to drug economic evaluations
- *Information Technology*—Pharmacy computer system development, health plan website development, performance report generation, and interface with electronic prescribing and data interchange trading partners

Numerous professional clinical and business opportunities exist for pharmacists, with more positions developing every year as managed care expands and broadens its service offerings. Outside of health plans and PBMs but within managed care, pharmacists have unlimited entrepreneurial opportunities in related companies and activities including disease management, specialty pharmacy, information technology, health education, and health outcomes research.

Evolution of Health Care Management

Health care in the U.S. is a market driven business.

Commercial and government payers have many choices when selecting health plans, PBMs, and other venders and customizing health, pharmacy, and ancillary benefits for their members. We have seen a continuous evolution of managed care organizations and benefit design driven in concert by health plans (attempting to develop novel health care benefits with richer benefits yet at a competitive price) and payers who make demands on the market and offer their business to health plans and PBMs that best satisfy their unique cost and quality demands.

While there are many trends within managed care, perhaps the following will have the greatest impact on pharmacy benefit management in the coming years.

Continuing Pressure on Health Plans and PBMs to Contain Costs

This will result in higher member prescription copayments and greater number of employers adopting a tiered copayment structure. Approximately 75% of commercial managed care lives are now subject to a three-tier copayment structure today, and this will increase as payers attempt to contain and shift costs to utilizing members. Opponents claim that higher copayments will present financial barriers for some members, and may result in nonadherence of prescriptions. Several high cost, high utilization drugs will lose patent protection over the next few years, which will provide opportunities for pharmacy benefit cost savings. This is balanced by the increasing availability of expensive biotechnology products that, for some patients, provide outcomes not realized with existing medications, but at a higher cost.

Lower Member Drug Copayments for Specific Diseases

In contrast to the above trend, there is emerging interest by some employers groups, such as Pitney-Bowes, to reduce the prescription copayment for cost-effective drugs to treat several high cost and high prevalence medical conditions, including diabetes, asthma, CHF, and dyslipidemia. The market is curious and cautiously watching the impact on drug adherence and, more importantly, medical and economic outcomes of these benefit design changes.

Availability and Acceptance of Health Savings Accounts (HSAs)

These novel mechanisms, actually tax-deferred medical savings accounts, allow members to save and spend a fixed amount of tax-deferred dollars for an array of customized health benefits. For example, members (or their dependents) who use several high-cost drugs may allocate a greater portion of their personal HSA for pharmacy benefits to minimize their out-of-pocket spending. HSAs can be confusing for members but when understood are likely to be quite popular and will give the member more freedom of choice. This presents opportunities for pharmacists to counsel their patients on the most cost-effective drug use.

Growth in the Acceptance of Health Outcomes Data

Over the past 20 years, managed care has evolved from managing health care components (e.g., hospital, physician, pharmacy benefits) in isolation without evaluating the impact of the appropriate use of cost-effective drugs on reducing hospitalizations, diagnosis tests, and physician visits. Partially due to the AMCP Format for Formulary Submissions and published health outcomes data, P&T Committees are selecting formulary products with overall value in total direct medical cost containment and quality of life. Payers, unfamiliar with health outcomes methodologies, have traditionally encouraged cost-minimization in pharmacy benefit management and are beginning to understand the impact of cost-effective drugs in member (employee) quality of life, absenteeism, and productivity. As a result, enlightened payers are focusing on direct, as well as indirect, health outcomes and encouraging health plans and PBMs to provide adherence intervention.

Medicare Modernization Act of 2003

The most sweeping changes in Medicare since its inception were signed into law by President Bush in December 2003. The Medicare Modernization Act (MMA) adds outpatient prescription drug benefits for 41 million Medicare recipients beginning in January 2006 under Medicare Part D. The MMA also makes important changes in reimbursement of injectable drugs currently covered through Medicare Part B. The Congressional Budget Office predicts 87% of eligible Medicare recipients will enroll to receive outpatient medical and pharmacy benefits through Medicare Advantage (MA) provider (formerly Medicare+Choice plans) or pharmacy benefits alone from a Prescription Drug Program (PDP) provider. MA plans must be a health plan or insurer, but PDPs may be MA plans (called MA-PDP) or PBMs (PDP). Current Medicaid

dual eligible beneficiaries will be auto-enrolled into a Medicare provider to obtain pharmacy benefits. At this writing, many regulations and policies remain undecided, but the final benefits, formulary guidance, reimbursement levels, and selected health plans and PDPs will be determined throughout 2005.

Electronic Prescribing

As described above, electronic prescribing will increase as pilot programs are successful and demonstrate cost efficiencies and improve the quality of care. Dispensing pharmacists will likely realize time savings and obtain more drug history and clinical information to allow a more meaningful interaction with the patient. If these objectives are realized, electronic prescribing may provide further support of pharmacist reimbursement for pharmacotherapy management counseling.

Transition from Managing Costs to Care Management

We have described the development, management, and future trends of managed care pharmacy benefits. In the 31 years since the HMO Act was signed into law, managed care has grown to be the primary method of financing and delivery health care in the U.S., although managed care organizations are quite diverse in how they meet customer expectations.

Managed care has continuously evolved since its inception, although the fundamental tenets on which managed care was founded remain the same—delivery of cost-effective and high quality health care with an emphasis on preventive medicine. The role of pharmacy benefit management has evolved from being a cost center to a source of significant value, contributing to clinical, economic, and humanistic outcomes. The transition from managing costs to managing care through appropriate use of cost-effective pharmaceuticals is largely the result of health outcomes data demonstrating the link between pharmaceutical use and health outcomes.

Managed care has presented many opportunities for pharmacists in population-based pharmacy benefit management, health outcomes research, and entrepreneurial adventures. The future indicates even greater opportunities will be present for pharmacists to demonstrate the value of medicines as well as the profession of pharmacy.

References

1. Fox, PD. An overview of managed care. In: Kongstvedt, PR, ed. *Essentials of Managed Health Care*. 4th ed. Gaithersburg, MD: Aspen Publishers; 2001:4–8.

2. Interstudy Publications. Available at: www.hmodata.com and the American Association of Preferred Provider Organizations, www.aappo.org.

3. Academy of Managed Care Pharmacy: Format for Formulary Submissions. Version 2.0. Available at: http://www.amcp.org/data/nav_content/formatv20%2Epdf. 2002:12.

4. eHealth Initiative. Electronic Prescribing toward Maximum Value and Rapid Adoption. Recommendations for Optimal Design and Implementation to Improve Care, Increase Efficiency and Reduce Costs in Ambulatory Care. Available at: http://www.ehealthinitiative.org/initiatives/erx/document.aspx?Category=249&Document=270. 2004:11.

5. Center for Information Technology Leadership. The Value of Computerized Provider Order Entry in Ambulatory Settings. 2003.

6. eHealth Initiative. Electronic Prescribing toward Maximum Value and Rapid Adoption. Recommendations for Optimal Design and Implementation to Improve Care, Increase Efficiency and Reduce Costs in Ambulatory Care. Available at: http://www.ehealthinitiative.org/initiatives/erx/document.aspx?Category=249&Document=270. 2004:11.

7. Agency for Healthcare Research and Quality. MEPS Highlights #11: Distribution of Health Care Expenses. 1999.

8. eHealth Initiative. Electronic Prescribing toward Maximum Value and Rapid Adoption. Recommendations for Optimal Design and Implementation to Improve Care, Increase Efficiency and Reduce Costs in Ambulatory Care. Available at: http://www.ehealthinitiative.org/initiatives/erx/document.aspx?Category=249&Document=270. 2004:11, 32.

9. Institute for Safe Medication Practices. A Call to Action: Eliminate Hand-Written Prescriptions within 3 Years. Available at: http://www.ismp.org/msaarticles/whitepaper.html. 2000.

10. http://www.rxhub.net/.

Chapter 7

Home Care

Mary R. Monk-Tutor

Introduction

Home care is a diverse field encompassing many services provided in a patient's place of residence, including nursing care, infusion therapy, durable medical equipment (DME; also called Home Medical Equipment or HME), respiratory care, physical therapy, and other supportive care.[1–11] These services may be provided in a variety of health care practice settings, including hospitals, private corporations, community pharmacies, home health agencies, and ambulatory infusion centers. In addition, home care may be provided to long-term care (LTC) patients who reside in nursing or assisted living facilities rather than in their own homes.[4,12,13]

Home Infusion Therapy (HIT) is one of the most challenging and interesting areas of pharmacy practice simply because there is no *standard* patient population. Patients of all ages across a wide range of disease states and acuity levels may be candidates for HIT.[4,14] In addition, some patients require only acute care while others need either continuous or intermittent care across their lifespan for chronic conditions such as nutritional deficiencies, multiple sclerosis, cystic fibrosis, pancreatitis, diabetes, heart failure and cancer.[4–7,10,15–20] HIT also represents a site of care in which all components of the model of Total Pharmacy Care are present: drug information, patient self-care, clinical pharmacy practice, pharmaceutical care, and product distribution services.[21]

The home health care industry has experienced dramatic growth since the early 1980s and continues to provide a strong job market for pharmacists who have the skills to work in this environment. In 1999 and 2000, annual expenditures in the United States on home care exceeded $33 billion and approximately 7.6 million patients (about 3% of the total population) were treated with some form of home care by one of over 642,000 health care professionals.[22] Spending on home care increased from $2.4 billion in 1980 to $34.5 billion in 1997, $45.3 billion in 2001, and is expected to reach $87 billion by 2010 with continued annual growth predicted at 7% through at least 2013.[23–24] Of this, home infusion therapy represents $4 to $5 billion or just over 10% of the entire home care market and has a projected annual growth rate of 5% to 9%.[25–26] In 1999, home infusion medications accounted for about 1% of the total U.S. pharmaceutical prescription drug market, with 76% of sales as injectable drug products (see Table 7-1).[27]

Table 7-1
Market Estimates (2003)[24–26,28]

Sector	Market Size (in billions of dollars)
Home Health Nursing	30–33.3
Specialty Pharmacy	10–15
Respiratory Therapy/Home Medical Equipment	4.5–10
Home Medical Supplies	4–6
Home Infusion Therapy	4–5
Hospice	4–5

Although the annual growth rate for home care services has dropped from a phenomenal 64% a year between 1982–86 to 24% a year between 1986–93, it is expected to remain at about 14% annual growth through at least 2009.[5,10,17,29] As such, this market will remain a viable one for pharmacists who wish to practice in an environment that allows them to use many varied skills, work within an interdisciplinary health care team, and have direct interaction with patients.

Definitions

It should be noted that the terms *home care* and *home health care* refer to a wide array of services that may be provided in the home while *home infusion therapy* refers specifically to the provision and clinical monitoring of infusions and other injectable therapies or enteral nutrition.[1,5] Knowledge of the following definitions is also important for a basic understanding of this practice environment:

Ambulatory Infusion Centers (AICs)—Physical facilities to which a patient comes to receive injectable therapies rather than having these services provided in the home. AICs are often located in a physician's office, hospital emergency room, outpatient clinics, and rarely, inside HHAs or pharmacies.[4,6]

Clinical Respiratory Services—Services that include diagnostic testing and the provision and clinical monitoring of inhaled respiratory medications and related equipment and are provided by registered respiratory technicians (RRTs).[4] Services and equipment typically provided in clinical respiratory care include apnea monitors, nebulizers, oxygen concentrators, portable oxygen, ventilators, suction machines, phototherapy, and continuous positive airway pressure (CPAP) machines.[32]

Durable Medical Equipment (DME) or **Home Medical Equipment (HME)**—Services that include the set up, delivery, and maintenance of prescribed medical equipment in a patient's place of residence as well as patient education and ongoing monitoring of both equipment and clinical outcomes of the care provided. Equipment such as ambulatory aides (canes, walkers, wheel chairs, scooters), bedside commodes, and hospital beds are considered to be *low tech* DME.[4,32] *High tech* DME includes infusion pumps for the delivery of either enteral solutions or injectable medications and respiratory aides such as medication compressors, oxygen, ventilators, and apnea monitors.[4,9,18,32]

High-Tech Home Care—Care that includes the provision and clinical monitoring of complex products and services such as physical or respiratory therapy, nursing care, home infusion therapy, and other services requiring the skills of a nurse, pharmacist, or other licensed health care professional.[4,9,19]

Home Care—The provision of health-related products or services provided to a patient in his or her place of residence that substitutes to some extent for acute inpatient care.[1,9] Although traditionally thought of as only home nursing services, home care now includes a wide array of products and services provided by a variety of professionals and paraprofessionals such as nurses, home health aides, pharmacists, pharmacy technicians, and equipment and delivery personnel. Other types of staff that may work in home care or hospice programs include social workers, occupational therapists, speech therapists, physical therapists, respiratory therapists, dieticians, and volunteers, as well as financial and business personnel.[4,6]

Home Health Agencies (HHAs)—Nursing agencies that provide a variety of services to acute or chronically ill patients in their place of residence according to a plan of treatment prescribed by a physician. While HHAs may also employ physical therapists, occupational therapists, dieticians, or social workers as well as personal care aides, they rarely employ pharmacists or pharmacy technicians.[4]

Home Health Services—Services that are provided by HHAs and typically include skilled nursing services such as administration and monitoring of both oral and injectable medication, wound care management, and patient education.[4,30]

Home Infusion Therapy—Therapy that includes the provision (compounding and delivery) and clinical management of injectable medications in the patient's place of residence by health care professionals, primarily, pharmacists and nurses.[1,4,5] These medications are usually administered by intravenous, subcutaneous, intramuscular, intrathecal, epidural or intra-arterial routes via central or peripheral vascular access devices.[31] Services provided by home infusion pharmacists include compounding and dispensing, clinical monitoring, care coordination, management of medical supplies, equipment, venous access devices, and practice and facility management.[31]

Hospice Services—Services that provide palliative care such as the management of pain and other symptoms to individuals with terminal illnesses who are expected to live no longer than 6 months. Care is usually provided in the home; however, some free standing and hospital-based hospice facilities do exist in the United States. An interdisciplinary team that usually includes physicians, nurses, social workers, pharmacists, clergy, and volunteers work together to meet the physical, psychosocial and spiritual needs of the patient and his or her family. Hospice programs often contract with pharmacies to provide needed oral or injectable medications for their patients.[4]

Personal Care and Support Services—Services that include assistance with activities of daily living such as cleaning, shopping, meal preparation, and helping patients to self-administer oral medications. These services are provided by paraprofessionals such as home health aides, home attendants, or homemaker aides.[4,6]

Background

Table 7-2 presents a summary of the major historical development of home health care services in the United

States since 1796. Thus far, two changes in Medicare reimbursement have provided the greatest incentive for growth of home care services. First, passage of the Medicare (Title XVIII) and Medicaid (Title XIX) Amendments to the Social Security Act of 1965 allowed for limited reimbursement of home therapies, including respiratory therapy, physical therapy, and home total parenteral nutrition (TPN) solutions.[5,8,9,19,33,34] Second, Medicare's implementation of a prospective payment reimbursement system for inpatients in 1983 with reimbursement based on diagnosis related groups (DRGs) created pressures to reduce inpatient length of stay and prompted many hospitals to develop home care programs.[5,36,37] As a result, in 1985 the home health care market was described as "the fastest growing segment of the health industry."[11]

The success of early hospital-based home infusion services led to the development of more hospital-based services and private, for-profit home infusion vendors (including community pharmacy-based franchises) as well as to the development of services provided out of the offices of private physicians.[5,6,37] Home infusion therapy in particular grew out of a need for treatment options other than inpatient care for patients with *chronic acute* conditions such as Crohn's disease and cystic fibrosis.[39]

In the 1990s, changes in Medicare reimbursement again had the most significant effect on home care practice as introduction of the Balanced Budget Act of 1997 (BBA) changed reimbursement for home health services (but not infusion therapy) from a traditional fee-for-service system to prospective payment. This change resulted in multiple acquisitions, mergers, and bankruptcies of home care programs as they tried to stay in business under significant decreases in reimbursement payments and, thus, drastically decreased the total number of home health agencies and home infusion providers in the United States. At its peak in 1997, more than 10,000 Medicare-certified HHAs were in business; however, with the implementation of prospective payment for home care services, the number of HHAs declined to around 7,000 and seems to be remaining steady around this number.[29] As a result of the BBA, 30–40% of the total number of HHAs in the United States closed during the late 1990s alone.[40,41]

Finally, the implementation of Medicare Part D benefits is expected to stimulate another significant increase in the home infusion market beginning in 2006 because reimbursement for home infusion by Medicare will no longer be tied to the use of durable medical equipment, such as an infusion pump.

Drivers of Home Care

The most influential drivers of the HIT market are an aging population and a related increase in chronic disease, technology, and rising costs of health care.[4–6] By 2030, the baby boomers, then aged 66 to 84, will make up 20% of the U.S. population.[42] Decreased usage of traditional inpatient acute care and further reimbursement limitations that promote more cost-effective sites of care are expected to result in continued growth of the home health and home infusion markets.[14,43] Improvement in the innovative designs of infusion pumps and telehealth diagnostic and monitoring equipment will also provide natural areas of expansion for home care.

Although cost savings provided by home care services have not been well-documented in the literature, use of home infusion therapy rather than traditional inpatient care has the potential to result in drastic savings for patients, health systems, and third party payers. For example, while the average hospital stay in 2003 was estimated to cost $1,872 per day for an average of 5.4 days for those aged 45 and above, the cost of an average home health care visit was only $88.[28,44] Home infusion therapies have been reported to save 18% to 75% for IV anti-infective therapies and 60% to 76% for TPN therapies over inpatient costs.[45] In addition, a comparison of estimated inpatient versus home care costs for a single patient over a 9-month period of treatment with an inotropic agent for congestive heart failure resulted in a cumulative savings of $20,500 with the use of home infusion therapy.[46]

Another faculty influencing the growth of the home infusion industry is the number of inpatient pharmacies that are choosing not to provide their own comprehensive IV admixture services. In 2002, 52.4% of hospitals outsourced the preparation of total parenteral nutrition solutions, 16.7% outsourced the preparation of patient-controlled analgesia and epidural analgesia, 15.7% outsourced the preparation of large and small volume IV admixtures, and 9.1% outsourced the preparation of IV heparin and saline to use as flushes.[47] These preparations were most likely outsourced to home infusion pharmacies or organizations that provide central admixture services such as Central Admixture Pharmacy Services (CAPS).

Table 7-2
Historical Development of Home Care Services[5,8,9,19,27,30,33–35]

1796	First recorded home health care services—Boston Dispensary
1850	Visiting nursing services established
1911	Insurance policies began covering home nursing service (Metropolitan Life)
1941	Syracuse University Hospital began offering home care services for its discharged patients, primarily nursing
1947	Montefiore Hospital opens *Hospital without Walls* program
1950s	Polio epidemic in United States resulted in addition of physical and occupational therapy and home care services to traditional nursing services
1965	Medicare legislation establishes reimbursement for limited home services, including home TPN
1973	Medicare coverage of home care services extended to disabled patients of all ages
1978	National Hospice Organization founded
1980s	Advances in high technology infusion devices, growth of the self-care movement, implementation of cost-containment strategies by hospitals and third party payers, growth of the elderly population, increasing numbers of patients with cancer and AIDS
1982	National Association of Home Care founded
1983	Tax Equity and Fiscal Responsibility Reform Act leads to prospective payment and Medicare DRGs for inpatient care
1988	Medicare Catastrophic Coverage Act (PL 100-360) introduced and repealed (allowed for reimbursement of home antibiotic infusions)
1988	Home Care Accreditation Program developed by JCAHO
1990s	Continuing advancement in infusion technology, focus on therapy outcomes and quality improvement in health care, possible changes in infusion reimbursement schedules, continued growth of the AIDS and cancer populations
1991	National Home Infusion Association (NHIA) established by National Community Pharmacists Association (NCPA)
1993	*Pharmacy Only* Home Care Accreditation by JCAHO begins
1994	Section of Home Care Practitioners established by American Society of Health-System Pharmacists (ASHP)
1996	Health Insurance Portability and Accountability Act (HIPPA) passes, requiring protection of electronic patient data and a standardized coding system for home infusion billing
1997	Balanced Budget Act (BBA) authorizes a change in home care reimbursement under Medicare from fee-for-service to a prospective payment system (phased in over 3 years using an interim payment system [IPS])
1998-99	Medicare IPS drastically cuts reimbursement for home care services; approximately 3,000 home health agencies go out of business as a result
1999	Medicare-certified home care providers begin required collecting of OASIS data
1999	Olmstead vs. L.C. affirms patients' right to home health care services under the Americans with Disabilities Act
2000	Medicare prospective payment systems (PPS) begin for home care services
2006	Medicare Prescription Drug, Modernization, and Improvement Act of 2003, Pub.L. No. 108-173 (2003) goes into effect and will for the first time allow the majority of home infusion therapies to be reimbursed under Medicare

AIDS = Acquired Immunodeficiency Syndrome; DRGs = Diagnosis Related Groups; JCAHO = Joint Commission on Accreditation of Healthcare Organizations; OASIS = Outcomes and Assessment Information Set; TPN = Total Parenteral Nutrition

Source: Adapted from Reference 5.

Common Home Infusion Therapies

As mentioned previously, there is no standard population of patients who receive home infusion therapy. However, certain categories of therapies are used more often than others in this setting. The most commonly provided infusion therapies include parenteral and enteral nutrition, anti-infectives, pain management, cardiovascular agents, tocolytics, antineoplastic chemotherapy, biotechnology agents, and related therapies such as antiemetics and hydration fluids with or without electrolyte replacements.[5,6,46,48] Table 7-3 provides an overview of the home infusion market by most commonly dispensed types of therapy.

Table 7-3
United States Home Care Market by Therapy Type 2003[31]

Therapy Type	Percent of Market
Anti-infectives	47.0
Other	28.1
Hydration Fluids	8.2
Pain Management	6.9
Parenteral Nutrition	4.2
Chemotherapy	3.6
Enteral Nutrition	1.2
Biologicals	0.8
TOTAL	100%

Common Practice Settings

Home infusion programs may differ in business structures, depending on the services provided and type of organization.[4,6] Most are licensed as pharmacies and some are also licensed as home nursing agencies; however, other home infusion programs are provided through physician's offices or clinics. The home infusion market is highly competitive with only a few large, national providers and many smaller local and regional providers.[5] Of the approximately 4,000 home infusion sites (sites, not companies) in the United States in 2000, 62.5% were independent companies, 25.0% were hospital-affiliated, and 10.0% were national company sites, including franchise organizations.[4]

As of 2004, there were approximately 1,000 providers of home infusion among all settings; however, only five companies (Apria, Lincare, Option Care, Coram Healthcare, and American Home Patient) still accounted for almost 25% of the total market share.[25,26] The most common organizational structures are discussed in more detail below, including hospital-based programs, corporate programs, community pharmacy-based programs, ambulatory infusion centers, home health agency-based programs, and specialty pharmacies.

Hospital-Based Programs

Hospital-based programs provide additional revenue to their health systems and also help to decrease inpatient costs by allowing an earlier discharge to the home environment.[10,49,50] These programs may either be developed internally within a health system or formed via partnerships with external home infusion providers, such as national corporations or community pharmacies.[6,51,52] Hospital-based home infusion services sometimes employ nurses or work with a home health agency owned by the same health system. However, it is more common for pharmacies to work with external home health agencies to provide patient care via formal contracts or referral agreements with each other.[6]

The number of hospitals providing home care services has fluctuated greatly over time with a high of 40% reported in 1985.[52] Less than 5% of all home infusion providers filling third party claims in 1996 were hospital-based programs; however, in 2001 69% of hospitals reported having pharmacists involved in some type of home care service although the specific nature of the service was not identified.[17,54]

Corporate Systems

The corporate landscape of the home infusion industry has changed dramatically over the last 10–15 years. In 1990, there were 10 large, national players in the market.[10] However, by 1992 eight national infusion providers represented 60% of the market, and by 1995 only five national corporations remained but jointly held just over 50% of the market share.[5,10,20] However, in the same time period, both hospital-based programs and regional or local programs more than doubled, growing from 250 to 530 and from 1,500 to 3,500, respectively.[5]

Community Pharmacy-Based Programs

Little information has been published on community pharmacy-based infusion programs. Despite this lack of documentation, there is evidence that this field has grown considerably since it was reported that 11% of community pharmacies offered such services in 1984.[55]

For example, the average community pharmacy annual sales from infusion therapies was recorded to be $47,000 in 2002.[28] In 2003, 9% of independent community pharmacies reported offering home infusion therapy, 69% offered durable medical goods and 41% participated in hospice programs.[56] At least one national chain pharmacy (Walgreens) has offered home infusion therapy, home respiratory therapy and equipment, and durable medical equipment since 1995 and currently operates accredited home infusion facilities in at least five states.[32,57]

Infusion programs based in community pharmacies are governed by state boards of pharmacy and regulations specific to the states in which patients are served. Some states require special licenses as either parenteral, home health, or home infusion pharmacies. This information changes often, however, so the pharmacist practicing in home infusion therapy should regularly check with the board of pharmacy in all states in which he or she practices. While community pharmacy sometimes employs nurses, it is more common for pharmacies and home health agencies to work together to provide care via formal contracts or referral agreements with each other.[6]

Community pharmacists have a number of options available to them for the provision of infusion services, including independent businesses, partnerships, joint ventures, or contracted relationships with hospitals or other alternative infusion providers, or franchise membership.[4,5,17,58] Several franchise organizations are available to provide support for community pharmacies that wish to provide home infusion services, including Option Care, Inc. (Buffalo Grove, IL) and Vital Care, Inc. (Meridian, MS). These organizations provide services such as personnel training, corporate policies and procedures, and centralized billing in exchange for an initial start-up fee plus a percent of royalties.[6]

Ambulatory Infusion Centers

Ambulatory Infusion Centers (AICs) may be found in physician's offices, hospital emergency rooms or outpatient clinics, cancer centers, infectious disease centers, and sometimes in pharmacies or HHAs.[59] AICs specialize in providing infusion therapy and nursing care to noninstitutionalized, nonhome bound patients in an environment where the cost of care can be minimized while maintaining a high quality of care.[5] This model of care is appropriate for many ambulatory patients who self-administer some or all of their injectable medications but still need blood work, replace-

ment of infusion access devices, or additional education. Patients may also come to an AIC to pick up their home infusion medications and supplies and be counseled by a pharmacist.[5]

Although many AICs are freestanding organizations, they are increasingly becoming a physical component of home infusion providers, often to maintain managed care contracts.[22,60] The AIC model can be more efficient than home care in that more patients can be seen per day by fewer staff members.[59] There may also be a financial benefit to the patient and provider, based on a patient's third party payer. In addition, AICs are often used for the infusion of chemotherapy regimens that are not safe for a patient to receive in the home environment. It is not likely that AICs will replace home care services, but they may be a cost-efficient alternative for some appropriate patients.[18] Because there are special Medicare reimbursement guidelines as well as special licensure and accreditation guidelines for AICs, pharmacists interested in this practice model should seek additional information on these topics.[6] In addition, one should determine any limitations for pharmacist-provided care in an AIC under the state Pharmacy Practice Act.[59]

Hospice

As of 2002, approximately 3,200 hospice programs cared for 885,000 patients annually in the United States and the majority of expenditures (70.2%) were covered by Medicare.[61] Hospice programs provide palliative and supportive care, rather than curative therapies, for patients who are terminally ill.[62] The majority of these programs are freestanding organizations or HHA-based services that send caregivers into patients' homes; however, hospice services may also be based inside physical facilities such as hospitals or skilled nursing facilities where care is provided on site.[62] Hospice services include social, spiritual, and emotional care as well as medical care and allow patients to remain in the comfort of their own home among family members until the time of death.[62] It should be noted that most hospice programs do not accept patients who are receiving parenteral or enteral nutrition, chemotherapy, or anti-infectives, because these are considered to be curative rather than palliative therapies. Many patients, however, do receive pain management therapy, including continuous infusions of morphine or hydromorphone that require preparation and monitoring by a home infusion pharmacist. Practice in the hospice environment is discussed in more detail in Chapter 10.

Home Health Agency-Based Providers

While some HHAs do own an infusion pharmacy and employ pharmacists, as mentioned earlier, most nursing agencies have formal contracts or informal referral agreements with separately owned infusion pharmacies. When more than one organization is caring for a patient (such as an HHA with contracted pharmacy services at a community pharmacy), it is crucial that the pharmacist be involved in all care planning and coordination of care activities.[6]

Specialty Pharmacies

Although the niche market of *specialty pharmacies*, which includes primarily self-injectable, high-cost biotechnology products, is not considered to be traditional home infusion therapy, it does involve the delivery of drug products to patients' homes using a mail-order based business structure.[26] During the 1990s, increased availability of biotechnology agents that were safe for home use led to the development of specialty pharmacies that deal with this specific market niche.[63,64] Examples of such specialty products include blood factors, growth hormone, and Prolastin (alpha 1-proteinase inhibitor) and other drugs used for the treatment of conditions such as Fabry's and Gaucher's disease, multiple sclerosis, and chronic granulomatous disease.[63,65] Appropriate storage and delivery of these biological agents is a challenge because many of them cannot be shaken or must be kept within a narrow temperature range.[64] Some specialty pharmacies solely dispense products while others also provide some limited clinical monitoring by pharmacists as well.[6,64] As of 2004, there were 12 national specialty pharmacy corporations in the United States as well as many local providers.[64] These patient are typically taught to self-inject their medications and do not require home nursing services.

Standards of Practice in Home Infusion Therapy

Published guidelines related to the provision of home infusion therapy are available to assist pharmacists in the development and maintenance of a high quality practice from several national organizations and regulatory agencies. Those standards of practice most relevant to pharmacy practice are summarized in Table 7-4.

Table 7-4
Professional Guidelines and Standards of Practice Related to Home Infusion Practice[66-71]

Publisher	Document and Focus
ASHP	Technical Assistance Bulletin on Quality Assurance of Pharmacy Prepared Sterile Products (1999) (currently being revised)—Standards of practice for quality assurance and quality control related to the compounding of sterile preparations
ASHP	Guidelines on Minimum Standards for Home Care Pharmacies (1999)—Describes standards for practice management as well as clinical management of patients in the home
ASHP	Guidelines on the Pharmacist's Role in Home Care (2000)—Identifies the competencies required of pharmacists practicing in this setting
ASPEN	Standards for Home Nutrition Support (1999)—Addresses the interdisciplinary management of both TPN and enteral therapies in the home by pharmacists, nurses, physicians, and dieticians
ASPEN	Standards for Nutritional Support Pharmacists (2001)—Describes the pharmacist's role in nutritional support therapies administered in the home
AMA	Guidelines for the Medical Management of the Home Care Patient (1997)—Describe the physician's role and responsibility in the home care setting

Compounding Sterile Products for Home Use

Quality assurance is a critical component of the provision of home infusion therapy, and it is the pharmacist's responsibility to prepare and dispense products that are safe for patient use.[71-75] As in other settings that compound sterile preparations, guidelines must be followed closely to assure the integrity, sterility, and correct beyond-use dating of all sterile solutions. In January 2004, new United States Pharmacopeia (USP-NF) <797> guidelines were published outlining specific procedures to follow in the compounding of sterile preparations.[76] These guidelines are enforceable by state boards of pharmacy, the FDA, and accrediting bodies.[77] A major focus of the guidelines is the identification of three risk levels for sterile compounding (low, medium, and high) and the type of clean room facility, polices and procedures, and quality assurance testing that must be in place for compliance at each risk level. These issues are especially important in home infusion practice because many infusions are compounded with the intent that they will be used over days or weeks rather than hours as is typically the case in the inpatient environment. See Chapter 16 for a more detailed look at the requirements imposed on all compounding pharmacies by the new USP standards. Other professional resources available on the sterility and stability of home infusions include Trissell's *Handbook on Injectable Drugs*, King's *The King® Guide to Parenteral Admixtures*, McEvoy's *American Hospital Formulary Service Drug Information*, and Bing's *Extended Stability for Parenteral Drugs*.[78–81]

How Home Care Differs from Other Types of Pharmacy Practice

Home infusion pharmacists have many responsibilities that are not typically provided in other practice settings, including caring for patients 24 hours a day, seven days a week, complying with additional regulatory, legal, and accreditation requirements, managing infusion equipment and vascular access devices, negotiating reimbursement for products and services, and benchmarking clinical outcomes.[31] Some of the major differences between practice in this environment and other pharmacy settings are discussed below, including the primary disease states treated and therapies used, the role of the pharmacist, legal and regulatory requirements, facility requirements, and typical reimbursement policies.

Drug Therapies and Disease States

While the drug therapies that may be given in the home are usually limited only by safety or stability concerns the most commonly used categories include nutritional therapies (total parenteral nutrition (TPN), hydration fluids with or without electrolytes, enteral formulas), anti-infectives, pain management therapies, and chemotherapy.[6,48,82–84] In the past few years biotechnology agents have also developed as a strong and growing presence in the home care market.[5,63] The most common diagnoses of patients receiving home infusion therapy are skin and soft tissues infections, osteomyelitis, septicemia, cancer, fluid or electrolyte disorders, and other miscellaneous infections.[32,83] For example, Table 7-5 presents a summary of patient and therapy characteristics gathered in a study of 815 consecutive patients treated with home antimicrobial

therapy (representing 1,000 parenteral doses in the home).[48] Although limited in number and scope, the literature continues to report that home infusion therapies are safe, efficacious, and cost-effective, and that this is an environment in which pharmacists can use clinical, operational, and managerial skills to provide individualized patient care.[14,30,46,48,82,83]

Table 7-5
Characteristics of Patients Receiving Home Anti-infective Infusions[48]

Characteristic	Value
Age range	<1 to 99 (median range: 40–49)
Average duration of therapy	15.48 days (range: 1–191 days)
Most common diagnoses	19.0% Cellulitis 17.9% Sepsis 15.0% Osteomyelitis
Most common antimicrobial regimens	20.7% Antibiotic combination 18.4% Ceftriaxone 16.8% Vancomycin
Most common infusion system	58.5% Gravity drip 19.9% Syringe (IV push or IM) 13.0% Ambulatory infusion pump
Most common clinical outcomes	89.9% Completed therapy as expected

The Pharmacist's Role in Home Infusion Therapy and Home Care

Although typically less visible to the public than other pharmacy settings, practice in the home infusion setting is a team approach with the goal of providing patient-focused care as a member of an interdisciplinary team and the pharmacist must be available to provide care around the clock.[4,50,85] Therefore, the pharmacist working in home care needs a wide range of skills. Table 7-6 provides a summary of responsibilities of various home care team members, including that of the pharmacist and the pharmacy technician.

Typical job functions of a home care pharmacist include patient assessment and training, preparation and delivery of medications, equipment and supplies, clinical evaluation of prescribed therapies and moni-

Table 7-6
Team Functions[4-6,50]

Team Member	Primary Responsibilities
Physician	Provide prescriptions and orders for care at home; follow patient's progress via communication with rest of team and at clinic visits
Pharmacist	Conduct patient assessment and education, make recommendations for changes in medications based on clinical monitoring (includes review of laboratory values), infusion pump maintenance care plan development, coordination of care with nurses, sterile preparation design, compounding, and delivery to the home, documentation of care and services provided, on call services, communication with patient and physician on regular basis
Nurse	Conduct patient assessment and education, train patient to administer therapy, clinical monitoring, care plan development, coordination of care with pharmacist and physician, documentation of care and services provided, on call services
Patient/Caregiver	Learn to infuse solutions independently in the home; understand signs and symptoms of complications and who to call for assistance with problems

toring for desired outcomes, and supervision of technicians and other personnel.[4,6,8,50,86] In some practices the pharmacist may also take an active role in the marketing of the service including working closely or with referral sources, making sales calls to physician's offices and providing educational materials or presentations to other health care professionals.[6]

While most home care programs do not have a physician on staff, medical orders from each patient's attending physician are required for services to be provided in the home. Other team members, primarily nurses and pharmacists, are responsible for coordinating and providing direct patient care, monitoring the patient for improvement, and reporting outcomes back to the physician.[4,6] Clinical services are usually provided from a team of health care providers including pharmacists, technicians, service representatives, skilled nurses, licensed practical nurses, and respiratory therapists, who often work independently of each other but in a coordinated fashion.

The pharmacist in a home infusion pharmacy is responsible for working with nurses, physicians, and

patients in the areas of care coordination, care planning, education, and the provision and clinical monitoring of injectable medications.[4,6,87] Some infusion pharmacies also dispense oral medications; however, even if they do not supply such medications to their patients, home care pharmacists typically monitor oral therapies as well. Such monitoring can range from simply reviewing the current medication profile for interactions to evaluating the outcomes of therapy. In addition, pharmacists working in home infusion provide on call services 24 hours a day.[4,6,87]

The pharmacist has an especially important role in the evaluation and acceptance of new patient referrals. The patient medical history and current data, including reimbursement options, must be carefully reviewed in order to determine whether or not he or she is an appropriate candidate for home infusion therapy. In addition, the pharmacist must review the physician's orders for the prescribed therapy as well as the entire medication profile and confirm that the medication, schedule, route of administration, vascular access device, and infusion device are all appropriate for the patient and his or her diagnosis.[6] The pharmacist must also determine that the patient and caregiver are willing to receive the therapy, can be taught to administer the infusion (if necessary), and that the home environment is safe and appropriate for the care that is needed.[6] Some considerations for the home environment include the presence of electricity, running water, and telephone service and access to emergency or 911 services.

Some pharmacists also visit the homes of patients who are enrolled in home health nursing services but who are not prescribed parenteral therapies. In this situation, the pharmacist's role is to evaluate the appropriateness of drug therapy, take medication histories, assist patients in improving compliance and preventing drug-related problems, and simplify therapy.[39,88-90] Although neither Medicare nor Medicaid currently provides reimbursement for pharmacist interventions that are unrelated to dispensing, there is a role for the pharmacist in HHA.[39,89] Many VA hospitals offer opportunities for pharmacists to participate in such a service, which they call Hospital-Based Primary Care.[4]

Pharmacy technicians in the home care setting are primarily responsible for compounding intravenous medications and may also be involved in scheduling mixing, monitoring patient supply needs, coordinating deliveries, and billing.[4,86,91] However, technicians have additional responsibilities such as assistance with patient education, laboratory value monitoring, maintaining infusion devices for home use, quality control activities, and discharge planning.[91] Medications are typically delivered to the patient's home by a staff member or by a common courier such as Federal Express or United Parcel Service. In addition to pharmacists, pharmacy technicians and delivery drivers working in home infusion may sometimes provide on call services.[4]

Law and Regulation

As with other health care settings, numerous laws and regulations guide the practice of home infusion pharmacy. A summary of the major national regulations affecting practice are listed in Table 7-7. In addition to federal guidelines, home infusion practice is also regulated differently by the Board of Pharmacy in each state. For example, while many infusion pharmacies are licensed under traditional community pharmacy guidelines, as of 1999 almost 60% of states had pharmacy practice acts that specifically addressed home infusion pharmacy practice, but less than 10 states had special licensure requirements for home infusion pharmacies. Pharmacists practicing in home infusion should regularly check with their Board of Pharmacy for updated requirements, both for the state(s) in which the pharmacy is licensed and the state(s) in which their patients actually reside.[4]

The legality of faxing orders for controlled substances in schedule II (CII) is of particular concern because many infusion pharmacies dispense a large volume of injectable controlled substances. State laws vary considerably regarding the ability to accept a faxed copy of a CII prescription and whether or not a hard copy of the prescription with an original signature must be obtained and kept on file.[4,52] Pharmacists practicing in home infusion need to research this issue for the state(s) in which they are licensed as well as for all states in which the HIT pharmacy services home infusion patients.[4]

Home infusion pharmacists also need to understand how the Health Insurance Portability and Accountability Act of 1996 (HIPAA) affects their practice. In addition to requirements for confidentiality and security of electronic patient records, HIPAA guidelines also require home infusion providers to adopt a single standard coding system for the electronic submission of insurance claims in which all medications provided to patients can be identified by a specific National Drug Code (NDC) number.[4]

Table 7-7
Regulatory Factors Affecting HIT Practice[6,93–101]

Related to Sterile Product Preparation
- State-specific board of pharmacy regulations
- United States Pharmacopeia-National Formulary (USP-NF) Chapters <797>

Related to Infection Control and Safety
- United States Occupational Safety and Health Administration (OSHA) requirements related to hazardous substances, prevention of blood borne pathogrens, preventions and reporting of needle stick injuries
- United States Centers for Disease Control (CDC) Guidelines for the Prevention of Intravascular Catheter-Related Infections related to frequency of IV tubing changes and catheter flushing protocols

Related to Drug Control and Safety
- United States Drug Enforcement Administration (DEA) licensure and policies
- Health Insurance Portability and Accountability Act of 1996 (HIPAA) requirements for patient confidentiality, privacy and security

Related to Reimbursement
- Medicare and Medicaid rules and regulations for providing care and submitting claims
- Health Insurance Portability and Accountability Act (HIPAA) requirements for standardized electronic claiming procedures
- False Claims Act requirements to prevent fraud and abuse (Medicare only)
- Federal Antifraud and Abuse Laws (Anti-Kickback Laws) requirements to prevent illegal remuneration (Medicare)
- Stark Legislation requirements to prevent physician self-referrals to home care (Medicare)

Accreditation Requirements

Along with reimbursement trends, pharmacy accreditation has played an important role in shaping the home infusion market.[6] While accreditation is currently voluntary, it is required by a number of insurance providers in order to gain contracts, is required by the federal government for health systems that receive federal funding under Medicare, and will be required for home infusion providers under Medicare Part D benefits.[6,102]

Three accrediting bodies are currently available for providers of home infusions, including the Accreditation Commission for Health Care (ACHC) (Raleigh,

NC), the Community Health Accreditation Program (CHAP) (New York, NY), and the Joint Commission on Accreditation of Healthcare Organizations (JCAHO) (Oakbrook Terrace, IL) (see Table 7-8).[4,6] Each of these three programs is based on standards of practice and requires a site inspection by trained surveyors from the accrediting organization. Although accreditation is a voluntary process, some third party payers do require that a home care provider to be accredited in order to receive reimbursement or preferred provider contracts.[4,6]

Table 7-8

Comparison of Accrediting Bodies for Home Infusion Providers[103–105]

Organization	Services Eligible for Accreditation
ACHC (Raleigh, NC)	Home infusion pharmacies, HME services, hospice programs, pharmacy disease state management, specialty pharmacies select ambulatory services
CHAP (New York, NY)	Home health nursing, hospice, home infusion pharmacies, public health nursing, community nursing centers, physical therapy, speech therapy, occupational therapy, nutritional counseling, respiratory therapy, social work, homemakers, home health aides, hospice, management services, home medical equipment, infusion nursing
JCAHO (Oakbrook Terrace, IL)	Home infusion programs based in all settings, hospitals, ambulatory care clinics, clinical laboratories, home health nursing, home respirtory therapy, durable medical equipment

ACHC = Accreditation Commission for Home Care; CHAP = Community Health Accreditation Program; JCAHO = Joint Commission on Accreditation of Healthcare Organizations; DME = Durable Medical Equipment.

Some accreditation programs require that home care organizations participate in external benchmarking of clinical outcomes of care such as number of medication errors, vascular access device infections, or unplanned hospital readmission. In general, home infusion providers have demonstrated excellent outcomes, with one national benchmarking organization reporting that in over 4.3 million days of home infusion therapy since 1999, less than 1% of the patients have experienced vascular access device infections, medication errors, or unplanned hospitalizations sec-

ondary to complications of infusion therapy, and less than 2% have experienced adverse drug reactions related to infusion therapy.[31]

Physical Facilities

Regardless of the setting of a home infusion practice (hospital-based, community-pharmacy based, etc.), certain physical facilities are needed that are different from that of most other types of pharmacies. Under USP 797, a clean room with positive pressure air flow and an anteroom are required in addition to horizontal and vertical laminar flow hoods.[76] In addition, space is needed for each of the following: a business office for reimbursement activities and billing; an area for pharmacy staff to review charts and call patients; a temperature controlled warehouse area to store drugs, medical supplies, parenteral and enteral solutions, and DME; a staging area to stage products and equipment for delivery; a *dirty* area for receiving and cleaning DME that has been in the home; an area for equipment maintenance; and an area for the storage of hazardous waste.

Reimbursement

Changes in reimbursement patterns have had the greatest effect on the growth of the home infusion industry, and they will continue to shape this market in the future.[4,5] Reimbursement for home infusion therapies varies by third party payer as well as by geographic region. While most private commercial insurance companies do provide benefits for this type of care, Medicare and Medicaid currently only provide limited reimbursement. Tables 7-9 and 7-10 provide a summary of the current general benefits provided for home care by Medicare, Medicaid, and most commercial insurance plans for home care.

It is common for HIT to be reimbursed at a *per diem* or single daily rate rather than by each individual item.[4,6] In this system, payment rates per day of therapy are negotiated with the insurance provider, either by therapy type or for specific patients. In 2002, the Centers for Medicare and Medicaid Services (CMS) introduced an extensive set of standardized per diem codes as part of the Healthcare Common Procedure Coding System (HCPCS codes), which is now used to process HIT reimbursement claims by most providers and is also expected to be used by Medicare Part D beginning in 2006.[97]

It is important to note that Medicare is the largest single payer for home care services (other than patients). In 2002, 28.1% of all home care services

Table 7-9
CMS Guidelines for Home Health Care Reimbursement under Medicare[106]

Home care services must do the following:

- Require skilled nursing services (i.e., no custodial care or homemaker services)

- Be intermittent in nature (i.e., no daily care)

- Be deemed medically necessary by physician

- Be performed according to a physician's treatment plan, which must be reviewed by the physician at least every 60 days

- Be provided with the expectation that the patient will have defined endpoints of care (i.e., no care for patients with chronic diseases)

- Be provided only to homebound patients

were paid for out-of-pocket by patients while Medicare paid for 26%, private insurance paid for 18.9%, state and local governments paid for 12.3%, and Medicaid paid for 9.3%.[22,23] Under the Medicare Prescription Drug Improvement and Modernization Act of 2003 (MMA), Part D benefits will begin to cover numerous outpatient infusion therapies in January, 2006.[102] Because the new Part D coverage for prescription drugs is not linked to a requirement for DME (as is currently the case under Medicare Part B), more

options for home therapies will be available to patients. However, pharmacists have some concerns about the new Part D benefits regarding home infusion therapy. Some practitioners are concerned that the patient requirement to make a copayment on home infusion therapies will be cost-prohibitive for many because of the overall expense of these types of therapies, and, thus, continue to limit the utilization of home infusion therapy under Medicare.[25] Other concerns for home infusion pharmacists include how per diem rates will be determined, requirements for accreditation, changes in claims formatting and coding, introduction of formulary limitations, revisions to average wholesale price (AWP), requirements for competitive bidding for infusion drugs and equipment, restricted reimbursement for blood clotting factors, and increased competition with outpatient clinics resulting from improved physician reimbursement for administration of injectable chemotherapy.[31,108] Pharmacists working in the home care environment should continue to monitor Medicare Part D reimbursement policies in the future.

Preparation for a Career in Home Care

Education and Training

In addition to a pharmacy degree, a pharmacist seeking a job in home infusion therapy typically needs to complete a residency, complete specialized training, or

Table 7-10
Comparison of Current Reimbursement for Home Infusion Therapy by Third Party Payers[4,31,106,107]

Third Party	General Benefit	Special Requirements
Medicare	Under Part B (prosthetic device benefit): 80% of allowable charges but varies by therapy; therapy must require use of durable medical equipment (eg, infusion pump)	Medicare provider number Patient must be *homebound* Therapy must be *medically necessary*
Medicaid	Varies by state	Usually, only drug covered (no supplies, IV fluids, or equipment) and prior authorization is required; nutritional therapies are not covered in all states
Private	Usually, 80–100% once annual deductibles are met	May require use of preferred provider networks or require that HHA be provided by a specific organization; clinical case management may be required

have a minimum of 3 years of practice experience in a home infusion or hospital or ambulatory infusion setting.[4] Those students interested in pursuing a residency should contact ASHP and the American College of Clinical Pharmacy (ACCP) for additional information about home care residencies and talk with faculty members at their school or college of pharmacy to identify other nonaccredited residency programs. Many professional organizations provide ongoing continuing education related to home care (Table 7-11) and National Home Infusion Association (NHIA) also offers a specialized certificate training program in home infusion therapy.[6,109–116]

Table 7-11

National Organizations Providing Education about Home Infusion Therapy

- American Society of Health-System Pharmacy (ASHP) Section of Home, Ambulatory and Chronic Care Practitioners

- National Home Infusion Association (NHIA)

- American Society for Parenteral and Enteral Nutrition (ASPEN)

- National Association for Home Care (NAHC)

- Intravenous Nursing Society (INS)

Competencies Required for Home Infusion Practice

Pharmacists who choose to practice in the home infusion setting need a broad range of competencies that may not be required for all of those who practice in other environments. According to a task analysis, most HIT pharmacists must demonstrate distributive skills (78%), clinical skills (67%), administrative skills (59%), and operational skills (42%).[115] Figure 7-1 summarizes the patient care process in HIT from the time of referral until discharge. The pharmacist's role in the initial patient assessment is particularly important as it has been reported that up to 49% of the patients referred for home care are rejected because of psychological, physical, medical, or financial reasons.[32,116]

After a patient has been accepted for home infusion therapy, the home care pharmacist develops a comprehensive plan of care that focuses on the patient's specific needs and desired outcomes of therapy. It should be noted that laboratory tests are rarely done more than once or twice a week (if a patient requires more acute monitoring than this, he or she is probably not a good candidate for home care). The home care phar-

macist also plays a crucial role in the patient's multidisciplinary care team by actively participating in patient assessment, education and monitoring activities, and coordinating communication and service provision.[4,117]

The pharmacist's most important role is related to the provision and monitoring of drug therapy; therefore, the ability to select the most appropriate infusion device, medication formulation, and monitoring criteria is extremely important. A thorough knowledge of sterile product preparation, including sterility, stability, and compatibility issues, is required.[4,6,117] Successful HIT practice also includes the ability to manage operational issues such as inventory, hazardous waste, and delivery of goods to the patient's residence 24 hours a day, 7 days a week.[4,117] Skills in human resources management, financial management, and quality improvement processes are also crucial.[4,6,117]

Knowledge of Vascular Access and Infusion Devices

Pharmacists practicing in home infusion must also be familiar with infusion devices and venous access devices (VADs), as well as their specific uses. The most commonly used infusion delivery systems are summarized in Table 7-12. Electronic infusion pumps allow for the accurate infusion via positive pressure at various rates.[118] Many allow programming of the pump to infuse either intermittent, continuous, or keep-vein-open rate or patient controlled analgesia. These devices may also accommodate the infusion of multiple infusions at the same time at independent rates. Gravity drip systems are designed for use with nonviscous fluids whose infusion rate does not require precise control.[118] The drug prescribed and the duration, osmolarity, and pH and solution must all be considered by the pharmacist when recommending the most appropriate device to other members of the home infusion team.[119] The most commonly used VADs are described in Table 7-13, including the types of intravenous solutions that are recommended for use.

Future Trends

While the home health care industry will continue to be influenced by many factors, the most significant are likely to be changes in reimbursement and advancements in technology such as improved infusion devices and telemedicine and telepharmacy.[4,6,27,120] Examples of telemedicine include monitoring patients with cardiac disease via the telephone by assessing blood pressure or edema or educating patients about changes in

Figure 7-1
Patient Care Process in Home Infusion Therapy

Source: Reprinted with permission from Reference 4.

PATIENT CARE PROCESS IN HOME INFUSION (SOURCE)

Collect and document patient data

Demographics	Type of infusion therapy
Reimbursement	Patient willingness
Venous access device	Diagnosis
Equipment needs	Other care providers
Prescriber information	Home environment

Evaluate data against admission criteria

Appropriate drug?	Appropriate home environment?
Patient agreeable?	Care givers available?
Adequate reimbursement?	All criteria has been met?

Conduct and document initial patient assessment
Medication history and current use
Nutritional and pain level screening
Functional, physical, psychosocial assessment
Verify treatment orders with physician

Develop pharmaceutical care plan

Identify potential problems:

Drug-related	Environment-related
Equipment-related	Patient-related
Disease-related	Reimbursement-related
Delivery-related	Begin discharge planning

Establish desired outcomes of care:

Therapeutic goals	Functional goals
Educational goals	Psychosocial goals

Determine needed pharmaceutical interventions:

Services and products	Equipment and supplies
Laboratory work	Clinical monitoring
Patient education	Community resources

Communicate recommendations to:

Physician	Patient
Nurses	Other care providers

Implement care plan

Evaluate pharmaceutical response to infusion therapy

Lab work	Therapeutic response
Compliance	Signs and symptoms of disease
Patient satisfaction	Drug delivery system
Psychosocial response	Functional response

Revise care plan as necessary

Identify new goals	Identify new interventions
Adjust treatment orders	Provide additional education

Communicate changes to:

Physician	Patient
Nurses	Other care providers

Document information in patient record

Discharge patient

Determine if goals were met	Complete discharge summary
Notify physician, others	Pick up and maintain equipment

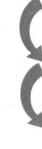

Table 7-12
Commonly Used Infusion Delivery Systems in Home Infusion Therapy[4,31]

Delivery System	Percent of Market
Electronic ambulatory pump	28.9
Gravity flow device (Controllers)	27.8
IV Push	15.7
Electronic stationary pump	15.3
Other Mechanical Device[a]	7.8
Other System	4.5
Total	100%

IV = intravenous

[a] Other mechanical device; includes implantable pumps and syringe pumps.

prescribed medications and providing counseling interventions when needed.[121] Examples of telepharmacy include the use of personal digital assistants, laptop computers, and the Internet to provide information and counseling to patients at a distance.[120]

Table 7-14 contains a summary of the factors that are expected to influence the home health care market in the future. However, as mentioned earlier, the availability of reimbursement for home health and home infusion services is the major limitation on the growth of this market. So, while telemedicine is expected to provide new oportunities for linking patients at home with health care professionals, these devices are not currently reimbursed by CMS (equipment may only be reimbursed if it is *durable* and if it is primarily used to treat, rather that prevent, disease or complications), which may limit the use of these innovative products among elderly patients.[122]

Table 7-13
Overview of Vascular Access Devices Used in Home Infusion Therapy[4,31,119]

Type of Device	Placement	Primary Use
Peripheral ($\frac{1}{2}$" to 3")	Forearm or hand with catheter tip located in a peripheral vein	Short-term therapy of 5 days or less with an isotonic, nonirritating and nonvesicant solution
Midline (>3")	Antecubital fossa with catheter tip located in the cephalic or basilica vein inferior to the shoulder	Short-term therapy of 5 days to 4 weeks of an isotonic solution not over 500 mOsm and with a pH of 5–9
PICC	Basilic or cephalic vein with catheter tip located in the superior or inferior vena cava	Any type of medium-term therapy lasting 11–12 weeks
Nontunneled Subclavian	Subclavian or internal jugular vein with catheter tip located in the superior vena cava	Any time of acute therapy lasting 2 weeks or less
Tunneled	Surgically inserted into the external jugular vein, the cephalic vein at the delto-pectoral groove, or the axillary-subclavian vein with catheter tip positioned at the junction of the superior vena cava and right atrium and the catheter exit site on the chest wall	Long-term continuous or intermittent therapy requiring 12 weeks to years
Implantable Port	Surgically placed subcutaneously in chest wall with catheter tip located in the subclavian vein or superior vena cava; device is accessed by placing a special needle with a 90° bend (a *right-angle* needle) through the skin and into the permeable membrane of the port below	Long-term intermittent therapy requiring 12 or more weeks

PICC = Peripherally inserted central catheter.

Table 7-14

Factors Expected to Influence Future Growth of the Home Infusion Market[4–6,13,112,120]

- Continued changes in reimbursement policies, especially, Medicare Part D

- Expansion of services to include nonhome bound patients

- Decrease in home chemotherapy and some home injectables because of Medicare Part D reimbursement that will increase payment to physician's for these services

- Increased use of telehealth and telepharmacy, including use of electronic records, video patient conferencing, web services, Internet services

- Increased infusion services provided to patients in long-term nursing facilities

- Increased use of home infusion to prevent hospitalization all together

Summary

Changing patterns of reimbursement and an aging U.S. population with an increased incidence of chronic disease have increased the need for the provision of both acute and chronic medical care in a patient's place of residence.[4–6] Despite slowed growth of the home care market in the last 10 years and declining reimbursements under managed care, the infusion industry will continue to be a strong market for years to come.[5] Pharmacy practice in home infusion therapy offers a unique practice environment for those who are interested in providing individualized care, including preparing and monitoring sterile preparations, to those patients who receive such therapy in their places of residence.

References

1. American Society of Health-System Pharmacist. ASHP guidelines on the pharmacist's role in home care. *Am J Hosp Pharm.* 1993;50:1940–4.

2. Lucarelli CD, Miller RJ. The pharmacist's role in the expanding home health care system. *NY St J Pharm.* 1986;6(3):7175.

3. McAllister JC. Home health care and the hospital pharmacist. *Am J Hosp Pharm.* 1985;42(11):2518–20.

4. Monk-Tutor MR, Powers T. Home Care. In: *Pharmacotherapy Self-Assessment Program. Book 2: Systems of Care. Sites of Care.* 4th ed. Kansas City, MO: American College of Clinical Pharmacy; 2000:257–75.

5. Monk-Tutor MR. The U.S. home infusion market. *Am J Health-Syst Pharm.* 1998;55:2019–25.

6. Flores K, Wilder G. *Module 1: Introduction to Home Infusion Practice.* Alexandria, VA: National Home Infusion Association; 2003.

7. Nutt RE. Carving a niche in intravenous therapy services. *Consult Pharm.* 1987;2(2):103–16.

8. Pierpaoli PG, McAllister JC. The evolution of home health care in hospital pharmacy. In: McAllister JC, ed. *A Hospital Pharmacist's Guide to Home Health Care.* Bethesda, MD: ASHP; 1986:2–9.

9. Warhola CF. *Planning for Home Health Services: A Resource Handbook.* Washington, DC: U.S. Bureau of Health Planning, U.S. Department of Commerce, National Technical Information Service (HPR-0102001); 1980:8–9.

10. Winters RW, Conners, RB. The future of the home infusion industry. In: Winters RW, Conners RB, eds. *Home Infusion Therapy: Current Status and Future Trends.* Chicago, IL: AHA Publishing, Inc.; 1995:247–58.

11. Zilz DA. Current trends in home health care. *Am J Hosp Pharm.* 1985;42:2520–5.

12. Bernstein LH. Epstein D. The long-term care invasion. *Infusion.* 1997;3(6):35–9.

13. Bernstein LH. Nursing facilities: the next frontier for IV providers. *Infusion.* 1995;1(10):52–4.

14. Triller DM, Hamilton RA, Briceland LL, et al. Home care pharmacy: extending clinical pharmacy services beyond infusion therapy. *Am J Health-Syst Pharm.* 2000;57:1326–31.

15. Cherney A. Alternative delivery sites: where does home health care fit? *Home Health Care Manage Prac.* 1997;10(1):1–9.

16. Boesch D. The changing home infusion market: staying ahead of the game. *Infusion.* 1994;1(1):12–5.

17. Henke C. IV therapy: home care's fastest growth market. *Homecare.* (Infusion supplement.) 1990;3:6–8.

18. Kaplan LK. The infusion therapy market: today and tomorrow. *Infusion.* 1996;2(10):18–24.

19. Monk-Tutor MR. Factors influencing the diffusion of a health care innovation: adoption of home infusion therapy services by community pharmacists (dissertation). Oxford, MS: University of Mississippi; 1993.

20. Report provides profile of home infusion services, patients. *Am J Hosp Pharm.* 1993; 50:846–9.

21. Holland R, Nimmo CM. Transitions. Part 1: beyond pharmaceutical care. *Am J Health-Syst Pharm.* 1999;56:1758–64.

22. National Association for Home Care. Basic statistics about home care 2001. Available at: http://www.nahc.org/Consumer/hcstats.html. Accessed November 1, 2004.

23. Rosenau PV, Linder SH. The comparative performance of for-profit and nonprofit home health care services in the U.S. *Home Health Care Services Quarterly.* 2001;20(2):47–59.

24. Centers for Medicare and Medicaid Services, Office of the Actuary. Exhibit 5: out-of-pocket expenditures, per capita amounts, and distribution by service, selected calendar years 1993–2013. 2001. Available at: http://content.healthaffairs.org/content/vol0/issue2004/images/data/hlthaff.w4.79v1/DC1/Hef. Accessed August 2, 2004.

25. Centers for Medicare and Medicaid Services. Health care industry market update, 9/22/03. Available at: http://www.cms.gov. Accessed September 12, 2004.

26. Ewing Bemiss & Co Healthcare Group. Home health-care leader, March 2004. Available at: http://www.ewingbemiss.com/new/Home%20IV%20mailer.pdf. Accessed October 8, 2004.

27. IMS. Home health care in the USA. Available at: http://www.ikms-global.com//insight/news_story/0008/news_story_000811.htm. Accessed September 20, 2004.

28. Wertheimer AI, Chaney NM, Popomaronis WT. Increasing profits, improving care. *America's Pharmacist.* 2004;August:13–6.

29. MEDPAC. Home health services: assessing payment adequacy and updating payments. In: *Home Health Services Report to the Congress: Medicare Payment Policy Home health services Section 3D.* Available at: http://www.medpac.gov/publications/congressional_reports/Mar03_Entire_report.pdf. Accessed October 8, 2004:142.

30. Triller DM, Clause SL, Domarew C. Analysis of medication management activities for home-dwelling patients. *Am J Health-Syst Pharm.* 2002;59:2356–9.

31. Kaplan LK. Comments on CMS-4068-P, proposed rule for the Medicare prescription drug benefit. October 4, 2004. Available at: http://www.nhianet.org/members/nhia_part_d_comments.pdf. Accessed November 1, 2004.

32. Walgreens. Scope of services. Available at: http://www.walgreenshealth.com/whc/hcare/jsp/hc_professionals_scopre_svcs.jsp. Accessed November 4, 2004.

33. Gerson CK. The team approach to home health care. *Am Pharm.* 1978;NS18(11):37–40.

34. Jackson BN. Home health care and the elderly in the 1980s. *Am J Occ Ther.* 1984;8(11):717–20.

35. Koren MJ. Home care—who cares? *New Eng J Med.* 1986;314(14):917–20.

36. Spivak D, Keith K. Joint ventures in home health care. In: Fisher K, Gardner K, eds. *Quality and Home Health Care: Redefining the Tradition.* Chicago, IL: JCAHO; 1987:124–7.

37. Balinsky W. Home care prescription drug reimbursement: a case for intravenous antibiotics. Nutley, NJ: Hoffman-LaRoche Inc.; 1986.

38. Kasmer RJ, Hoisington LM, Yukniewicz S. Home parenteral antibiotic therapy, Part I: an overview of program design. *Home Healthc Nurs.*1987;5(1)12–8.

39. Klotz RS. Past, present, and future of home infusion services in the United States. *Cal J Health-Syst Pharm.* 1997:23–6.

40. Levin Associates. Home health care: on the road back to profits and growth. Available at: www.levinassociates.com/publications/jenks/jenksheadlines/01%20henkshead/03jenksh. Accessed September 20, 2004.

41. Levit K, Cowan C, Braden B, et al. National health expenditures in 1997: more slow growth. *Health Affairs.* 1998;17(6):99–110.

42. Walker G. The market is out there. *Homecare.* April 1, 2004. Available at: http://homecaremag.com/mag/medical_market/index.html. Accessed September 2, 2004.

43. Schaeffer C, House K. The big boom industry. *Infusion.* 1996;2(12):21–31.

44. DeFrances CJ, Hall MJ. 2002 *National Hospital Discharge Survey. Advance Data No. 342.* U.S. Department of Health and Human Services Centers for disease Control and Prevention, National Center for Health Statistics: May 21, 2004.

45. Thickson ND. Economics of home intravenous services. *PharmacoEconomics.* 1993;3(3):220–7.

46. Ryan LM. Homecare therapy: a cost-effective alternative approach to the management of advanced heart failure. *Am J Man Care.* 1996;2(10):1351–5.

47. Pederson CA, Schneider PJ, Scheckelhoff DJ. ASHP national survey of pharmacy practice in hospital settings: dispensing and administration—2002. *Am J Health-Syst Pharm.* 2003;60:52–68.

48. Britton K, Powers T, Gordon A. Home antimicrobial therapy: a study of demographics and clinical outcomes. *Infusion.* 1997;3(8):28–33.

49. Cerne F. The fading stand-alone hospital. *Hospital & Health Networks.* 1994;(Jun 20):27–33.

50. Engert EB, Emery DW. Integrated delivery systems: non fait accompli. *Managed Care Quarterly.* 1999;7(1):29–38.

51. McAllister JC. Evaluating alternatives for providing home health-care services. *Am J Hosp Pharm.* 1985;2:2533–9.

52. McAllister JC. Home health care services: collaboration alternatives, vendor selection and program implementation. *Topics in Hospital Pharmacy Management.* 1984;11:56–71.

53. Stolar MH. ASHP national survey of hospital pharmaceutical services—1985. *Am J Hosp Pharm.* 1985;42:2667–78.

54. Knapp KK, Blalock SJ, Black BL. ASHP survey of ambulatory care responsibilities of pharmacist in managed care and integrated health systems—2001. *Am J Health-Syst Pharm.* 2001;58:2151–66.

55. Chi J. Home health care: how sweet it can be. *Drug Top.* 1984;April 2:23–36.

56. National Community Pharmacy Association. *NCPA-Pfizer Digest 2003.* Alexandria, VA: NCPA; 2003.

57. Walgreens. Home care services. Available at: http://www.walgreenshealth.com/whc/hcare/jsp/hc_home.jsp. Accessed November 4, 2004.

58. U.S. Congress, Office of Technology Assessment. *Home Drug Infusion Therapy under Medicare.* OTA-H-509. Washington, DC: U.S. Government Printing Office; May 1992.

59. Home infusion vs. ambulatory infusion centers. *Homecare.* April 1, 1999. Available at: http://home-caremag.com/mag/medical_home_infusion_vs/index.html. Accessed October 27, 2004.

60. Schleis TG. Ambulatory infusion centers: opportunities for the future. Presented at: ASHP Midyear Clinical Meeting. 1995;30(Dec):PI–52.

61. NHPCO. National hospice and palliative care organization facts and figures. February 2004. Available at: http://www.nhpco.org/facts. Accessed November 1, 2004.

62. NAHC. Hospice facts and statistics. November 2002. Available at: http://www.nahc.org/Consumer/hpcstats.html. Accessed November 1, 2004.

63. Lima HA. Looking down the pipeline: a biotech market update. *Infusion.* 2000:7(1):14–9.

64. National specialty pharmacies focus on rare, chronic diseases. *Am J Health-Syst Pharm.* 2004;61:133. News.

65. National Home Infusion Association. Bayer direct: new distribution program creates unanswered questions. *Infusion.* 1999;6(3):16–21.

66. American Society of Health-System Pharmacists. ASHP guidelines on minimum standards for home care pharmacies. *Am J Health-Syst Pharm.* 1999;56:629–38.

67. American Society of Health-System Pharmacists. ASHP guidelines on quality assurance for pharmacy-prepared sterile products. *Am J Health-Syst Pharm.* 2000;57:1150–69.

68. American Society for Parenteral and Enteral Nutrition. Standards for home nutrition support 1999. Available at: http://www.nutritioncare.org/membersonly/index.asp. Accessed November 5, 2004.

69. American Society for Parenteral and Enteral Nutrition. Standards of practice for nutrition support pharmacists 2001. Available at: http://www.nutritioncare.org/membersonly/index.asp. Accessed November 5, 2004.

70. American Medical Association. Guidelines for the medical management of the home care patient. Chicago, IL: AMA Press; 1997.

71. Kastango ES, Bradshaw BD. USP chapter 797: establishing a practice standard for compounding sterile preparations in pharmacy. *Am J Health-Syst Pharm.* 2004;61:1928–38.

72. O'Neal BC, Schneider PJ, Pedersed CA, et al. Compliance with safe practices for preparing parenteral nutrition formulations. *Am J Health-Syst Pharm.* 2002;59(3):264–9.

73. A primer on USP chapter 797. *Int J Pharm Compound.* 2004;8(4);251–63.

74. Kastango ES. ASHP discussion guide for compounding sterile preparations 2004. Available at: http://ashp.org/SterileCpd/797guide.pdf. Accessed June 7, 2004.

75. Morris AM, Schneider PJ, Pedersen CA, et al. National survey of quality assurance activities for pharmacy-compounded sterile preparations. *Am J Health-Syst Pharm.* 2003;60:2567–76.

76. United States Pharmacopoeia-National Formulary (USP-NF). Sterile drug products for home use. USP 24-NF 19, Chapter <797>. 1999:2130–69.

77. USP publishes enforceable chapter on sterile compounding. *Am J Health-Syst Pharm.* 2003;1814–7. News.

78. Trissell LA. *Handbook on Injectable Drugs.* 11th ed. Bethesda, MD: ASHP; 2001.

79. King JC, Catania PN. *The King® Guide to Parenteral Admixtures.* Napa, CA: King Guide Publications, Inc.; 2003.

80. McEvoy, GK, ed. *American Hospital Formulary System Drug Information.* Bethesda, MD: ASHP; 2004.

81. Bing CM. *Extended Stability for Parenteral Drugs.* Bethesda, MD: ASHP; 2001.

82. Pait EP, Pallesen BJ. Fundamental consideration in home chemotherapy administration. *Infusion.* 1996;2(12):24–34.

83. Barnadas G. Navigating home care: enteral nutrition—part 1. *Pract Gastroenterology.* 2003;(Oct):13–35.

84. Tice AD, Schleis TG, Nolet B, et al. U.S. outcomes registry for outpatient IV antimicrobial therapy. *Infusion.* 2000;6(7):27–35.

85. Cox K. Home care is the answer. *Homecare.* October 1, 2004.

86. Johnson K. Identifying and calculating activity-based pharmacy costs. *Infusion.* 1998;(Mar):15–21.

87. Monk-Tutor MR. Home care practice as a model for providing pharmaceutical care. *Am J Health-Syst Pharm.* 1998;55:486–90.

88. Schrecengost-Kibbey MA. Impact of pharmacist home visits on drug therapy. *Am J Health-Syst Pharm.* 2002;59:1293–4.

89. Triller DM, Clause SL, Briceland LL, et al. Resolution of drug-related problems in home care patients through a pharmacy referral service. *Am J Health-Syst Pharm.* 2003;60:905–10.

90. Audette CM, Triller DM, Hamilton R, et al. Classifying drug-related problems in home care. *Am J Health-Syst Pharm.* 2002;59:2407–9.

91. Henderson D, Hohnson-Choong S, Wiles S. Pharmacy technician's role in an ambulatory care infusion clinic. *Am J Health-Syst Pharm.* 2000;57(Sept 15):1664–5.

92. Franklin DM. Compliance defined. *Infusion.* 2003 Mar/Apr;9(2):43–6.

93. Weber P. Electronic claims under HIPAA. *Infusion.* 2003 Jul/Aug;9(4):16–20.

94. Berliner, Marie C .Legal issues in managed care contracting: home health care in the1990s. *Home Health Care Manage Prac.* 1997;9(2):22–8.

95. U.S. Department of Labor Occupational Safety and Health Administration. Occupationalexposure to blood borne pathogens. 1992, OSHA 3127. Available at: www.oshaslc.gov?oshStd_toc/OSHA_Std_toc.html. Accessed November 5, 2004.

96. Center for Disease Control. Guidelines for prevention of intravascular catheter-related infections. 2003. Available at: http://www.ded.gov/ncidod/hip?IV/lv.htm. Accessed November 5, 2004.

97. National Home Infusion Association. Available at: http://www.nhianet.org/natlcodingstd.htm. Accessed October 31, 2004.

98. United States Department for Health and Human Services. Office for Civil Rights—HIPAA. Available at: http://www.hhs.gov/ocr/hipaa/. Accessed November 5, 2004.

99. U.S. Department of Justice. Office of the Deputy Attorney General. Guidance on the use of the federal false claims act in civil health care matters. Available at: http://www.usdoj.gov/04foia/readingrooms/chcm.htm. Accessed November 5, 2004.

100. Federal Anti-Kickback Statute: if you know the rules you can avoid civil and criminal penalties—the legal corner—medical referral laws. Available at: http://www.findarticles.com/p/articles/mi_m0LMB/is_2_22/ai_97995728. Accessed November 5, 2004.

101. Stark Medicare Regulatory and Contracting Reform Act. Available at: http://www.house.gov/stark/documents/107th/contractsumm.html#Anchor-47857. Accessed November 5, 2004.

102. Medicare Prescription Drug, Modernization, and Improvement Act of 2003. Pub.L. No. 108–73 (2003). Available at: http://www.cms.hhs.gov/medicarereform/. Accessed November 5, 2004.

103. Community Health Accreditation Program. Available at: http://www.chapinc.org/chap-info.htm. Accessed November 2, 2004.

104. Joint Commission on Accreditation of Healthcare Organizations 2004. Available at: http://www.jcaho.org/htba/index.htm. Accessed November 4, 2004.

105. Accreditation Commission for Home Care. Available at: http://www.achc.org/A%20Quick%20Look.htm. Accessed November 4, 2004.

106. Centers for Medicare and Medicaid. Medicare provider reimbursement manual 2001. State Medicaid manual, part 4, services. Available at: http://www.cms.hhs.gov/manuals/45_smm/sm_04_4_toc.asp. Accessed November 5, 2004.

107. Centers for Medicare and Medicaid. Medicare coverage issues manual 2000. Available at: http://www.cms.hhs.gov/providers/fqhc/. Accessed November 5, 2004.

108. Meyer BM, Cantwell KM. The Medicare prescription drug, improvement, and modernization act of 2003: implications for health-system pharmacy. *Am J Health-Syst Pharm.* 2004;61:1042–51.

109. Franklin D. Module 2: overview of home infusion reimbursement. In: Monk-Tutor MR, ed. *NHIA Home Infusion Pharmacy Certificate Program.* Alexandria, VA: National Home Infusion Association; publication pending 2005.

110. Cain D, Kelley L. Module 3: overview of infusion devices, vascular access devices, and ancillary supplies. In: Monk-Tutor MR, ed. *NHIA Home Infusion Pharmacy Certificate Program.* Alexandria, VA: National Home Infusion Association; 2003.

111. Rollins C. Module 4: introduction to home infusion therapies: nutritional therapies. In: Monk-Tutor MR, ed. *NHIA Home Infusion Pharmacy Certificate Program.* Alexandria, VA: National Home Infusion Association; 2004.

112. Yocom S. Module 5: introduction to home infusion therapies: antibiotics, chemotherapy, and other therapies. In: Monk-Tutor MR, ed. *NHIA Home Infusion Pharmacy Certificate Program.* Alexandria, VA: National Home Infusion Association; publication pending 2005.

113. Thoma L. Module 6: compounded sterile preparations in home infusion. In: Monk-Tutor MR, ed. *NHIA Home Infusion Pharmacy Certificate Program.* Alexandria, VA: National Home Infusion Association; 2004.

114. Dillon R, Petroff B, Riddell M. Module 7: overview of financial and operational issues in infusion therapy. In: Monk-Tutor MR, ed. *NHIA Home Infusion Pharmacy Certificate Program.* Alexandria, VA: National Home Infusion Association; 2003.

115. Bemus AM, Lindley CM, Sawyer WT, et al. Task Analysis of home care pharmacy. *Am J Health-Syst Pharm.* 1996;53:2831–9.

116. Rehm SJ, Weinstein AJ. Home intravenous antibiotic therapy: a team approach. *Ann Intern Med.* 1983 Sept;99(3):388–92.

117. Reid, S. The role of the pharmacist in-home infusion therapy. In: Conners RW, Winters RB, eds. *Home Infusion Therapy: Current Status and Future Trends.* Chicago, IL: American Hospital Pub.; 1995.

118. Kwan JW. High-technology IV infusion devices. *Am J Hosp Pharm.* 1991;48(suppl 1):S36–51.

119. Moureau N. Vascular access with a focus on safety. *Infusion.* 1999;(6(1);16–26.

120. Focus group on telepharmacy. *Am J Health-Syst Pharm.* 2001:58:167–9. ASHP Report.

121. Rice R. Telecaring in home care: making a telephone visit. *Geriatr Nurs.* 2000;21(1):56–7.

122. Arcarese, JS. Medical devices in the home healthcare community. FDA Center for Devices and Radiological Health. November 1, 2002. Available at: http://www.fda.gov.cccdrh/CDRHHHC/091202report.html. Accessed September 20, 2004.

Chapter 8

Hospice and Palliative Care

Mary Lynn McPherson

Introduction

Hospice is a philosophy of care that recognizes death as the final stage of life. The primary goals are relief from pain and other symptoms, allowing the terminally ill patient to spend their last days with dignity, surrounded by their loved ones. With hospice care, the patient and family are the unit of care, and the emphasis is on enhancing the quality of remaining life, rather than length of life. The judicious use of medications is extremely important in achieving these goals, and pharmacists are recognized as highly valued members of the hospice team.

> *You matter because you are you, and you matter until the last moment of your life. We will do all we can, not only to help you die peacefully, but also to live until you die.*
>
> Dame Cicely Saunders,
> *founder of the modern day hospice movement*

End-of-life care in the United States embraces two evolving models: *traditional hospice care* as defined by the Medicare Hospice Benefit, and *palliative care*. Some authorities argue specific characteristics that differentiate between the two, while others in the United States and certainly abroad regard any differences as essentially a matter of semantics.

While it would not be incorrect to speak of offering palliative care to your child suffering from a skinned knee after falling off their bicycle, generally palliative care refers to an approach to managing life-limiting illnesses with a focus on symptom control and support, in lieu of cure or prolonging life. Palliative care has been defined by the authors of *The Oxford Textbook of Palliative Medicine* as "the study and management of patients with active, progressive, far-advanced disease for whom the prognosis is limited and the focus of care is the quality of life."[1]

In what ways are palliative care and hospice care similar? Many would say that in the United States, hospice is a governmentally regulated organization or program for dying persons and their families, which largely embraces the concept of palliative care.[2] The hospice philosophy, however, has a long and rich history.

Hospice care has been recorded as early as 400 A.D. when weary travelers in Europe were cared for until they rested or died. Frequently provided by religious orders, hospices provided care designed to meet physical, social, emotional, and spiritual needs of the weary and dying. As medical care advanced over subsequent centuries, care focused more on curative interventions and less on holistic care.

The modern hospice movement began in 1879, when Sister Mary Aikenhead founded Our Lady's Hospice for the Dying in Ireland. Cicely Saunders, trained eventually as a nurse, social worker, and physician, began her life's work at this organization, eventually opening St. Christopher's Hospice in Sydenham, London in 1967. This world-renowned hospice is still operational today, and Dr. Saunder's work has paved the way for hospice practice as we know it today.

Hospice care came to the United States as an alternative to the increasing medicalization and institutionalization of death. The first inpatient hospice program in the United States opened in 1974 in New Haven, Connecticut. In 2003, there were approximately 3,300 operational hospices in the United States, providing care to over 950,000 patients. Of these, approximately 95% were "Medicare-certified."[3]

The Hospice Medicare Benefit, initiated in 1983, is covered under Medicare Part A (hospital insurance). Medicare beneficiaries who choose hospice care receive noncurative medical and supportive care during their terminal illness, and support of the family during the patient's illness and bereavement period. The Medicare Hospice Benefit provides medical, nursing, social work, and home health aide care; supplies and medications related to terminal diagnosis necessary to achieve pain relief and symptoms control; and counseling, spiritual care, volunteer services, and bereavement. There are three eligibility criteria for the Medicare Hospice Benefit. These include the following:

1. The patient's primary care physician and the hospice medical director certify the patient is terminally ill with a life expectancy of 6 months or less, if the disease runs its normal course;

2. The patient chooses to receive hospice care rather than curative treatments for their illness, and

3. The patient enrolls in a Medicare-approved hospice program.

Medicare pays the hospice program a per diem rate to cover all expenses related to the patient's terminal illness. The per diem rate is increased if the patient requires general inpatient care, the family requires respite care for the patient (a brief admission to an inpatient facility), or if the patient requires continuous care in his or her home for up to several days. Hospice services are also covered by private health insurance and Medicaid in most states, using a compensation structure similar to that described under the Medicare Hospice Benefit.

Hospice care may be provided in the patient's home, wherever the patient is residing (e.g., single-family home, long-term care facility, assisted-living facility), a hospice unit, free-standing inpatient hospice facility, or hospital (Table 8-1). Regardless of the setting of care, the patient and family are the unit of care, as discussed previously. Emphasis is on controlling the patient's pain and other symptoms, and maximizing quality of life. The patient and family are central in the decision-making process regarding all aspects of care. Care is provided to the patient and family 24 hours a day, seven days a week.

Hospice care focuses not just on pain and other physical symptoms but also promotes psychological and spiritual growth and development. To accomplish these goals, hospice care is provided by an interdisciplinary team of professionals. Medicare-certified hospice programs must have a core interdisciplinary team that includes a doctor of medicine or osteopathy, a registered nurse, a social worker, and a pastoral or other counselor. In the majority of hospice programs, however, this core team is complemented by the addition of a pharmacist, certified nursing assistant, bereavement professional, volunteers, and others. Each discipline brings a different set of skills to the team, allowing total care of the patient and family.

Even though Medicare and other payers do not mandate the pharmacist as a core member of the interdisciplinary team, Medicare regulations state that the

Table 8-1
Locations of Deaths in 2003[3]

In 2003, for all Americans who died:

- About 25% died at home

- About 25% died in a nursing facility

- About 50% died at a hospital
  - 15% in the emergency room and
  - 35% in acute care

For those patients who died under hospice care:

- 50% died at home

- 23% died in a nursing facility

- 7% died in a hospice unit

- 9% died in a hospital

- 7% died in a free-standing inpatient facility operated entirely by the hospice

- 4% died in a residential care setting

Source: Reference 3.

hospice must "employ a licensed pharmacist; or have a formal agreement with a licensed pharmacist to advise the hospice on ordering, storage, administration, disposal, and record keeping of drugs and biologicals." Many hospices see the value of including the pharmacist as a full and integral member of the hospice team.

Palliative care is associated with the hospice philosophy but includes a broader approach to care. Provision of palliative care does not require adherence to a 6-months' prognosis or less, as is required for the Medicare Hospice Benefit. Increasingly, hospitals are offering the services of a palliative care team to patients in the intensive care unit or any patient requiring pain or symptom relief.

Experts in this field advocate that palliative care should be provided in conjunction with curative interventions at the time of diagnosis of a potentially terminal illness. This paradigm may shift increasingly toward palliative care and less so toward curative care as the disease progresses and may culminate in admission to a hospice program. In 2003, the average length of service in a hospice program was 55 days; the median length of stay was 22 days.[3] Unfortunately, many patients are referred to a hospice program only when they have extremely advanced disease, which limits the effectiveness of hospice services. In 2003, 36.9% of those served by a hospice program died in 7 days or less after admission.[3]

A significant intervention used to treat pain and other end-of-life symptoms in hospice and palliative care is the use of medications. The appropriate use of medications is critically important in this medically frail and frequently unstable population, which points to the importance of the pharmacist in this practice setting. The balance of this chapter will focus on the role of the pharmacist in hospice and palliative care.

It is not death or pain that is to be dreaded,
but the fear of pain or death.

Epictetus

Practice Opportunities

There are many opportunities for pharmacists to be involved in end-of-life care and to varying degrees. Most pharmacists will encounter patients with a life-limiting illness at some point regardless of the practice setting; therefore, it is reasonable to expect all pharmacists to possess a core body of end-of-life care knowledge.

Other pharmacists have incorporated the routine provision of end-of-life pharmaceutical care into their practice, ranging from a few hours per week to a full-time position. Many hospitals have developed an inpatient palliative care unit and/or team, which frequently includes a pharmacist member. Inclusion of the pharmacist on both inpatient and outpatient palliative care teams has been characterized in other countries and is a growing phenomenon in the United States.[4-7]

Two surveys have been conducted in the United States to determine pharmacist involvement in hospice care. Berry et al. surveyed 75 hospice organizations in 1981.[8] Of the 48 responses, 37 reported affiliation with a pharmacist, and an additional 10 anticipated using pharmacist's services in the future. The second survey conducted in 1991 queried 577 pharmacists who had indicated involvement or interest in providing pharmaceutical services to hospice patients.[9] Despite a low response rate of 9%, results showed a much larger range of servies provided by pharmacists to hospice programs, and a growing desire to include pharmacists as full members of the hospice team.

While many pharmacists volunteer as a consultant to hospice programs or provide pharmaceutical care solely as an extension of their role in providing medications, a growing number of pharmacists are considered integral to the hospice team and are paid for their services. Larger hospices, such as home-based programs with an average daily census of 200 or higher, or larger inpatient hospice programs can support their own pharmacy. Data provided from the National Hospice and Palliative Care Organization (NHPCO) National Data Set provides hospice program statistics.[10] In 2003, 51% of hospice programs were free-standing; 29.2% were hospital-based; 18.9% were home health based; and less than 1% were nursing home based.

As mentioned previously, all hospice programs are required to have a contractual arrangement with a pharmacist for the provision of drugs and biologicals. This pharmacist may be accessible to hospice staff to respond to drug information questions or even attend regular hospice interdisciplinary team meetings. Other pharmacists may serve solely as a consultant pharmacist to the hospice program, independent of providing pharmaceuticals. Other pharmacists provide services to hospices affilitated with a home health agency, or a long-term care facility. As shown in Table 8-1, approximately 25% of all Americans who died in 2003 were in a nursing facility, as well as 23% of hospice patients who died in 2003. Pharmacists who work as consultants to nursing facilities must also be knowledgeable about end-of-life care, enabling them to appropriately determine the goals of drug therapy and assess outcomes in terminally ill patients.

Because pharmacists are the most accessible health professional and are often asked for advice by the general public, pharmacists in all practice settings need to have a basic understanding of pharmaceutical palliative care.

The desire to take medicine is perhaps the greatest
feature which distinguishes man from animals.

Sir William Osler

Pharmacist's Responsibilities in Hospice and Palliative Care

As discussed above, there are a variety of functions and services pharmacists can provide in hospice and palliative care. Some pharmacists may provide a few selected services to end-of-life patients, while others may fully embrace this role and be involved in a range of palliative pharmaceutical care. Sometimes the extent of pharmacist involvement depends on the practice setting.

The American Society of Health-System Pharmacists (ASHP) is supportive of pharmacist involvement in hospice and palliative care, and they have published a position statement to this effect.[11] This position paper should be required reading for all pharmacists, particularly those involved in hospice and palliative care. The background of hospice and palliative care is described, as well as proposed pharmacist's responsibilities (see Table 8-2).

Responsibility #1—Assessing the appropriateness of medication orders and ensuring the timely provision of effective medications for symptom control.

Hospice and palliative care pharmacists are responsible for maintaining an accurate medication profile for the terminally ill patient and assuring the appropriateness of drug therapy. Literature supports the role of pharmacists in managing chronic pain and working collaboratively with other hospice professionals to enhance the quality and cost-effectiveness of drug therapy in this patient population.[12,13]

While end-of-life care may be considered a specialty practice, hospice and palliative care practitioners must be familiar with the presentation, associated symptoms, and disease progression of the most commom medical conditions seen in this patient population. Data from NHPCO from the year 2003 shows that cancer diagnoses accounted for 49% of hospice admissions. The remaining 51% of hospice admissions encompass a variety of noncancer diagnoses (see Table 8-3).[3] For example, it is important to be knowledgeable about commom metastatic patterns of various cancers. Prostate cancer frequently metastasizes to bone; breast cancer frequently spreads to bone and brain. Anticipitating disease progression allows the pharmacist to recommend appropriate drug therapy that is more likely to achieve the therapeutic goal.

To best evaluate a patient's drug regimen, the pharmacist must have a clear understanding of the purpose and therapeutic goal of every medication the patient is receiving. For example, the goal of an analgesic regimen is to reduce the pain score to a level that the patient finds acceptable and enable the patient to perform their desired activities of daily living (e.g., sleep through the night, socialize with family). The therapeutic goal may change as the patient's prognosis changes. For example, a patient with a long-standing history of hypercholesterolemia may have had an LDL-cholesterol goal of <100 mg/dL for the past 3 years. Now that the patient has a prognosis of 3 months, for example, comfort measures are of primary importance, and the burden of continuing to take medication for hypercholesterolemia may outweigh any benefit from continued therapy.

In addition to maximizing the cost effectiveness of the medication regimen (see responsibility number 5),

Table 8-2

Pharmacist Responsibilities in Hospice and Palliative Care[11]

ASHP Statement on the Pharmacist's Role in Hospice and Palliative Care

- Assessing the appropriateness of medication orders and ensuring the timely provision of effective medications for symptom control
- Counseling and educating the hospice team about medication therapy
- Ensuring that patients and caregivers understand and follow the directions provided with medications
- Providing efficient mechanisms for extemporaneous compounding of nonstandard dosage forms
- Addressing financial concerns
- Ensuring safe and legal disposal of all medications after death
- Establishing and maintaining effective communication with regulatory and licensing agencies

Source: Reference 11.

Table 8-3

Terminal Diagnoses of Hospice Patients in 2003[3]

Diagnoses	Percentage of Hospice Patients in 2003
Cancer	49%
End-stage heart disease	11.0%
Dementia	9.6%
Lung disease	6.8%
End-stage kidney disease	2.8%
End-stage liver disease	1.6%

Source: Reference 3.

the pharmacist should systematically review the medication regimen for appropriateness as well as detecting and resolving drug-related problems. A critical thinking process that includes consideration of both the financial implications of drug therapy, and appropriateness is shown in Figure 8-1. Pharmacists, physicians, and nurse case managers who admit patients to hospice and palliative care can use this critical thinking process to optimize the medication regimen. The following is a discussion of drug-related problems and examples from hospice and palliative care practice.[14,15]

- *Need for Additional Drug Therapy*—Patients may require drug therapy to treat a previously untreated indication, to add synergistic or potentiating drug therapy, or to fill the need for prophylactic or preventive drug therapy. Examples in a hospice or palliative care practice may include the need to treat unrecognized pain (e.g., misdiagnosed behavioral disturbance), failure to include an angiotensin converting-enzyme inhibitor in the drug regimen of a patient with chronic heart failure, or the need for a bowel regimen in a patient receiving an opioid.

Figure 8-1
Critical Thinking Process—Medication Regimen Review

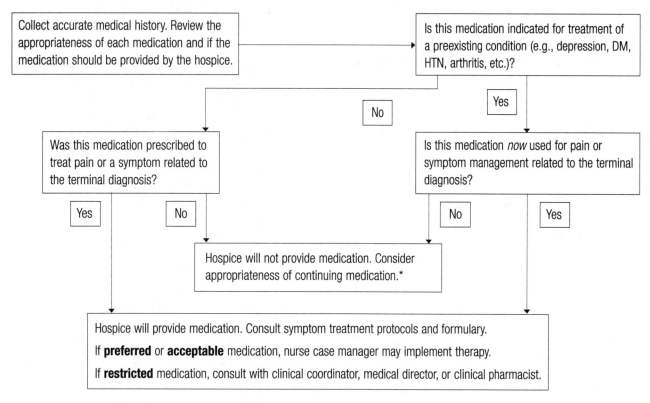

Review medication regimen at the time of admission, and at the beginning of every recertification period.

Collect accurate medical history. Review the appropriateness of each medication and if the medication should be provided by the hospice.

Is this medication indicated for treatment of a preexisting condition (e.g., depression, DM, HTN, arthritis, etc.)?

No

Yes

Was this medication prescribed to treat pain or a symptom related to the terminal diagnosis?

Is this medication *now* used for pain or symptom management related to the terminal diagnosis?

Yes   No

No   Yes

Hospice will not provide medication. Consider appropriateness of continuing medication.*

Hospice will provide medication. Consult symptom treatment protocols and formulary.

If **preferred** or **acceptable** medication, nurse case manager may implement therapy.

If **restricted** medication, consult with clinical coordinator, medical director, or clinical pharmacist.

*Consider appropriateness of continuing medications hospice will not be providing:
- What is the therapeutic goal for this medication, and is the goal being achieved?
- Does the dose need to be increased or decreased? Is the dosing interval correct?
- Is the route of administration and dosage formulation appropriate? Is the patient able to take the medication?
- Can this medication be discontinued without causing the patient pain or other symptom?
- Is the patient experiencing any adverse effects from this medication, or is it potentially interacting with another medication?
- Are there any symptoms currently not beng managed? Should a new medication be ordered?

- *Unnecessary Drug Therapy*—As discussed above, the therapeutic goal for the patient's medications may change as they continue on the disease trajectory. For example, at some point, continuing antihypertensive and antidiabetes medications may cause more harm than good (e.g., hypotension or hypoglycemia) as the patient declines.

  Another example of unnecessary drug therapy is the use of two drugs from the same therapeutic class (e.g., two nonsteroidal anti-inflammatory agents or two benzodiazepines). A patient may be receiving one antidepressant for depression and another as an adjunctive agent for the treatment of neuropathic pain. The pharmacist is in an excellent position to recommend simplification of the medication regimen.

- *Incorrect Medication*—This category describes a case where a medication is indicated, but the patient is receiving a less than optimal drug. For example, the patient may be taking a less effective medication than other therapeutic options, they may have a contraindication to therapy or perhaps are using an inappropriate dosage formulation. An example of an incorrect medication is the use of diphenhydramine to treat insomnia in a terminally ill patient. A thorough assessment of the patient's complaint may disclose pain that prevents a full night's rest. The preferred treatment in this case would be an appropriate analgesic, instead of sedating the patient.

  This category may also include the use of inappropriate dosage formulations, even though the medication may be appropriate. For example, if a terminally ill patient has persistent pain, it would be inappropriate to administer a short-acting opioid analgesic (e.g., immediate release morphine tablets) every 4 hours around the clock. To optimize quality of life, it would be preferable to use an oral, long-acting formulation of the drug (e.g., MS Contin).

- *Dosage Too Low*—Examples in this category include administration of a dosage too low, an inappropriately long dosing interval, or too short a duration of therapy. A classic example of subtherapeutic dosing in terminal care is the misconception that opioids have a "ceiling dose." In fact, pure mu-opioid agonist agents, such as morphine, do not have a maximum daily dose. The dose that controls the patient's pain complaint,

without causing unacceptable toxicity, is the appropriate dose. For some patients it may be 30 mg of oral morphine per day. For other patients it may be 3,000 mg of oral morphine per day.

- *Adverse Drug Reaction*—Adverse drug reactions include events described as side effects, unwanted pharmacologic effects, drug-induced illness, and drug interactions. Pharmacists must be vigilant in screening for the presence of adverse drug reactions or the potential for such with the addition of new medications to the regimen. Some medications cause adverse effects to which tolerance develops, while others do not. For example, opioids frequently cause nausea and sedation when therapy is initiated, but patients generally develop tolerance within 36–48 hours. Patients will never develop tolerance to constipation associated with opioid therapy; therefore, this should be anticipated and the patient started on an appropriate bowel regimen.

- *Dosage Too High*—When a patient receives an excessively high dose of a medication, this increases the risk for toxicity and diminishes patient tolerability of the regimen. Pain patients may inadvertently take in excess of the recommended total daily dose of acetaminophen (4 g) by using additional doses of combination analgesics (e.g., hydrocodone/acetaminophen; oxycodone/acetaminophen), in addition to over-the-counter products.

  Patients with reduced liver or kidney function may require medication dosage adjustment or selection of an alternate agent. For example, all opioids are metabolized by the liver, and the risk of toxicity is increased in patients with liver dysfunction. Some opioids are metabolized to active drug products (e.g., morphine, meperidine, propoxyphene), which could be problematic in patients with impaired renal function.

- *Nonadherence to Drug Therapy*—There are many causes of nonadherence to drug therapy including unavailability of medication, patient's inability to pay for the medication, patient inability to utilize the dosage formulation, inappropriate health beliefs, patient not understanding directions for using medication, or the patient forgetting to take the medication, or chosing not to. It is important to discuss the patient's beliefs about medication use and pain/symptom management, and to dispell commonly held myths and misconceptions (opioids cause addiction, etc.).

As patients' near the end of their life, they may require the pharmacist's expertise in selecting, and sometimes crafting, appropriate dosage formulations to facilitate drug administration. Some patients cannot swallow tablets or capsules as they decline and may benefit from an intensol (concentrated liquid formulation of a drug) formulation. Up to 1 mL of an intensol liquid may be instilled in the buccal cavity of a patient propped up to avoid aspiration with good success. Some medications may be compounded as rectal or transdermal formulations to eliminate the need for the patient to swallow drugs.

Pharmacists may review a patient's medication regimen during hospice team meeting (see next section), when the admission orders are submitted to the pharmacy, or respond to specific requests for information as needed by the other hospice professionals. Many pharmacists are "on call" for pain and symptom consult questions 24 hours a day.

Pharmacists who work with a hospice program to provide pharmaceuticals must have the appropriate inventory of medications and dosage formulations. For example, for pain management it would be important for the provider pharmacist to have immediate release tablets or capsules as well as intensol oral solution of morphine available in addition to oral long-acting tablets.

Many patients will require a liquid formulation of their medications prior to death as they grow too weak to swallow. Hospice nurse case managers are very skilled at anticipating a patient's inability to swallow in coming days and will order appropriate medications to adjust. However, occasionally the patient's clinical condition changes rapidly or a new symptom develops suddenly. It is important that the provider pharmacy be prepared to deliver medications within a few hours as necessary. Many pharmacies have developed a *starter kit* or *comfort kit* that is placed in the home of each hospice patient. Typically, these kits include three to five doses of the most commonly used medications such as morphine, lorazepam, haloperidol, and hyoscyamine, usually as oral solutions. The pharmacy generally charges the hospice a fee for each comfort kit, ranging from $10 to $25 dollars. When you consider patient and family satisfaction and avoidance of emergency drug delivery fees, comfort kits are generally very cost effective for the hospice program.[16]

Responsibility #2—Counseling and educating the hospice team about medication therapy.

Pharmacists are able to offer a tremendous amount of valuable information about pain and symptom management and the appropriate use of medications in managing these symptoms. As discussed above, pharmacists are able to detect drug-related problems and advise the hospice team on appropriate drug selection and monitoring. Increasingly, the pharmacist is a regular member of the hospice interdisciplinary team, which meets at least once every 2 weeks to review every patient in the hospice program.

In addition to providing drug information during hospice team meeting, the pharmacist may provide regularly scheduled educational sessions on a variety of topics to hospice health care providers. For example, the pharmacist may give an inservice on new therapeutic interventions and dosage formulations or review the pharmacotherapeutic management of pain or a variety of symptoms.

Some hospices maintain a formulary, or preferred drug list, which the pharmacist has likely helped to develop. The pharmacist may give an annual update on the status of the formulary and update the formulary as new drugs and drug products become available. The pharmacist may also conduct regular drug use evaluation audits and educate the staff on the outcomes of these audits.

Pharmacists are also frequently called upon to educate other members of the hospice team, including certified nursing assistants, psychosocial professionals, and volunteers about drug therapy in hospice. It's not uncommon for a patient to share a concern or question about his or her drug therapy with the nursing assistant or volunteer, and an educated professional will know to direct the questions to the nurse case manager.

Responsibility #3—Ensuring that patients and caregivers understand and follow the directions provided with medications.

Pharmacists are charged with the responsibility of ensuring that all labeling of drug products is complete and accurate and understandable by the patient, family, and caregiver. Some patients may require special tools to measure, dose, or administer medications, which the pharmacist can supply and explain. Some pharmacists make home visits to meet with patients, families, and caregivers and to explain how to appropriately use medications.

The pharmacist is in an excellent position to dispell myths and misconceptions about medication use, particularly opioids. Many patients (and health professionals) do not understand the difference between addiction, tolerance, and physical dependence (see Table 8-4).[17] Some patients and families are fearful of morphine because the patient may become addicted to the medication. Another popular misconception is that if the patient starts taking morphine (or another opioid analgesic), there will be no alternative analgesic for when the "pain really gets bad." The pharmacist would need to explain that there is no maximum dosage of pure mu-opioid agonists such as morphine, and the dosage would be increased as needed.

It is important for pharmacists working in end-of-life care to appreciate the sensitive and emotional issues that may arise. Not only must pharmacists possess expert pharmacotherapeutic knowledge, but they should aslo be empathetic and caring, able to listen to patients and families, and respond appropriately. This type of situation may make some health practitioners uncomfortable, including pharmacists. Working with patients who are dying is a sacred trust, and a truly caring attitude and a commitment to prompt and accurate service is critical. Having said that, the ability to participate in providing comfort to patients at this juncture in their lives is one of the greatest contributions a pharmacist can make.

Table 8-4
Definitions of Addiction, Physical Dependence, and Tolerance[17]

Addiction

Addiction is a primary, chronic, neurobiologic disease with genetic, psychosocial, and environmental factors influencing its development and manifestations. It is characterized by behaviors that include one or more of the following: impaired control over drug use, compulsive use, continued use despite harm, and craving.

Physical Dependence

Physical dependence is a state of adaptation that is manifested by a drug class specific withdrawal syndrome that can be produced by abrupt cessation, rapid dose reduction, decreasing blood level of the drug, and/or administration of an antagonist.

Tolerance

Tolerance is a state of adaptation in which exposure to a drug induces changes that result in a diminution of one or more of the drug's effects over time.

Source: Reference 17.

Responsibility #4—Providing efficient mechanisms for extemporaneous compounding of nonstandard dosage forms.

Pharmacists should maintain the appropriate inventory to accommodate a terminally ill patient's need for alternate dosage formulations. Sometimes, however, the patient requires a dosage formulation that is not commercially available. This may be the need for a liquid, rectal, or transdermal dosage formulation that is not otherwise available or preparation of a different or higher concentration of a medication. Whenever possible, pharmacists should compound products for which stability and bioavailability data are available.

Responsibility #5—Addressing financial concerns.

Under the Medicare Hospice Benefit, the hospice program is obligated to provide drugs and biologicals as needed for the palliation and management of the terminal illness and related conditions. It is important that the hospice program provide the most cost effective drug therapy possible to maximize pain and symptom control. Drug costs are one of the fastest rising health care expenses, and inappropriate drug coverage can imperil a hospice program's financial situation. Pharmacists are in an excellent position to help review the literature and determine the most cost effective pharmacotherapeutic interventions to manage terminal symptoms.[18,19] This is not to say the least expensive medication is always the best medication to use. Sometimes the more expensive medication provides better symptom control, or less toxicity.

As shown in Figure 8-1, this author has developed symptom-based treatment protocols, and a formulary or preferred drug list for use by hospices. All medications are classified as either preferred, acceptable, or restricted. A *preferred* medication is one where evidence exists demonstrating efficacy in treating a symptom commonly experienced by a terminally ill patient. *Acceptable* medications are just that; acceptable for alternatives to the preferred medication for treating a specific symptom. The nurse case manager may suggest the use of a preferred or acceptable medication to the prescribing physician or continue therapy with one of these medications at the expense of the hospice program if the symptom is related to the terminal diagnosis, without additional approval. Some medications are considered to be *restricted* either because evidence is lacking regarding their efficacy, the medication causes significant toxicity, or expense of the drug renders it an agent of second or third choice. If the nurse case manager feels the need to use a restricted medication, or a restricted medication is ordered by the primary care physician, the nurse case manager must discuss the case with the clinical pharmacist, the clinical coordinator, or medical director of the hospice program. If after considering the goals of therapy the team feels the medication is appropriate, then the medication is ordered at the expense of the hospice program. Medications that are not related to the terminal diagnosis (e.g., medications for diabetes, hypertension, or hypercholesterolemia), or are not used to treat pain or other symptom may be continued if appropriate and desired by the patient. These medications would be procured by the usual process used by the patient prior to admission to hospice.

If the patient is taking medications that are not provided by the hospice program, the pharmacist and hospice team is still charged with the responsibility of assessing the appropriateness of continuing these medications and addressing financial concerns of the patient or family. For example, a patient with amyotrophic lateral sclerosis (ALS) may be admitted to hospice receiving riluzole (Rilutek). This medication has been shown to slow disease progression for several months, early in the disease process. If the patient is truly appropriate for hospice referral (prognosis less than 6 months) then it is unlikely the medication is offering any therapeutic benefit at that point. The patient may have difficulty swallowing the medication, and this is an extremely expensive medication. The pharmacist, nurse, or physician should have a gentle conversation with the patient and family about their perceptions regarding the benefits of continuing this medication and the advantages of discontinuing therapy. For those medications that the patient chooses to continue and receives benefit but has financial difficulty obtaining, the pharmacist can assist by investigating alternate resources such as assistance program from pharmaceutical manufacturers.

Responsibility # 6—Ensuring safe and legal disposal of all medications after death.

Once medications are dispensed, the patient owns the medications. At the time of death, most states would disallow the use of these medications for another patient or family member. Therefore, medications that remain at the time of the patient death must be disposed of to avoid diversion or inappropriate use. Pharmacists are able to assist hospice programs to design policies to deal with the disposal of medications at the time of death that are in keeping with federal and state regulations, as well as environmental rules and regulations.

Responsibility #7—Establishing and maintaining effective communication with regulatory and licensing agencies.

Hospice patients frequently use large quantities of controlled substances; therefore, it is important that the pharmacist maintain open and effective communication with state and federal controlled-substance agencies. The pharmacist can also advise the hospice program regarding their role in dealing with controlled substances, such as policies on emergency drug use, and drug disposal (as above).

Pharmacists may also serve the hospice in a variety of administrative roles, such as serving on the Board of Directors, the Quality Assurance Committee, the Medication Policies and Procedures Committee, and the Ethics Committee. Minimally the pharmacist should be involved in the creation and annual review and editing of policies and procedures pertaining to medication use. According to 2003 data from NHPCO, 63.7% of hospice programs are accredited (45.6% by JCAHO, 9.6% by CHAP, 6.1% by state organizations, and 2.7% by other accrediting groups).[10] Every accrediting organization is likely to have standards pertaining to medication use; the pharmacist is in an excellent position to participate in activities designed to meet these standards.

Although the world is full of suffering, it is full also of the overcoming of it.

Helen Keller, 1880–1968

Preparation for a Career in Hospice and Palliative Care

Pharmacists who wish to practice in hospice and palliative care need to have a fairly comprehensive understanding of common terminal diagnoses, such as those shown in Table 8-3. For each terminal diagnosis, it is important to know what symptoms the patient is likely to experience prior to death. For example, pain is highly prevalent in all terminally ill patients. Patients with end-stage obstructive lung disease or pulmonary malignancy are very likely to experience dyspnea. It is important to be familiar with the most current therapies used to palliate these symptoms, how to select the most cost effective therapy and to monitor therapeutic and potentially adverse outcomes from drug therapy. The pharmacist's knowledge of dosage formulations and compounding is a critical part of drug therapy in end-of-life patients. Very often pharmacists are called on to perform opioid conversion calculations (e.g., calculate how to switch from morphine to methadone, etc.). These calculations can be complex, and mistakes may cause unnecessary suffering, or disastrous outcomes (e.g., overdosage and potential death). As discussed earlier, the pharmacist must use good communication skills and develop a caring, empathetic attitude to work with this patient population.

Do pharmacy students acquire these skills to an acceptable degree during their didactic and experiential training? A survey sent to 83 schools and colleges of pharmacy in the United States in 2001 queried end-of-life care education offered at their respective institutions.[20] Sixty-two percent of institutions who responded offer didactic education on end-of-life care, with a mean of 3.89 lecture hours of instruction per year. Sixty-one percent of these lectures were required, 17% were elective, and 22% were both required and elective. The most common lecture topics included grieving and death, pharmacotherapy, and physician-assisted suicide. Over half of the institutions responding (58%) provide experiential rotations in end-of-life care. Experiential rotations sites included hospice organizations, oncology services, and long-term care facilities. Thirty-eight percent of the institutions that offered any instruction in hospice or palliative care have a faculty member that specialized in this area. An impressive 93% of respondents reported that end-of-life care issues were either necessary or of interest to them for curriculum inclusion, and 60% perceived a need to increase content in the curriculum.

An earlier study reported results from surveying 3,762 hospice programs in the United States regarding their participation in training pharmacy students.[21] There were 907 responses, and 10% reported participating in the training of pharmacy students (27% participated in training medical students, 39% trained social work students, and 69% trained nursing students).

Bookwalter et al. evaluated the content on end-of-life care in eight major pharmacy textbooks in 2003.[22] Their results showed inadequate coverage of end-of-life care in these references, and that which was present was of overall low quality. The authors noted that these findings were consistent, however, with that found in medicine and nursng textbooks.

A more recent survey evaluated the extent to which pain management is taught in schools of pharmacy in the United States.[23] Given the media attention given to pain in recent years, it would be expected that pain management would be addressed to a greater extent than palliative care in these curricula. While pain management was covered to some extent in schools of pharmacy who responded, it was covered in a fragmented fashion (e.g., part of the cancer therapeutics segment or pharmacology of analgesics). Only two schools of pharmacy offered a stand-alone course in pain management and they were both electives. Most respondents felt that content on the diagnosis of pain, patient assessment and physical assessment was "minimal" in their respective curricula. The authors concluded that the topic of pain management is poorly presented and inadequately developed in the curricula of many U.S. schools of pharmacy.

Given that much of the content on pain management and hospice or palliative care in schools of pharmacy is elective, students who are interested in a career in this area should seek those opportunities. Even if a school of pharmacy does not offer an experiential rotation in hospice or pallative care, most schools will entertain a proposal for a specialty rotation, which the student can arrange with a pharmacist practicing in this area.

Advanced training opportunities in hospice and palliative care are fairly scarce in the United States. There are two or three specialty residents in hospice and palliative care and a few additional residencies or fellowships in pain management. Graduates of these programs have gone on to extremely rewarding careers.

Practicing pharmacists can certainly seek opportunities to enhance their skills in hospice and palliative care such as participating in practice-intensive continuing education opportunities, including pain and palliative care traineeships and certificate programs. There are many excellent reference textbooks, journals, and websites that interested pharmacists should investigate (see Table 8-5). Practitioners may wish to join associations, such as the American Academy of Hospice and Palliative Medicine and the National Hospice and Palliative Care Organization, and attend annual conferences to increase skill level.

A newly formed organization, the American Society of Pain Educators, is seeking to develop a multidisciplinary credential certifying practitioners are pain educators. Perhaps in the future a specialty designation will be established for pharmacists who practice in end-of-life care through the Board of Pharmaceutical Specialties.

Table 8-5

Recommended Textbooks, Journals, Websites, and Organizations on Hospice and Palliative Care

Websites:

American Academy of Hospice and Palliative Medicine. Available at: http://www.aahpm.org/.

National Hospice and Palliative Care Organization. Available at: http://www.nhpco.org.

Journals:

American Journal of Hospice and Palliative Medicine. Available at: http://www.pnpco.com/pn01000.html.

Journal of Pain and Palliative Care Pharmacotherapy. Available at: https://www.haworthpress.com/store/product.asp?sku=J354.

Journal of Pain and Symptom Management. Available at: http://www.elsevier.com/wps/find/journaldescription.cws_home/505775/description#description.

Journal of Palliative Medicine. Available at: http://www.liebertpub.com/publication.aspx?pub_id=41.

Textbook:

Oxford Textbook of Palliative Medicine, 3rd Edition. Edited by Derek Doyle, Geoffrey Hanks, Nathan Cherny, and Sir Kenneth Calman. Available at: http://www.oup.co.uk/academic/medicine/palliative_medicine/otpm3e/.

Do not go gentle into that good night, Old age should burn and rave at close of day; Rage, rage against the dying of the light.

Dylan Thomas, 1914–1953

Summary

A career in hospice and palliative care can be incredibly rewarding. Pharmacists who practice in this area either on a full-time or part-time basis can witness first hand the impact they have on a patients' quality of life, providing pain and symptom relief. Students as well as new and seasoned practitioners are encouraged to learn more about this practice opportunity.

References

1. Doyle D, Hanks GWC, MacDonald N. Introduction. In: Doyle D, Hanks GWC, MacDonald N, eds. *Oxford Textbook of Palliative Medicine*. Oxford, England: Oxford University Press; 1993:3.

2. Field MJ, Cassel CK, eds. Committee on Care at the End of Life, Division of Health Care Servicew, Institute of Medicine. *Approaching Death: Improving Care at the End of Life*. Washington, DC: National Academy Press; 1997:31.

3. National Hospice and Palliative Care Organization. Hospice facts and figures from the National Hospice and Palliative Care Organization. Available at: http://www.nhpco.org/files/public/Hospice_Facts_110104.pdf. Accessed February 27, 2005.

4. Dean TW. Pharmacist as a member of the palliative care team. *Can J Hosp Pharm.* 1987;40(3):95–6.

5. Lucas C, Glare PA, Sykes JV. Contribution of a liaison clinical pharmacist to an inpatient palliative care unit. *Palliat Med.* 1997;11(3):209–16.

6. Austwick RA, Brown LC, Goodyear KH, et al. Pharmacist's input into a palliative care clinic. *The Pharmaceutical Journal.* 2002;268:404–6.

7. Gilbar P, Stefaniuk K. The role of the pharmacist in palliative care: results of a survey conducted in Australia and Canada. *J Palliat Care.* 2002;18(4):287–92.

8. Berry JI, Pulliam CC, Calola SM, et al. Pharmaceutical services in hospices. *Am J Hosp Pharm.* 1981;38:1010–4.

9. Arter SG, Berry JI. The provision of pharmaceutical care to hospice patients: results of the National Hospice Pharmacist Survey. *J Pharm Care Pain Sympt Control.* 1993;1:25–42.

10. National Hospice and Palliative Care Organization. 2003 NHPCO National Data Set Summary Report—Demographics and Operations. Available at: http://www.nhpco.org/files/public/NDS00_03Trends Stats101904.pdf. Accessed February 27, 2005.

11. American Society of Heath-System Pharmacists. ASHP statement on the pharmacist's role in hospice and palliative care. *Am J Health-Syst Pharm.* 2002;59:1770–3.

12. Gammaitoni AR, Gallaher RM, Welz M, et al. Palliative pharmaceutical care: a randomized, prospective study of telephone-based prescription and medication counseling services for treating chronic pain. *Pain Med.* 2000;1(4):317–31.

13. Knowlton CH. Collaborative pharmacy practice enters hospice care. *Caring.* June 2004;26–9.

14. Strand LM, Morley PC, Cipolle RJ, et al. Drug-related problems: their structure and function. *Annals Pharmacother.* 1990;240:1093–7.

15. McPherson ML. Performing a medication regimen review in hospice and palliative care. *Am J Hosp Palliat Care.* 2001;18(3):193–9.

16. Herbert KA, McPherson ML. Utilization of medication starter kits in Maryland hospice programs. 37th ASHP Midyear Clinical Meeting and Exhibits: Atlanta, GA; December 2002.

17. American Academy of Pain Medicine. American Pain Society and American Society of Addiction Medicine. Definitions related to the use of opioids for the treatment of pain. Available at: http://www.aahpm.org/. American Academy of Hospice and Palliative Medicine. March 31, 2005.

18. Snapp JN, Kelley D, Gutgsell TL. Creating a hospice pharmacy and therapeutics committee. *Am J Hosp Palliat Care.* 2002;19(2):129–34.

19. Lycan J, Grauer P, Mihalyo M, et al. Improving efficacy, efficiency and economics of hospice individualized drug therapy. *Am J Hosp Palliat Care.* 2002;19(2):135–8.

20. Herndon CM, Jackson K, Fike DS, et al. End-of-life care education in United States pharmacy schools. *Am J Hosp Palliat Care.* 2003;20(5):340–4.

21. Herndon CM, Fike DS, Anderson AC, et al. Pharmacy student training in United States hospices. *Am J Hosp Palliat Care.* 2001;18(3):181–6.

22. Bookwalter TC, Rabow MW, McPhee SJ. Content on end-of-life care in major pharmacy textbooks. *Am J Health-Syst Pharm.* 2003;60:1246–50.

23. Singh RM, Wyant SL. Pain management content in curricula of U.S. schools of pharmacy. *JAMA.* 2003;43(1):34–40.

Chapter 9

Pharmaceutical Industry

Carriann E. Richey

Introduction

The ethics and economics of the pharmaceutical industry receive regular comment by the media, politicians, and patients. The focus of this chapter is to review the role of pharmaceutical industry professionals and their interactions with health-system pharmacists. Specifically, this chapter will address job characteristics and guidelines managing these interactions. Many career opportunities in industry exist for pharmacists, including drug discovery, manufacturing, marketing, medical information, product development, quality assurance, sales, regulatory, project management, health outcomes research, legal, information technology, training and development, and scientific communications.[1] This chapter will mention these career options; however, the list provided is not meant to be all inclusive.

Monaghan et al. completed a survey of pharmacy, medical, and nurse practitioner students to evaluate their knowledge and opinion of "four domains associated with the pharmaceutical industry: (a) pharmaceutical marketing techniques and expenditures, (b) professional position statements regarding ethical interactions with the pharmaceutical industry, (c) use of evidence-based information resources versus Pharmaceutical Sales Representatives (PSRs) as a source for appropriate therapeutic decision making, and (d) strategies to address patient requests for specific medications (e.g., prompted by Direct To Consumer (DTC) marketing)."[2] This survey as well as other studies, editorials, and commentaries on the pharmaceutical industry will be presented in this chapter. As with this survey, the sales and marketing initiatives of the pharmaceutical industry come first to one's mind. This chapter will expand on these interactions. Interactions involving investigational drugs, education programming, and business decisions further exemplify the complex interrelationship between health-system pharmacists and their industry counterparts.

Definitions

Descriptions of each role are provided with current titles used in the profession. Evolution of these roles and their identifiers is likely and discussions with current professionals may provide the best source for relating the information provided here to current career opportunities. Different corporations now and over time may use unique terminology or combine tasks based on their operational processes.

Advisory boards contain experts from practice or research. These boards support pharmaceutical development at various stages and provide the company with feedback and guidance based on their clinical experience.

Business-to-business representatives are involved with formulary and price negotiations for private and government contracts. They may also support development of best practice models.

Clinical research professionals including clinical research monitors and administrators are responsible for the oversight of clinical trials. Some companies may combine these roles or separate them such that clinical research monitors regularly visit the site to complete data verification and clinical research administrators reside internally to link the external and internal team members. Data provided by institutions are recorded onto collection sheets commonly referred to as case/clinical report forms (CRFs). It is these CRFs which are reviewed by clinical research monitors.

Detailing occurs when a PSR meets with a health care practitioner to deliver their marketing message and provide product details.

Drug safety professionals monitor serious adverse events and respond to Medwatch (spontaneous adverse event) reports. These professionals are involved with global safety surveillance. They may be involved with clinical trial safety surveillance or postmarketing surveillance. In some countries, postmarketing surveillance includes regular tracking of events, whereas other countries may rely on spontaneous reporting.

A **formulary** is a preferred drug list for a specific institution. Each institution may implement its own procedures for execution of formulary restrictions.

Health outcomes specialists may interact with health-system practitioners to exchange ideas related to pharmacoeconomic modeling and outcomes trial data. This exchange may guide design of pharmacoeconomic trials.

Investigational review boards review and approve research proposals for a specific institution.

Medical or drug information specialists will address specific questions by patients and health care practitioners that require review of data on file or address topics not directly related to the marketing mission. Global medical or drug information specialists assist worldwide company personnel.

Medical Liaisons (MLs) have the responsibility of building relationships with key health care practitioners in a given area. These key practitioners may be referred to as thought leaders or opinion leaders. MLs are often separate from the sales and marketing function of a company supporting medical and research interest due to their medical training and/or experience. These individuals may also be referred to as scientific liaisons or clinical liaisons.

Pharmaceutical Sales Representatives (PSRs) or Pharmaceutical Drug Representatives have the primary responsibility of reaching out to providers and prescribers within a defined area. Often assigned to a therapeutic area, these professionals deliver the marketing message for pharmaceutical products based on training received by the pharmaceutical manufacturer. According to McCabe, there are three general categories of representatives in pharmaceutical sales: primary sales or mass-market representatives; specialty pharmaceutical sales representatives; and hospital or institutional representatives. Entry level sales positions are typically in primary sales.[3]

PhRMA is the Pharmaceutical Research and Manufacturers of America. It is a nonprofit association that represents the country's leading research-based pharmaceutical and biotechnology companies.

Pharmaceutical company also identified as the manufacturer or sponsor identifies the member company who develops, manufactures, and supplies medications for patients.[4]

Pharmaceutical products or **pharmaceuticals** are the terms for the drug therapies developed by pharmaceutical companies.

Pharmacovigilence or **safety surveillance** refers to the monitoring of adverse events for a pharmaceutical product.

Protocols are documents designed to communicate the study design, inclusion and exclusion criteria, and other study procedures to medical personnel administering the trial at their institutional location.

Regulatory agencies throughout the world function to approve or deny applications for new molecular or chemical entities.

Regulatory scientists or **regulatory managers** in a pharmaceutical company serve as a liaison with these regulatory agencies and are experts in the regulations for drug development.

Speaker panels or **speaker bureaus** are groups of practitioners who have experience with pharmaceutical products through participation in clinical research or experience with special patient populations. These practitioners may be asked to speak on behalf of a pharmaceutical company.

Types of Interactions with Industry Professionals

The above section of definitions includes roles in the pharmaceutical industry. Each role serves on a continuum of two functions: (1) product development and (2) business operations. Interactions generally imply business operations, which is where this section will begin.

Zarowitz et al. summarizes several types of interactions between the pharmaceutical industry and health systems. The objective of their review was to analyze the pros and cons of the relationship with their health system and the pharmaceutical industry and to develop recommendations for other health-systems. The suggestions offered in this reference may be useful to anyone who is new to practice or desires to improve relationships with the industry.[5]

Pharmaceutical Sales Representatives and Health Care Practitioners

The marketing and sale of pharmaceuticals to legal prescribers of medication is a common goal of each PSR. Although each pharmaceutical company may differ in their philosophical approach to these tasks, there are common traits that each company seeks in hiring someone to represent them. Since the individual must interact on a regular basis with health professionals and must convey information in an appropriate fashion, basic communication skills are essential. Interpersonal skills that are sufficiently flexible to conform to differing personalities also play an important role in daily associations. Other traits that are likely common among pharmaceutical company hires are patience, diligence, an ability to understand basic medical and pharmaceutical terminology, organization skills, an acceptable appearance, and the ability to accept criticism and deal with it constructively.

During regular interactions with health practitioners, PSRs offer the latest marketing information about their product. Product information is often distributed in the form of professional brochures, medical literature reprints, or multimedia presentations. Brand reminders such as pens and paper have come under scrutiny and further guidance related to gifts is outlined below. They may also provide greater support through medication vouchers, which may be distributed to patients. Vouchers may allow for patient prescription rebates or discount access to over-the-counter medications.

It is not uncommon for a pharmaceutical company to advertise for a PSR through any one of a number of media. Following is a recent job posting from the Internet[6]:

> The role of the Sales Representative is to expand the sales of our products and to convert [use of] competitive products in a manner that is commensurate with company policy and sales direction. In this role, the Sales Representative will be trained to understand & demonstrate our products to our customers. They will also need to demonstrate the ability to handle customer product questions and objections in a way that is consistent with sales training methodology. Additionally, they will be expected to execute the selling cycle in a manner that is concise, professional, ethical and persuasive, and which leads the customer to action.

Since the marketing and sale of pharmaceuticals demands the provision of information as a central responsibility for the PSR, research has been done to determine their effectiveness in carrying out this role. Lexchin comments on published reports of what type of information providers receive from PSRs. The information requested includes (1) indications, (2) therapeutic benefits, (3) safety data, (4) comparative data with new and old drugs, and (5) drug prices. Unfortunately, little data may be supplied about product safety,

comparable data, and product prices. A review of four studies conducted in Australia, Finland, and the U.S. all suggested that sales representatives primarily focused on indications. Respondents in these surveys perceived that safety data, when it was provided, was done with a positive perspective for the particular product.[7] Pharmacists may assist prescribers by providing additional information related to safety, comparisons, and product prices.

PSRs may also distribute drug samples. A drug sample is defined as "a package containing a limited quantity of a pharmaceutical product sufficient to evaluate clinical response, distributed to authorized health care practitioners free of charge, and for patient treatment."[8] Samples may increase sales, ultimately benefiting the pharmaceutical manufacturer. However, there are definite benefits to practitioner and patients. Both positive and negative considerations related to drug samples include the following:

- Treatment options for indigent populations
- Immediate response for a suffering patient
- Opportunity for experience with a new product by a physician
- Convenience
- Detailed written patient education
- Encourage prescribing behavior in accordance with new clinical guidelines. In addition to the potential benefits of drug samples, an ASHP position statement regarding drug sampling suggests the following concerns with this distribution technique.[9]
- May lack components of pharmaceutical care
- Poor drug control including incorrect labeling and packaging
- Access to prescription drugs by inappropriate personnel
- Encouragement of poor prescribing practices
- Contributes to the cost increase for all patients

Practitioners must evaluate the potential benefits and risks associated with drug sampling and evaluate their current practice procedures. Pharmacists who successfully engage in dialog with their patients can evaluate the use of drug sampling by physicians in their practice setting and encourage appropriate use and prescribing. PSRs may educate pharmacists about manufacturer-sponsored patient-assistance programs, which is an alternative to drug sampling. This allows patients to register with the manufacturer to receive medications at a discounted rate or no cost. An ASHP position statement suggests that these programs may present fewer risks to the patient than drug sampling.[10]

Pharmaceutical Sales Representatives and Pharmacy/Therapeutic Committees

Health-system pharmacists are often involved with or influenced by a therapeutics or pharmacy review committee at their institution. Many health systems have a preferred formulary list of drugs which are to be prescribed by physicians within the health system. Formularies have proven valuable to institutions because, in addition to promoting rational therapy, they may enhance purchasing power and lower drug costs.

Sales or medical field staff from the pharmaceutical company may provide information upon request to address specific concerns of such a committee. Formulary adoption of a particular medication can be extremely valuable to PSRs. The logic is that once a drug is successfully introduced to a patient in an organized health setting which utilizes a formulary, it is more likely that they will remain on that therapy as an outpatient. This in turn will increase the market share of a particular product in that area beyond the institutional setting.

Medical Liaisons and Thought Leaders

Medical liaisons (MLs) deliver medical educational messages as opposed to a marketing message. Lawrence explains that as a ML he was responsible for establishing and maintaining relationships with thought leaders (also known as opinion leaders). MLs share scientific information about drug products with customers and marketing and sales peers and instruct them on key points.[11] They may also give presentations to practitioners. These may be presented during grand rounds or in committee meetings. MLs often have a more extensive medical background, allowing them to provide more information about comparison products and off-label uses.

Medical Liaisons and Health Care Practitioners

In addition to the activities mentioned above, MLs may support continuing education. This is generally done in the form of unrestricted educational grants. These grants allow health-system pharmacists to meet licensing requirements, review drug classes, and support their own lifelong learning. Many continuing education providers rely on pharmaceutical company

financial support. Due to limited availability and time-consuming application process, government and private foundations subsidize only a small portion of the need.

Clinical Research Personnel and Investigational Practitioners

Figure 9-1 diagrams the basic interaction between health care investigators, the medical community, investigational review boards, and the pharmaceutical industry regarding clinical research. Health-system pharmacists who manage or participate in investigational drug departments have regular contact with industry individuals with regard to upcoming, ongoing, and completed research. Practitioners who interact with pharmaceutical companies as investigators, speakers, or in an advisory capacity provide health-systems a conduit for early release of valuable information regarding new drug indications, effectiveness, toxicity, and dosage forms. Pharmaceutical sponsors may select investigational sites for clinical trials based on relationships, investigator experience, and appropriate patient populations. These field clinical research agents and/or medical liaisons build relationships with practitioners separate from the sales and marketing professionals.

Health-system practitioners "who participate in clinical trials can contribute to the evidentiary base for practice and can offer their patients a chance to receive cutting-edge therapies and the close follow-up that often accompanies a trial protocol. In addition, trial participation can benefit physicians themselves through research opportunities for those holding faculty appointments and, where trials are sponsored by industry, a flow of income outside the public health insurance system." This viewpoint by Ferris et al. outlines the potential benefits to both patients and health-system practitioners with regard to clinical human research.[12] As mentioned previously in this chapter, the potential for unethical behavior exists in this system.

The specific interaction between the pharmaceutical industry, clinical research investigators, and investigational drug departments at institutions balances several unique situations. Provider participation in clinical research allows patients a chance to receive innovative therapies. This includes both clinical trial involvement and the opportunity for compassionate or emergency-use therapies. Clinical trials require more rigorous patient monitoring and documentation than that employed in current practice. Clinical research

Figure 9-1
Basic Industry Interactions— Clinical Research Diagram

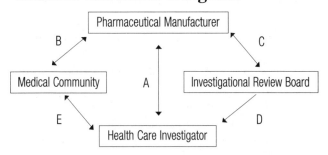

A. Pharmaceutical industry provides investigators with protocols, draft informed consent documents, and fees to cover study costs. Investigators provide the pharmaceutical manufacturer data collected from patient experiences in clinical trials.

B. Pharmaceutical manufacturers provide medications and information to the medical community. In return the medical community accepts the clinical research process and supports their business.

C. Investigational review boards may seek information from pharmaceutical manufactures in determining whether to approve or deny their institutions participation in clinical trials. When investigational review boards approve clinical trials, pharmaceutical manufacturers are able to move forward with clinical trials.

D. Investigational review boards respond to the ethical issues of clinical trials and support investigators in selecting appropriate trials. Investigators provide data and information regarding adverse events to the investigational review board.

E. The medical community provides a peer assessment for investigators related to their clinical research. As well it provides alternatives to patients when investigational studies are not appropriate.

professionals monitor and guide the activities of physicians, pharmacists, and staff at participating clinical research sites (hospitals, clinics, etc.) to collect quality data in accordance with the protocol. Poor quality data might cause rejection of significant patient information prohibiting the company from demonstrating efficacy and/or safety. Recreating quality data is costly, both in terms of time and money. Industry professionals regularly visit, evaluate and train research personnel on research practices that are more stringent than general clinical practice standards. These research practices are dictated not only by individual company policies and procedures but by national and international regulations.

Medical or Drug Information Specialists and Health Care Practitioners

Pharmaceutical companies hire a staff of individuals to answer complicated questions by health care practitioners. Call centers generally have multiple tiers of individuals, with varying experience and training. The first responder will provide answers to questions frequently asked or directly inline with the marketing message. If a question extends beyond this information, it will be forwarded to a medical or drug information specialist. The individual can search clinical trial data and competitor information to formulate an answer to the specific question.

Pharmaceutical manufacturers also communicate with health care practitioners in writing via package inserts and other patient education materials. Package inserts (sometimes referred to as labels) are strictly regulated, and therefore pharmacists employed in the role of label development are contained within the regulatory department. Information contained includes chemical structure, pharmacological data from clinical trials, dosing, risks, contraindications, drug interactions, and patient information. Information provided by medical information specialists should support statements on the package insert in order to avoid regulatory conflicts.

Pharmaceutical Marketing and Patients

A discussion of the pharmaceutical industry would not be complete without mention of a practice that indirectly affects practitioners. This is industry communications involving DTC advertising. As noted below, DTC advertising causes patients to request, or even demand, new and often more expensive drugs. The ASHP position statement on DTC advertising, last reviewed in 2001, is provided below.

> To support direct-to-consumer advertising that is educational in nature about prescription drug therapies for certain medical conditions and appropriately includes pharmacists as a source of information; further,

> To oppose direct-to-consumer advertising of specific prescription drug products; further,

> To support the development of legislation or regulation that would require nonprescription drug advertising to state prominently the benefits and risks associated with product use that should be discussed with the consumer's pharmacist or physician.[13]

Pharmacists may assist patients by answering questions about DTC advertisements and therapeutic options.

Pharmaceutical Marketing and Students

A survey of student understanding of the relationship between the health professions and the pharmaceutical industry outlined similarities and differences between student practitioners with regard to their perspectives of the pharmaceutical industry.[1] Specifically, the authors sought to evaluate student perception of marketing, advertising, and sales activities. The survey instrument used in this study identified 55 items composed of multiple choice and true/false questions and multistructured problems using different forms of resources, clinical cases, etc. Students were selected from the following disciplines: medicine, pharmacy, and nurse practitioner. Fifty-nine students were currently studying medicine, 94 pharmacy students were included, and 17 were enrolled in a nurse practitioner program.

The mean scores of all the student groups were less than 50% with regard to knowledge of marketing expenditures. All students expressed some knowledge of the ethical principles governing interactions with PSRs, represented by mean scores in the 60th percentile. Within this category, students indicated the greatest knowledge related to acceptance of gifts. However, additional understanding was needed with regard to continuing education subsidies and payments.

When comparing PSR interactions with drug information resource utilization, pharmacy students reported less confidence in clinical drug manuals and accuracy of information from PSRs than medical or nursing students. Pharmacy students reported significantly less interaction with PSRs than the other two groups.

After students evaluated six hypothetical cases involving patients requesting medications that may not be medically necessary, the authors evaluated the students confidence in influencing a patient to a more appropriate agent and confidence in satisfying the patient. Pharmacy students were more confident than the other groups with regard to both influence and satisfaction.

The results of this study suggest that pharmacy and other professional students have baseline knowledge of the pharmaceutical industry before graduation. However, their activities and instruction within the curriculum might modify these opinions and address only specific factors related to the relationship between the pharmaceutical industry and health care practitioners.

Guidance of Interactions by Industry Professionals

Institutional Policies and Procedures

Health institutions generally have policies and procedures related to the activities of a PSR within their facility. ASHP offers a document titled *Guidelines for Pharmacists on the Activities of Vendors' Representatives in Organized Health Care Systems*. Table 9-1 outlines suggested PSR Policy and Procedure Language and components from this document.[14] Different facilities may choose different elements to form their policy and procedures on interactions with representatives.

Office of the Inspector General

The federal Office of Inspector General (OIG) has published eleven guidance documents since 1998 to support compliance efforts related to pharmaceutical manufacturer fraud and abuse.[15] The federal office imposes financial and legal penalties to providers and pharmaceutical manufacturers who are determined to participate in fraud or abuse. Providers include hospitals, home health agencies, nursing facilities, individual practitioners, and small group practice. Specifically, three areas which the OIG carefully scrutinizes are identified as: (1) integrity of data for state and federal payments; (2) kickbacks and other illegal remuneration; and (3) drug samples laws and regulations. Integrity of data for state and federal payments applies to pricing and rebates. For example, pharmaceutical companies who attempt to hide pricing concessions provided to some purchasers to avoid passing on the same discount to the states may be guilty of criminal conduct. With regard to relationships with PSRs, OIG focuses on training and compensation. Training guidelines include regular training of sales force on OIG suggestions, industry standards, and PhRMA code. Generally pharmaceutical manufacturers are encouraged to design a set of disciplinary actions, regularly communicate with the OIG for guideline clarification, and a tracking system for sales force activities. The guidance documents also indicate that the company may violate the law if it offers a salesperson extraordinary incentive bonuses and expense accounts.

Drug sample guidance is provided by individual legislation referred to as the Prescription Drug Marketing Act (PDMA); however, OIG suggests training the sales force regularly, careful labeling of samples, and specific notes on packaging indicating that samples are subject to the PDMA statute. PDMA was enacted in 1988 to

Table 9-1
PSR Policy and Procedure Language

Elements of Policy and Procedure Language	What Information Is Included	Sample Language
A defined scope of applicability	Definition of who the policies and procedures are applicable to	Representatives of manufacturers providing products for the prevention, diagnosis, or treatment of disease
Orientation of representatives	Orientation to the facility, director of medical staff, review of policy and procedure, and/or discussion of the formulary	When the data sheet is initially completed, the representative will receive two copies of the Hospital and Health Services Pharmaceutical Representatives Policy. One copy must be signed and kept in the pharmacy. By signing this policy, the representative acknowledges that he/she has read, understands, and agrees to abide by the policies and procedures outlined. The representative should retain the other copy of this policy for his/her records. The representative will also receive orientation to pharmacy purchasing procedures and will be informed of the formulary status of his/her respective products.
Directory	Process for recording information about the representative and what information is to be contained. Suggested information includes name, address, company contact, product lines, manager contact information, distribution information and medical director information.	Pharmaceutical Sales Representative's Data Sheet Name: Company: Address: Telephone Number: Name of District Manager: Address of District Manager: Telephone Number of District Manager: I have reviewed the policies and procedures governing the activities of pharmaceutical sales representatives within the hospital and do hereby agree to abide by such. Failure to do so may result in loss of display privileges and/or being expelled from the hospital and restricted from doing business on hospital property.
Availability of vender-contact information to professionals in the setting	How/if the information above will be available to the medical staff	Vender contact information will be maintained in the inpatient pharmacy
Registration while on premises	Representatives may be required to register each time they visit the institution and required to wear appropriate name and company identification	All PSRs will be required to sign into the PSR book in each respective pharmacy whenever visiting hospital premises. The entry will include PSR name, company, time in/time out, purpose of visit, and with whom an appointment is scheduled. At the time of registration, each representative will be given a badge that is to be worn visibly at all times that identifies them as a PSR. PSRs who do not display the badge maybe challenged and required to obtain a badge immediately.

Table 9-1, continued

Locations permitted	Ability to access patient versus nonpatient care areas	During all visits, PSRs must not interfere in patient care, family privacy, or health care professionals' practice. PSRs may conduct business in the following areas, when appointments or advance arrangements have been made: designated display areas, the cafeteria or other areas designated by the department of pharmacy and/or the Pharmacy and Therapeutics Committee. At no time shall PSRs be in direct patient care areas.
Appointments and purposes	Representatives may be encourages to schedule appointments or enter the facility for a specific predefined purpose	Any and all appointments must be scheduled in advance including to support staff and other personnel. Unscheduled visits to this medical center are prohibited. Contact with physicians and other providers will be limited to the provider's request and will be by advance appointment only.
Exhibits	Ability to distribute informational materials and the details guiding these activities	No advertisements should be posted on walls, doors, windows, and cabinets or placed in reception area(s). Any bona fide educational items to be posted on bulletin boards (e.g., for lectures) should be left with the charge nurse or practice manager for display in employee-only areas (i.e., break room).
Dissemination of promotional materials	Ability to disseminate information for formulary versus nonformulary products as well as guidelines related to on-label and off-label uses	PSRs may provide information, literature or reprints on their products to the staff at the convenience or request of the staff. Only company approved, labeled material and reprints from major peer reviewed journals may be utilized in product promotion. Any materials on nonformulary or formulary restricted products must clearly be labeled as nonformulary or formulary restricted. A verbal statement to the recipient as to formulary status is insufficient. A written notice, as to formulary status, must be placed on all materials.
Samples	Guidelines for the distribution of product and/or drug samples	The use of pharmaceutical samples within the hospital is prohibited. Pharmaceutical samples may be used in out-patient areas when they are considered to be a medical necessity that is of benefit to the patient. Additional policies may apply in specific out-patient areas. It is the responsibility of the representative to read, understand, and abide by any additional policies and procedures in the area they are visiting.
Noncompliance	Outline assessment and actions of failure to follow policy and procedures	First offense PSRs will receive an oral warning from the pharmacy team leader (or his/her designee) with a request for corrective action. The oral warning will remain on record for 1 year. Second offense PSRs will receive a written warning from the P&T chairperson to the PSR with a copy to either regional manager or company professional affairs department. The written warning will remain on record for 1 year. Third offense PSR privileges will be revoked for 1 year. The company represented by the PSR will not be permitted to display, make appointments or provide in-services, or other related marketing activities for a minimum of 1 year. Reinstatement will be at the discretion of the pharmacy team leader. A list of all PSRs who have received a written warning or who have lost hospital privileges will be submitted to the P&T Committee on a quarterly basis. Other disciplinary actions will take place, when appropriate, at the discretion of the pharmacy team leader.

establish requirements for distribution, storage, disposal, record-keeping, security and violations related to pharmaceuticals.

PhRMA Code

On April 18, 2002, the PhRMA executive committee voted unanimously to adopt a code on the interactions with health care professionals. This voluntary code took effect in July, 2002, and outlines guidelines for how PSRs and others involved in marketing should interact with health care professionals. The reasons cited for PhRMA developing this code are: (1) to voluntarily and proactively refocus the pharmaceutical industry to its purpose of scientific medical research and education; (2) to remove the need for government regulation or legislation; (3) to improve the industry's image and reputation; and (4) to regain the public's trust. The key points of PhRMA code are outlined in Table 9-2. The PhRMA code defines the term health care professional as those who interact with patients and who may affect purchasing or prescribing decisions and formulary status of pharmaceutical products. This includes health-system pharmacists who can affect purchasing, prescribing behavior, or formulary status. All members of PhRMA have agreed to implement this new code.[16]

Pharmaceutical manufacturers are implementing the PhRMA code by developing a process of quality communications with their sales force by providing training on the code, company specific ethics and compliance tools, and OIG guidance. These changes should create a focus on quality medical science and education.

Accreditation Council for Continuing Medical Education and Accreditation Council for Pharmacy Education

The Accreditation Council for Continuing Medical Education (ACCME), the accrediting body for continuing physician education, approved rules relating to physician speakers with ties to pharmaceutical companies. Under these regulations, physicians are not able to present anecdotal experience with that company's drug at continuing medical education classes. Specifically, this ruling suggests that systematic clinical trials would replace anecdotal observations and any review of scientific literature would have to include both positive and negative studies.[17]

Accreditation Council for Pharmacy Education (ACPE) empowers continuing education providers to closely monitor the quality of programs for licensed pharmacists. Twenty-six criteria direct providers on program management, preparation, announcement, content, and format.

Food and Drug Administration

In addition to other responsibilities, the Food and Drug Administration (FDA) regulates direct to consumer advertising, mandating that these advertisements portray a fair balance of risks and benefits for medica-

Table 9-2
Key Points of PhRMA Code

Category	Description/Guidance
General interaction	These interactions should focus on informing health care professionals about scientific and educational information and supporting medical research to maximize patient benefits
Entertainment	Entertainment should not be included in interactions. Exceptions are allowed at venues conducive to providing scientific and educational information however spouses and guests are not allowed.
Continuing Education	Sponsors can provide support for conferences but not individual participants. Sponsors should not be involved specifically with the content.
Consultants	Legitimate consulting should utilize practitioners for their expertise to address a specific need but not as a token for prescribing
Gifts	Gifts with personal benefit only are not allowed. Items for health care benefit of patients are allowed if less than $100. Examples of allowable gifts might include office pens, notepads, and anatomical models.

tions. This includes information about the major risks of the product in accordance with the package insert.[18] The FDA also regulates the conduct of manufacturer sponsored clinical research in organized health-care settings. Specific regulations relating to these activities include Title 21 Code of Federal Regulations (CFR) Part 50, Protection of Human Subjects; Title 21 CRF Part 56, Institutional Review Boards; and Title 21 CRF Part 312, Investigational New Drug Application. The FDA publishes the Good Clinical Practice Consolidated Guideline with reference to the International Conference on Harmonisation of Technical Requirements for Registration of Pharmaceutical for Human Use. These guidelines address standards for designing, conducting, recording, and reporting clinical trials in the U.S., Japan, and the European Union. One additional regulation related to clinical research is overseen by the Department of Health and Human Services. This federal regulation, Title 45 CRF Part 46, outlines guidance for the protection of human subjects.[19]

Internal Industry Careers

Beyond the industry professions that practitioners see and interact with are thousands of employees. Pharmacists may fill not only the careers listed above that interact with health care practitioners, but also many other roles. The remainder of this chapter will provide some insight into these careers.

Business-to-business associates receive drug utilization and market share data to determine rebates based on business contracts with pharmaceutical companies. Individuals employed in this setting have an interest and background in business negotiation, managed care, formulary management, and/or pharmacoeconomics.

Clinical research administrators may oversee clinical trial activity from in-house either communicating directly by phone with the institutional site or by communications to the field monitor. Clinical or product development professionals while similar to clinical research professionals may be more involved with study design, communication of design to regulatory agencies, writing of patient summaries, and study result reporting. A variety of skills are useful for this position including verbal and written communication, time management, and medical knowledge.

Drug discovery begins with the early stages of molecular and chemical identification. Professionals in drug discovery may utilize skill sets such as organic and medicinal chemistry, pharmacology, pharmaceutics, pharmacogenomics, etc.

Health outcomes professionals utilize pharmacoeconomic backgrounds to create models and studies to investigate the benefits of a given pharmaceutical product. Health care practitioners might participate in Phase IV postmarketing studies, discuss economic considerations at their institution, or utilize this information when making formulary decisions.

Marketing professionals are generally unique when compared to their sales counterparts because they serve an internal function within their company. They may complete market research studies and analysis, develop branding and advertising materials, and/or design exhibit presentations. These professionals must understand competitors and be able to think creatively. Management positions also are open to health care practitioners including pharmacists who have strong leadership skills.

Project management is not unique to the pharmaceutical industry. Project management involves management of objectives, timelines, responsibilities, and final production for individual projects. Health-system pharmacists are prepared to interact with a variety of science and medical professionals including physicians, statisticians, research scientists, toxicologists, medical writers, etc., which prepare them for successful careers in project management within the pharmaceutical industry.

Quality assurance professionals serve a different function from individuals in quality control. Quality assurance involves working with clinical development, training and development, and regulatory components of the company to assure business operations function at an acceptable level of quality. The quality assurance departments may also include ethics, advisories, or other standards committees. Quality control professionals test chemical products and evaluate manufacturing processes.

Regulatory professionals interact with regulatory agencies throughout the world. Unlike a legal department, which contains mostly individuals with a doctor of jurisprudence degree (JD), regulatory professionals are more likely to have a science or medical background. These individuals must have an understanding of the medical environment and how a product might position itself in the market. They must also be able to communicate scientific and medical information to regulators to support positive product approval.

Scientific communications professionals are responsible for developing communication materials for scientific and medical information. Often this suggests a medical writing function including completion of study reports, regulatory documents, and protocols. These professionals may also be involved with scientific poster design for medical conferences and meetings.

Deciding If Industry Is for You?

When determining if a career in industry is an appropriate fit, individuals must evaluate their specific skills set. Each career track has a specific set of skills which must be matched with the pharmacist's background and experience. In light of this, a few general characteristics might apply to pharmacists who are successful and satisfied in the pharmaceutical industry. First, individuals should be comfortable with operating in the business environment. Professionals who are able to recognize the value of developing prescription medications in light of business standards can survive corporate competition and appropriately balance scientific and business needs. Second, one should be comfortable and confident even if the medical community might believe that all information provided by industry professionals is tainted and biased. Third, teamwork is often required especially for internal positions. Individuals who enjoy contributing to a team goal through communication and adaptability will fair well in an industry career.

Summary

Haines et al. expressed concern for the extent of relationships between the pharmaceutical industry and pharmacy practitioners. These authors suggest that while a pen may start as a trivial gift, it is easy to see the potential for more influence and eventual effect on advertising.[20] This position is not uncommon and has driven changes including the PhRMA Code of Ethics and OIG compliance monitoring. Negative public perceptions could force a series of legislative and regulatory changes, which might limit or eliminate the profits of pharmaceutical manufacturers. However, as health care professionals, we must consider how this could stifle innovation. This includes innovation for advances in therapies, roles for health care pharmacists, and a quality health care system.

By being informed professionals and consumers, pharmacists can manage the role a pharmaceutical company has in influencing potentially inappropriate care. Pharmacists' who seek guidance on management of relationships with the pharmaceutical industry can utilize ASHP's *Guidelines on Pharmacists' Relationships with Industry*. This document addresses topics such as gifts and hospitality, continuing education, consultants and advisory arrangements, clinical research, disclosures, etc.[21] We should consider the education and skills of individuals employed by the pharmaceutical industry and afford them the same opportunity to prove their ability to balance their business and medical responsibilities to produce medications that improve many lives.

References

1. Riggins JL. Pharmaceutical industry as a career choice. *Am J Health-Syst Pharm.* 2002;59:2097–8.

2. Monaghan MS, Galt KA, Turner PD, et al. Student understanding of the relationship between the health professions and the pharmaceutical industry. *Teaching and Learning in Medicine.* 2003;15(1):14–20.

3. How do pharmaceutical companies choose sales representatives? Marysville, WA; 2004. Available at: www.medzilla.com. Accessed April 4, 2005.

4. Dwyer P. The duty of the pharmacist and the pharmaceutical industry. *Med Law.* 2003:495–516.

5. Zarowitz BJ, Muma B, Coggan P, et. al. Managing the pharmaceutical industry-health system interface. *Ann Pharmacother.* 2001;35:1661–8.

6. www.medzilla.com. Accessed April 4, 2005.

7. Lexchin J. Interactions between doctors and pharmaceutical sales representatives, editorial. *Can J Clin Pharm.* 2001;8(2).

8. Groves KE, Sketris I, Tett SE. Prescription drug samples—does this marketing strategy counteract policies for quality use of medicines? *Journal of Clinical Pharmacy and Therapeutics.* 2003;28:259–71.

9. American Society of Health-System Pharmacists. Position statement 9702: Drug Samples. Available at: www.ashp.org. Revised 2001.

10. American Society of Health-System Pharmacists. Position statement 9703: Manufacturer-Sponsored Patient-Assistance Programs. Available at: www.ashp.org. Revised 2001.

11. Ferris LE, Naylor CD. Physician remuneration in industry-sponsored clinical trials: the case for standardized clinical trial budgets. *CMAJ.* 2004;171(8):883–6

12. Lawrence KR. Journey to the pharmaceutical industry and back: my experience as a medical liaison. *Am J Health-Syst Pharm.* 2002;59:2098–9.

13. American Society of Health-System Pharmacists. Position statement 9701: Direct-to-Consumer Advertising of Pharmaceuticals. Available at: www.ashp.org. Revised 2001.

14. American Society of Hospital Pharmacists. ASHP guidelines for Pharmacists on the Activities of Vendors' Representatives in Organized Health Care Systems. *Am J Hosp Pharm.* 1994;51:520–1.

15. Office of Inspector General. Department of Health and Human Services. OIG compliance program guidance for pharmaceutical manufacturers. May 5, 2003. Available at: http://oig.hhs.gov.

16. PhRMA. PhRMA code on interactions with healthcare professionals. July 1, 2002. Available at: www.phrma.org.

17. Accreditation Council for Continuing Medical Education (ACCME). *The 2004 Updated ACCME standards for Commercial Support: Standards to Ensure the Independence of CME Activities.* September 2004.

18. Viale PH. What nurse practitioners should know about direct-to-consumer advertising of prescriptions medications. *Journal of the American Academy of Nurse Practitioners.* 2003;15(7):297–304.

19. American Society of Health-System Pharmacists. ASHP guidelines on clinical drug research. *Am J Health-Syst Pharm.* 1998;55:369–76.

20. Haines ST, Dumo P. Relationship between the pharmaceutical industry and pharmacy practitioners: undue influence? *Am J Health-Syst Pharm.* 2002:59:1871–4.

21. American Society of Hospital Pharmacists. ASHP guidelines on pharmacists' relationships with industry. *Am J Hosp Pharm.* 1992;49:154.

Chapter 10

Medication Therapy and Patient Care

Jannet M. Carmichael, William N. Jones

Introduction

You have arrived for your 10-hour pharmacist shift when new orders come from the Intensive Care Unit (ICU). The patient is being admitted with a diagnosis of acute coronary syndrome (ACS). A 75-year-old white male had substernal chest pain ("Feels like and elephant sitting on my chest"), radiating down his left arm for about 6 hours, called 911, and was brought to the hospital.

His past medical history includes hypertension, type 2 diabetes mellitus, hyperlipidemia, and cigarette smoking (35 pack-years). The medications continued from home were lisinopril 5 mg daily, metoprolol 12.5 mg twice daily, glyburide 5 mg bid, metformin 850 mg bid, rosiglitazone 4 mg bid, lovastatin 10 mg qd; added were enoxaparin 30 mg twice daily, nitroglycerin IV 5 mcg/min and titrated to relief of chest pain, clopidogrel 300 mg once and then 75 mg daily, antacid prn, $Mg(OH)_2$ prn, and acetaminophen prn. As the pharmacist, you quickly make sure the orders are filled accurately and are sent to the ICU by runner.

Later, while making rounds you review the medical chart and see the patient. The patient's physical examination shows an older man who looks his stated age, appears ashen, and diaphoretic. The vital signs on admission were the following: blood pressure (BP) 150/100 mm Hg, heart rate 102, temperature 98.6°F, weight 100 kg. Pertinent physical findings are bilateral rales in lung fields, 3+ pitting edema to mid-calf, heart is regular rate and rhythm, no murmurs, S3 noted, no S4. His ECG shows he did not have a myocardial infarction (MI). Laboratory tests are normal except his serum glucose is 211 mg/dL, and a lipid profile performed 3 months ago revealed a total cholesterol of 230 mg/dL, triglycerides 150 mg/dL, HDL cholesterol 40 mg/dL, and LDL cholesterol 160 mg/dL, and HbA1c performed 3 months ago was 9.5%.

Although he is ruled out for a MI, he is taken to the cardiac catheterization laboratory and found to have a 70% occlusion of proximal left main coronary artery and an 80–90% occlusion of the left anterior descending coronary artery. Two stents were inserted after the patient was given abciximab 0.25 mg/kg once and 0.125 mg/kg/hr for 12 hours. His chest pain was completely relieved and did not recur over the next 36 hours. His echocardiogram shows an ejection fraction (EF) of 35%.

He was discharged from the hospital several days later, with a diagnosis of ACS, hypertension, diabetes, hyperlipidemia and prescribed the following medications: lisinopril 5 mg daily, metoprolol 25 mg bid, glyburide 5 mg bid, metformin 850 mg bid, rosiglitazone 4 mg bid, lovastatin 10 mg qd, clopidogrel 75 mg daily. His BP is now 145/90 mm Hg and HR 80. He was still short of breath and had 2+ pitting edema and mild S3.

Definitions

Clinical Pharmacy—A health science specialty that embodies the application by pharmacists of the scientific principles of pharmacology, toxicology, pharmacokinetics, and therapeutics to the care of patients.[1]

Collaborative Drug Therapy Management—The provision of pharmaceutical care in a collaborative and supportive practice environment allowing a qualified pharmacist legal, regulatory and ethical responsibility to solve drug related problems when discovered.[2]

Medication Therapy Management (MTM)—A distinct service or group of services that optimize therapeutic outcomes for individual patients. MTM services are independent of, but can occur in conjunction with, the provision of a medication. (Defined for provisions of the Medicare Prescription Drug, Improvement and Modernization Act of 2003.)[3]

Pharmaceutical Care—A patient centered practice in which the practitioner assumes responsibility for a patient's drug-related needs and is held accountable for this commitment.[1]

Importance of Medication to Patient Care

An Institute of Medicine (IOM) report, *To Err is Human: Building a Safer Health System,* pointed out a serious problem faced by the entire health care system.[4] Between 44,000 and 98,000 Americans die each year in hospitals due to medication errors. A second IOM report, *Patient Safety: Achieving a New Standard of Care,* promoted comprehensive patient safety programs in all health care settings.[5] Others have shown that iatrogenic injury is common and that drugs are the largest contributor to injury.[6]

More than 1 million serious medication errors occur every year in U.S. hospitals.[7] Such errors include administration of the wrong drug, drug overdoses, and overlooked drug interactions and allergies. They occur for many reasons, including illegible handwritten prescriptions and decimal point errors. Computerized physician order entry (CPOE) is one means that assists in eliminating these latter errors. Pharmacy services should implement such CPOE programs. However, these systems should be integrated with the entire medical record to reduce the chance of a myriad of other errors.[8]

Not only are drug-related problems common, but they also tend to keep patients in the hospital longer and have a higher total cost of care. These events have a large total direct cost to the health care system. One adverse drug event adds more than $2,000 on average to the cost of hospitalization.[9] Schneider et al. found a total additional cost related to drug errors of about $1.5 million between 1992 and 1994.[10] Bates et al. estimated the cost to be nearly $2 million dollars per year for a 700-bed academic hospital.[11] Investigators have also shown that about one-third to more than one-half of the events are preventable and that outcomes are improved when pharmacists are actively and directly engaged in direct patient care.[11–13] Because of concerns about patient safety and the quality of health care, in particular about drug therapy, pharmacists have unprecedented opportunities to increase their value and significance. This chapter will address how individual pharmacists working in collaboration with other health care providers can contribute to improved patient outcomes.

Components of Medication Therapy in Patient Care

The roles of the pharmacist are to prevent disease, control symptoms of disease, slow disease progress, and cure disease.[14] Beginning in May 2005, the updated North American Pharmacist Licensure Examination (NAPLEX) examination will include the following domains of practice to become a registered pharmacist:

Area 1: Assess Safe and Effective Pharmacotherapy and Optimize Therapeutic Outcomes (54% of the exam)

Area 2: Assure Safe and Accurate Preparation and Dispensing of Medications (35% of the exam)

Area 3: Provide Health Care Information and Promote Public Health (11% of the exam)

It seems clear that the public should rely on pharmacists to assist in making sure their medication therapy is safe and effective. However, using a systematic approach to the delivery of this care is critical to optimizing the outcome for each patient.[15,16] The case presentation above is used to provide a backdrop to discuss how pharmacists in institutional practice can contribute to positive clinical outcomes.

Preventative Care

Recently, potential preventable hospitalizations, or hospitalizations that may be preventable with high quality primary and preventive care, have gained more attention.[17] The patient above was admitted to the hospital and had an invasive procedure at great emotional and monetary expense. Could this all have been prevented? It may have been possible to avoid this event by treating his blood pressure, diabetes, and hyperlipidemia more aggressively before admission. Health-system pharmacists need to consider how continuity can be improved or optimized between the hospital and home to prevent future problems.

Patient admission (entry), discharge (exit), or transfers from one level of care to another are always problem-prone points in the medication-use process. These transitions occur in all types of health systems—ambulatory care, behavioral health care, home care, office-based or outpatient surgery, long-term care as well as acute care facilities. These transition points allow an assessment of the patient's drug related needs to determine if drug related problems can be identified and resolved. Common causes for medication problems at this time include inaccurate or incomplete medication histories, such as not knowing the medication's name, dose, and use, and omission of herbal and OTC products a patient is taking.[18] If a patient is seeing several physicians and using many medications from several pharmacies this confounds the complications. In our patient above, the seriousness of his medical condition prevented direct patient interviews.

The Joint Commission on Accreditation of Healthcare Organizations (JCAHO) recognizes these weak links in the medication-use system. As a result they have included a new National Patient Safety Goal in their list of goals for 2005. Goal 8 states that medications must be accurately and completely reconciled across the continuum of care.[19] This represents just one of many important steps to assess patients at critical points to improve medication therapy and patients care.

Upon admission the above patient's medications were continued and others were added. All of these medications are common to the formulary of hospitals for treatment of ACS. Were the medications prescribed needed? Did the patient need any drugs that were not ordered? Were the doses selected appropriate for the patient's conditions?

The initial step in providing pharmaceutical care is to assess the patient's drug related needs by gathering and analyzing patient-specific information. In this case the patient has multiple problems including hypertension, diabetes, hyperlipidemia, and coronary artery disease. Hospitalizations resulting from poor outpatient control of all these problems are common and preventable. It also appears he has evidence of congestive heart failure. Cigarette smoking is a preventable health and social issue that has negative health effects.

Transfer from one level of care to another and discharge from the hospital create other potential opportunities for the pharmacist to assist in preventing medication problems and/or preventing future hospitalizations through identification and documentation of improved patient outcomes, goals, and endpoints. The Health Insurance Portability and Accountability Act of 1996 (HIPAA) supports this confidential communication of shared patient health information.[20]

Information describing your patient's presenting signs and symptoms, illness, conditions, or problems will focus much of the remaining pharmacotherapy assessment. Your patient's primary and most urgent complaint, questions, or illness serves as the beginning of that assessment.

Evidence-Based Medicine

The committee on Quality of Healthcare in America was formed in June 1998 and charged with developing a strategy that would substantially improve the quality of health care over the next 10 years. The report of that group, *Crossing the Quality Chasm*, states the goals of health care must be patient-centered, safe, effective, timely, efficient, and equitable.[21] The assessment of evidence-based medicine relies heavily on their safe and effective use. Drug therapy is increasingly complex, and pharmacists are uniquely trained to analyze reports

and guidelines to determine individual needs of their patients.

Our patient above has obvious health care needs at the time of admission since his blood pressure, diabetes, and cholesterol are all uncontrolled. There are clearly indications for drug therapy and he is taking medications for these diseases, but they are not effective in meeting optimum goals. These are problems that need to be addressed, but they may take a lower priority at the time of admission.

What should the initial goals of therapy and care plan be for a patient with ACS? Since high-risk patients can die, preventing death takes the highest priority. Although the pharmacist rapidly filled the orders, several issues related to appropriate drug selection could have been addressed. The first one is that aspirin was not prescribed for this patient. This is one of the key components to the evidence-based treatment guidelines of ACS recommended by the American College of Cardiology and American Heart Association (ACC/AHA).[22] A second issue is that full anticoagulation is needed for patients with ACS and the dose of enoxaparin given was one to prevent a thromboembolism.[23] A third issue is the dose of metoprolol taken upon admission and continued at discharge. Clearly, beta-blockers are part of optimal therapy in treating patients with a myocardial infarction. However, the doses used in clinical trials were high (i.e., target of 200 mg daily of metoprolol). Anderson et al. found that 15% of veterans discharged after a myocardial infarction reached the target dose at discharge and the dose was about half the target dose for the following 12 months. In 65% of the patients no evidence could be found to limit the dose.[24] All of these treatments are associated with reducing the morbidity and mortality of ACS. These types of omission errors can be resolved by all pharmacists.

Hypertension, hyperlipidemia, and diabetes are areas that were not addressed further on admission when outpatient medications were continued. His lower blood pressure might indicate that the patient was not taking his medications prior to admission. Despite this lower blood pressure, he is not at the minimum evidence-based goal blood pressure of <140/<90 mm Hg. The Joint National Committee for the Detection Evaluation and Treatment of High Blood Pressure (JNC-7) has the recommendation for the blood pressure to be <130/<80 mm Hg for patients with diabetes.[25] Patients with diabetes often have concurrent hyperlipidemia and the National Cholesterol Education

Program Adult Treatment Panel III recommendations for diabetic patients is to have an LDL cholesterol <100 mg/dL.[26] Diabetes leads to coronary heart disease, renal failure, and blindness. Controlling diabetes also needs to be undertaken. Despite three drugs, the patient has poorly controlled diabetes. Although the doses of glyburide and rosiglitazone are low, the chance of reaching the target HbA1c is low without treating the patient with insulin. Finally, no consideration was given to his heart failure possibly being related to rosiglitazone.

It is clear that comprehensive and current evidence-based drug information is critical to the practice of patient care. However, no individual can expect to continually keep pace with all the areas of clinical practice. It is, therefore, important that each provider adopt a philosophy and ability to remain a life-long learner. In addition we must create systems in institutions where health care providers can develop the skills needed to access and apply needed drug information. This means not only having the current drug information but also knowing how to apply it to each patient under care. Institutional pharmacists should consider developing their own journal clubs to help each other keep pace with the rapidly expanding knowledge base being published. Publishing newsletters regarding new therapy or improving therapy is another way to share information within the hospital that will help optimize patient outcomes.

The implementation and application of evidence-based care to patients may be even more complex. Even after the information is known and determined to be appropriate for a patient, getting the patient the correct therapy and assuring that he/she takes it regularly requires many additional steps. Therefore, it is not enough to identify a drug related problem, but the problem must be solved and change implemented for long enough to see a positive outcome. In addition, if the original outcome is not optimal the patient will need additional assessment.

Returning to the concepts of pharmaceutical care and how they relate to medication therapy of a hospitalized patient, one may observe that the immediate symptoms were relieved. However, the missed opportunities to slow disease progression and possibly prevent disease in the future were inadequately addressed. Except for not prescribing aspirin, this patient did have other therapy prescribed that would meet the qualitative elements of the ACC/AHA guidelines for ACS.

This demonstrates the continuous nature of the care process. Once acute outcomes are met for the patient's most immediate needs, the process of assessment, establishing additional goals of therapy and follow-up begins again.

Pharmacist's Role to Provide Patient Care

The pharmacist's role in providing drug therapy includes many elements. "Assess Safe and Effective Pharmacotherapy and Optimize Therapeutic Outcomes" and "Assure Safe and Accurate Preparation and Dispensing of Medications" are the two largest domains of pharmacy practice as defined by NAPLEX.

Pharmacists can improve the quality of drug therapy by

1. identifying and resolving drug therapy needs through direct patient care
2. improving the organizational structures through which drug therapy is provided
3. creating medication-use systems that regularly evaluate the performance of 1 and 2

Pharmacists will take a leadership role to continuously improve and redesign the medication-use process with the goal of achieving significant advances in patient safety, health-related outcomes, prudent use of resources, and efficiency. Other chapters of this text will cover improved organizational structures in detail. However, the institution's role to support patient centered practice by pharmacists should not be overlooked or underestimated. Without timely, safe, and accurate drug distribution the best direct patient care services will be compromised. Developing and managing medication distribution and control systems that maximize the use of technology and technicians is essential to free the pharmacist to perform direct patient care functions. In addition, the management of medication-use systems such as a formulary, contracting, criteria for drug use, and medication-use evaluation to improve quality and cost effective care is also essential.[27] Re-engineering hospitals to position pharmacists to solve drug related problems and evaluate outcomes is just as important as providing that care.

Individual pharmacist's clinical functions must be organized around patient needs and directed at outcomes.[28] The professional practice of pharmacy has been described as clinical pharmacy, pharmaceutical care, collaborative drug therapy management, and medication therapy management.[29–31] All these terms add essential clarity about the process components of a pharmacist's participation in a team of health care professionals working together to provide quality care in health systems.

Pharmaceutical Care

The concept of patient centered care practiced by pharmacists in institutional practice was introduced in 1980: "Pharmaceutical care includes the determination of the drug needs for a given individual and the provision not only of the drug required but also the necessary services (before, during or after treatment) to assure optimally safe and effective therapy. It includes a feedback mechanism as a means of facilitating continuity of care by those who provide it."[32]

For pharmaceutical care to occur, individual practitioners must take personal responsibility for optimal outcomes of drug therapy. Although pharmacists developed the idea of pharmaceutical care it is not *about* pharmacists. It is an idea about a system for the delivery of patient care that can be done by any qualified practitioner. Clinical pharmacy is an essential component in the delivery of pharmaceutical care. The biggest difference from traditional pharmacy practice in hospitals and the pharmaceutical care model is the former is often indirectly providing products and services to patients that support care. Pharmaceutical care requires direct interaction by pharmacists with patients and health care professions to focus on improved outcomes of care. Clinical practice by pharmacists should constitute the main practice of pharmacy rather than an add-on service or some optional service offered to only a few patients. Pharmacists must be creative in finding ways to maximize the time they have to interact directly with patients and health care professionals.

Great, so how do individual pharmacists practice pharmacy clinically? It is important to have a systematic practice process so that all steps in the process are included. Table 10-1 provides an overview of the activities and responsibilities in the patient care process. This includes patient assessment, developing a care plan, and a follow-up evaluation.[33] This process requires that the pharmacist accept responsibility for identifying the patient's drug-related problems (Table 10-2). It is also requires activities that are practiced and steps that are followed so many times repetitively, that they become ingrained into all the pharmacist's activities. This is particularly important for pharmacy interns, students during clerkships, and residents completing clinical experiences. To improve skills in delivering pharmaceutical care requires repetition and practice.

Patient Pharmacotherapy Assessment

It may seem obvious, but the type of relationships required to deliver patient care by a pharmacist requires the pharmacist to see and assess the patient. The first activity in the assessment process is to make contact with and commit to the patient. The initial assessment occurs when the pharmacist interviews the patient personally either on admission or transfer, when a medication is needed, or at other times when the patient is stable and alert. At these times relevant patient-specific information used in making decisions about drug therapy is collected, analyzed, and documented. Additional patient contact should continue throughout the stay and at the time of discharge.

The needs of the patient require gathering information from the patient, other health care professionals, and the medical record. Activities of assessment require a pharmacist to collect, synthesize, and interpret the relevant information available.

Obviously, patient demographics, past medical history, the medication history, and past and current laboratory data are critical elements. Physical examination and imaging data are important elements that the pharmacist needs to understand and integrate into the treatment plan. For example, the pharmacist should know that a patient with pneumonia being treated with an antibiotic has had a chest radiograph and be able to understand the radiologist's impression noting consolidation. In Table 10-3 are questions that help to systematically assess drug therapy and to optimize care.

Identification and Resolution of Drug-Related Problems

The pharmacist's goal is to identify, prevent, and resolve any potential or actual drug-related problem. If we again refer to the case above, major types of drug related problems can be observed. Drugs were not given that were indicated (as in our case with aspirin). Patients may be prescribed a drug that is not indicated (giving rosiglitazone which created additional fluid accumulation in a heart failure patient). This patient may have been given ineffective drug therapy (based on the admission blood pressure, lipid levels, and glucose results). The dose can be too low (as in our patient with metoprolol and enoxaparin) or too high. Adverse drug reactions can occur as a result of taking the wrong drug or having a drug-drug or drug-food interaction (a patient taking antacids at the same time as an oral fluoroquinolone). Not taking the drug prescribed could be a persistence and adherence to drug

Table 10-1

Activities and Responsibilities in the Patient Care Process

	Activities	Responsibilities
Assessment	Meet the patient	Establish the therapeutic relationship
	Elicit relevant information from the patient	Determine who your patient is as an individual by learning about the reason for the encounter, the patient's demographics, medication experience, and other clinical information
	Make rational drug therapy decisions using the Pharmacotherapy Workshop	Determine whether the patient's drug-related needs are being met (indication, effectiveness, safety, compliance), identify drug therapy problems
Care plan	Establish goals of therapy	Negotiate and agree upon endpoints and timeframe for pharmacotherapies with the patient
	Select appropriate interventions for: resolution of drug therapy problems achievement of goals of therapy prevention of drug therapy problems	Consider therapeutic alternatives Select patient-specific pharmacotherapy Consider nondrug interventions Educate patient
	Schedule a follow-up evaluation	Establish a schedule that is clinically appropriate and convenient for the patient
Follow-up evaluation	Elicit clinical and/or lab evidence of actual patient outcomes and compare them to the goals of therapy to determine the effectiveness of drug therapy	Evaluate effectiveness of pharmacotherapy
	Elicit clinical and/or lab evidence of adverse effects to determine safety of drug therapy	Evaluate safety of pharmacotherapy Determine patient compliance
	Document clinical status and any changes in pharmacotherapy that are required	Make a judgment as to the clinical status of the patient's condition being managed with drug therapy
	Assess patient for any new drug therapy problems	Identify any new drug therapy problems and their cause
	Schedule the next follow-up evaluation	Provide continuous care

therapy drug related problem (noncompliance). This last drug therapy problem is an extremely common one and critical to medication management. The best pharmacological treatment plan will be ineffective if patients do not continue to take medications. In one large database analysis, only 52% of patients prescribed lipid-lowering therapy continued to fill prescriptions 5 years after the initial prescription.[34] Other studies show similar low persistence rates over time.[35–38] Ensuring medication compliance is an essential role for all members of the health care team, but especially the pharmacist. At the time of hospital discharge, pharmacists should educate their patients about the impor-

tance of the long-term need for medications. Once in the community, the issues of persistence again become evident. If patients fail to continue medications they may have recurrence of disease. The pharmacist has a unique position in monitoring persistence and adherence. This requires more than the traditional model of practice that is often indirectly interacting with patients and health care providers.

Once the data are gathered, they should be organized such that all the important elements are connected. The pharmacist will make rational drug therapy decisions using the information gathered, list and rank the patient's drug related problems, and prioritize them.

Table 10-2
Categories and Common Causes of Drug Therapy Problems

Drug Therapy Problem	Common Causes of Drug Therapy Problems
Unnecessary drug therapy	▪ There is no valid medical indication for the drug therapy at this time ▪ Multiple drug products are being used for a condition that requires single drug therapy ▪ The medical condition is more appropriately treated with nondrug therapy ▪ Drug therapy is being taken to treat an avoidable adverse reaction associated with another medication ▪ Drug abuse, alcohol use, or smoking is causing the problem
Need for additional drug therapy	▪ A medical condition requires the initiation of drug therapy ▪ Preventive drug therapy is required to reduce the risk of developing a new condition ▪ A medical condition requires additional pharmacotherapy to attain synergistic or additive effects
Ineffective drug	▪ The drug is not the most effective for the medical problem ▪ The medical condition is refractory to the drug product ▪ The dosage form of the drug product is inappropriate ▪ The drug product is not an effective product for the indication being treated
Dosage too low	▪ The dose is too low to produce the desired response ▪ The dosage interval is too infrequent to produce the desired response ▪ The drug interaction reduces the amount of active drug available ▪ The duration of drug therapy is too short to produce the desired response
Adverse drug reaction	▪ The drug product causes an undesirable reaction that is not dose-related ▪ A safer drug product is required due to risk factors ▪ A drug interaction causes an undesirable reaction that is not dose-related ▪ The dosage regimen was administered or changed too rapidly ▪ The drug product causes an allergic reaction ▪ The drug product is contraindicated due to risk factors
Dosage too high	▪ Dose is too high ▪ The dosing frequency is too short ▪ The duration of drug therapy is too long ▪ A drug interaction occurs resulting in a toxic reaction to the drug product ▪ The dose of the durg was administered too rapidly
Noncompliance	▪ The patient does not understand the instructions ▪ The patient prefers not to take the medication ▪ The patient forgets to take the medication ▪ The drug product is too expensive for the patient ▪ The patient cannot swallow or self-administer the drug product appropriately ▪ The drug product is not available for the patient

Table 10-3
Drug Therapy Assessment Worksheet

Question	Assessment
Correlation between medical illness and drug therapy?	Treated for hypertension, diabetes, and hyperlipidemia. Smoking cessation not addressed (or do not know).
Appropriate drug selection?	Three oral hypoglycemic drugs are not controlling diabetes. Aspirin was not prescribed.
Correct dosing regimen?	Dose of lisinopril, lovastatin, metoprolol, glyburide, rosiglitazone are low. Targets not reached. Dose of enoxaparin is too low to fully anticoagulate the patient.
Therapeutic duplication?	Three drugs for diabetes. This could be acceptable.
Allergy or ADR?	More information is needed. Does the patient have heart failure induced by rosiglitazone?
Drug interaction? (actual or potential)	No problem
Failure to receive therapy?	No aspirin ordered on admission. More information is needed. Pharmacist does not have enough information to assess persistence.
Cost-effective?	Clearly not cost-effective to prescribe drugs that fail to manage disease. Can he afford medication copay? Does he even have insurance?
Patient's knowledge of therapy?	More information is needed. Pharmacist has not talked to the patient.

Source: Reference 15.

The drug therapy assessment (Table 10-3) is an organized way to address each of the problems of a patient.

Developing a Care Plan and Goals of Therapy

Establishing goals of therapy and a care plan for the patient is important to implement the patient's drug therapy needs. The treatment goals in our patient should include reducing the symptoms of heart failure in the short-term (and having the patient discharged home) and a long-term goal of prolonging life (hopefully a high quality lifestyle). Parameters to measure for a patient with congestive heart failure (on the flow sheet) include the weight, blood pressure, serum electrolytes, some physical examination notes (e.g., edema notes from the physician), and the specific drug therapy that would include the doses of medication. The endpoints are specific targets to reach and may change for each individual. The rationale to have all of these elements on a flow sheet is to visualize changes that are occurring over time. An example of a patient's flow sheet having congestive heart failure is included in Table 10-4.

Next the pharmacist will determine feasible pharmacotherapeutic alternatives to achieve these goals. A list of therapeutic modalities that could achieve the desired outcomes for this patient is needed. Selection of the *best* pharmacotherapeutic alternative with this patient in mind brings us face-to-face with the evidence-based approach to medicine. Part of this process involves selection of appropriate plans that will resolve identified drug therapy problems, achieve new goals of therapy, and prevent new drug therapy problems.

Follow-Up Evaluation

Developing a care plan requires that a monitoring plan be in place to determine if the pharmacotherapeutic plan is reaching the desired outcomes. In the example, one can observe the changes that occurred over time in the patient's blood pressure, weight, symptoms, and signs of heart failure as the drug therapy changed. Often, flow sheets developed by pharmacists only include laboratory data but may not include information related to the treatment. The flow sheets can

Table 10-4

Example of Congestive Heart Failure Patient Flow Sheet

Date	Admission	Day 1	Day 2	Day 3	Day 4	Day 5	Day 6	Day 7
WT (kg)	87	87	86.5	85	84	83	82	81
BP	120/80	120/80	115/75	115/75	115/75	115/75	115/75	115/75
Na/Cl	141/100	141/100	140/100	139/98	140/98	139/97	140/96	139/95
K/CO$_2$	4.5/25	4.4/26	4.3/25	4.3/26	4.2/26	4.1/27	4.0/27	4.0/28
Furosemide	0	20 mg	40 mg	80 mg	80 mg	80 mg	80 mg	80 mg
Lisinopril	0	2.5 mg	5 mg	10 mg	10 mg	10 mg	10 mg	10 mg
Edema	4+	3+	3+	2+	2+	1+	1+	1+
Symptoms	SOB rest	SOB rest	SOB↓	SOB↓↓	SOB↓↓	SOB↓↓	SOB 0	SOB 0

integrate the laboratory data with signs and symptoms of a specific disease and the drug therapy. Placing all of the data into the columns allows the authors to easily observe changes that are temporally related to the drug therapy. It might be suggested that many times pharmacists take snapshots of drug therapy rather than observing the entire video. Especially in an acute care setting, continually monitoring therapy is critical to prioritization of drug related problems.

It is easily noted that the weight and the signs and symptoms decreased temporally related to the increase in diuretic dose. Adding the angiotensin converting enzyme inhibitor made a small change in the blood pressure but not enough to alter the plan to reach a dose of 10 mg daily. Finally, as the dose of furosemide increased over time, the serum potassium fell slightly. By integrating all of the components of care into one flow sheet, the pharmacist minimizes the fragmentation that may happen by only observing the drugs or only the laboratory tests. Since the goal of therapy includes reducing symptoms, it is important to know that specific diuretic and angiotensin receptor antagonist doses reduced symptoms. The long-term outcomes of optimal drug therapy should slow disease progression. It is also possible to predict when an intervention is needed by comparing the changes in laboratory tests in association with the drug therapy.

It may seem evident that forming a drug-monitoring plan is necessary to determine if the pharmacotherapeutic plan is meeting the desired outcomes. In our example the patient is in an acute care setting with constant monitors and probes to provide feedback. All too often in chronic therapy or in transfer to a less

acute care model, this step is never performed. Practitioners often loose patients to follow-up or fail to identify the therapeutic outcome expected at the time a new drug is added to address a new problem. This has led to a growing problem of adding but never stopping medication, multiple drug use, drug interactions, and additional drug related problems especially in the elderly.

The pharmacist should reconcile a complete list of medications, identify drug related problems, document care, and expected outcomes for the next pharmacist or other health care providers. Providing the patient with a written list of medications at the time of discharge is helpful for the patient and all community health care providers. Just as important is documenting the expected outcomes from therapy and where in the continuum of follow-up and monitoring the process has come.[39]

Permission from the physician or others responsible for the patient's care may also be required to implement changes that resolve problems found. A collaborative relationship with all those who participate in the patient's care is beneficial. This type of pharmacist practice is aimed at the patient but can also benefit physicians and others caring for the patient as well.

Note the pharmacist need not perform all the steps in the pharmaceutical care process independently.[40] Many are done in collaboration with the entire health care team and system. However, the relationship established with the patient to provide that care assumes the pharmacist will take responsibility to make sure all steps are performed in a timely fashion to improve the patient's quality of life.

Selected nondisease factors can impact the pharmaceutical care plan and should be considered. Since the kidneys or liver metabolize most drugs, monitoring commonly addressed by pharmacists include renal and/or hepatic dysfunction. Other issues that could impact the pharmaceutical care plan include ethnicity and religion (e.g., patient not wanting a blood transfusion), cognitive function, patient preferences, and health beliefs/insurance coverage. These issues cannot be ignored in a patient-centered model of care delivery. Pharmacists may have evidence to support a particular treatment, but the patient may have selected not to accept that course of action. The evolving view of health care places the patient at the center of a new system with more integration and collaboration, as opposed to fragmentation. The requirements for pharmacist participation include a collaborative practice environment with access to patients, access to all pertinent medical records, knowledge, skills and abilities to manage drug therapy, time to document activities of care, and compensation. When all these systems are present patients will achieve better drug therapy outcomes.

Many barriers are in place that prevent pharmaceutical care from occurring. These include allocation of pharmacists' time to distributive functions; inadequate manpower or technology; location of the pharmacist in relationship to the patient (e.g., the pharmacist might be inside the satellite pharmacy behind the locked door rather than on the patient wards); and legal and regulatory issues that fail to maximize the pharmacist's time with patients.

It will take leadership and vision to continuously improve and redesign the medication-use process and meet the drug therapy needs of our patients. Meeting our goals of achieving advances in patient safety, improving health-related outcomes from therapy, prudent use of resources, and improving efficiency need to be the measures of our success.

Value of Clinical Pharmacy Services

There is little doubt that pharmacists provide cost-effective care. The American College of Clinical Pharmacy (ACCP) has summarized the value of the pharmacist. Over approximately 25 years, three different ACCP task forces have reviewed 131 original articles regarding the clinical and economic value of pharmacists' clinical services.[41-43] These articles have clearly demonstrated improved clinical outcomes at the same or a lower cost. The categories of clinical and economic impact were categorized into disease state management, general pharmacotherapy management, target drug programs, patient education, and prescribe education programs. Areas such as improved antibiotic utilization, pharmacokinetic services, making rounds with physicians, improved analgesia, and reducing laboratory tests are examples of the numerous studies. The cost savings and avoidance were measured in some of these studies and the mean ratio of savings/avoidance compared to the pharmacist cost ranged from 1.1 to 75. These studies do fit the model of Kissick in that pharmacists have documented the quality of the care provided and the lower costs associated with the services, programs, and interventions.[44]

Two surveys of over 1,000 hospitals have been completed addressing the practices of pharmacists in hospitals. Mortality is statistically lower among the hospitals with clinical research programs, drug information services, programs where medication histories are actively obtained, and where CPR teams include a pharmacist.[45,46] In one of the earliest studies assessing outcomes, Bjornson et al. demonstrated that the duration of hospitalization was shorter and the mortality was lower when medicine and surgery teams had pharmacists participate in rounds.[12]

Summary

Pharmacists can improve the quality of drug therapy by improving the organizational structures through which drug therapy is provided and by providing direct patient care. The clinical, societal, and economic case to prevent and resolve drug-related morbidity and mortality is very strong. Pharmacists are uniquely positioned and trained to work collaboratively with other health professionals to address the drug related needs of patients and improve outcomes from therapy. However, changes to the current system of health care delivery are needed to maximize outcomes.

Direct patient care functions of the pharmacist should be the goal of all pharmacy practice. The ability to use the unique knowledge, skills, and ability of the contemporary pharmacist to work within the health care system is a prerequisite for success. Success lies in redesign of the medication-use process by the institution to support patient centered care and position all pharmacists to meet the drug therapy needs of patients by identifying and resolving drug related problems and preventing drug related mortality. Pharmacists should use the evidence of benefit to justify the broad implementation of pharmaceutical care to improve medication use in society.

References

1. Cipolle RJ, Strand LM, Morley PC. *Pharmaceutical Care Practice*. New York: McGraw-Hill; 1998:1.

2. Carmichael JM. Collaborative practice agreements (collaborative drug therapy management). *Encyclopedia of Clinical Pharmacy*. New York: Marcel Dekker, Inc.; 2003:199–206.

3. American Pharmacist Association website. Additional information on MTMS. Available at: http://www.aphanet.org/AM/Template.cfm?Section=APhA_Resources_Medicare&Template=/CM/ContentDisplay.cfm&ContentID=1681. Accessed February 5, 2005.

4. Kohn LT, Corrigan JM, Donaldson MS, eds. Errors in health care: a leading cause of death and injury. In: *To Err is Human: Building a Safer Health System*. Committee on Quality of Health Care in America, Institute of Medicine. Washington, DC: National Academy Press; 1999:26–48.

5. Institute of Medicine. *Patient Safety: Achieving a New Standard of Care*. Washington DC: National Academy Press; 2004.

6. Leape LL, Brennan TA, Laird N, et al. The nature of adverse events in hospitalized patients. Results of the Harvard Medical Practice Study II. *N Engl J Med*. 1991;324:377–84.

7. Birkmeyer JD, Dimick JB. *Leapfrog Safety Standards: Potential Benefits of Universal Adoption*. Washington, DC: The Leapfrog Group; 2004.

8. American Society of Health-System Pharmacists. ASHP guidelines on preventing medication errors in hospitals. *Am J Health-Syst Pharm*. 1993;50:305–14.

9. Classen DC, Pestotnik SL, Evans RS, et al. Adverse drug events in hospitalized patients: excess length of stay, extra costs and attributable mortality. *JAMA*. 1997;277:301–6.

10. Schneider PJ, Gift MG, Lee YP, et al. Cost of medication-related problems at a university hospital. *Am J Health-Syst Pharm*. 1995;52:2415–8.

11. Bates DW, Spell N, Cullen DJ, et al. The costs of adverse drug events in hospitalized patients. Adverse Drug Events Prevention Study Group. *JAMA*. 1997;277:307–11.

12. Bjornson DC, Hiner WO Jr, Potyk RP, et al. Effect of pharmacists on health care outcomes in hospitalized patients. *Am J Hosp Pharm*. 1993;50:1875–84.

13. Leape LL, Cullen DJ, Clapp MD, et al. Pharmacist participation on physician rounds and adverse drug events in the intensive care unit. *JAMA*. 1999;282:267–70. Erratum in: *JAMA*. 2000;283:1293.

14. American Society of Health-System Pharmacists. ASHP statement on pharmaceutical care. *Am J Health-Syst Pharm*. 1993;50:1720–3.

15. Campbell S, Jones WN. *How to Develop a Treatment Plan. Clinical Skills Module #4*. Bethesda, MD: American Society of Health-System Pharmacists; 1994.

16. American Society of Health-System Pharmacists. ASHP guidelines on a standardized method for pharmaceutical care. *Am J Health-Syst Pharm*. 1996;53:1713–6.

17. Preventable hospitalizations: window into primary and preventive care. 2000. Available at: http://www.ahrq.gov/data/hcup/factbk5/factbk5a.htm. Accessed December 21, 2004.

18. Gleason KM, Groszek JM, Sullivan D, et al. Reconciliation of discrepancies in medication histories and admission orders of newly hospitalized patients. *Am J Health-Syst Pharm*. 2004;61:1689–95.

19. Joint Commission on Accreditation of Healthcare Organizations. National patient safety goals for 2005. Rationale and interpretive guidelines. Issued September 10, 2004. Available at: http://www.jcaho.org/accredited+organizations/patient+safety. Accessed February 2005.

20. U.S. Department of Health and Human Services. Protecting the privacy of patients' health information HHS Fact Sheet. April 14, 2003. Available at: http://www.hhs.gov/news/facts/privacy.html. Accessed December 20, 2004.

21. Institute of Medicine (IOM). *Crossing the Quality Chasm: A New Health System for the 21st Century*. Washington, DC: National Academy Press; 2001.

22. Braunwald E, Antman EM, Beasley JW, et al. ACC/AHA 2002 guideline update for the management of patients with unstable angina and non-ST-segment elevation myocardial infarction—summary article: a report of the American College of Cardiology/American Heart Association task force on practice guidelines (Committee on the Management of Patients With Unstable Angina). *J Am Coll Cardiol*. 2002;40:1366–74.

23. Hirsh J, Raschke R. Heparin and low-molecular-weight heparin: the seventh ACCP conference on antithrombotic and thrombolytic therapy. *Chest*. 2004;126:188S–203S.

24. Anderson SC, Jones WN, Evanko TM. Dosage of beta-adrenergic blockers after myocardial infarction. *Am J Health-Syst Pharm*. 2003;60:2471–4.

25. Chobanian AV, Bakris GL, Black HR, et al. The seventh report of the Joint National Committee on Prevention, Detection, Evaluation, and Treatment of High Blood Pressure: the JNC 7 report. *JAMA*. 2003;289:2560–72. Epub 2003 May 14. Erratum in: *JAMA*. 2003;290:197.

26. Executive summary of the third report of The National Cholesterol Education Program (NCEP) Expert Panel on detection, evaluation, and treatment of high blood cholesterol in adults (adult treatment panel III). *JAMA*. 2001;285:2486–97.

27. American Society of Health-System Pharmacists. ASHP guidelines: minimum standards for pharmacies in hospitals. *Am J Health-Syst Pharm*. 1995;52:2711–7.

28. Hepler CD. Clinical pharmacy, pharmaceutical care, and the quality of drug therapy. *Pharmacotherapy.* 2004;24:1491–8.

29. Bosso JA. Clinical pharmacy and pharmaceutical care. *Pharmacotherapy.* 2004;24:1499–500.

30. Hepler CD, Strand LM. Opportunities and responsibilities in pharmaceutical care. *Am J Pharm Ed.* 1989;53(suppl):S7–15.

31. Carmichael JM, O'Connell MB, Devine B, et al. Collaborative drug therapy management by pharmacists: a white paper from the American College of Clinical Pharmacy. *Pharmacotherapy.* 1997;17(5):1050–61.

32. Brodie DC, Parish PA, Poston JW. Societal needs for drugs and drug related services. *Am J Pharm Ed.* 1980;44:276–8.

33. Cipolle RJ, Strand LM, Morley, PC. *Pharmaceutical Care Practice: The Clinician's Guide.* 2nd ed. New York: McGraw Hill; 2004.

34. Avorn J, Monette J, Lacour A, et al. Persistence of use of lipid-lowering medications: a cross-national study. *JAMA.* 1998;279:1458–62.

35. Benner JS, Glynn RJ, Mogun H, et al. Long-term persistence in use of statin therapy in elderly patients. *JAMA.* 2002;288:455–61.

36. Morgan SG, Yan L. Persistence with hypertension treatment among community-dwelling BC seniors. *Can J Clin Pharmacol.* 2004 Fall;11(2):e267–73. Epub 2004 Dec 13.

37. Osterberg L, Blaschke T. Adherence to medication. *N Engl J Med.* 2005;353:487–97.

38. American Society of Health-System Pharmacists. ASHP guidelines on documenting pharmaceutical care in patient medical records. *Am J Health-Syst Pharm.* 2003;60:705–7.

39. Carmichael JM. Do pharmacists need prescribing privileges to implement pharmaceutical care? *Am J Health-Syst Pharm.* 1995;52:1699–701.

40. Willett MS, Bertch KE, Rich DS, et al. Prospectus on the economic value of clinical pharmacy services. *Pharmacotherapy.* 1989;9:45–56.

41. Schumock GT, Meek PD, Ploetz PA, et al. and the Publications Committee of the American College of Clinical Pharmacy. Economic evaluations of clinical pharmacy services: 1988–1995. *Pharmacotherapy.* 1996;16:1188–1208.

42. Schumock GT, Butler MG, Meek PD, et al. for the 2002 Task Force on Economic Evaluation of Clinical Pharmacy Services of the American College of Clinical Pharmacy. Evidence of the economic benefit of clinical pharmacy services: 1996–2000. *Pharmacotherapy.* 2003;23:113–32.

43. Kissick W. *Medicine's Dilemma Infinite Needs Versus Finite Resources.* New Haven, CT: Yale University Press; 1994.

44. Bond CA, Raehl CL, Pitterle ME, et al. Health care professional staffing, hospital characteristics, and hospital mortality rates. *Pharmacotherapy.* 1999;19:130–8.

45. Bond CA, Raehl CL, Franke T. Clinical pharmacy services, pharmacy staffing, and the total cost of care in U.S. hospitals. *Pharmacotherapy.* 2000;20:609–21.

Chapter 11

Institutional Accreditation and Pharmacy Guidelines

Charles P. Coe, John P. Uselton

Introduction

This chapter describes and discusses institutional accreditation programs and pharmacy guidelines (including laws, rules, regulations, pharmacy professional standards, national codes and guidelines, and organization-specific requirements). Their use in improving performance and quality of care is emphasized. Major entities that are sources of standards affecting pharmacy practice are identified. (Table 11-1). The information is an overview and is not sufficient to ensure compliance. Sources for additional information and resources to assist in compliance are indicated.

Definitions

A number of terms are closely associated with institutional accreditation and pharmacy guidelines. Many are defined in context in the chapter; others are defined here. Definitions of some terms vary or are evolving. To assure currency and consistency, most of the following definitions are those of the Joint Commission on Accreditation of Healthcare Organizations® (Joint Commission™ or JCAHO®). The unreferenced definitions are those of the authors.

Accreditation—Determination by an accrediting body that an eligible health care organization complies with the accrediting body's applicable standards.[1]

Accrediting Body—An organization or entity that establishes standards for accreditation and determines that a health care organization complies with the standards.

Assessment—"For performance improvement, the systematic collection and review of patient-specific data."[2]

Certification—Confirmation by an entity that an organization complies with the entity's predetermined standards.

Certifying Body—An organization or entity that establishes standards for certification and determines that a health care organization complies with the standards.

Table 11-1
Some Major Entities That Are Sources of Standards Affecting Pharmacy Practice

Accrediting and Certifying Bodies

> Joint Commission on Accreditation of Healthcare Organizations
> American Osteopathic Association
> Centers for Medicare and Medicaid Services

Federal and State Government Entities

> Food and Drug Administration
> Drug Enforcement Administration
> Occupational Safety and Health Administration
> National Institute for Occupational Safety and Health
> Centers for Disease Control and Prevention
> Office for Civil Rights
> Agencies with Shared Responsibilities
> State Boards of Pharmacy

Nongovernmental Standards-Setting Entities

> United States Pharmacopeia
> National Fire Protection Association

Pharmacy Professional Organizations

> American College of Clinical Pharmacy
> American Pharmacists Association
> American Society of Consultant Pharmacists
> American Society of Health-System Pharmacists

Compliance—Meeting or adhering to the requirements of a standard, law, rule, or regulation.

Measurement—"The systematic process of data collection, repeated over time or at a single point in time."[3]

Outcome Measure—"A measure that indicates the result of the performance (or nonperformance) of a function(s) or process(es) such as the health outcome of a patient."[4] A pharmacy outcome measure might reflect the reduction of adverse events.

Performance Improvement—"The continuous study and adaptation of a health care organization's functions and processes to increase the probability of achieving desired outcomes and to better meet the needs of individuals and other users of services."[5]

Practice Guidelines—"Tools that describe processes found by clinical trials or by consensus opinion of experts to be the most effective in evaluating and/or treating a patient who has a specific symptom, condition, or diagnosis, or tools that describe a specific procedure. Synonyms include practice parameter, protocol, preferred practice pattern, and guideline."[6]

Process Measure—"A measure that focuses on a process that is designed to achieve a certain outcome."[4] A pharmacy process measure might focus on simplifying the steps in a medication distribution process.

Quality Control—"The performance of processes through which actual performance is measured and compared with goals and the difference is acted on."[7]

Quality Improvement—"...the collaborative and interdisciplinary approach to the continuous study and improvement of the processes of providing health care services to meet the needs of consumers and others." "Quality improvement involves identifying measuring, implementing, monitoring, analyzing, planning, and maintaining processes to ensure they function effectively."[8]

Quality of Care—"The degree to which health services for individuals and populations increase the likelihood of desired health outcomes and are consistent with current professional knowledge."[7]

Standard—"A statement that defines the performance expectations, structures, or processes that must be in place for an organization to provide safe and high quality care, treatment, and services."[9] Standards often reflect best practices (i.e., "recognized by a majority of professionals in a particular field.").[10] Best practices "are typically evidenced based and consensus driven."[10] This chapter uses standards in a broad context to include requirements and practice guidelines of accrediting bodies, governmental agencies, professional organizations, and other entities.

Structure Measure—"A measure that assesses whether organizational resources and arrangements are in place to deliver health care, such as the number, type, and distribution of medical personnel, equipment, and facilities."[4] A pharmacy structure measure might focus on ensuring adequate deployment of staff.

Survey—"A key component in the accreditation process, whereby a surveyor(s) conducts an on-site evaluation of an organization's compliance with … standards."[9]

Surveyor—"… a physician, nurse, administrator, laboratorian, or any other health care professional … who evaluates standards compliance, and provides education and consultation regarding standards compliance to surveyed organizations or networks."[9]

Institutional Accreditation and Certification Programs

Accreditation acknowledges that a hospital or other health care organization has met or exceeded the requirements of an accrediting body (e.g., the Joint Commission and the American Osteopathic Association [AOA]). Health care organizations stress the importance of maintaining their accredited status. Loss of accreditation can severely affect an organization's prestige and the organization may find it difficult to attract qualified staff. Many states consider accreditation in state licensure and may exempt accredited organizations from inspections. Accreditation standards sometimes become the expected legal standards of care and failure to comply might present legal difficulties for an organization.[11]

Organizations must be certified by the Centers for Medicare and Medicaid Services (CMS) to participate in the federal Medicare program. CMS confers *deemed status* on a health care organization when that organization is judged or determined to be in compliance with relevant Medicare requirements because it has been accredited by a voluntary organization whose standards and survey process are determined by CMS to be equivalent to those of the Medicare program.[12] Joint Commission and AOA accredited organizations are eligible automatically to participate in the Medicare program. Note that the Joint Commission and AOA accredit; Medicare certifies. Joint Commission accreditation, AOA accreditation, or CMS certification qualifies an organization to participate in the Medicare program.[13]

Joint Commission Accreditation

The Joint Commission is "An independent, not-for-profit organization dedicated to improving the safety and quality of care in organized health care settings. Founded in 1951, its members represent the American College of Physicians-American Society of Internal

Medicine, the American College of Surgeons, the American Dental Association, the American Hospital Association, the American Medical Association, the public, and the nursing profession. The Joint Commission engages in issues and activities concerning the advancement of health care safety and quality, including public policy initiatives, standards development, and accreditation and certification programs."[14] The Joint Commission is the principal accrediting body for the operation of hospitals and other health care organizations. The Joint Commission Internet website is http://www.jcaho.org.

Joint Commission Standards

The Joint Commission has established standards for acute care hospitals and other health care organizations. Acute care standards relevant to pharmacy include medication management, infection control, safety and security, education, and performance improvement. Each standard includes one or more elements of performance (i.e., "The specific performance expectations and/or structures or processes that must be in place in order for a hospital to provide safe, high-quality care, treatment, and services)."[15]

National Patient Safety Goals (NPSGs)

The Joint Commission's National Patient Safety Goals (NPSGs) are "...critical initiatives that health care organizations must examine to ensure patients are receiving safe, quality care."[16] "...all organizations are required to comply with the National Patient Safety Goals in which relevant services are provided."[17] NPSGs are established annually.[18]

Joint Commission Surveys

Any health care organization may request a survey (i.e., an evaluation) to determine its level of compliance with Joint Commission standards. Surveyors review key systems, assess compliance with relevant standards, and determine how well the organization provides care, treatment, and services. Surveyors also evaluate compliance with the requirements for the Joint Commission's NPSGs. If the Joint Commission finds an organization compliant with the standards, it lists the organization as *accredited*. Accreditation is for about 3 years. Note that the Joint Commission accredits health care organizations—not departments and services. Pharmacists must work with other departments and services in their organization to ensure that their organization complies with the standards.

Resources

ASHP's *Continuous Compliance with Joint Commission Standards* provides complete guidelines for compliance with standards relating to pharmacy and guidance in preparing for surveys.[19] The Joint Commission's *Accreditation Process Guide for Hospitals* helps hospitals understand the Joint Commission's accreditation process, how to apply for accreditation, what to expect during a survey, sample survey agendas, and other information needed to assure a smooth survey experience.[20] The Joint Commission publishes its standards in the *Comprehensive Accreditation Manual for Hospitals: The Official Handbook (CAMH)*. The *CAMH* includes accreditation policies and procedures, accreditation participation requirements, the latest standards, compliance information, how to gauge compliance, and a glossary of terms.[21] The Joint Commission also publishes standards for ambulatory care, behavioral health care, home care, long-term care, and other health care organizations. ASHP's *Continuous Compliance with Joint Commission Standards* provides complete guidelines for compliance with the NPSGs relating to pharmacy and medication use.[22]

AOA Accreditation

The American Osteopathic Association (AOA) "...is a member association representing more than 54,000 osteopathic physicians (D.O.s). The AOA serves as the primary certifying body for D.O.s, and is the accrediting agency for all osteopathic medical colleges and health care facilities. The AOA's mission is to advance the philosophy and practice of osteopathic medicine by excellence in education, research, and the delivery of quality, cost-effective healthcare within a distinct, unified profession."[23] Osteopathic hospitals and other health care organizations desiring accreditation by the AOA must comply with the requirements of the AOA's Healthcare Facilities Accreditation Program (HFAP).[24] The AOA Internet website is http://www.aoa-net.org.

AOA Standards

AOA HFAP standards address all departments and functions including pharmacy services and medication use. Some AOA standards are more prescriptive than Joint Commission standards. Therefore, compliance with Joint Commission standards is not necessarily sufficient to meet AOA standards (and vice versa).[25]

AOA Surveys

Any health care organization may request a survey (i.e., an evaluation) to determine its level of compliance with AOA HFAP standards. Surveyors review key systems, assess compliance with relevant standards, and determine how well the organization provides care, treatment, and services. If the AOA finds an organization compliant with the standards, it lists the organization as *accredited*. Accreditation is for three years.

Resources

ASHP's *Continuous Compliance with Joint Commission Standards* provides complete guidelines for compliance with AOA HFAP standards relating to pharmacy and medication use.[19] The AOA publishes its standards in the *Accreditation Requirements for Healthcare Facilities*.[26]

CMS Certification

CMS is a federal agency that …"administers the Medicare program and works in partnership with the States to administer Medicaid, the State Children's Health Insurance Program (SCHIP), and health insurance portability standards."[27] "CMS maintains oversight of the survey and certification of nursing homes and continuing care providers (including hospitals, nursing homes, home health agencies [HHAs], end-stage renal disease [ESRD] facilities, hospices, and other facilities serving Medicare and Medicaid beneficiaries)…."[28] The CMS Internet website is http://cms.hhs.gov.

Conditions of Participation (CoPs) and Standards

"CMS develops Conditions of Participation (CoPs) … that health care organizations must meet to participate in the Medicare and Medicaid programs." Each CoP consists of one or more standards that define the requirements for compliance. "These standards are used to improve quality and protect the health and safety of beneficiaries."[29]

The standards take into consideration that health care organizations are subject to state and federal laws and undergo substantial state inspection through licensure programs (hospital, pharmacy, fire and safety, health department, etc.). Therefore, CMS standards encourage practices in accordance with generally recognized principles and avoid conflict with state and federal laws, state licensure requirements, and Joint Commission and AOA standards.[30]

Although CMS conditions and standards are uniform throughout the country, interpretation and stringency of application vary considerably from state to state. However, if you meet your state board of pharmacy rules and regulations and your practices are gen-erally in accordance with Joint Commission standards, you should be in compliance with the conditions in most states.[30]

CMS Surveys

CMS surveys are conducted by a state agency (often the state health department) under contract to CMS. CMS surveys are usually conducted annually. Organizations do not need to comply with all standards to comply with a condition. However, they must comply with all conditions to be certified.[30]

Joint Commission and AOA accredited organizations are deemed eligible to participate in the programs and do not need additional CMS certification.[13] CMS selects a small percentage of Joint Commission and AOA accredited organizations to undergo validation surveys. Validation surveys are conducted to ensure that Joint Commission and AOA surveys are equivalent to CMS surveys.

Resources

ASHP's *Continuous Compliance with Joint Commission Standards* provides complete guidelines for compliance with CMS CoPs and standards relating to pharmacy.[19] The CoPs, survey protocol, and interpretative guidelines for the CoPs are available on the CMS Internet website.[31]

Federal and State Government Entities

Laws, regulations, and rules are closely related legal requirements. Laws are often imposed by an authority (e.g., federal or state government), regulations are governmental orders having the force of law, and rules address specific, limited situations. The legal requirements of federal and state entities may directly or indirectly affect the practice of pharmacy. Some examples are described below.

Food and Drug Administration (FDA)

The federal Food and Drug Administration (FDA) "…is responsible for protecting the public health by assuring the safety, efficacy, and security of human and veterinary drugs, biological products, medical devices, our nation's food supply, cosmetics, and products that emit radiation. The FDA is also responsible for advancing the public health by helping to speed innovations that make medicines and foods more effective, safer, and more affordable; and helping the public get the accurate, science-based information they need to use medicines and foods to improve their health."[32] The FDA implements and enforces the federal Food, Drug, and Cosmetic Act, sets labeling requirements for food, prescription and over-the-counter drugs and cosmetics, sets standards for investigational drug studies and product approval, and regulates and oversees the manufacturing and marketing of drugs.[33] The FDA Internet website is http://www.fda.gov.

Drug Enforcement Administration (DEA)

The Drug Enforcement Administration (DEA) enforces the federal controlled substances laws and regulations. The DEA investigates and prepares for the prosecution of those who violate controlled substances laws and regulations and enforces provisions of the controlled substances act relating to the manufacture, distribution, and dispensing of legally produced controlled substances.[34] Most states have a similar agency that enforces controlled substances laws at the state level. Security and accountability for controlled substances are significant challenges for health care organizations. The DEA Internet website is http://www.dea.gov.

Occupational Safety and Health Administration (OSHA)

The mission of the Occupational Safety and Health Administration (OSHA) "… is to assure the safety and health of America's workers by setting and enforcing standards; providing training, outreach, and education; establishing partnerships; and encouraging continual improvement in workplace safety and health."[35] OSHA standards affecting health-system pharmacies include those dealing with hazardous materials. ASHP's *Continuous Compliance with Joint Commission Standards* provides an overview of OSHA's Hazard Communication Standard.[36] ASHP's *Competence Assessment Tools for Health-System Pharmacies* contains materials for assessing pharmacy staff competence in handling hazardous materials.[37] The OSHA Internet website is http://www.osha.gov.

National Institute for Occupational Safety and Health (NIOSH)

"The National Institute for Occupational Safety and Health (NIOSH) is the federal agency responsible for conducting research and making recommendations for the prevention of work-related injury and illness."[38] Some NIOSH recommendations are of concern to health-system pharmacies. For example, a NIOSH alert "Preventing Occupational Exposure to Antineoplastic and other Hazardous Drugs in Healthcare Settings" warns of the health risks to workers exposed to these drugs and recommends protection procedures for minimizing the potential adverse health effects.[39] Pharmacies should ensure that their policies and procedures for handling these drugs reflect the NIOSH recommendations. The NIOSH Internet website is http://www.cdc.gov/niosh.

Centers for Disease Control and Prevention (CDC)

The Centers for Disease Control and Prevention (CDC) promotes "… health and quality of life by preventing and controlling disease, injury, and disability."[40] CDC guidelines address hand-hygiene, standard (or universal) precautions, and other infection control issues that must be considered when developing organization and department practices. The CDC Internet website is http://www.cdc.gov.

Office for Civil Rights (OCR)

The responsibilities of the Office for Civil Rights (OCR) include enforcement of certain provisions of the Health Insurance Portability and Accountability Act of 1996 (HIPAA). HIPAA aims to assure health insurance portability, reduce health care fraud and abuse, enforce standards for health information, and guarantee security and privacy of health information.[41] Compliance with the security and privacy provisions of the act may be particularly challenging for pharmacies. The OCR Internet website relating to HIPAA is http://www.hhs.gov/ocr/hipaa.

Agencies With Shared Responsibilities

Some government agencies share responsibilities associated with certain legal requirements. For example, the Department of Health and Human Services, Department of Justice, Department of Labor, Department of Transportation, Equal Opportunity Employment Commission, Federal Communications Commission, and other government agencies share responsibilities associated with the Americans with Disabilities Act (ADA). The ADA protects the rights of Americans with physical and mental disabilities.[42] Pharmacy departments must be aware of the provisions of the act and be prepared to make reasonable accommodations for disabled individuals. Pharmacy standards of performance must not impose an undue hardship on these individuals. The ADA Internet website is http://www.ada.gov.

State Boards of Pharmacy

States regulate pharmacy practice through their state boards of pharmacy (although the actual name of the agency may vary). Board of pharmacy responsibilities include setting licensure requirements for individuals, pharmacies, and some health care organizations. Boards of pharmacy also establish and enforce the rules and regulations of the state's pharmacy practice act and discipline pharmacists and pharmacies. Some boards of pharmacy enforce their state's controlled substances act. Specific responsibilities differ from state to state. State requirements may be less stringent or more stringent than accreditation and certification requirements. In all cases, the most stringent requirements take precedence. Pharmacists should contact their state board of pharmacy for specific information relating to licensure and pharmacy practice in their state.

Nongovernmental Standards-Setting Entities

Nongovernmental organizations often set standards that are enforced by government agencies (e.g., the FDA and boards of pharmacy) and other entities (e.g., the Joint Commission). Two examples are described below.

United States Pharmacopeia (USP)

"The United States Pharmacopeia (USP) is a non-governmental, standards-setting organization that advances public health by ensuring the quality and consistency of medicines, promoting the safe and proper use of medications, and verifying ingredients in dietary supplements…. Currently, USP provides standards for drugs, dietary supplements, and health care products. These standards are published in the *United States Pharmacopeia* and *National Formulary* (*USP–NF*)…."[43] USP Chapter 797 sets standards for pharmaceutical compounding of sterile preparations (including expiration dating, storage conditions, design of facilities, personnel cleaning and gowning, and suggested standard operating procedures).[44] The USP Internet website is http://www.usp.org.

National Fire Protection Association (NFPA)

The National Fire Protection Association (NFPA) aims "… to reduce the worldwide burden of fire and other hazards on the quality of life by providing and advocating scientifically-based consensus code and standards, research, training and education."[45] Organization and department standards must be consistent with NFPA codes. The NFPA Internet website is http://www.nfpa.org.

Pharmacy Professional Organizations

Pharmacy professional organizations have established standards of practice, guidelines, and codes for their specialty areas. Through their efforts, these organizations have raised the expectations for pharmacy practice. Pharmacy organizations are prepared to educate pharmacists about the standards and assist them in implementing and maintaining practices that meet the standards. When necessary, pharmacy organizations work with accrediting bodies, governmental agencies, and other groups to assure consistency and currency.

American College of Clinical Pharmacy (ACCP)

"The American College of Clinical Pharmacy (ACCP) is a professional and scientific society that provides leadership, education, advocacy, and resources enabling clinical pharmacists to achieve excellence in practice and research."[46] ACCP practice resources are the foundation of clinical pharmacy standards. The ACCP Internet website is http://www.accp.com.

American Pharmacists Association (APhA)

The American Pharmacists Association (APhA) is a national professional society of pharmacists. "The Association is a leader in providing professional information and education for pharmacists and an advocate for improved health of the American public through the provision of comprehensive pharmaceutical care."[47] The APhA's Code of Ethics for Pharmacists states the principles that "… guide pharmacists in relationships with patients, health professionals, and society."[48] The APhA Internet website is http://www.aphanet.org.

American Society of Consultant Pharmacists (ASCP)

The American Society of Consultant Pharmacists (ASCP) is a professional association representing senior care pharmacists. ASCP' Standards of Practice for Long-Term Care Pharmacy "… are not considered minimum standards, but rather focus on optimum provision of pharmaceutical care to patients residing in institutional settings. The standards focus on the pharmacy or organization providing the pharmaceutical services and on the role of the pharmacist in relating to the patient and to other health care professionals."[49] The ASCP Internet website is http://www.ascp.com.

American Society of Health-System Pharmacists (ASHP)

The American Society of Health-System Pharmacists (ASHP) is a professional organization for pharmacists practicing in health-systems. ASHP has adopted professional policy positions, statements, and guidelines that foster improvement in pharmacy practice and patient care. They "… represent a consensus of professional judgment, expert opinion, and documented evidence."[50] Since ASHP policy positions, statements, and guidelines are often more stringent, more explicit, and less subject to misinterpretation than Joint Commission, AOA, and CMS standards, they can help an organization meet or exceed accreditation and certification requirements.[51] The ASHP Internet website is http://www.ashp.org.

ASHP is also the accrediting body for practice sites that conduct pharmacy residency programs. ASHP residency standards are available for pharmacy practice and specialty residencies as well as for pharmacy technicians.[52] Meeting ASHP requirements for residency accreditation can help the pharmacy raise the quality of its services.

Organization and Department Standards

Although accrediting bodies, regulatory agencies, professional organizations, and other standards setting entities define external requirements and expectations, health care organizations must develop internal requirements (i.e., standards) that are specific to their needs. Organization and department standards must establish the management framework to ensure compliance and quality of care. External and internal requirements must be integrated into organization and department policies and procedures, competence requirements, performance evaluations, and performance improvement programs. Pharmacy assessments should include compliance with their organization and department standards.

Bylaws, Rules, Regulations, Policies and Procedures

An organization's bylaws, rules, and regulations provide the framework for governing the organization. Policies and procedures are "The formal, approved description of how a governance, management, or clinical care process is defined, organized and carried out."[6] Pharmacy departments must comply with their organization's bylaws, rules, and regulations. Departmental policies and procedures must be consistent with the organization's requirements and should be developed with the input of pharmacists and support staff. Policies and procedures should be used in orientation, education and training of staff.

Competence Assessment and Performance Evaluation Programs

Health care organizations should have programs for determining that individuals are competent (i.e., have the "… skills, knowledge, and capability to meet defined expectations."[10] The Joint Commission requires its accredited organizations to have a competence assessment program that "… is systematic, and allows for a measurable assessment of each person's ability to perform required activities." Organizations define the competencies that are required, how the competencies will be assessed, the assessment frequency, and actions to be taken when a person does not meet the competency requirements.[53]

Performance evaluation programs are ongoing processes "… for providing positive and negative feedback to staff and students as well as volunteers who work in the same capacity as staff providing care, treatment, and services." The Joint Commission requires performance expectations (standards) to be described in the person's job description. Some organizations conduct performance evaluations concurrently with competence assessments.[54] Performance expectations must be reasonable, achievable, measurable, and reflect the person's job responsibilities, adherence to policies, and predefined behavioral requirements. Pharmacy leadership and staff should work together to develop expectations that are mutually agreeable. ASHP's *Competence Assessment Tools for Health-System Pharmacies* contains job descriptions, performance evaluations, study materials, tests, skills assessment checklists, and guidelines for assessing the competence of pharmacists and support staff.[55]

Performance Improvement Programs

Most health care organizations have active performance improvement (PI) programs designed to improve processes related to care, treatment, and services. PI programs are evolving. Although approaches vary, most contain elements of quality control and quality improvement.

The Joint Commission's approach to PI includes outcome, process, and structure measures and reflects current standards of practice. The Joint Commission's PI standards require a proactive, organizationwide program that includes the following:

- monitoring performance and collecting data,
- aggregating and analyzing data,
- analyzing undesirable patterns and trends in performance,

- identifying and managing sentinel events,
- using information from data analysis "… to make changes that will improve performance and patient safety and reduce the risk of sentinel events" and
- "… identifying and reducing unanticipated adverse events and safety risks to patients…."[56]

Many organizations coordinate their PI program with their risk management activities (i.e., "Clinical and administrative activities … to identify, evaluate, and reduce the risk of injury to patients, staff, and visitors and the risk of loss to the organization."[57] PI activities (i.e., activities that improve performance and the quality of care) must take precedence over risk management activities.

Summary

Institutional accreditation and certification requirements and pharmacy guidelines form a basis for setting pharmacy standards. Compliance with accreditation and certification standards, while voluntary, is essential for an organization. Meeting the minimum requirements of state and federal legal entities is mandatory. Certain nongovernmental organizations set standards that are enforced by governmental agencies or other entities. Standards established by pharmacy professional organizations are often optimal and may be more challenging than accreditation and legal requirements. Internal requirements (e.g., organization and department standards) must be consistent with external requirements. Whatever the source and whether voluntary or mandatory, compliance with these requirements raises the level of pharmacy services and improves the quality of patient care.

References

1. Joint Commission on Accreditation of Healthcare Organizations (JCAHO). *Comprehensive Accreditation Manual for Hospitals: The Official Handbook.* Oakbrook Terrace, IL: Joint Commission on Accreditation of Healthcare Organizations; 2004:GL-1.

2. Joint Commission on Accreditation of Healthcare Organizations (JCAHO). *Comprehensive Accreditation Manual for Hospitals: The Official Handbook.* Oakbrook Terrace, IL: Joint Commission on Accreditation of Healthcare Organizations; 2004:GL-3.

3. Joint Commission on Accreditation of Healthcare Organizations (JCAHO). *Comprehensive Accreditation Manual for Hospitals: The Official Handbook.* Oakbrook Terrace, IL: Joint Commission on Accreditation of Healthcare Organizations; 2004:GL-13.

4. Joint Commission on Accreditation of Healthcare Organizations (JCAHO). *Comprehensive Accreditation Manual for Hospitals: The Official Handbook.* Oakbrook Terrace, IL: Joint Commission on Accreditation of Healthcare Organizations; 2004:SV-18.

5. Joint Commission on Accreditation of Healthcare Organizations (JCAHO). *Comprehensive Accreditation Manual for Hospitals: The Official Handbook.* Oakbrook Terrace, IL: Joint Commission on Accreditation of Healthcare Organizations; 2004:GL-17.

6. Joint Commission on Accreditation of Healthcare Organizations (JCAHO). *Comprehensive Accreditation Manual for Hospitals: The Official Handbook.* Oakbrook Terrace, IL: Joint Commission on Accreditation of Healthcare Organizations; 2004:GL-18.

7. Joint Commission on Accreditation of Healthcare Organizations (JCAHO). *Comprehensive Accreditation Manual for Hospitals: The Official Handbook.* Oakbrook Terrace, IL: Joint Commission on Accreditation of Healthcare Organizations; 2004:GL-20.

8. Joint Commission on Accreditation of Healthcare Organizations (JCAHO). *Comprehensive Accreditation Manual for Hospitals: The Official Handbook.* Oakbrook Terrace, IL: Joint Commission on Accreditation of Healthcare Organizations; 2004:SV-17-8.

9. Joint Commission on Accreditation of Healthcare Organizations (JCAHO). *Comprehensive Accreditation Manual for Hospitals: The Official Handbook.* Oakbrook Terrace, IL: Joint Commission on Accreditation of Healthcare Organizations; 2004:GL-22.

10. Joint Commission on Accreditation of Healthcare Organizations (JCAHO). *Comprehensive Accreditation Manual for Hospitals: The Official Handbook.* Oakbrook Terrace, IL: Joint Commission on Accreditation of Healthcare Organizations; 2004:GL-4.

11. Coe CP, Uselton JP. *Preparing the Pharmacy for a Joint Commission Survey.* 5th ed. Bethesda MD: American Society of Health-System Pharmacists; 2003:1–2.

12. Joint Commission on Accreditation of Healthcare Organizations (JCAHO). *Comprehensive Accreditation Manual for Hospitals: The Official Handbook.* Oakbrook Terrace, IL: Joint Commission on Accreditation of Healthcare Organizations; 2004:GL-6.

13. Coe CP, Uselton JP. *Preparing the Pharmacy for a Joint Commission Survey.* 5th ed. Bethesda MD: American Society of Health-System Pharmacists; 2003:1.

14. Joint Commission on Accreditation of Healthcare Organizations (JCAHO). *Comprehensive Accreditation Manual for Hospitals: The Official Handbook.* Oakbrook Terrace, IL: Joint Commission on Accreditation of Healthcare Organizations; 2004:GL-12.

15. Joint Commission on Accreditation of Healthcare Organizations (JCAHO). *Comprehensive Accreditation Manual for Hospitals: The Official Handbook.* Oakbrook Terrace, IL: Joint Commission on Accreditation of Healthcare Organizations; 2004:GL-7.

16. Joint Commission on Accreditation of Healthcare Organizations (JCAHO). *Comprehensive Accreditation Manual for Hospitals: The Official Handbook.* Oakbrook Terrace, IL: Joint Commission on Accreditation of Healthcare Organizations; 2004:SV-16.

17. Joint Commission on Accreditation of Healthcare Organizations (JCAHO). *Comprehensive Accreditation Manual for Hospitals: The Official Handbook.* Oakbrook Terrace, IL: Joint Commission on Accreditation of Healthcare Organizations; 2004:QR-2.

18. Joint Commission on Accreditation of Healthcare Organizations (JCAHO). *Comprehensive Accreditation Manual for Hospitals: The Official Handbook.* Oakbrook Terrace, IL: Joint Commission on Accreditation of Healthcare Organizations; 2004:APR-8.

19. Coe CP, Uselton JP. *Continuous Compliance with Joint Commission Standards.* 6th ed. Bethesda MD: American Society of Health-System Pharmacists; 2006.

20. Joint Commission on Accreditation of Healthcare Organizations (JCAHO). *Accreditation Process Guide for Hospitals.* Oakbrook Terrace, IL: Joint Commission on Accreditation of Healthcare Organizations; 2004:1–2.

21. Joint Commission on Accreditation of Healthcare Organizations (JCAHO). *Comprehensive Accreditation Manual for Hospitals: The Official Handbook.* Oakbrook Terrace, IL: Joint Commission on Accreditation of Healthcare Organizations; 2004:iii.

22. Coe CP, Uselton JP. *Continuous Compliance with Joint Commission Standards.* 6th ed. Bethesda MD: American Society of Health-System Pharmacists; 2006.

23. American Osteopathic Association. About the AOA. Available at: http://www.osteopathic.org/index.cfm?PageID=aoa_main. Accessed September 8, 2004.

24. American Osteopathic Association. Accreditation and program approval. Available at: http://do-online.osteotech.org/index.cfm?PageID=acc_main. Accessed September 8, 2004.

25. Coe CP, Uselton JP. *Preparing the Pharmacy for a Joint Commission Survey.* 5th ed. Bethesda MD: American Society of Health-System Pharmacists; 2003:257.

26. American Osteopathic Association (AOA). *Accreditation Requirements for Healthcare Facilities.* Chicago: American Osteopathic Association; 2001.

27. Centers for Medicare and Medicaid Services. Facts about the Centers for Medicare & Medicaid Services. Available at: http://www.cms.hhs.gov/researchers/projects/APR/2003/facts.pdf. Accessed September 8, 2004.

28. Centers for Medicare and Medicaid Services. Survey and certification. Available at: http://www.cms.hhs.gov/medicaid/survey-cert. Accessed September 8, 2004.

29. Centers for Medicare and Medicaid Services. Conditions of participation (CoPs). Conditions for coverage (CfCs). Available at: http://www.cms.hhs.gov/cop. Accessed September 8, 2004.

30. Coe CP, Uselton JP. *Preparing the Pharmacy for a Joint Commission Survey.* 5th ed. Bethesda MD: American Society of Health-System Pharmacists; 2003:284.

31. Centers for Medicare and Medicaid Services (CMS), Department of Health and Human Services. *State Operations Manual Appendix A-Survey Protocol, Regulations and Interpretive Guidelines for Hospitals.* 1st rev. Washington, DC: Government Printing Office; 2004. Available at: http://www.cms.hhs.gov/manuals/107_som/som107ap_a_hospitals.pdf. Accessed September 8, 2004.

32. U.S. Food and Drug Administration. FDA's mission statement. Available at: http://www.fda.gov/opacom/morechoices/mission.html. Accessed September 8, 2004.

33. U.S. Food and Drug Administration. What FDA regulates. Available at: http://www.fda.gov/comments/regs.html. Accessed September 8, 2004.

34. U.S. Drug Enforcement Administration. DEA mission statement. Available at: http://www.dea.gov/agency/mission.html. Accessed September 8, 2004.

35. Occupational Safety and Health Administration. OSHA mission statement. Available at: http://www.osha.gov. Accessed September 8, 2004.

36. Coe CP, Uselton JP. *Continuous Compliance with Joint Commission Standards.* 6th ed. Bethesda MD: American Society of Health-System Pharmacists; 2006.

37. Murdaugh LB. *Competence Assessment Tools for Health-System Pharmacies.* 3rd ed. Bethesda MD: American Society of Health-System Pharmacists; 2005:129–45.

38. National Institute for Occupational Safety and Health. About NIOSH. Available at: http://www.cdc.gov/niosh/about.html. Accessed September 8, 2004.

39. National Institute for Occupational Safety and Health. NIOSH alert: preventing occupational exposures to antineoplastic and other hazardous drugs in healthcare settings. Available at: http://www.cdc.gov/niosh/docs/2004-HazDrugAlert. Accessed September 8, 2004.

40. Centers for Disease Control and Prevention. About CDC. Available at: http://www.cdc.gov/aboutcdc.htm#mission. Accessed September 8, 2004.

41. United States Department of Health and Human Services (HHS). Medical privacy—national standards to protect the privacy of personal health information. Available at: http://www.hhs.gov/ocr/hipaa. Accessed September 8, 2004.

42. U.S. Department of Justice. ADA home page. Available at: http://www.ada.gov. Accessed September 8, 2004.

43. United States Pharmacopeia (USP). U.S. Pharmacopeia fact sheet. Available at: http://www.usp.org/aboutusp/uspfactsheet.html. Accessed September 8, 2004.

44. The United States Pharmacopeial Convention (USPC). Pharmaceutical compounding—sterile preparations. In: *The United States Pharmacopeia.* 27th rev. ed., and the *National Formulary,* 22nd ed. Rockville, MD: USPC; 2004:2350–70.

45. National Fire Protection Association. About NFPA. Available at: http://www.nfpa.org/catalog/home/ AboutNFPA/index.asp. Accessed September 8, 2004.

46. American College of Clinical Pharmacy. About ACCP. Available at: http://www.accp.com/about.php#mission. Accessed September 8, 2004.

47. American Pharmacists Association. About the American Pharmacists Association. Available at: http:www.aphanet.org. Accessed September 8, 2004.

48. American Pharmacists Association. Code of ethics for pharmacists. Available at: http://www.aphanet.org. Accessed September 8, 2004.

49. American Society of Consultant Pharmacists. Practice standards for long term care pharmacy. Available at: http://www.ascp.com/public/pr/practice/ascpstandards. shtml. Accessed September 8, 2004.

50. American Society of Health-System Pharmacists (ASHP). ASHP policy positions, statements, and guidelines. Available at: http://www.ashp.org/bestpractices/ index.cfm?cfid=2502094&CFToken=94711049. Accessed September 8, 2004.

51. Coe CP, Uselton JP. *Preparing the Pharmacy for a Joint Commission Survey.* 5th ed. Bethesda MD: American Society of Health-System Pharmacists; 2003:5.

52. American Society of Health-System Pharmacists (ASHP). Residency and accreditation information. Available at: http://www.ashp.org/rtp/index.cfm? cfid=628218&CFToken=14004614. Accessed September 8, 2004.

53. Joint Commission on Accreditation of Healthcare Organizations (JCAHO). *Comprehensive Accreditation Manual for Hospitals: The Official Handbook.* Oakbrook Terrace, IL: Joint Commission on Accreditation of Healthcare Organizations; 2004:HR-10.

54. Joint Commission on Accreditation of Healthcare Organizations (JCAHO). *Comprehensive Accreditation Manual for Hospitals: The Official Handbook.* Oakbrook Terrace, IL: Joint Commission on Accreditation of Healthcare Organizations; 2004:HR-11.

55. Murdaugh LB. *Competence Assessment Tools for Health-System Pharmacies.* 3rd ed. Bethesda MD: American Society of Health-System Pharmacists; 2005.

56. Joint Commission on Accreditation of Healthcare Organizations (JCAHO). *Comprehensive Accreditation Manual for Hospitals: The Official Handbook.* Oakbrook Terrace, IL: Joint Commission on Accreditation of Healthcare Organizations; 2004:PI-1-2.

57. Joint Commission on Accreditation of Healthcare Organizations (JCAHO). *Comprehensive Accreditation Manual for Hospitals: The Official Handbook.* Oakbrook Terrace, IL: Joint Commission on Accreditation of Healthcare Organizations; 2004:GL-21.

Using Practicing Standards to Improve Patient Safety, Quality of Care, and Advance Pharmacy Practice in Hospitals and Health Systems

Kasey K. Thompson

Introduction

This chapter will provide a broad overview of the use of practice standards to help guide professional decision making and advance pharmacy practice in hospitals and health systems.

Hospital pharmacy has a long and rich history in the area of practice standards development. As early as 1935 concerns about the status of drug dispensing in hospitals garnered the attention of the American College of Surgeons (ACS), which asked pharmacists Edward Spease and Robert Porter to produce the first set of minimum standards for hospital pharmacy.[1] ASHP continues to revise and publish an updated set from the 1935 version of the minimum standards for pharmacies in hospitals.[2]

For more than 60 years, the American Society of Health-System Pharmacists (ASHP) has been the leader in developing standards to help pharmacists who practice in hospitals and health systems improve medication use and enhance patient safety.

This chapter will explain why this dedication to the development of standards by hospital and health-system pharmacists has served a vital role through the provision of a national evidence-based framework that has helped to guide local, state, and federal regulators and national accrediting bodies in their enforcement activities, as well as providing pharmacy practitioners, hospitals and health systems, and other health care professionals with a strong sense of direction on the best approaches to ensuring patient safety, quality, and optimal medication-use outcomes.

This chapter will provide the reader with insights into how standards are developed, implemented, and adhered to in the hospital and health-system setting, as well as commentary on the future of evidence-based practice standards. Examples of similarities and differences will be provided regarding how various pharmacy practice settings approach and use standards. At the conclusion of this chapter, the reader should have a strong appreciation for why practice standards are necessary to ensure medication-use safety and quality and to advance pharmacy practice in hospitals and health systems.

Definitions

Evidence-Based Medication Use—A systematic method that draws on the results of controlled clinical trials and consensus advice on best practices.[3]

Guideline—Provides voluntary guidance and direction to practitioners and other audiences based on consensus of professional judgment, expert opinion, and documented evidence. Guidelines are written to establish reasonable goals, to be progressive and challenging, yet attainable as "best practices" in applicable settings.[4]

Standard—A Standard sets forth performance expectations for activities that affect the safety and quality of patient care.[5]

Importance of Standards

Standards are *not* instruction manuals or cookbooks. Standards do *not* typically provide step-by-step instructions on how every step in the process gets accomplished and by whom. Standards describe *what* needs to be done and provide enough detail for professionals to make decisions on *how* best to accomplish any given standard in their individual organizations. Standards are valuable because they establish common expectations for common settings, such as hospitals, and they provide a framework by which safe and effective processes of care can be established, implemented, maintained, and improved. Approaches to achieving common standards might differ from one organization to another, but the common elements of the standards remain the same.

It can be correctly stated that without standards everything is right. It is vital for common performance expectations to be created and agreed on regarding how similar systems, such as medication use in hospitals, should consistently perform.

Evidence-based standards that are developed though a recognized, credible, and comprehensive process can provide common and adaptable expectations for individual hospitals and health systems to implement safe and effective practices. Organizations such as the Joint Commission on Accreditation of Healthcare Organizations (JCAHO), the National Quality Forum, and ASHP are examples of organizations that develop credible standards and guidance to ensure high quality—safe and effective—patient care.

The 1999 Institute of Medicine (IOM) report, *To Err is Human: Building a Safer Health System*, recognized ASHP as an organization that publishes extensively on safe medication practices. The IOM noted that ASHP has developed many standards and guidelines and has widely disseminated a list of top priority actions for preventing adverse drug events in hospitals.[6] The point to be made is that by the time the IOM published its seminal report on medical errors that essentially launched the "patient safety movement," ASHP had, in fact, been publishing and developing standards on safe medication practice for nearly 60 years.

Adaptability of standards is important because services and the types of patients served differ from one organization to another. Difference, for example, might include the types of services a large university hospital provides (e.g., transplant and other complex procedures, nuclear medicine, etc.,) with 24-hour pharmacy services as compared to a small community hospital that might only have pharmacists on duty for a limited number of hours. However, adaptability does not imply that standards should be different or do not apply to one setting but not another. The endpoint of the standard remains the same, but the methods and intervening steps to achieving the standard may differ. For example, it is essential to have a pharmacist review all medication orders against the patients profile for appropriateness before the medication is administered to the patient. However, in the case of some small and rural hospitals that do not have 24-hour services, the order might be reviewed through the use of technology that allows a pharmacist in a remote location (from home or another hospital) to access the patient record and review and approve the order. In this example the standard is the same, but the approach to achieving the standard is different.

Ideally, consistency associated with evidence-based practices is enhanced, and patient care outcomes are ultimately improved, through standardization. The practice standards, *Best Practices for Hospital and Health-System Pharmacy: Position and Guidance Documents of ASHP*, developed by ASHP represent a rich source of information on virtually every area in hospital and health-system pharmacy practice. Topics include the following:

- Automation and Information Technology
- Drug Distribution and Control
- Education and Training
- Formulary Management
- Government, Law, and Regulation
- Medication Safety
- Medication Therapy and Patient Care
- Pharmaceutical Industry
- Human Resources

The ASHP compendium of *Best Practices for Hospital and Health-System Pharmacy: Position and Guidance Documents of ASHP* is an invaluable resource that is available free on the web to anyone who seeks to design safer and more effective medication-use systems.[4]

The important roles that ASHP practice standards have played can be observed in virtually every hospital in the United States and abroad. This distinction makes the point ever so clear that regardless of controversies or the time it takes from a standard to move from development to widespread adoption into practice, the endeavor itself is one that has unquestionable benefit to patients.

How Standards Are Developed

Standards development occurs in a variety of ways depending on the type of standard being developed and the processes employed by the developing organization. An important point related to standards development is that the best standards are developed in a voluntary fashion by the practitioners and organizations that will be using the standard. It stands to reason that pharmacists, who practice in hospitals and health systems, as medication management experts, would be the most qualified and appropriate professionals to develop medication-use related standards. However, it is important to recognize that health care is an interdisciplinary activity that includes patients and their families, other health professionals, organizations, and regulators.

Therefore, for a standard to be effective beyond the philosophical confines of one group of professionals, it is important that consensus be developed throughout the standards development process to ensure that the perspectives and insights of others are considered. The following process used by ASHP to develop guidance documents serves as a good example of how an organization that represents a distinct group of professionals approaches standards development.

An ASHP member council or commission recommends the development of a guidance document after considering whether the topic has the following:

- Generates a need among practitioners for authoritative advice

- Achieves some stability and there is sufficient experience upon which to base a guideline

- Is relevant to the practice of a significant portion of ASHP's members

- Is within the purview of pharmacy practice in hospitals and health systems

- Is without other sufficient guidance

- Does not pose significant legal risks to ASHP

Another consideration is whether ASHP leadership believes that there is room for improvements in practice and that an ASHP document would foster that improvement.[4]

The development of ASHP guidelines generally includes the following steps:

1. A group of experts (usually ASHP members) on a given topic volunteer to develop a preliminary draft. Drafters are selected based on demonstrated knowledge of the topic and their practice settings.

2. The draft is sent by ASHP to reviewers who have interest and expertise in the given topic. Reviewers consist of hospital and health-system pharmacists and selected individuals, such as other health care professionals, who are knowledgeable in the content area, representatives of various ASHP bodies, and other professional organizations. A strength of ASHP's guidelines resides in the public comment process ASHP employs that allows anyone who is interested in commenting to do so, as well as active outreach by ASHP to other interested individuals and organizations.

3. Based on the comments, a revised draft is submitted to the appropriate ASHP policy-recommending body for action. When the draft meets the established criteria for content and quality, that body recommends that the ASHP Board of Directors approve the document.

The guidance documents developed by ASHP are voluntary and have no basis in law or regulation. However, it is sometimes the case that a state board of pharmacy or federal regulator such as the FDA or national accrediting body such as JCAHO, might look to ASHP guidelines to provide a framework for the development of laws, regulations, and enforceable standards, respectively. A comparison of ASHP guidelines to the JCAHO Medication Management Standards published in the *Comprehensive Accreditation Manual for Hospitals* provides an excellent example of where ASHP practice standards have provided a framework for the development of enforceable standards by other organizations.[7]

The previous example of the rigorous process used by ASHP to identify and develop practice standards is achieved in a similar fashion by other prominent standards-developing organizations such as JCAHO. Important points are that the best standards are ones that are developed by those working in the area in which the standards will be used, and standards benefit by broad-based external review and the inclusion of all stakeholder groups that have expertise in the area in which standards are being considered.

Implementation and Adherence to Standards

The challenges of practice standards reside to a lesser degree in the development of the standard and to a greater degree in the implementation of the standard into mainstream practice. It has been reported that the lag between the discovery of more efficacious forms of treatment and their incorporation into routine patient care is unnecessarily long, in the range of about 15 to 20 years.[8] Although the previous example may not be precisely analogous to the time it takes for a practice standard to be adopted into practice, it does provide a clue to the general rate at which health care providers and organizations recognize and implement the best evidence into routine practice. A survey conducted in 2003 assessed the compliance of quality assurance practices in hospitals for pharmacy compounded sterile preparations with the *ASHP Guidelines on Quality Assurance for Pharmacy-Prepared Sterile Products*. The

CHAPTER 12: USING PRACTICING STANDARDS TO IMPROVE PATIENT SAFETY, QUALITY OF CARE, AND ADVANCE PHARMACY PRACTICE IN HOSPITALS AND HEALTH SYSTEMS

167

survey findings supported the fact that progress had been made on adherence to the guidelines but still noted that hospital pharmacies were not in full compliance with the ASHP guidelines that were published in 2000.[9]

In the area of patient safety, it has been suggested that regulations through the efforts of JCAHO have resulted in the most progress toward improving patient safety.[11] Ideally, professionals and organizations would voluntarily adopt practice standards that have been proven to improve patient safety without the need for government regulation, but the fact remains that competing demands, culture, and available resources play major roles in determining whether the right things happen and when.

Distinguishing Practice Settings

Pharmacy practice settings differ significantly regarding the extent to which practice is standards-based. Since inception hospital pharmacy has worked diligently to ensure that patient care and medication management services are standards-based. From the first set of minimum standards for hospital pharmacy in 1935 to the development of minimum standards for pharmacy internships in hospitals in the 1950s, hospital pharmacists have been leading advocates for standards-based practices.[11]

Most hospitals and health systems must be accredited by JCAHO in order to receive payment from Medicare, Medicaid, and most health plans. JCAHO standards and surveys focus a great amount of attention on the safety and quality of the medication-use system. Those JCAHO standards that address medication management reflect many complementary adaptations of the core principles and practices described in ASHP guidelines. JCAHO accreditation represents another important layer of standards-based oversight to help ensure the achievement of optimal safety, quality, and patient care outcomes.

Hospital and health-system pharmacies must also comply with laws and regulations that are promulgated and enforced by states boards of pharmacy and federal authorities. There is an important distinction to be made between the minimum requirements of state boards of pharmacy that all pharmacy practice settings must meet, and the more comprehensive sets of quality guidelines and standards established by organizations such as ASHP and JCAHO. Hospital and health-system pharmacy has benefited by adopting a self-regulatory

mandate to ensure safety and quality and has consistently opened itself to external review by multiple agencies to validate that the right things are happening through the use of standards.

Evolution of Standards

Since the establishment of the first set of minimum standards for hospital pharmacies in 1935, the area of standards and guidelines development has expanded and evolved. New challenges and opportunities have arisen in areas such as automation and information technology; infection control; the provision of direct patient care services by pharmacists in acute and ambulatory settings; biological and chemical terrorism; the expanding roles of pharmacy technicians; pharmacogenomics; formulary management; patient safety; population-based medication use; and many others.

Many of the evolving areas for standards development listed above provide fertile ground for hospital and health-system pharmacists who already benefit by significant experience in the development and application of practice standards, to continue to forge new ground and advance their practice beyond what was imaginable in 1935 when Spease and Porter developed the first set of minimum standards.

The growing attention and interest in using computerized prescriber order-entry, clinical decision support, and electronic medical records provides unique opportunities for incorporating the most important practice standards into information systems, to more efficiently and effectively drive the implementation and ongoing use of standards. The challenges presented by incorporating practice standards into information systems reside in ensuring that those standards remain up-to-date. Current revision cycles and approaches used by standards developing organizations such as ASHP will need to be adapted to meet the needs of the end user and the requirements imposed by the technology. Efforts are currently underway by ASHP to prepare guidance documents in a way that is readily applicable to current and future health information technology (IT) systems.

An important new horizon to apply standards and accreditation processes is in the area of ensuring better continuity of care from acute to ambulatory settings. Physician office practices and community pharmacies have a unique opportunity and responsibility to develop, adopt, and/or adapt, practice standards that consistently meet the needs of the patients they serve as transitions are made from one care setting to the next. Fruitful opportunities will exist to use technology to connect care settings in a highly-integrated and standards-based fashion to ensure optimal medication use.

Summary

Standards for the practice of pharmacy in hospitals and health systems are, and continue to be, integral to the safe and effective use of medications. More important than gaining an understanding of how practice standards are developed and used, is for individual pharmacy practitioners to contribute to the practice standards development process throughout their entire careers, remembering that the best standards are those that are developed by the professionals who are engaged in the practice and will be most affected by the standards once they are implemented.

The American Society of Health-System Pharmacists is still one of the few pharmacy or health care professional organizations that dedicate significant resources to the development of practice standards to advance overall public health related to medication use and the practice of pharmacy in hospitals and health systems. It can be difficult to judge at the time a standard is conceptualized and developed whether that standard will ultimately have an impact on improving patient care or advancing pharmacy practice. However, evidence to date suggests that most issues rising to the level of standards development are ones that either immediately, or over a period of time, have made a measurable difference in the lives of the patients we serve.

References

1. Harris RR, McConnell WE. The American Society of Hospital Pharmacists: a history. *Am J Hosp Pharm.* 1993;50:S7.

2. American Society of Health-System Pharmacists (ASHP). ASHP guidelines: minimum standard for pharmacies in hospitals. *Am J Health-Syst Pharm.* 1995;52:2711–7.

3. ASHP Leadership Agenda.

4. Hawkins BH, ed. *Best Practices for Hospital and Health-System Pharmacy: Position and Guidance Documents of ASHP.* Bethesda, MD: American Society of Health-System Pharmacists; 2004–2005.

5. Joint Commission on the Accreditation of Healthcare Organizations (JCAHO) website. Available at: http://www.jcaho.org/about+us/index.htm.

6. Kohn LT, Corrigan JM, Donaldson MS, eds. *To Err Is Human: Building A Safer Health System.* Washington, DC: National Academy Press; 1999.

7. Joint Commission on the Accreditation of Healthcare Organizations (JCAHO). Comprehensive Accreditation Manual for Hospitals: The Official Handbook (CAMH). Oakbrook Terrace, IL: JCAHO; 2005.

8. Balas EA, Boren SA. Managing clinical knowledge for health care improvement. *Yearbook of Medical Informatics.* 2000:65–70.

9. Morris AM, Schneider PJ, Pedersen CA, et al. National survey of quality assurance activities for pharmacy-compounded sterile preparations. *Am J Health-Syst Pharm.* 2003;60:2567–76.

10. Wachter RM. The end of the beginning: patient safety five years after 'to err is human.' *Health Aff.* 2004;Jul–Dec (suppl web exclusives):W4,534–45.

11. American Society of Hospital Pharmacists (ASHP). Revised minimum standard for pharmacy internship in hospitals. *Am J Hosp Pharm.* 1958;15:228–31.

Chapter 13

Residency Training for Practice

Wayne F. Conrad

Introduction

The purpose of this chapter is to familiarize the reader with various aspects of pharmacy residency training. The importance and impact of residency training is emphasized. The evolution of residency standards and role of ASHP are discussed. Processes for practice sites to plan and initiate a residency program are outlined. The chapter also contains important information for students on how to find and select a residency program of their choice.

A pharmacy residency is an organized, directed, postgraduate training program in a defined area of pharmacy practice. It is intended to provide residents with the knowledge and skills that pharmacy practitioners need to face the challenges of today's complex health care environment, while also providing experiences which will help meet practice demands and opportunities of the future.

Residency training is experiential learning. Residents acquire skills by actually performing tasks and by sharing accountability for outcomes. They are guided by experienced, model practitioners. Mentoring between a competent and experienced preceptor and a resident is a critical element of resident training. It provides exponential returns to both parties through coaching, critiquing, encouraging, and knowledge sharing.[1]

Over the years pharmacy residency programs have had a major impact on pharmacy practice and training. Residency training programs have been recognized as the most effective means of developing the knowledge and skills necessary to become competent to provide pharmaceutical care and to develop and manage the systems and programs in which pharmaceutical care is delivered.[2] Residency training programs and their graduates have been cited as being unrivaled in influencing the profession by providing the following:

- An unparalleled capacity for self-renewal for practitioners and the profession
- Both an intellectual and emotional commitment to the achievement of excellence in the profession
- A perpetuation of leadership and meaningful values for the practice community[1]

Residency training program graduates have served the profession as a critical mass of leaders who have continually served as change agents for innovation. Given the unprecedented challenges of today's health care environments as well as the compelling need to amalgamate the concept of pharmaceutical care into mainstream practice, it would appear that the residency training/professional leadership linkage phenomenon is now even more critical to the profession's future.[3]

Accreditation and the Evolution of Residency Standards

The profession of pharmacy has a long tradition of postgraduate training. In 1948, the American Society of Health-System Pharmacists (ASHP) developed formal training guidelines for hospital pharmacy internship programs, the precursors of residency training.[4] ASHP designed these internships to produce a body of practitioners who could maintain the high practice standards of hospital pharmacy practice. By 1962, the desire for consistency in the quality of graduates led to adoption of an accreditation process by ASHP and the development of the Hospital Pharmacy Residency Accreditation Standard.[4]

Accreditation is the process by which an agency or organization evaluates and recognizes a program of study or an institution as meeting certain predetermined requirements.[5] ASHP is the accrediting agency for pharmacy residencies. Requirements for pharmacy residency training, as reflected in accreditation standards, have always attempted to challenge programs to be at the vanguard of practice.[6] Over the years, changes in health care delivery have required changes in residency training. During the early years postgraduate training, as reflected in ASHP accreditation standards, focused primarily on the manufacture and preparation of pharmaceutical products and on systems that could be implemented to ensure the integrity of those products up to the point of administration. Moreover, substantial effort was placed on providing trainees with leadership skills needed to pursue leadership roles in the hospital pharmacy community.[6]

The clinical pharmacy movement of the 1970s led to the creation of two additional hospital-based pharmacy practice residencies. The standards for these were the ASHP Accreditation Standard for Residency in Clinical Pharmacy and the ASHP Standard for Specialized Residency.[7,8] The purpose of these residencies was to develop skills to enable graduates to deliver more *clinical* and/or more specialized pharmacy services.[6] Since that time, ASHP has created 17 specialty supplemental standards that are in use today.

In 1991, the ASHP Accreditation Standard for Residency in Pharmacy Practice (with emphasis in Pharmaceutical Care) replaced both the hospital and clinical pharmacy standards.[9] Its purpose was to train entry-level practitioners to meet the increasingly complex pharmaceutical care needs of patients in four core areas of pharmacy practice—acute care, ambulatory care, drug information, and practice management. Adoption of the term *pharmacy practice* in this standard was significant. Clear consensus was established that the time had come to no longer distinguish between *clinical pharmacy practice* and *pharmacy practice* since the practice of pharmacy is inherently clinical.[10]

As the concept of pharmaceutical care became widely accepted throughout the profession, it became evident that residency training programs were needed to develop change agents and future leaders in other areas of practice besides hospital pharmacy. To meet this need ASHP partnered with other national professional organizations to develop residency training standards in home care, long-term care, community care, and managed care pharmacy practice.[11–14]

In 1993, the ASHP Research and Education Foundation funded a 3-year demonstration project to develop and study a systematic approaching to residency training which was termed *Residency Learning System* (RLS).[15] The RLS Model that was developed as part of the project had four components: goal statements and educational objectives, instruction by preceptors, assessment, and a decision process.[16] The concepts associated with the systematic approach to residency training were subsequently incorporated into the ASHP Accreditation Standard for Residencies in Pharmacy Practice, which was approved by the ASHP Board of Directors in 2001 and is used today.[17]

Types of Residencies

There are two general types of accredited pharmacy residency programs—pharmacy practice residencies, which may be termed *postgraduate year one* (PGY1) and *specialized or advanced residencies* (PGY2).[18] Residents in pharmacy practice (PGY1) are provided the opportunity to accelerate their growth beyond entry-level professional competence in direct patient care and in practice management and to further the development of leadership skills that can be applied in any position and in any practice setting.[17] Pharmacy practice residency training takes place in a variety of settings including hospitals, community pharmacies, home care and long-term care facilities, ambulatory care settings, and managed care facilities.

Specialized or Advanced Residencies (PGY2) are intended to take place after the successful completion of a pharmacy practice residency. PGY2 residency programs must be designed to develop accountability, practice patterns, habits, and expert knowledge, skills, attitudes and abilities in the respective advanced area of pharmacy practice, far beyond the broad skills and competencies that might be expected from a PGY1 residency.[19]

Since the inception of residency standards in the 1960s, the number of residency programs and number of residency graduates has continued to grow. In 2004, there were almost 700 ASHP-accredited residency programs. Figure 13-1 illustrates growth in residency programs from 2000 to 2004. Approximately 420 of these were pharmacy practice programs while 280 were specialty programs.

The Commission on Credentialing

The Commission on Credentialing is the body within ASHP structure responsible for administering its accreditation program.[5] The Commission is comprised of 14 practitioners who are directors of pharmacy or program directors of accredited residency programs, two public members, and a staff secretary (ASHP Director of Accreditation Services). Representatives of the Academy of Managed Care Pharmacy, American Pharmacists Association, and the American College of Clinical Pharmacy are invited guests, as are staff members of the ASHP Department of Accreditation Services, contract surveyors, and the ASHP Board Liaison. The Commission meets twice per year. Among its charges, the Commission develops standards for pharmacy training programs, considers new programs for

Figure 13-1
Accredited Residency Program Growth over Time 1990–2004

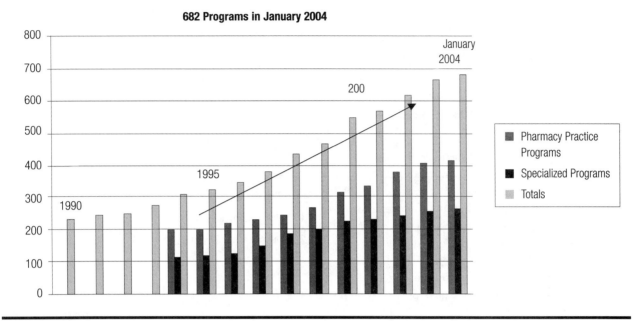

682 Programs in January 2004

accreditation and reviews programs for reaccreditations. Members of the Commission typically serve, along with a member of the staff of Accreditation Services or a contract surveyor, on accreditation survey teams.

Applying for Accreditation

The procedures for making application for accreditation of a pharmacy residency program are given in the ASHP document *ASHP Regulations on Accreditation of Pharmacy Residencies*.[20] The application may be submitted after the first resident has completed at least 9 months of training. After all of the application materials have been received by ASHP, arrangements are made with the training site for an on-site evaluation by an accreditation survey team.

The Accreditation Survey

A typical accreditation site survey visit is completed in 2 days and includes interviews with designated individuals (e.g., chief executive officer of the training site, chair of the pharmacy and therapeutics committee and other physicians, nurses, the director of pharmacy, and members of the pharmacy staff, including residents). There is also intensive review of the pharmacy service, residency training program documentation, and the site's facilities with primary emphasis on the pharmacy

department and the areas it serves. The survey is conducted by a two-member team, as described above.

The site evaluation is conducted in the spirit of quality improvement. Its purposes are to determine the degree of compliance with the requirements of the appropriate accreditation standard and to offer recommendations and advice for meeting the requirements of the accreditation standard.

The Accreditation Survey Report

Following the site evaluation the survey team prepares a report summarizing its findings, listing significant items of noncompliance or partial compliance with the appropriate standard and offering specific recommendations on improving pharmacy services and the residency training program. The report is sent to the chief executive officer of the training site with a copy to the residency program director for review. The site is requested to respond to the survey report, outlining any progress that has been or is planned to be made in overcoming deficiencies listed in the report. The report, along with the comments submitted by the training site, is considered by the Commission on Credentialing when it acts on the application.

Reaccredidation and Interim Self-Audit

Accredited residency programs are expected to continue to improve their services and training program during the accreditation cycle. Accreditation is granted for from 1–6 years depending on the extent of compliance with accreditation standards and when the Commission wants to receive an additional report documenting continued improvement. Programs accredited for 6 years are expected to submit a status report after 3 years. A reaccreditation survey is scheduled every 6 years.

How to Design and Conduct a Residency Program

The RLS Decision Process (Appendix 13-1) has been developed by ASHP to assist programs to plan and conduct residency training programs.[16] The steps may be subdivided into four stages: planning the overall program, customizing the residency program plan for each resident, instructing the resident, and monitoring resident progress. In devising the program's plan, the program director together with the program's preceptors should initially determine the purpose of the residency and the broad educational outcomes that a resident must achieve. The outcomes must address development of the resident's competence in patient care and practice management according to the appropriate accreditation standard.

As part of the RLS Model, ASHP has developed a comprehensive set of goals and objectives that represent the skills and abilities that might be learned in pharmacy practice residencies.[16] Rather than attempting to write their own educationally sound goals and objectives, program directors and preceptors should select those goals and objectives in the RLS Model that relate to the purpose and outcomes of the residency being planned.

Training structure refers to the organization, length, and timing of discreet learning units within residency programs.[16] Residency programs should structure their programs in such a way as to make maximum benefit out of the strengths of their program and preceptors. Learning rotations (generally 4-week experiences) have been the traditional mechanism used by most programs to train residents to provide care to different patient populations. Recently, longer time periods and longitudinal experiences have been found to be advantageous in some circumstances for developing resident competence, independence, and self-confidence.

Preceptor evaluation of each resident's performance must be done during (formative) and at the end (summative) of each learning experience. The primary pur-

pose of these evaluations should be to provide specific and qualitative feedback to help residents improve their performance. As part of its program plan residencies should develop an assessment strategy that also includes resident evaluation of the preceptor and resident self-evaluation.

The residency program plan is a predetermined process for how the program director and preceptors will conduct their residency training. However, in order to meet the needs of individual residents, the program director must customize the program plan for each resident. The individualized plan should focus on how to address the resident's weaknesses and strengths while also taking into account the resident's interests.

One-on-one teaching by a preceptor in the practice environment is probably the most effective and time-honored method for transmitting the profession's problem solving skills to colleagues and to the next generation of pharmacists.[16] It is the hallmark of residency training. Preceptor roles in practice based instruction include direct instruction, modeling, coaching, and facilitation. The role used depends on the resident's stage of learning as depicted in the Learning Pyramid (see Figure 13-2).[15] The Learning Pyramid captures the learner's progression to skill in problem solving and the preceptor's role in furthering that goal.[23] Foundation skills and knowledge form the base of the pyramid. One cannot solve a problem without under-

---

Appendix 13-1
RLS Decision Process

1. Identify program outcomes
2. Write program purpose statement
3. Establish program goals
4. Structure learning experiences
5. Categorize goals for evaluation
6. Assign goals and assessment points
7. Design learning activities
8. Establish assessment strategy
9. Customize plan
10. Orient resident to RLS
11. Deliver instruction
12. Monitor resident progress

Source: Reference 16.

standing the content knowledge the mind needs to draw upon in its search for a solution. The teaching strategy for content is direct instruction such as one-on-one discussions between the resident and preceptor or provision of content directed reading assignments.

In practical application the resident moves from understanding to doing. Modeling and coaching are two teaching strategies that help the resident accomplish this level. When modeling, the preceptor solves one or more patient cases, talking about his or her thinking process as it unfolds so that the resident hears the preceptors strategy, how he or she makes decisions, and in what order. The preceptor's strategy becomes the model that the resident attempts to emulate in the second stage of application, in which the preceptor steps aside and coaches the resident through similar problems, providing feedback as the resident attempts to solve the cases.

During culminating integration the resident moves toward putting together strategic content and procedural knowledge into an independent problem-solving process that takes place in a real-life learning situation. The preceptor's role shifts to deciding what cases the resident is ready to solve and acting as a resource if the resident needs assistance.[23]

The final step in conducting a residency program is to monitor the progress of the resident throughout the training year. The program director and residency program preceptors should meet on a regular basis (at least quarterly) to discuss each resident's progress. Adjustment should be made in the resident's customized plan as appropriate. The program director and preceptors should also revaluate the residency program on an annual basis so that opportunities for improvement may be identified and implemented.

Financial Aspects of Conducting a Residency Program

Costs to conduct a residency program include development and administrative costs, personnel time associated with precepting residents, resident's travel allowance, project expenses, and resident's stipend and fringe benefits. Residency stipends are generally less than 50% of a staff pharmacist salary. Since residency training is most effective when residents actively participate in the delivery of pharmacy services, most of the cost of residency training may be offset by considering the replacement costs for personnel time associated with residents providing direct patient care serv-

Figure 13-2
The Learning Pyramid

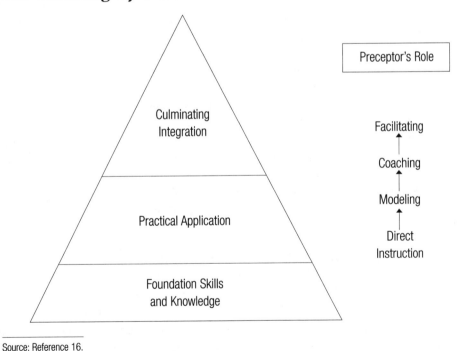

Source: Reference 16.

ices, practice management functions, and staffing associated with drug distribution. In addition, the costs associated with conducting an accredited residency program in an institution may be offset by Medicare pass-through funding.[24,25]

Additional Information for Students

An accredited pharmacy practice residency program is recommended for any graduating pharmacy student with an interest in institutional pharmacy practice, clinical practice, clinical teaching, or a leadership role in a defined area of practice. Because of the concentrated nature of residency training, it may be anticipated that residency graduates will develop a level of competence equivalent to several years of practice as a pharmacist.[12] There are several other reasons to consider residency training. Many pharmacist positions in practice and academia require 1 or even 2 years of residency training as a minimum credential. Completion of a residency training program will increase employment opportunities and upward mobility. Accreditation ensures that the residency program has undergone external review and that the program is in substantial compliance with accreditation standards. Therefore, nonaccredited programs should be viewed more cautiously.

Residency programs provide residents with a stipend while they are training. The amount of the stipend varies from program to program, depending on such factors as the value of fringe benefits, geographic area (cost of living), and related factors. Cash stipends are significantly less than the starting salary of most pharmacist positions. However, total income over the length of a career in a specific area of practice will likely be greater for those that have completed residency training.

Accredited pharmacy practice residencies differ in many ways such as practice setting, training emphasis, sophistication of practice, size of training site, number of preceptors, number of residents in training, geographic location, stipend, etc. Students should find out as much information as possible about individual programs to help them determine their choice of residency program. The ASHP Residency Directory lists a description of each program and is an excellent starting point for information.[24] Students would be well-advised to also obtain information from faculty advisors, clerkship preceptors, employers, and current residents before applying to individual programs. The ASHP Residency Showcase, which is held each year at the ASHP Midyear Clinical Meeting and regional residency showcases

held by colleges of pharmacy and professional organizations offer a unique opportunity to talk directly with program directors, preceptors, and residents of several different residency programs.

The ASHP Resident Matching Program provides an orderly process to help applicants obtain positions in residency programs of their choice, and to help programs obtain applicants of their choice.[25] With the Match, applicants must still apply directly to programs they are interested in, and applicants and programs interview and evaluate each other independently of the Match. However, no offers are made by programs during the interview period. Applicants and programs can fully evaluate each other before the programs must decide on their preferences for applicants and before applicants must decide on their preferences for programs. After all interviews are completed, each applicant submits a Rank Order List on which the applicant lists the desired programs, in numerical order of the applicant's preference. Similarly, each program submits a Rank Order List on which the program lists the desirable applicants, in order of the program's preference. The Match then places individuals into positions based entirely on the preferences stated in the Rank Order Lists. The result of the Match is that each applicant is placed with the most preferred program on the applicant's Rank Order List that ranks the applicant and does not fill all its positions with more preferred applicants. Similarly, each program is matched with the most preferred applicants on its list, up to the number of positions available, who rank the program and who do not receive positions at programs they prefer.

Summary

The increasing emergence of integrated health care delivery systems and advances in drugs and drug-delivery technology have resulted in greater complexity and diversity in the delivery of pharmaceutical care. Therefore, meeting the needs of patients will require more highly trained practitioners than ever before. Clearly, the most efficient method for pharmacists to receive such training is through postgraduate residencies.[6] There is support among professional practice associations and the American Association of Colleges of Pharmacy for residency training as a means of meeting future manpower needs.[26–28] However, the number of residency programs in existence currently is not sufficient to meet the demand for residency programs. Hence, substantially more residencies must be developed in a variety of practice settings. Continued cooperation among pharmacist practitioners, pharmacy associations, and colleges of pharmacy will be needed to achieve this objective.

References

1. Pierpaoli PG, Flint NB. Residency training-the profession's forge for leadership development. *Pharm Pract Manage Q.* 1995;15(2):44–6.

2. Guerrero RM. Restructuring postgraduate training programs for survival. *Pharm Pract Manage Q.* 1995;15(2):65–71.

3. Pierpaoli PG. Mentors and residency training. *Am J Hosp Pharm.* 1990;47:112–3.

4. Letendre DE. Introduction and summary: directions for postgraduate pharmacy residency training proceedings of the 1989 national residency preceptors' conference. *Am J Hosp Pharm.* 1990;47:85–8.

5. Lazarus H. Hospital pharmacy residency programs. In: *Handbook of Institutional Pharmacy Practice.* 2nd ed. Baltimore, MD: Williams & Wilkins; 1986.

6. Letendre DE, Brooks PJ, Degenhart ML. The evolution of pharmacy residency training programs and corresponding standards of accreditation. *Pharm Pract Manage Q.* 1995;15(2):30–43.

7. ASHP accreditation standard for residency training in clinical pharmacy. *Am J Hosp Pharm.* 1980;37:223–8.

8. ASHP accreditation standard for specialized pharmacy residency training. *Am J Hosp Pharm.* 1980;37:1229–32.

9. ASHP accreditation standard for residency in pharmacy practice. *Am J Hosp Pharm.* 1992;49:146–53.

10. Letendre DE. Reflections on the future of pharmacy residency programs: an ASHP perspective. *Am J Pharm Ed.* 1992:56:298–300.

11. Goal statements, objectives, and instructional objectives for pharmacy practice (with emphasis in home care) residency training. American Society of Health-System Pharmacists. Available at: www.ashp.com/rtp/Starting/practice-residencies. Accessed November, 2004.

12. Goal statements, objectives, and instructional objectives for pharmacy practice (with emphasis in long term care) residency training. American Society of Health-System Pharmacists. Available at: www.ashp.com/rtp/Starting/practice-residencies. Accessed November, 2004.

13. Goal statements, objectives, and instructional objectives for pharmacy practice (with emphasis in community care) residency training. American Society of Health-System Pharmacists. Available at: www.ashp.com/rtp/Starting/practice-residencies. Accessed November, 2004.

14. Goal statements, objectives, and instructional objectives for pharmacy practice (with emphasis in managed care) residency training. American Society of Health-System Pharmacists. Available at: www.ashp.com/rtp/Starting/practice-residencies. Accessed November, 2004.

15. Conrad WF, Nimmo CM, Brooks PJ. *ASHP Model for Pharmacy Residency Learning Demonstration Project Final Report.* Bethesda, MD: American Society of Health-System Pharmacists; 1996.

16. *The Residency Learning System (RLS) Model.* 2nd ed. Bethesda, MD: American Society of Health-System Pharmacists; 2001.

17. ASHP accreditation standard for residencies in pharmacy practice. Approved by ASHP Board of Directors April, 2001. American Society of Health-System Pharmacists. Available at: www.ashp.com/rtp/Starting/practice-residencies. Accessed November, 2004.

18. ASHP accreditation standard for specialized pharmacy residency training (with guide to interpretation). Approved by the ASHP Board of Directors, April 27, 1994. Developed by the ASHP Commission on Credentialing. American Society of Health-System Pharmacists. Available at: www.ashp.com/rtp/Starting/practice-residencies. Accessed November, 2004.

19. ASHP supplemental accreditation standard for postgraduate year two (PGY2) residency programs. Unpublished draft. Bethesda, MD: ASHP Commission on Credentialing; November, 2003.

20. ASHP regulations on accreditation of pharmacy residencies. Approved by the ASHP Board of Directors on September 26, 2003. American Society of Health-System Pharmacists.

21. Miller DE, Woller TW. Understanding reimbursement for pharmacy residents. *Am J Health-Syst Pharm.* 1998;55:1620–3.

22. Medicare program: changes to the hospital inpatient prospective systems and fiscal year 2004 rates. Department of Health and Human Services, Centers for Medicare and Medicaid Services. *Federal Register.* 2003;68:45346–71.

23. Nimmo CM. Staff development for pharmacy practice. In: *Developing Training Materials and Programs: Facilitating Staff Development.* Bethesda, MD: American Society of Health-System Pharmacists; 2000.

24. ASHP residency directory. American Society of Health-System Pharmacists. Available at: www.ashp.com/rtp/Starting/practice-residencies. Accessed November, 2004.

25. Residency matching program. American Society of Health-System Pharmacists. Available at: www.ashp.com/rtp/Starting/practice-residencies. Accessed November, 2004.

26. ASHP long-range position on pharmacy manpower needs and residency training. *Am J Hosp Pharm.* 1980;37:1232–4.

27. The strategic plan of the American College of Clinical Pharmacy. American College of Clinical Pharmacy. *The ACCP Report.* 2002;Oct S1–6.

28. AACP commission to implement change in pharmaceutical education: position paper 4. American Association of Colleges of Pharmacy. Available at: www.aacp.org. Accessed November, 2004.

Chapter 14

Interprofessional Teams/Collaborative Practice Models

Cynthia Brennan

Case Study

Mr. Newman, a 66-year-old patient with diabetes, comes for his 15-minute visit with Dr. Jackson. After evaluating Mr. Newman's acutely painful hip and treating his gastroesophageal reflux disease, Dr. Jackson has 3 minutes left to assess the patient's diabetic control. Having unsuccessfully searched Mr. Newman's medical records to find the last eye examination results, hemoglobin A_{1c} (HbA_{1c}) and lipid levels, Dr. Jackson orders another round of tests and schedules a return visit for the patient. Mr. Newman does not keep a log of his home glucose readings.

Definitions

Interdisciplinary—Refers to communication within a profession.

Interprofessional—Refers to communication across the health care professions.

Clarion Call for Health Care Reform

In 2001, the Institute of Medicine's (IOM) Committee on Quality of Health Care in America published their report, *Crossing the Quality Chasm: A New Health System for the 21st Century*.[1] This report identified six aims for the improvement of the health care system in order to provide high quality care. The following is what the Committee agreed that health care must be:

1. *Safe*—Avoiding injuries to patients from the care that is intended to help them

2. *Effective*—Providing services based on scientific knowledge to all who could benefit and refraining from providing services to those not likely to benefit (avoiding underuse and overuse, respectively)

3. *Patient-Centered*—Providing care that is respectful of and responsive to individual patient preferences, needs, and values and ensuring that patient values guide all clinical decisions

4. *Timely*—Reducing waits and potentially harmful delays for both those who receive and those who give care

5. *Efficient*—Avoiding waste, including waste of equipment, supplies, ideas, and energy

6. *Equitable*—Providing care that does not vary in quality because of personal characteristics such as gender, ethnicity, geographic location, and socioeconomic status. The IOM Report also provides a set of *rules* for the redesign of health care processes

This report establishes a foundation for the structure and function of a redesigned health care system that promotes team-based practice models and recommends that "Private and public purchasers, health care organizations, clinicians, and patients should work together to redesign health care processes in accordance with the following rules:

1. *Care based on continuous healing relationships.* Patients should receive care whenever they need it and in many forms, not just face-to-face visits. This rule implies that the health care system should be responsive at all times (24 hours a day, every day) and that access to care should be provided over the Internet, by telephone, and by other means in addition to face-to-face visits.

2. *Customization based on patient needs and values.* The system of care should be designed to meet the most common types of needs but have the capability to respond to individual patient choices and preferences.

3. *The patient as the source of control.* Patients should be given the necessary information and the opportunity to exercise the degree of control they choose over health care decisions that affect them. The health system should be able to accommodate differences in patient preferences and encourage shared decision-making.

4. *Shared knowledge and the free flow of information.* Patients should have unfettered access to

their own medical information and to clinical knowledge. Clinicians and patients should communicate effectively and share information.

5. *Evidence-based decision making.* Patients should receive care based on the best available scientific knowledge. Care should not vary illogically from clinician to clinician or from place to place.

6. *Safety as a system property.* Patients should be safe from injury caused by the care system. Reducing risk and ensuring safety require greater attention to systems that help prevent and mitigate errors.

7. *The need for transparency.* The health care system should make information available to patients and their families that allows them to make informed decisions when selecting a health plan, hospital, or clinical practice, or choosing among alternative treatments. This should include information describing the system's performance on safety, evidence-based practice, and patient satisfaction.

8. *Anticipation of needs.* The health system should anticipate patient needs, rather than simply reacting to events.

9. *Continuous decrease in waste.* The health system should not waste resources or patient time.

10. *Cooperation among clinicians.* Clinicians and institutions should actively collaborate and communicate to ensure an appropriate exchange of information."

Based upon the IOM blueprint for overhauling the health care system, effective interprofessional teams that include pharmacists are ideally suited for providing high quality patient care.

Developing Effective Health Care Teams

The Role of Team Members

Interprofessional or multidisciplinary teams have demonstrated their value with improved patient outcomes and safety while reducing health care costs. These teams can be found in various settings including primary care, disease-specific care settings, critical acute care (intensive care unit, trauma units, operating rooms and emergency rooms) as well as geriatric and end-of-life care. The complexity of care encountered in these settings requires highly functional teams supported by clinical information and decision support systems to provide safe, effective, patient-centered, timely, efficient, equitable care. Pharmacist team members improve safety, efficacy (monitoring and adjusting medications), efficiency (filling medication-related roles that physicians may not perform well), and contribute their unique skills and body of knowledge to the team as health care decisions are being made.

Nurses are trained to evaluate the patient's responses to actual and potential health problems and therapy, provide care coordination, and are key members of any health care team. Other team members may include social workers to address the patient's psychosocial and economic issues, physical and occupational therapists to help patients maintain their functionality and independence, and nutritionists to focus on dietary issues and other ancillary health care personnel. The exact composition of the team depends upon the health care setting, the practice environment, and the patient population.

Characteristics of Effective Teams

Successful teams share specific characteristics that enhance their functionality and lead to improved patient outcomes. These include the following:

1. *Structure*—Appropriate size and composition to meet the needs of the patient population

2. *Process*—Effective communications, goals, expectations, and conflict management

3. *Function*—Matching roles, training and experience to the needs of the team

4. *External Support*—Obtaining resources and rewards for team successes

Outcomes Related to Coordination of Care as a Measure of Effective Team-Based Care

Coordination of care or clinical integration has been defined as "the extent to which patient care services are coordinated across people, functions, activities, and sites over time so as to maximize the value of services delivered to patients."[2] Effective coordination of care requires functional health care teams supported by clinical information systems and organizational structure to facilitate care that is patient-centered, timely, and efficacious. Patient care that is well coordinated across disciplines and settings has demonstrated improved patient outcomes and greater efficiency for the health care system.[1] Pharmacists unique contributions to the health care team around the medication use process play a significant role in care coordination for patients who move between the acute care, ambulatory care, home care and alternative care settings. Often, the only point of care coordination is the pharmacist who manages medication-related requests from a variety of specialty and primary care providers.

In 2005, the Joint Commission of Accreditation of Health Care Organizations (JCAHO) added *Medication Reconciliation* to its list of patient safety goals further validating the unique contributions of pharmacists:

"Goal: Accurately and completely reconcile medications across the continuum of care.

- During 2005, for full implementation by January 2006, develop a process for obtaining and documenting a complete list of the patient's current medications upon the patient's admission to the organization and with the involvement of the patient. This process includes a comparison of the medications the organization provides to those on the list.

- A complete list of the patient's medications is communicated to the next provider of service when it refers or transfers a patient to another setting, service, practitioner or level of care within or outside the organization."[3]

Although JCAHO does not specifically require a pharmacist to perform this activity, Bond et al. evaluated 429,827 medication errors from 1,081 hospital over 1 year and demonstrated 17,638 fewer medication errors when pharmacists performed medication admission histories.[4] Clearly, pharmacists are the logical health care team member to provide verification of appropriate medications at each transitional point of care in order to reduce or eliminate therapeutic duplications and other drug misadventures and to improve the coordination of care around medication use.

Workforce Preparation

The IOM report also called for the restructuring of clinical education as well as a review of regulatory and legal system issues. Although it is beyond the scope of this chapter to detail the educational and training requirements needed to prepare an interprofessional workforce as well as laws and regulations governing health care professionals, we will briefly review some of these issues to set a context for overcoming barriers inherent in our current health care system for establishing effective teams.

Clinical Training and Education

The IOM *Crossing the Quality Chasm* Recommendation 12 states: "A multidisciplinary summit of leaders within the health professions should be held to discuss and develop strategies for (1) restructuring clinical education to be consistent with the principles of the 21st-century health system throughout the continuum of undergraduate, graduate, and continuing education for medical, nursing, and other professional training programs; and (2) assessing the implications of these changes for provider credentialing programs, funding, and sponsorship of education programs for health professionals."[1]

A new skill set will be required for all clinicians who provide patient care in a health care system that is moving into team-based care. The delivery of health care has shifted from acute to chronic care that establishes a new care delivery paradigm. In order to prepare health care professionals to respond to this new model, professional schools will need to focus on building competence to do the following:

- Work effectively in teams with shared responsibility

- Manage an ever-expanding base of evidence, critically evaluate new information, and determine how to incorporate it into practice

- Respond to a variety of approaches to the delivery of health care including collaborative practice models, group visits, and the use of electronic communication for follow-up care[5,6]

- Create changes in the patient-clinician relationship that include communicating in an open manner to support decision making and self-management skills as the patient becomes a partner with the health care team[7-9]

- Implement best practices through the design and measurement of the quality of care provided in terms of both process and outcomes[10]

- Utilize decision support tools to improve utilization in the health care system

- Understand and implement safety design principles such as standardization, simplification, and technological innovations to reduce errors[11,12]

Regulation of the Health Professions

The IOM report also commented on regulatory and legal system barriers in Recommendation 13: "The Agency for Healthcare Research and Quality should fund research to evaluate how the current regulatory and legal systems (1) facilitate or inhibit the changes needed for the 21st-centrury health care delivery system, and (2) can be modified to support health care professionals and organizations that seek to accomplish the six aims set forth in Chapter 2."[1]

Scope-of-practice acts attempt to establish minimum practice standards to assure patient safety but can limit effectiveness of team-based care. Since these acts reside at the state level, there are inconsistencies across the country. In most states, medical practice acts are broadly written, but other health care professionals are narrowly defined, usually by carving out responsibilities from the medical practice act. Additionally, a separate governance structure for each profession and the complexity of rules across disciplines and settings have shown to be significant barrier to use of multi-disciplinary teams.

There has been some discussion around proposed nationally uniform scopes of practice that have coordinated, publicly accountable policies to assure competence; however, current licensure and scope-of-practice laws offer no assurance of continuing competency. A novel approach has been suggested that involves an additional level of oversight in which teams of practitioners in addition to individuals are licensed or certified to provide care.[13] Clearly, this is an issue that will require attention as we move into new practice models of care.

Legal Liability Issues

Innovative care models can contribute to the threat of litigation due to changes from previous practice models. Risk occurs when applying novel methods of care that may not be completely tested. Similarly, organizational support for changes in practice models requires good educational efforts and communication with patients to prepare them for an unfamiliar care model. Legal decisions are often based on *standards of practice in the relevant medical community* from expert testimony. Thus far, evidence-based practice standards have had little effect on litigation; however, organizations that are implementing novel practice models should consider alternate approaches to liability.

Economic, Clinical, and Safety Outcomes Associated with Pharmacist-Provided Patient Care Services

Economic Value of Pharmacist-Provided Patient Care Services

The first publication to report a cost-benefit analysis of a clinical pharmacy service was published in 1979 looking at a hospital-based pharmacokinetic service. Its purpose was to evaluate benefits and costs of clinical pharmacy services as one possible "solution to increasing acceptance of such services by the medical profession, third-party payers, and consumers."[14] From that insightful beginning, the pharmacy profession has experienced multiple successes with these stakeholders through the provision of direct patient care and collaborative practice models throughout the health care system. However, the need to justify the value of patient care services provided by the pharmacist continues to play a major role in today's health care world.

Published articles on the economic impact of pharmacist-provided direct patient care are indispensable tools for the pharmacy manager, clinical coordinator, and clinician who may be developing, implementing, or defending such services. Two landmark articles have summarized and evaluated the body of literature that assessed the economic impact of clinical pharmacy services and provided guidance on research methods and future research needs.[15,16] The reviewers used five major categories to describe the type of service or intervention as follows:

1. "*Disease Management*—A clinical pharmacy service primarily directed at patients with a specific disease state or diagnosis like asthma.

2. *Pharmacotherapeutic Monitoring*—A clinical pharmacy service that encompassed a broad range of activities based primarily on the needs of an assigned group of patients with services provided such as patient drug regimen review and recommendation, adverse drug reaction monitoring, drug interaction assessment, formulary compliance, and rounding with physicians.

3. *Pharmacokinetic Monitoring*—A clinical pharmacy service that primarily involved evaluation of anticipated or actual serum drug concentrations and provision of subsequent dosing recommendations.

4. *Targeted Drug Program*—A clinical pharmacy service that primarily focused on a single drug or class of drugs and may have included predefined guidelines for provision of alternative therapy or dosing recommendations, such as intravenous to oral switch recommendations for antibiotics.

5. *Patient Education Program or Cognitive Service*—A clinical pharmacy service that primarily instructed patients on the proper administration of drugs and/or identified drug-related problems."[15]

The results from the 2003 publication reviewed 59 evaluable studies and demonstrated that pharmacists provided a positive economic impact in 85% of these. Sixteen of these studies calculated the benefit: cost ratio, which ranged from 1.74:1–17.0:1 with a median of 4.68:1. In other words, for every dollar invested in pharmacist services, the health care system realized over four dollars of cost savings. These studies occurred in multiple settings and the pharmacists involved provided various clinical services.

Although these are impressive results, there has been relatively little published on the economic value of the pharmacist as part of an inter-professional health care team. In the hospital setting, we have seen that pharmacist participation in the patient care team can reduce length of stay, prescription costs, and hospital costs; avoid drug costs; and reduce costly, avoidable adverse drug events.[17–22] In the ambulatory care setting, pharmacists have contributed to reduced drug costs and reduced costs associated with clinic visits.[23–25] In the managed care setting, numerous studies have demonstrated cost savings as a result of reduced drug costs and use of other health services.[26]

Clinical Value of Pharmacist-Provided Patient Care Services

Many published reports have demonstrated improved health outcomes with pharmacist-provided patient care services across the continuum of care. Pharmacist-run anticoagulation services have shown improved anticoagulation control, reduced bleeding and thromboembolic events, provided cost savings of $1,600 per patient per year in reduced emergency room visits and hospitalizations, and reduced length of stay.[27–29] Pharmacists have also been shown to improve clinical outcomes for patients with various chronic conditions such as asthma, HIV/AIDS, dislipidemia, diabetes, congestive heart failure, and multiple chronic condi-

tions within primary care settings.[30–40]

An excellent series of articles have been published since 2000 that describe, analyze, and interpret the results of the IMPROVE (Impact of Managed Pharmaceutical Care on Resource Utilization and Outcomes in Veterans Affairs Medical Centers) study. This study is one of the largest pharmaceutical care studies conducted. It was an intervention study that looked at global outcomes following management by pharmacists and demonstrated effective methods of identifying patients who could benefit the most from pharmacist interventions. The first article described the types of interventions made by clinical pharmacists, the second publication described the economic analysis of these interventions, and the third publication sought to interpret the findings of the pharmacist interventions.[41–43]

A total of 1,045 patients were randomized to either a control group (n=531) and received usual care or the intervention group (n=523) and were referred to clinic-based pharmacists for care. Study pharmacists documented a total of 1,855 contacts with the intervention group patients and made 3,048 therapy-specific interventions over the 12-month study period. There was no meaningful difference in patient satisfaction or quality of life in the two groups. Selected disease-specific indicators found an improved rate of measurement of hemoglobin A1C tests and better control of total and low-density lipoprotein (LDL) cholesterol levels in the intervention group compared with the total control group. Total health care costs (clinic visits including pharmacist visits, hospitalizations, drugs, lab tests, imaging procedures) increased in both groups over the 12-month period. The mean increase in costs in the intervention group was $1,020, which was 29% lower than the control group's value of $1,313.

Medication Use Safety Value of Pharmacist-Provided Patient Care Services

In the hospital setting, pharmacist participation on the health care team was associated with lower mortality rates averaging 386 patient lives per hospital per year.[44] Medication admission histories in 30 hospitals resulted in 3,843 fewer deaths each year and participation on the Cardiopulmonary Resuscitation (CPR) Team in 282 hospitals resulted in 5,047 fewer deaths each year. A subsequent larger study by the same authors of 1,081 hospitals evaluated a total of 429,827 medication errors, a rate of 5.22% of patients admitted each year.[4] Factors associated with decreased medication errors per occupied bed per year included the presence of a drug information service, pharmacist-provided adverse drug reaction management, pharmacist-managed drug protocols, pharmacist participation on medical rounds, pharmacist-provided medication admission histories, and increased staffing of clinical pharmacists per occupied bed. Taken together, these landmark studies demonstrate the pharmacist's role as a member of the health care team to improve medication-related safety.

A 66% reduction in adverse drug events was seen when pharmacists participated in patient rounds in the intensive care unit of a large academic medical center.[22] During the 6-month study period, pharmacists intervened on about 400 safety-related issues primarily related to medication errors. These errors included incomplete orders, incorrect dosages and frequency, sub optimal drug choices, and duplicate therapy. Physicians responded positively to the pharmacist presence on rounds and accepted 99% of their recommendations. These authors projected $270,000 in annual cost savings related to the pharmacist prevention of adverse drug events as a result of their participation on the health care team.

Pharmacists in Collaborative Practice Models of Care

Collaborative Drug Therapy Management Activities

Collaborative drug therapy management (CDTM) authorizes pharmacists to enter into agreements with physicians to jointly manage a patient's medication therapy. In 2004, 40 states had passed CDTM laws allowing pharmacists to enter into these agreements. Although each state law is different with some requiring specific credentials or certifications to participate in CDTM, these activities may include the following:

- Selecting, initiating, modifying, continuing, and discontinuing a patient's drug therapy

- Ordering, performing, and interpreting medication-related laboratory tests as appropriate to monitor patient's response to medications

- Providing assessment of the patient's response to therapy

- Participating in disease state management for patients with chronic conditions that includes the coordination of care activities across the health care continuum

- Educating and counseling the patient and/or caregiver on medication use

- Administering medications and vaccines

Research Supporting Pharmacists in Collaborative Practice Models

Although it is implied in many of the articles cited in this chapter, there are relatively few published studies that look specifically at the role pharmacist collaboration plays in achieving improved patient outcomes. As part of a larger study, Isetts et al. reported their quality improvement and care process validation results of the therapeutic decisions made by pharmacists in a collaborative practice for several years.[45] A panel of 12 physicians and pharmacists reviewed 5,780 pharmacist-managed interventions for 2,524 patients. The rate of achieving therapeutic goals increased from 74% prior to the pharmacist intervention to 89% after the patients' latest encounters. Panelists agreed with the pharmacists' decisions in 94.2% of the cases, were neutral about their decisions in 3.6% of the cases, and disagreed in 2.2% of the cases. This study demonstrates the clinical credibility of drug therapy management services provided by pharmacists working in collaborative practices with physicians.

Pharmacists practicing in a medically underserved, limited English-speaking pediatric clinic designed and implemented collaborative protocols to evaluate and treat five acute conditions including cough/cold, fever, diaper rash, vomiting/diarrhea, and head lice.[46] During the first year of the program, 191 patients were evaluated and treated. Two physicians and four pharmacists reviewed each intervention for cough/cold (145 or 76% of patients) and found no unexpected or adverse outcomes. The conclusions from this study supported the clinical credibility of pharmacy-based evaluation and treatment under collaborative agreements to improve access to care for children with minor illnesses.

A study conducted in the Cincinnati, Ohio Department of Veterans Affairs Medical Center Lipid Clinic looked at the influence of an inter-professional team that included a clinical pharmacist, nurse practitioner, dietitian, clinical psychologist, and a consultant cardiologist in meeting the National Cholesterol Education Program (NCEP) goals.[33] The cardiologist reviewed laboratory data and confirmed the therapeutic decisions of the team each week during their preclinic meeting, adding quality assessment oversight to the team's decisions. The results demonstrated that after four clinic visits, patients in the lipid clinic group were four times more likely to reach NCEP goals than patients in a comparable general internal medicine clinic, thus supporting an interprofessional, goal-oriented collaborative practice model of care.

Other studies have looked at various care delivery models for providing collaborative drug therapy management and most describe the economic, clinical, and/or medication safety outcomes realized with the addition of the pharmacist as noted earlier in this chapter. To date, there are very few studies that have built quality assurance reviews into their model to the extent Isett, Kalister, and Shaffer did.

Characteristics of Effective Collaborative Practice Models

Characteristics that influence the development of collaborative relationships between physicians and pharmacists include role specification, trustworthiness, and relationship initiation.[47] In a study to develop a theoretical model of physician/pharmacist collaborative relationships, Zillich et al. looked at three groups of relationship characteristics to identify which most influenced the development of collaborative practice. The three groups included the following:

- *Participant Variables*—Demographics of the participants

- *Context Drivers*—Practice environment and professional interactions of the participants

- *Exchange Characteristics*—Describe the nature of the exchange and include relationship initiation, trustworthiness, and role specification

Their results demonstrated that the influential characteristics of physician/pharmacist collaborative relationships included mild influence from participant and context factors. The three domains of exchange factors were significantly associated with strong collaborative practices.

Establishing a Collaborative Drug Therapy Management Service

Kuo et al. reviewed regulatory and billing issues while providing a case study for establishing CDTM services within a clinic.[48] They recommend 10 steps for establishing a successful service:

1. Establish a working relationship with physician colleagues

2. Assess the needs of your patients

3. Draft collaborative CDTM protocols and agreements

4. Apply for credentialing/privileging status within your health organization

5. Consult the billing office staff at the clinic

6. Design a clinic-encounter form

7. Identify and train support personnel

8. Allocate resources

9. Advertise the CDTM

10. Evaluate and improve your service

Each organization should tailor their service to meet the expectations and culture of the practice the pharmacist will be joining. Employing the characteristics of successful physician/pharmacist collaboration as identified above should facilitate the implementation of a favorable CDTM service.

An excellent review of a model primary care pharmacy service that includes a program description, tools for the pharmacy practitioner, and economic and clinical outcomes related to pharmacists activities was published in 2004.[49] Carmichael et al. describe 8 years of experience in their Veterans Health Administration system site with insight on developing CDTM practice, justifying pharmacy staffing and data system support to assist in the implementation of their practice model. Additionally, the authors have included a copy of their scope of practice for their clinical pharmacy specialists.

Scope of Practice for Pharmacists in Collaborative Practice Models

A critical activity for establishing a collaborative practice is to define the scope of practice for pharmacists practicing within the organization. This sets the expectations for pharmacy staff as well as the members of the interprofessional team. The scope of practice should be broadly written to facilitate professional decision-making but may not exceed the state's scope-of-practice laws. Appendix 1 is an example of a scope of practice document from an academic medical center in Washington State where the CDTM laws are quite liberal.

The Pharmacist Privileging Process

Pharmacists who are practicing under CDTM agreements within an organization should undergo a credentialing/privileging process that aligns with the physicians and mid-level practitioners within their organization. At the Institute of Medicine's summit on interprofessional health care, it was recommended that certification and licensing groups establish performance-based assessment standards to ensure the

Scope of Practice: Ambulatory Clinical Pharmacy Specialists

Harborview Medical Center, Seattle, Washington

Purpose

Identify scope-of-practice privileges for the clinical pharmacy specialists (CPS) at Harborview Medical Center (HMC) and define criteria for the qualifications for these privileges. The CPS will be qualified and authorized to perform specific clinical duties to ensure that cost-effective, high-quality health care and appropriate pharmaceutical care are provided to patients.

Policy

Scope-of-practice guidelines for CPSs shall be delineated in writing and will follow established protocols approved by the HMC Clinic Medical Directors, Associate Medical Director for Ambulatory Care Services, Medical Director, and the Washington State Board of Pharmacy.

Qualifications

The CPS is trained in clinical therapeutics, pharmacokinetics, and pharmacology. He or she is a Doctor of Pharmacy (Pharm.D.) graduate, has completed an accredited pharmacy residency, specialty residency in primary care, is a specialty board-certified pharmacist, or has equivalent education, training, and experience functioning as a clinical pharmacist. The HMC Credentialing Committee credentials all ambulatory CPS practicing at Harborview Medical Center.

Structure and Process

In most cases, the CPS works in the clinic's Provider Room to facilitate consultations between the CPS and other providers including attending physicians, medical residents, mid-level practitioners and others. The CPS shall provide consultations and accept referrals from medical staff. The CPS role differs with attending physicians and medical residents. In the case of medical residents who are in training to manage various patient care issues, the CPS shall offer consultation (education) on medication therapy management.

In the case of attending physicians, the CPS shall provide consultation services and accept referrals for therapeutic disease state management activities that require intensive medication dosage titration, management and follow-up. In the vast majority of cases, patients referred to the CPS are identified as *high risk* for drug-related problems. These risks include the following:

- Five or more medications in a regimen
- 12 or more doses per day
- A medication regimen that changes often
- Three or more concurrent disease states
- A history of noncompliance
- The presence of drugs that require therapeutic drug monitoring

Key Functions

The CPS collaborates with physicians to provide safe, evidence-based, cost-effective medication therapy management that improves a patient's health related quality of life through the following actions:

- Conducts comprehensive health and drug histories and performing physical examinations necessary to assess drug therapy
- Documents relevant findings in the patient's medical record
- Evaluates drug therapy using subjective and objective findings related to patients' responses to drug therapy and communicates and documents the findings and recommendations to appropriate individuals and in the medical record
- Develops, documents, and executes therapeutic plans utilizing the most efficacious medications per national, Pharmacy and Therapeutics Committee or HMC-specific guidelines or protocols including the Preferred Drug Formulary
- Orders and analyzes laboratory and diagnostic test data to monitor and adjust drug therapy as necessary
- Initiates, adjusts, and discontinues medication therapy to meet therapeutic goals established by protocol
- Provides care coordination for chronic disease states as well as self-limiting acute conditions per protocol
- Identifies and takes specific corrective action for drug-related problems
- Provides patient and health care professional education and medication education
- Evaluates and documents patients' and caregivers' ability to understand medication instructions and provide oral and written counseling on their medications
- Completes facility billing for all CPS visits
- Administers medication according to pre-established protocols (pediatric asthma/vaccines)
- Serves as a clinical manager of drug-related programs in clinics in conjunction with the attending physician

Common Conditions Identified for CPS Disease State Management

- Attention Deficit Hyperactivity Disorder (ADHD)
- Anticoagulation therapy including the Pharmacist-run VT Program
- Asthma/COPD
- Cardiovascular (CHF, HTN, Lipids, MI, CAD)
- Diabetes
- Emergency contraception
- Hepatitis
- Home antibiotic care
- Highly active antiretroviral therapy (HAART) for HIV infection
- Iron supplementation for children
- Medication assessment and adherence
- Over-the-counter (OTC) triage protocols
- Pain management (acute post-op pain and chronic nonmalignant pain)
- Pharmacokinetic consultation
- Smoking cessation
- Travel medicine

Supervision

The ultimate responsibility for CPS staff rests with the Assistant Director, Ambulatory Pharmacy; however, a collegial relationship with mutual consultation and referral exists between physicians and the CPS. Consultation with the physician or referring practitioner is outlined, and cosignature is required for practice outside approved procedures and protocols. The CPS will provide patient care as a nonphysician clinician. A physician is available at all times by telephone or in person for consultation. Periodic chart and peer reviews by pharmacy and medical colleagues and annual evaluations provide ongoing quality assurance and medication-use evaluation. The CPS practices are included in the medication-use evaluation process.

Patient Outcomes

When possible, HMC-specific patient outcomes will be assessed using the Value Compass (HMC's internal quality improvement) methodology. When this is not possible, evidence-based literature on the effectiveness of clinical pharmacy services shall be used to predict the economic, clinical, operational, and humanistic outcomes of the service.

competence of health professionals.[50] Although each organization has its own standards for privileging, most review provider's credentials and performance prior to authorizing them to practice within the organization. Privileging is required to receive reimbursement for services from third party payers as well as Medicare. An excellent primer on pharmacist credentialing/privileging was published in 2004 and includes background material, a resource list, and several case studies demonstrating the privileging process in various types of health care systems.[51]

Medication Therapy Management Services

At the end of the 2003 legislative session, the United States Congress passed the *Medicare Prescription Drug, Improvement, and Modernization Act,* which included a provision known as Medication Therapy Management Services (MTMS). This part of the law was left to the Centers for Medicare and Medicaid Services (CMS) to implement and CMS asked the pharmacy profession for guidance on implementing MTMS. In July 2004, 11 national pharmacy organizations including the Academy of Managed Care Pharmacy, American Association of Colleges of Pharmacy, American College of Apothecaries, American College of Clinical Pharmacy, American Pharmacists Association, American Society of Health-System Pharmacists, American Society of Consultant Pharmacists, National Association of Boards of Pharmacy, National Association of Chain Drug Stores, National Community Pharmacists Association, and the National Council of State Pharmacy Association Executives approved the *Pharmacy Profession Stakeholders Consensus Document* to define MTMS:

> "Medication Therapy Management is a distinct service or group of services that optimize therapeutic outcomes for individual patients. Medication Therapy Management Services are independent of, but can occur in conjunction with, the provision of a medication product.
>
> Medication Therapy Management encompasses a broad range of professional activities and responsibilities within the licensed pharmacist or other qualified health care provider's, scope of practice. These services include but are not limited to the following, according to the individual needs of the patient:
>
> a. Performing or obtaining necessary assessments of the patient's health status;

b. Formulating a medication treatment plan;

c. Selecting, initiating, modifying, or administering medication therapy;

d. Monitoring and evaluating the patient's response to therapy, including safety and effectiveness;

e. Performing a comprehensive medication review to identify, resolve, and prevent medication-related problems, including adverse drug events;

f. Documenting the care delivered and communicating essential information to the patient's other primary care providers;

g. Providing verbal education and training designed to enhance patient understanding and appropriate use of his/her medications;

h. Providing information, support services and resources designed to enhance patient adherence with his/her therapeutic regimens;

i. Coordinating and integrating medication therapy management services within the broader health care-management services being provided to the patient.

A program that provides coverage for Medication Therapy Management services shall include:

a. Patient-specific and individualized services or sets of services provided directly by a pharmacist to the patient.* These services are distinct from formulary development and use, generalized patient education and information activities, and other population-focused quality assurance measures for medication use.

b. Face-to-face interaction between the patient* and the pharmacist as the preferred method of delivery. When patient-specific barriers to face-to-face communication exist, patients shall have equal access to appropriate alternative delivery methods. MTM programs shall include structures supporting the establishment and maintenance of the patient*-pharmacist relationship.

c. Opportunities for pharmacists and other qualified health care providers to identify patients who should receive medication therapy management services.

d. Payment for Medication Therapy Management Services consistent with contemporary provider payment rates that are based on the time, clinical intensity, and resources required to provide services (e.g., Medicare Part A and/or Part B for CPT & RBRVS).

e. Processes to improve continuity of care, outcomes, and outcome measures.

*In some situations, Medication Therapy Management Services may be provided to the caregiver or other persons involved in the care of the patient."[52]

Although there are many similarities between MTMS and CDTM, the pharmacist providing medication therapy management services may be constrained by their individual state's scope of practice law from fully implementing this service. In early 2005, CMS released their final rules around the implementation of Medication Therapy Management Services and determined that "insufficient standards and performance measures exist to support further specification" for the services. The agency noted in the final rule that before the definition of medication therapy management services had been crafted during the consensus conference, "no widely agreed upon definition...existed, let alone standards and measures" for the programs. The agency stated that it will collect details from plans on how they implement medication therapy management programs, with the goal of having the programs "evolve and become a cornerstone" of the Part D benefit.[53]

Innovations in Care: The Planned Care Model

A multidimensional solution to the complex issues around coordination of care has been implemented in a few organizations.[8] Known as the *Planned Care Model* (Figure 14-1), it was developed to bring health care resources to the patient in the right place and at the right time. It identifies six essential elements including community resources and policies, health care organization, self-management support, delivery system design, decision support, and clinical information systems.

Support from the health care organization is essential as all other elements are built upon that foundation. This usually entails organizational realignment and partnerships with payers to sustain the care model. Community linkages with senior centers and other community support groups leverage the organization's resources and commitment to the model. Within the health care organization, operational and structural elements are deployed to support health care providers as well as patients (the last four elements).

Self-management support is a collaboration between the patient and the health care team to build skills and confidence for patients to manage their chronic condition. Typically, the pharmacist's role

Figure 14-1
The Planned Care Model Developed by Improving Chronic Illness Care (ICIC)[a]

Planned Care Model

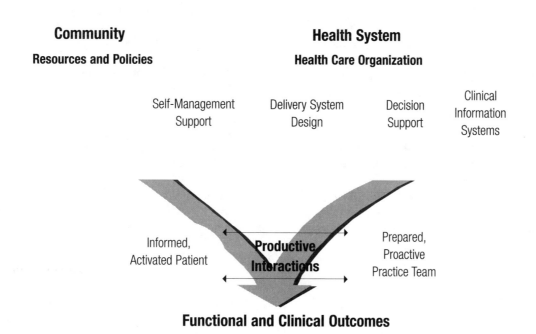

Community

Resources and Policies

Health System

Health Care Organization

Self-Management Support

Delivery System Design

Decision Support

Clinical Information Systems

Informed, Activated Patient

Productive Interactions

Prepared, Proactive Practice Team

Functional and Clinical Outcomes

[a] A national program supported by The Robert Wood Johnson Foundation with direction and technical assistance provided by Group Health Cooperative's MacColl Institute for Healthcare Innovation.

---

includes self-measurement and medication use (glucometer teaching, medication education, inhaler technique, using weight measurement to assess heart failure). Delivery system design refers to structural changes needed to support true team-based care where the roles and expectations of each member of the team are clear and optimize the contribution of each team member. Decision support uses evidence-based guidelines to standardize and integrate best practices into each patient visit. Finally, well-designed clinical information systems facilitate population-based standards of practice to be tailored to the individual patient through automatic reminder systems, performance measure feedback to the health care teams, and the development of registries to electronically sort and identify specific patient populations for interventions.

Ultimately, the planned care model seeks to build a practice team that is prepared for today's visit with an informed and empowered patient. The successful visit includes assessment and tailoring of therapy, colla-borative problem definition, evidence-based clinical management, collaborative goal setting and problem solving, shared care plan development, and active, sustained follow up. The pharmacist's role in this colla-borative model of care leverages his or her unique set of qualifications around optimizing medication use.

Case Study Revisited

Dr. Jackson recently joined a forward-thinking group of practitioners that includes nurse practitioners, a pharmacist, a nutritionist, and a social worker. Today Mr. Newman's visit is a different experience for him and his physician. Prior to this visit, the clinical pharmacist scheduled Mr. Newman for an educational session around the importance of keeping a blood glucose diary, told him to bring that information to each clinic visit, and taught him how to use a glucometer. This was documented in the electronic medical record (EMR) with an alert to download the patient's glucometer information upon check-in for today's appointment. When the patient is escorted to the exam room, the medical assistant logs into Mr. Newman's EMR in the room and instructs the patient to remove his shoes and socks to facilitate his routine diabetic foot check. Dr. Jackson greets the patient while she reviews the laboratory results, glucometer readings, and results of his recent eye exam. She notes that his blood glucose readings are very inconsistent and after questioning learns that the patient is having trouble with his insulin regimen. She refers the patient to the clinical pharmacist who adjusts the dosing schedule to meet Mr. Newman's daily routine and schedules follow-up phone calls to fine-tune the changes.

This case serves to demonstrate the differences in the quality of patient care received from a highly functional health care team compared with a more traditional care model. Pharmacists play an integral part in collaborative care models of practice bringing a unique set of knowledge and skills to the health care team and their patients.

Acknowledgements

I wish to thank Daniel Lessler, MD, MHA, Ambulatory Care Medical Director at Harborview Medical Center, for his vision and leadership in supporting team-based, collaborative care that leverages pharmacists' knowledge and skills to provide high quality patient care and to my clinical pharmacy specialists for making this vision a reality.

Suggested Readings

Bond CA, Raehl CL, Franke T. Clinical pharmacy services, hospital pharmacy staffing, and medication errors in United States hospitals. *Pharmacotherapy.* 2002;22: 134–47.

Carmichael JM, Alvarez A, Chaput R, et al. Establishment and outcomes of a model primary care pharmacy service system. *Am J Health-Syst Pharm.* 2004;61:472–82.

Carter BL, Malone DC, Billups SJ, et al. Interpreting the findings of the IMPROVE study. *Am J Health-Syst Pharm.* 2001;58:1330–7.

Ellis SL, Billups SJ, Malone DC, et al. Types of interventions made by clinical pharmacists in the IMPROVE study *Pharmacotherapy.* 2000;20:429–35.

Leape LL, Cullen DJ, Clapp MD, et al. Pharmacist participation on physician rounds and adverse drug events in the intensive care unit. *JAMA.* 1999;282(3):267–70.

Malone DC, Carter BL, Billups JS, et al. An economic analysis of a randomized, controlled, multicenter study of clinical pharmacist interventions for high-risk

veterans; the IMPROVE study. *Pharmacotherapy.*. 2000;20:1149–58.

Schumock GT, Butler MG, Meek PD, et al. Evidence of the economic benefit of clinical pharmacy services—1996–2000. *Pharmacotherapy.* 2003;23(1):113–32.

References

1. Committee on Quality of Health Care in America. *Crossing the Quality Chasm: A New Health System for the 21st Century.* Washington, DC: National Academies Press; 2001.

2. Shortell SM, Gillies RR, Anderson DA. Remaking health care in America. 2nd ed. San Francisco, CA: Jossey-Bass; 2000.

3. Joint Commission on Accreditation of Healthcare Organizations. National patient safety goals for 2004 and 2005. Available at: www.jcaho.org/ accredited+organizations/patient+ safety/ npsg.htm. Accessed December 10, 2004.

4. Bond CA, Raehl CL, Franke T. Clinical pharmacy services, hospital pharmacy staffing, and medication errors in United States hospitals. *Pharmacotherapy.* 2002;22:134–47.

5. VonKorff M, Gruman J, Schaefer J, et al. Collaborative management of chronic illness. *Ann Intern Med.* 1997;127(12):1097–102.

6. Wagner EH. More than a case manager. *Ann Intern Med.* 1998;129(8):654–6.

7. Bodenheimer T, Lorig K, Holman H, et al. Patient self-management of chronic disease in primary care. *JAMA.* 2002;288(19):2469–75.

8. Bodenheimer T, Wagner EH, Grumbach K. Improving primary care for patients with chronic illness. *JAMA.* 2002;288(14):1775–9.

9. Lorig KR, Sobel DS, Stewart AL, et al. Evidence suggesting that a chronic disease self-management program can improve health status while reducing hospitalization: a randomized trial. *Med Care.* 1999;37(1):5–14.

10. Cretin S, Shortell SM, Keeler EB. An evaluation of collaborative interventions to improve chronic illness care. Framework and study design. *Evaluation Review.* 2004;28(1):28–51.

11. Knapp KK, Ray MD. A pharmacy response to the Institute of Medicine's 2001 initiative on quality in health care. *Am J Health Syst Pharm.* 2002;59(23): 2443–50.

12. Kohn LT, Corrigan JM, Donaldson MD, eds. To err is human: building a safer health system. Washington, DC: National Academies Press; 2000.

13. Gragnola CM, Stone E. Considering the future of health care workforce regulation: responses from the field to the Pew Health Professions Commission's December 1995 report. Reforming health care workforce regulation: policy considerations for the 21st century. Available at: www.http://futurehealth.ucsf.edu/ pdf_files/futwkreg.pdf. Accessed December 10, 2004.

14. Bootman LJ, Wertheimer AI, Zaske D, et al. Individualizing gentamicin dosage in burn patients with gram-negative septicemia: a cost-benefit analysis. *J Pharm Sci*. 1979;168:267–72.

15. Schumock GT, Butler MG, Meek PD, et al. Evidence of the economic benefit of clinical pharmacy services—1996–2000. *Pharmacotherapy*. 2003;23(1):113–32.

16. Schumock GT, Meek PD, Ploetz PA, et al. Economic evaluation of clinical pharmacy service: 1988–1995. *Pharmacotherapy*. 1996;16(7):1188–208.

17. Boyko WL, Yurkowski PJ, Ivey MF, et al. Pharmacist influence on economic and morbidity outcomes in a tertiary care teaching hospital. *Am J Health-Syst Pharm*. 1997;54:1591–5.

18. Lata P, VanCourt B, Larson P. Pharmacist as a member of a hospital case management department. *Am J Health-Syst Pharm*. 2000:57:2202–6.

19. Yee DK, Veal JH, Trinh B, et al. Involvement of HMO-based pharmacists in clinical rounds at contract hospitals. *Am J Health-Syst Pharm*. 1997;54:670–3.

20. Baldinger SL, Chow MS, Gammon RH, et al. Cost savings from having a clinical pharmacist work part-time in a medical intensive care unit. *Am J Health-Syst Pharm*. 1997;54:2811–4.

21. White CM, Chow MSS. Cost impact and clinical benefits of focused rounding in the cardiovascular intensive care unit. *Hosp Pharm*. 1998;33:419–23.

22. Leape LL, Cullen DJ, Clapp MD, et al. Pharmacist participation on physician rounds and adverse drug events in the intensive care unit. *JAMA*. 1999;282(3):267–70.

23. Rodgers S, Avery AJ, Meechan D, et al. Controlled trial of pharmacist intervention in general practice: the effect on prescribing costs. *Br J Gen Pract*. 1999;49:717–20.

24. Beck JK, Dries TJ, Cook EC. Development of an interdisciplinary, telephone-based care program. *Am J Health-Syst Pharm*. 1998;55(5):453–7.

25. Grace KA, McPherson ML, Burstein AH. Diabetes care and cost of pharmacotherapy versus medical services. *Am J Health-Syst Pharm*. 1998;55:S27–9.

26. Borgsdorf LR, Miano JS, Knapp KK. Pharmacist-managed medication review in a managed care system. *Am J Hosp Pharm*. 1994;51(6):772–7.

27. Chiquette E, Amato MG, Bussey HI. Comparison of an anticoagulation clinic with usual medical care: anticoagulation control, patient outcomes, and health care costs. *Arch Intern Med*. 1998;158(15):1641–7.

28. Spalek VH, Gong WC. Pharmaceutical care in an integrated health system. *J Am Pharm Assoc (Wash)*. 1999 Jul–Aug;39(4):553–7.

29. Mamdani MM, Racine E, McCreadie S, et al. Clinical and economic effectiveness of an inpatient anticoagulation service. *Pharmacotherapy*. 1999 Sep;19(9):1064–74.

30. Pauley TR, Magee MJ, Cury JD. Pharmacist-managed, physician-directed asthma management program reduces emergency department visits. *Ann Pharmacotherapy*. 1995;29(1):5–9.

31. Simoni JM, Frick PA, Pantalone DW, et al. Antiretroviral adherence interventions: a review of current literature and ongoing studies. *Top HIV Med*. 2003;11(6):185–98.

32. Till LT, Voris JC, Horst JB. Assessment of clinical pharmacist management of lipid-lowering therapy in a primary care setting. *J Manag Care Pharm*. 2003;9(3):275–6.

33. Shaffer J, Wexler LF. Reducing low-density lipoprotein cholesterol levels in an ambulatory care system. Results of a multidisciplinary collaborative practice lipid clinic compared with traditional physician-based care. *Arch Intern Med*. 1995;155(21):2330–5.

34. Irons BK, Lenz RJ, Anderson SL, et al. A retrospective cohort analysis of the clinical effectiveness of a physician-pharmacist collaborative drug therapy management diabetes clinic. *Pharmacotherapy*. 2002;22(10):1294–300.

35. Whellan DJ, Gaulden L, Gattis WA, et al. The benefit of implementing a heart failure disease management program. *Arch Intern Med*. 2001;161(18):2223–8.

36. Gattis WA, Hasselblad V, Whellan DJ, et al. Reduction in heart failure events by the addition of a clinical pharmacist to the heart failure management team: results of the Pharmacist in Heart Failure Assessment Recommendation and Monitoring (PHARM) Study. *Arch Intern Med*. 1999;159(16):1939–45.

37. Luzier AB, Forrest A, Geuerstein SF, et al. Containment of heart failure hospitalizations and cost by angiotensin-converting enzyme inhibitor dosage optimization. *Am J Cardiol*. 2000;86(5):519–23.

38. Jameson J, VanNoord G, Vanderwoud K. The impact of pharmacotherapy consultation on the cost and outcome of medical therapy. *J Fam Prac*. 1995;41(5):469–72.

39. Galt KA. Cost avoidance, acceptance, and outcomes associated with a pharmacotherapy consult clinic in a VA Medical Center. *Pharmacotherapy*. 1998;18(5):1103–11.

40. Mason JD, Colley CA. Effectiveness of an ambulatory care clinical pharmacist: a controlled trial. *Ann Pharmacother*. 1993;27(5):555–9.

41. Ellis SL, Billups SJ, Malone DC, et al. Types of interventions made by clinical pharmacists in the IMPROVE study. *Pharmacotherapy*. 2000;20:429–35.

42. Malone DC, Carter BL, Billups JS, et al. An economic analysis of a randomized, controlled, multicenter study of clinical pharmacist interventions for high-risk veterans; the IMPROVE study. *Pharmacotherapy*. 2000;20:1149-58.

43. Carter BL, Malone DC, Billups SJ, et al. Interpreting the findings of the IMPROVE study. *Am J Health-Syst Pharm*. 2001;58:1330–7.

44. Bond CA, Raehl CL, Franke T. Clinical pharmacy services, hospital services and hospital mortality rate. *Pharmacotherapy*. 1999;19:556–64.

45. Isetts BJ, Brown LM, Schondelmeyer SW, et al. Quality assessment of a collaborative approach for decreasing drug-related morbidity and achieving therapeutic goals. *Arch Intern Med*. 2003;163(15):1813–20.

46. Kalister H, Newman RD, Read L, et al. Pharmacy-based evaluation and treatment of minor illnesses in a culturally diverse pediatric clinic. *Arch Pediatr Adolesc Med.* 1999;153:731–5.

47. Zillich AJ, McDonough RP, Carter BL, et al. Influential characteristics of physician/pharmacist collaborative relationships. *Ann Pharmacother.* 2004;38(5):764–70.

48. Kuo GM, Buckley TE, Fitzsimmons DS, et al. Collaborative drug therapy management services and reimbursement in a family medicine clinic. *Am J Health Syst Pharm.* 2004;61(4):343–54.

49. Carmichael JM, Alvarez A, Chaput R, et al. Establishment and outcomes of a model primary care pharmacy service system. *Am J Health-Syst Pharm.* 2004;61: 472–82.

50. Greiner AC, Knebel E, eds. Health professions education: a bridge to quality (2003). Available at: www.nap.edu/openbook/0309087236/html/. Accessed December 10, 2004.

51. Galt KA. Credentialing and privileging for pharmacists. *Am J Health-Syst Pharm.* 2004;61(9):661–70

52. American Society of Health-System Pharmacists. Summary of Executive Sessions, Medication Therapy Management Programs. Available at: http://ashp.org/gad/MTM_ExecSum.pdf. Accessed December 10, 2004.

53. 42 CFR Parts 400, 403, 411, 417, and 423 Medicare Program; Medicare Prescriptions Drug Benefit; Final Rule. *Federal Register.* January 28, 2005;70(18): 4193–585.

Chapter 15

Medication Management

Kathy A. Chase

Introduction

Medication safety and medication cost are two challenges for pharmacists. These two factors are not always in alignment with one another. Medication use management provides a mechanism to assure the safe and effective use of drugs in a cost conscious manner. Key to medication management in the health-system environment is the formulary system. The formulary system is a mechanism for ongoing assessment of medications that are available for use. The system is managed by a committee of experts, which includes pharmacists and physicians.

Historically, medication management has been limited to the formulary. More recently use of preprinted orders, evidence-based medication use guidelines, and outcomes assessment has become part of the medication management process. However, the principles of medication management remain constant. This chapter will discuss the medication management system with focus on the following:

- Formulary System
- Pharmacy and Therapeutics Committee
- Formulary Management
- Drug Use Evaluation
- Medication Use Policies
- Published Formulary

The Formulary System

A drug formulary is often described as a list of medications routinely stocked by the health care system. The formulary was developed by hospitals in the 1950s as a management tool. It was initially used to assure that physicians had an adequate and consistent supply of medications for their day-to-day needs. A key purpose of the formulary was to discourage the use of marginally effective drugs and treatments.

Over time, the formulary has evolved beyond a list of medications to a system that methodically evaluates medications on an ongoing basis for inclusion or exclusion, establishes guidelines for optimal medication use, and develops policies and procedures for prescribing, dispensing, and administering medications.

The formulary is now one element of the formulary system. It is a continually updated list of medications and related information, representing the clinical judgment of pharmacists, physicians, and other experts in the diagnosis and/or treatment of disease and promotion of health. The Pharmacy and Therapeutics Committee, or equivalent, is the organized team of experts that manages the formulary system.

There are advantages and disadvantages to a formulary system. The system does provide a systematic method to review scientific evidence on clinical effectiveness and cost effectiveness in drug selection decision, thus potentially improving health outcomes while reducing costs. Overly restrictive formulary systems may potentially reduce the quality of care by limited access to clinically indicated medications.

The Pharmacy and Therapeutics Committee

The Pharmacy and Therapeutics Committee (P&T Committee) has oversight for medication management in the health system. Specific regulatory or accrediting bodies may confirm this accountability. To be effective, the committee must have the support of the individual members as well as the health system and medical staff as a whole.

Organization

The committee is generally a policy recommending body to the medical staff through the Medical Executive Committee. More recently, in some organizations, the P&T Committee has reported directly to a health-system board rather than a local Medical Executive Committee. The committee is responsible to the medical staff as a whole, and its recommendations are subject to approval by the organized medical staff as well as the routine administrative approval process.

The frequency of the meeting, the length of the meeting, and sense of accomplishment of the meeting participant often limit meeting participation. The frequency of meetings should be often enough to conduct business in a reasonable time period. Often it is difficult for committee members to commit longer than 90 minutes to a meeting. Therefore, meetings should be limited to 60–90 minutes in length. Because drug products and medical literature are continually changing, meetings should occur at least four to six times per year. Generally, monthly meetings are needed to keep the meeting time to 60–90 minutes.

Subcommittees or task forces have been established to facilitate meeting efficiency. Examples of subcommittees include medication safety, drug review panels, and medication use review. The medication safety task force may be charged with review of adverse drug events and medication errors, their trending, and development of plans for prevention of future events. Drug review panels may be focused on a particular specialty such as cardiology or infectious disease and review drug products and guidelines in their area of specialty. The medication use review task force may monitor one or more medications use reviews, evaluate the data and development plans to optimize specific drug use. Figure 15-1 illustrates how these subcommittees relate to the organizational structure of the P&T Committee.

It is important to establish rules for a quorum. Such rules may establish a minimum number of members that must be present to conduct a meeting or a minimum number of member types that must be present to conduct a meeting. For example, a committee with 15 members must have at least five members present of which two must be physicians and one must be a pharmacist before a quorum has been established.

Committee Membership

P&T Committee membership should include pharmacists, nurses, physicians, administrators, risk or quality improvement managers, and others as appropriate. These members are selected with the guidance of the medical staff. Medication management is a multidisciplinary process. Committee membership should include nonphysician members such as nurses, respiratory therapists, and other health care professionals. While the voting members of the P&T Committee in many hospitals remains the physician members only, this is changing as the committee membership is evolving.

Figure 15-1
Formulary Management Process

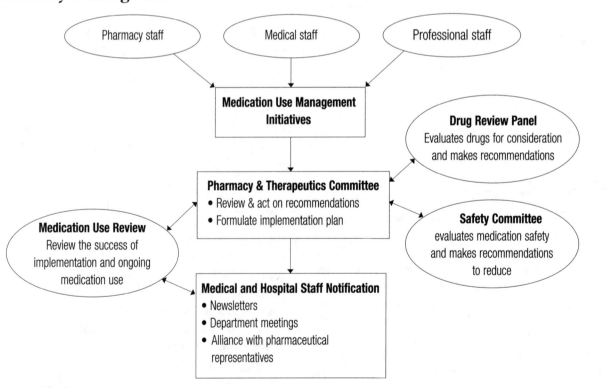

Responsibilities

The committee performs the following functions:

- Establishes and maintains the formulary system

- Selects medications for formulary inclusion by considering the relative clinical, quality of life, safety, and pharmacoeconomic outcomes. Decisions should be balanced to all of the above. Decisions should include consideration of continuity of care (e.g., local health plan formularies).

- Evaluates medication use and related outcomes

- Prevents and monitors adverse drug reactions and medications errors

- Evaluates or develops and promotes use of drug therapy guidelines

- Develops policies and procedures for handling medications to include their procurement prescribing, distribution, and administration

- Educates health professionals to the optimal use of medications

Formulary System Maintenance

The committee develops a list of medications for use in the organization. They may also develop guidelines for the optimal use of the medications and/or for specific disease management. They review the medication list and guidelines on a regular basis to assure that it is current and meets the needs of the medical staff and patients.

Medication Selection and Review

The committee should have established methods for medication selection and review. A written medication review is prepared from available literature. The review should be unbiased, as should the discussion of the review. Meeting participants (committee members and guests) should be required to discuss any conflict of interests prior to discussion of the drug or drug class. Medication selection criteria should include medication efficacy, safety, and cost.

- Is it a duplication of an existing formulary agent? If so, is it more effective? Safer? Less Costly?

- How should it be used?

- When should it be used?

- Who should use it?

- Are there any other special concerns?

Barriers to optimal formulary decisions may include physician experience with the drug under con-

sideration, physician preference for other agents, detailing by pharmaceutical company representatives, and unpublished or anecdotal studies and reports. Selection criteria should be such to minimize the effect of the aforementioned barriers.

Medication Use Evaluation

The committee should establish a regular process for reviewing how medications are used in the health-system. Medications may be considered for review based on their use, safety, cost or a combination of factors. For example, antibiotics represent a high use item; overuse of a particular antibiotic may place patients at risk for the development of resistant infections; and some antibiotics may also be costly. Establishment of specific criteria for use, review for compliance to the criteria, and routine review of the data is the foundation of the medication use process. Key to the process is timely data to review, action plan development, and follow-up.

Medication Safety Evaluation

Medication safety is evaluated through adverse drug reaction reports and medication error reports. Such reports may be local (i.e., from the health system) or global (i.e., literature, press releases). The impact of such reports should be considered relative to the health-system population, resources, and alternatives. A report of increased bleeding in patients over the age of 65 may not be critical in a pediatric hospital. However, reports of infusion rate reactions may require changes in nursing procedures in drug administration. Such reports should be used in considering whether a drug should be added to the formulary, retained on the formulary, or deleted from the formulary.

Drug Therapy Guidelines

The development of drug therapy guidelines is often the result of a medication use review or medication safety evaluation. A review of this data may indicate that the drug is not being used in an optimal manner with regard to patient selection, dosage, frequency, route, length of therapy, or a combination. The development and implementation of drug therapy guidelines may foster the safe, efficacious and cost effective use of selected drug products. Education of the professional and medical staff to these guidelines is critical to their success. Just as important is a method for routine review of the guidelines to assure they are current.

Policy and Procedure Development

The P&T Committee is responsible for medication use in the hospital. This includes the development of guidelines on historically pharmacy related topics of medication procurement, selection, and distribution. In addition, they are responsible for the medication administration process. This may include determining what medications are administered in specific locations for the hospital (i.e., intensive care unit) or under specific conditions (i.e., by chemotherapy certified nurse). Finally, they define the formulary management process. Specifically, guidelines for the evaluation of medications by the P&T Committee, frequency of such review, maintenance of the medication list, et cetera.

Education

The P&T Committee must communicate its actions to health-system staff and physicians. A newsletter is often employed to communicate these decisions. The newsletter may also include clinical information on drugs added to the formulary, drug therapy guidelines developed, and medication safety information available. The success of a newsletter may be limited by the format and content. The newsletter should be visually pleasing, easy to follow, and succinct. Optimally, it should be limited to two to four pages in length. The audience for the newsletter is generally broad and includes physicians, nurses, pharmacists, and other health care professionals. Other methods to communicate and educate others to P&T Committee actions are presentation at medical staff department meetings, nursing unit staff meetings, and pharmacy staff meetings and electronically through email or the health-system website. The P&T Committee may also assist in the development of programs to educate health care professionals or patients regarding medications.

Regulatory and Accrediting Bodies

Regulatory and accrediting bodies may require a P&T Committee and define its membership and responsibilities. Regulatory bodies requiring such activity include the State Department of Health or Board of Pharmacy; this varies by state. Accrediting bodies requiring this activity include the Joint Commission on Accreditation of Healthcare Organizations (JCAHO), the American Osteopathic Association (AOA), and Commission on Accreditation of Rehabilitation Facilities (CARF). The facility type will define the accrediting body; each has a slightly different interpretation of the term *formulary*. Regulations and accreditation standards are dynamic and require vigilance by the pharmacy to assure compliance.

Pharmacist Role

Pharmacists are essential to the formulary management process. Often pharmacists will guide the P&T Committee activities to assure optimal medication management. The pharmacist responsibilities may include the following:

- Establish P&T Committee meeting agenda
- Analyze and disseminate scientific, clinical, and health economic information regarding a medication or therapeutic class for review by the P&T Committee
- Conduct drug use evaluation and analyze data
- Record and archive P&T Committee actions
- Follow-up with research when necessary
- Communicate P&T Committee decisions to other health care professionals such as pharmacy staff, medical staff, and patient care staff

Formulary Management

The formulary is the foundation of the formulary system. Optimizing the number of medications, dosage forms, strengths, and packages sizes can have both patient care and financial benefits. Patient care benefits include safety and efficacy. Medication safety can be achieved by selecting agents with a positive side effect profile and limiting agents to reduce medication error risk. The selection of a single generic product will limit the number of agents available within the pharmacy stock. This minimizes the risk of selecting the incorrect agent for dispensing or administration. In addition, it reduces the carrying costs associated with stocking the medication.

Formularies can be categorized by their access to medications as *open* or *closed*. An open formulary has no limitation to access to a medication. Open formularies are generally large. A closed formulary is a limited list of medications. A closed formulary may limit drugs to specific physicians, patient care areas, or disease states via *formulary restrictions*.

Formulary restrictions do not necessarily translate to optimal medication management. For example, limitation of an antibiotic to a *restricted* status may result in cost shifting to a different antibiotic. While sometimes this change is desirable, that may not always be the case. The *new agent of choice* may be more expensive or less safe than the *restricted* agent. Careful consideration of the impact of the formulary product selection and/or restriction is critical to the process. Some authors have suggested that restricting formularies has resulted in increased health care costs by increasing utilization of physician visits and hospitalizations.[1,2] While this data has been criticized, it is important to note the impact of formulary decisions in total health care costs.[3] The Institute of Medicine (IOM) evaluated the Veterans Administration (VA) *National Formulary* impact on health care costs in six closed or *preferred* class of drugs.[4] The IOM concluded that the VA National Formulary was cost savings, probably generating savings of $100 million over 2 years and did not appear to have any effect on hospital admissions for selected heart or ulcer related conditions.

Drug product selection should be based on individual chemical entities. The Food and Drug Administration (FDA) defines the equivalence of individual chemical entities or generic equivalents. A list of such equivalents can be found in the Approved Drug Products with Therapeutic Equivalence Evaluation commonly known as the *Orange Book*. Policies for the use and dispensing of generically equivalent products should be set forth in the formulary system policy.

Many health systems have also established *therapeutic equivalents* and *therapeutic interchange* programs. Therapeutic equivalents are drug products with different chemical structure but are of the same pharmacologic and/or therapeutic class and are expected to have similar therapeutic effects and adverse effects. Examples of therapeutic equivalents include first generation cephalosporins and histamine-2 blockers. Therapeutic interchange is the authorized exchange of therapeutic alternatives in accordance with previously established and approved written guidelines. Establishment of therapeutic equivalents extends beyond the

chemical entity. It must include the dosage strength, dose frequency, and route of administration for the interchange. Examples of therapeutic interchanges are listed in Table 15-1.

The P&T Committee should established guidelines for generic substitution and therapeutic interchange. Such guidelines should include the following:

- The pharmacist is responsible for selecting generically equivalent products in concert with FDA regulations.

- Prescribers may specify a specific brand if clinically justified. The decision should be based on pharmacologic and/or therapeutic considerations relative to the patient.

- The P&T Committee determines therapeutic equivalents and how they are processed.

The pharmacist is responsible for the quality, quantity, and source of all medications, chemical, biologicals, and pharmaceutical preparations used in the diagnosis and treatment of patients. Such products should meet the standards of the United States Pharmacopeia and the Food and Drug Administration.

Formulary maintenance is the ongoing process of assuring relative safety and efficacy of agents available for use in the health system. Processes used in formulary maintenance include the following:

- New product evaluation
- Therapeutic class review
- Formulary changes (rationale for retaining or deleting an agent from the formulary)
- Nonformulary drug use review

New Product Evaluation

Pharmacists have the opportunity to assume a leadership role in the selection of agents to the formulary.

Table 15-1
Therapeutic Interchange Equivalence by Therapeutic Class

Therapeutic Class	Generic Name	Dosage	Dosage Frequency	Route
First Generation	Cefazolin	1 gm	Every 8 hr	IV
Cephalosporins	Cephalothin	1 gm	Every 6 hr	IV
	Cephapirin	1 gm	Every 6 hr	IV
H2 Blockers	Cimetidine	300 mg	Every 6 hr	IV
	Ranitidine	50 mg	Every 8 hr	IV
	Famotidine	20 mg	Every 12 hr	IV

The evaluation of an agent should consider the indications for use, pharmacokinetics, safety, and cost. Considerations to drug storage, mode of administration, special considerations, and drug-dispensing issues should also be included in the evaluation. Development of a standard format for new drug evaluations is useful in facilitating P&T Committee discussions. Standard elements include the following:

- *Generic Name*—List officially approved name of all chemical entities in the drug product.

- *Trade Name*—List common trade name(s) of the drug product.

- *Therapeutic or Pharmacologic Class*—State the pharmaceutical or therapeutic class to which the agent belongs. Similar agents within the class may be listed.

- *Pharmacology*—Describe the mechanism of action and related pharmacologic effects of the drug. If the mechanism is unknown, state this.

- *Pharmacokinetics*—Describe how the drug is handled by the body. Include onset of effect, serum half-life, metabolic considerations, and route of excretion as appropriate.

- *Indications for Use*—State the indications approved for use by the Food and Drug Administration. Include any additional uses under investigation.

- *Clinical Studies*—Briefly describe clinical study data supporting the indications for use. This review should be an unbiased, comparative review of studies, which identifies strengths and weaknesses as appropriate. Study description should include information about the patient populations, inclusion and exclusion criteria, study design and protocol, statistical analysis, outcomes, and conclusions.

- *Adverse Effects/Warnings*—List adverse effects associated with the drug and the frequency of occurrence. Describe methods to reduce or treat adverse effects. Discuss the risks and benefits of this drug therapy. Also, list any special precautions such as drug use in pregnancy, excretion of the drug into breast milk, et cetera.

- *Drug Interactions*—List drug-drug and drug-food interactions associated with this agent, significance of these interactions, and methods for prevention.

- *Dosage Range*—List a dosage range for different routes of administration and indications for the drug. Include special dosing considerations for renal disease, age, and hepatic function.

- *Dosage Form and Cost*—List the dosage form and strengths proposed for formulary addition. Include the cost of each dosage form and strength. A table listing comparable agents may be useful in determining the value of a formulary addition or modification.

- *Summary*—Summarize the information provided in a single paragraph.

- *Recommendation*—State the recommendation and rationale for the recommendation. Recommended actions may include formulary addition, formulary restriction, formulary deletion, or do not add to formulary.

- *References*—List references used. Reference materials useful in preparation of the formulary monograph should be unbiased and current. Peer-reviewed primary literature is optimal whenever possible. Other resources include textbooks such as American Hospital Formulary Service Drug Information and Drug Facts and Comparison. Electronic databases such as DrugDex (www.micromedex.com), Medline (www.ncbi.nlm.nih.gov/entrez/query.fcgi?), and National Guideline Clearinghouse (www.guideline.gov) are often useful.

In preparing the drug monograph, it is important to understand the P&T Committee needs. Some committees desire a detailed analysis of the points listed above, whereas others prefer an abbreviated monograph. Critical elements to both are efficacy, safety, and cost. To assist the P&T Committee membership, use of tables and comparative data within a therapeutic class or indication is useful. Knowing the cost of an agent is meaningless if the cost of comparator agents is unknown. The recommendation put forth by the pharmacist should be concise, include the rationale for the decision, any possible formulary deletions that might result by adding this agent, guidelines for use when appropriate, and consideration for future review. Some health systems add new agents to the formulary for a limited or *trial* period such as 3 or 6 months. This conditional approval allows the P&T Committee to further assess the use and safety of the product before *final* formulary addition.

Therapeutic Class Review

The regular review of drug classes by the P&T Committee is useful in assuring that optimal drug therapeutic options are available. Therapeutic class reviews should not be so broad or all inclusive so as to not be meaningful. The review of antimicrobials may be too broad whereas the review of quinolone antibiotics may prove to be more useful. The committee may set forth criteria for these reviews. Such criteria might include new medical information, adverse event profiles, purchase or use data and cost. Some P&T Committees conduct a therapeutic class review with each consideration for formulary addition. The objective is to have the optimal agents within a therapeutic class in terms of efficacy, safety, and cost. The end result of a therapeutic class review may be formulary modifications (i.e., additions or deletions), implementation of a drug use review or the development of therapeutic guidelines.

Formulary Changes

A process to continually update the formulary must be established. Such a process should include a method for making additions and deletions to the formulary. This process typically involves the submission of a request for formulary addition or deletion from the pharmacy or medical staff. This request may be written or verbal. Requests generally require specific information.

- Agent to be considered for addition or deletion
- Rationale for request. This should include the impact on the cost and quality of patient care.
- Alternative agents currently on the formulary

Some organizations require or permit the requesting individual to attend the P&T Committee to support their request.

Nonformulary Drug Review

The objective of a formulary is to have the most efficacious, safe, and cost effective agents available for routine use in the health system. On occasion, unique patient needs may require the use of a nonformulary agent. To prevent the erosion of the formulary system by overuse of nonformulary agents, a process for the management of nonformulary agents should be in place. Such a process should include a policy of the use of nonformulary drugs, procedure for procurement of nonformulary drugs, and regular review of nonformulary drug use by the P&T Committee. The policy

for use of nonformulary drugs should include pharmacist contact with the prescribing physician to offer alternatives. It may also include the completion of a nonformulary request form by the prescribing physician or authorization by the P&T Committee chair prior to dispensing. Procedure for drug procurement should be well-defined and communicated to the pharmacy, medical, and nursing staff so that expectations are appropriately understood. Such a procedure may indicate up to a 24-hour delivery time for nonformulary medications. The procedure may also permit the use of patient's own medications in concert with other hospital policies. The ongoing assessment of nonformulary drug use by the P&T Committee is an important part in managing the medication process. Critical information for the committee to consider includes agent used, formulary alternatives, number of times used in previous 6–12 months, patient safety, and cost impact. Understanding this information will allow the committee to determine an action plan. Such actions include reconsideration of an agent for formulary addition, development of guidelines for use of a drug within a therapeutic class or disease state, or individual physician intervention.

In the future, formulary management will include the impact of automating the medication prescribing process. This may include the establishment and/or review of order entry *rules*. Such rules may include weight based dosing, required laboratory tests, and allergy checks. In addition, the responses (*pop-ups*) to the rules may be determined by the P&T Committee through the formulary management process. Review of this information will be a key element in managing and monitoring medication use throughout the health system.

Drug Use Evaluation

Drug use evaluation is a tool to ensure that drugs are used appropriately, safely, and effectively. Drug use or medication use evaluation programs were first established in the 1980s. They provide an ongoing, structured, organized approach to ensure that drugs are used appropriately. More recently, the term *outcome assessment* has been used to describe such programs. The desired endpoint is the same—safe, efficacious drug therapy.

Drug use evaluation programs should be incorporated into the overall hospital performance improvement process. They should employ the performance improvement model used by the health system. There are multiple performance improvement models. A common model used in health systems is FOCUS-PDCA or (PDSA). The acronym is described below.

<u>F</u>ind process to improve

<u>O</u>rganize a team that knows the process

<u>C</u>larify current knowledge of the process

<u>U</u>nderstand causes of process variation

<u>S</u>elect process improvement

<u>P</u>lan

<u>D</u>o

<u>C</u>heck (or <u>S</u>tudy)

<u>A</u>ct

Figure 15-2 illustrates a drug use evaluation using the PDCA model for antibiotic prophylaxis for surgery.

Pharmacists can take a leadership role in designing the drug use evaluation programs. The program should measure and compare the outcomes of patients who received drug therapy in concert with approved criteria versus those that did not. Selection of agents for drug use evaluation programs should be based on whether a drug is high-use, high-cost, or high-risk. Many drugs fall into more than one category: thrombolytic agents are high-cost and high-risk; select antibiotics may be high-use. Drug use criteria may be diagnosis-related, prescriber-related, or drug-specific.

Diagnosis-related criteria identify indications for which select drug(s) may be appropriate for a given disease state. For example, the use of selected antibiotics for community acquired pneumonia. Use of other antibiotics would fall outside the approved list and require follow-up.

Prescriber-related criteria identify specific physicians whom the P&T Committee has determined may use certain drugs. For example, selected antibiotics may be limited to infectious disease specialists or drotrecogin alfa may be limited to critical care specialists.

Drug-specific criteria focus on specific aspects of a select drug such as the dose or dosing frequency. For example, the dosage regimen of a low molecular weight heparin might be reviewed. Dosage regimens outside the criteria would require action.

Pharmacists, working with key physicians, develop criteria for drug use evaluation. The criteria should be focused and limited. Select three to five criteria to evaluate that are meaningful and simple to collect. If possible, data should be collected during the patient visit (concurrent) rather than retrospectively (chart review). Concurrent review often is more complete. It allows the pharmacist to obtain information from the prescriber that may not have been clear in the medical record. It also provides timely information to act on. Because medical information is dynamic, the most meaningful drug use evaluations should reflect current practice patterns rather than those of 6–18 months ago. The criteria should also include a number of patients to be reviewed and the time period. For example, "20 patients each month" receiving the drug are reviewed. The drug use evaluation criteria are presented to the P&T Committee for their review and endorsement prior to commencing data collection.

Technology may be used to collect or screen data. Use of information systems to identify patients for review and collate the data will facilitate the process. Handheld computers or personal data assistants (PDAs) may be useful in the data collection process.

Once the data has been collected it should be compiled for review. The use of trend graphs or control charts are helpful in identifying opportunities for improvement. The result of a drug use evaluation may be validation that drug use is appropriate and safe. However, it may also indicate an opportunity for improving the way a drug is used. Once the data is collated, it may be beneficial to form a task force to develop an action plan. This task force should include key physicians, nurses, pharmacists, and other health care professional appropriate to the drug therapy under review. The task force should develop an action plan and criteria for ongoing monitoring. The action plan may include development of drug use guidelines, preprinted orders, medication order entry *rules*, professional staff education, formulary changes, or a combination of these actions. The drug use evaluation results and action plan are presented to the P&T Committee for consideration. The committee will review and endorse and/or modify the plan for implementation and follow-up. A single drug use evaluation should not continue indefinitely. Once the desired endpoint has been achieved, the review may be discontinued or the ongoing review may be less frequent (e.g., once or twice a year).

Medication Use Policies

Medication use policies are critical in the management of medications in the health care settings. Such policies should include the following:

- Formulary management

Figure 15-2
PDCA Model: Antibiotic Prophylaxis for Surgery Patients

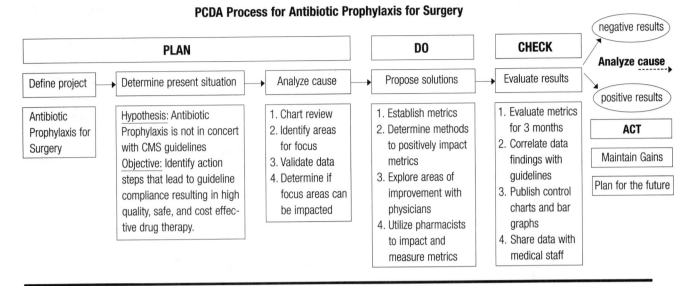

PCDA Process for Antibiotic Prophylaxis for Surgery

- Pharmacy and Therapeutics Committee
- Medication prescribing, dispensing, and administration

Formulary Management

Formulary policies should include information on who may use a specific agent (formulary restrictions), how a drug is added or deleted from the formulary, how a drug is stocked, and which drugs are stocked. The formulary restriction policy should specifically define how items are selected for formulary restriction, rationale for selecting approved prescribers, and a method for managing the process. A formulary policy should describe the method for drug addition and deletion as well as nonformulary drug use. A policy should describe how an agent is added to the pharmacy stock once it is added to the formulary and who gets to decide. For example, the P&T Committee approves the addition of a chemical entity added and the pharmacy manager selects dosage forms, strengths, et cetera, or the P&T Committee determines the chemical entity and dosage form(s) and the pharmacy manager selects the strengths or sizes to be stocked. The basic policies and procedures governing the formulary system should be incorporated in the medical staff bylaws or in the medical staff rules and regulations.

Pharmacy and Therapeutics Committee

The policy should address the committee membership, operation, and responsibilities.

Medication Prescribing, Dispensing, and Administration.

Organizational policies on the prescribing, dispensing, and administration of pharmaceuticals are required and necessary to ensure safe medication use. Such policies should address all aspects of the medication process.

- *Writing Medication Orders or Prescriptions*— Defines practitioners that may write medication orders or prescriptions in concert with state and federal regulations. This or related policies may also include the format for order writing and unacceptable abbreviations.

- *Verbal Orders*—Defines who may accept a verbal order and the transcription process of such an order. This policy should address the reading back of the order to confirm its accuracy.

- *Stop Orders*—Defines the orders that are automatically terminated, how the prescriber is notified, if appropriate, and the method for their reinstatement.

- *Investigational Drug Orders*—Defines how investigational drugs are managed in the health care system. This policy should include the review process as well as the method for prescribing, dispensing, administering, and monitoring investigational agents.

- *Controlled Substances*—Defines the flow of controlled substances through the health care system. This policy should include approved prescribers, the ordering process from the pharmacy and the vendor, the distribution and tracking of use, discrepancy tracking and follow-up, and management of diversion.
- *Generic and Therapeutic Substitution*—Defines how a drug is selected for generic substitution and therapeutic equivalents approved by the P&T Committee. It should describe how an alternative agent may be prescribed if deemed medically necessary.
- *Self-Administration of Medications*—Defines the conditions and process for the administration of medication by the patient in the hospital setting.
- *Medication Samples*—Defines the conditions and process for the use of medication samples in the hospital or clinic setting.
- *Floor Stock*—Defines the criteria for selecting agents for floor stock, process for modifying the stock, and the regular review of the stock by the P&T Committee.
- *Definition of Order Interpretation*—Defines the meaning of specific types of orders including sliding scale orders, range orders, as needed orders, tapering orders, and titrating orders.
- *Medication Administration Times*—Defines specific medication administration times and rules for interpretation. This may include the definition of *stat* and related terminology.
- *Adverse Drug Reactions*—Defines an adverse drug reaction, the reporting process, and monitoring methods.
- *Medication Errors*—Defines a medication error, the reporting process, and monitoring methods.
- *Others*—Other topics for policy consideration include pharmaceutical representatives, pharmacy hours of service, emergency medications, and medication delivery devices.

Published Formulary

The published formulary should provide information on the medications approved for use, basic therapeutic information about each item, information on medication use policies and procedures, and special information about medications such as dosing guidelines, et cetera.

Medication List

The key element of the published formulary is the list of medications approved for use. This section includes both entries for each medication and indexes to facilitate use.

Medication entries may be arranged alphabetically by generic name and trade (synonym) name, therapeutic class, or a combination. At a minimum, each drug entry should include the following:

- *Generic Name of Primary Active Ingredient*—Combination products may be listed by generic ingredients or trade name.
- *Trade or Synonym Name That is Commonly Used*—A disclaimer in the introduction to the formulary should explain that the presence or absence of a trade name does not imply that it is or is not the agent stocked by the pharmacy.
- *Dosage Form, Strength, and Size Stocked by the Pharmacy*
- *Active Ingredients (Formulation) for Combination Products*

Additional information that may be added:

- *DEA Schedule (C-II through C-V)*
- *Special Precautions*—Such as for IM use only and protect from light.
- *Pediatric or Adult Dosage Ranges*
- *Cost Information*—Some health systems have chosen not to publish actual purchase prices for confidentiality reasons but rather to list a cost scale to allow for price comparisons. Cost information is most useful when drugs are arranged within a therapeutic group or class to allow for easy comparison.

The medication list should include one or more indexes. The index should assist the user in locating the medication entry by generic name. The index should include both generic and trade name entries. The trade name entry may state "see generic name, page 123." Such an index may be incorporated into the formulary itself. If that is done, then the formulary listing should be alphabetical and include both generic and trade names. A second index type is the therapeutic index. This index arranges drugs generically by therapeutic or pharmacologic class. It is particularly useful for the prescriber that is not familiar with the formulary of a health system and desires to prescribe a certain type of drug (i.e., ACE inhibitor).

Medication Use Policy and Procedures

Inclusion of information on the prescribing, dispensing, and administration of medications in the published formulary provides a quick reference for health care providers. Either selected policies may be published or key information summarized in an abbreviated format. Policies for inclusion are the formulary policy, P&T Committee policy, and organizational regulations regarding medication use. Information on pharmacy operating procedures may be beneficial. These would include hours of services, prescription policies, medication distribution procedures, contact information and other pharmacy services such as anticoagulation monitoring or pharmacy newsletters.

Medication Use Guidelines

This section should detail guidelines for medication use, which are approved or endorsed by the P&T Committee. Such guidelines may include preprinted orders and clinical pathways that have been developed. Examples of medication use guidelines are provided below.

- Antibiotic use guidelines
- Antibiotic use in surgical prophylaxis
- Community acquired pneumonia clinical pathway
- Weight-based heparin orders
- Potassium replacement orders
- ICU sedation guidelines
- Thrombolytic therapy guidelines for stroke
- Alcohol detoxification orders

Special Information

The information in this section is health-system specific. It should be tailored to the needs of the professional and medical staff based on the services provided by the health system and the pharmacy. Examples of topics to include are below.

- Nutritional products approved for use
- Equivalent dosage tables (e.g., pain medications, corticosteriods)
- Parenteral nutrition formulas
- Pediatric dosages
- Potassium content of drugs or foods
- Antidote list
- Advanced Cardiac List Support (ACLS) or emergency medication list and dosages

- Metric conversion table
- Serum drug levels
- Standard concentrations of drugs in IV solutions
- Common equations used (e.g., ideal body weight, estimated creatinine clearance, anion gap)
- Antibiograms
- Drug dosing in renal or hepatic dysfunction
- Examples of forms that are routinely used such as nonformulary drug requests, adverse drug reaction reports

Publishing the Formulary

The formulary must be published regularly. The medication list should be readily available to all personnel involved in the medication process. It should be easy to use and visually pleasing. There is no standard format for formularies. Elements of the formulary often include the following:

- Title page
- Table of contents
- Medication list
- Medication use guidelines
- Special information
- Medication use policies
- Indexes

To facilitate the ease in use, each section may be printed in a different color. Printing the generic name in a bold face or other unique type will facilitate ease of use within the medication list section. Portability of the formulary may also facilitate use; making it pocket-sized may be beneficial. Electronic versions of the formulary may be preferable. The posting of the formulary on the health-system website allows for ease in updating and customization to the health system's needs. Electronic versions may be integrated with the medication order entry module of the health-system information system.

Distribution of the Formulary

Copies of the formulary should be made available where medications are prescribed, administered, and dispensed. This would include placement in patient care areas, such as nursing stations, clinics, emergency department, and other outpatient areas. Each pharmacist or pharmacy work area should also have a copy. Ideally, each health-system department head and administrator should have a copy as well as each member of the medical staff.

Maintaining a Current Formulary

Printed formularies are often revised and printed annually. This annual revision should include additions and deletions to the formulary, changes in drug products, removal of drugs from the market, changes in hospital policies, and additions, deletions, or modifications for medication use guidelines.

A method should be established for updating the formulary between editions. Methods to update the formulary include supplement sheets that are attached inside the cover of the formulary books, newsletters detailing changes to the formulary, and online changes for electronic formularies. All formularies should have the edition listed on the cover. The use of a different color cover each year reduces confusion between the current and previous editions.

Summary

The pharmacist plays a critical role in the management of medication use in the health system. As the drug expert, the pharmacist can assure safe, efficacious, and cost effective drug use through the formulary system. Ongoing formulary maintenance and routine drug use evaluations are key elements in this process. Focused consideration of medication safety in all medication related discussions optimizes formulary system management.

References

1. Foulke GE, Siepler J. Antiulcer therapy: an exercise in formulary management. *J Clin Gastroenterol.* 1990;12(suppl 2):S64–8.

2. Kozma CM, Reeder CE, Lingle EW. Expanding Medicaid drug formulary coverage. Effects on utilization of related services. *Med Care.* 1990 Oct;28(10):963–77.

3. Posey LM. Formularies and Quality of Care: Pharmacoeconomics drives revisionist thinking. *The Consultant Pharmacist.* 1996 May;11(5).

4. Blumenthal D, Herdman R, eds. *Description and Analysis of the VA National Formulary.* VA Pharmacy Formulary Analysis Committee, Division of Health Care Services, Institute of Medicine; 2000.

5. Formulary Management. The Academy of Managed Care Pharmacy's concepts in managed care pharmacy. Academy of Managed Care Pharmacy. Available at: http://www.amcp.org/data/nav_content/Formulary%20Management%20%2D%20Memohead%2Epdf.

6. Tanielian T, Harris K, Suárez A, et al. *Impact of a Uniform Formulary on Military Health System Prescribers: Baseline Survey Results.* National Defense Research Institute and Rand Health; 2003.

7. White paper: formulary development at express scripts. Available at: http://www.express-scripts.com/ourcompany/news/formularyinformation/development/formularyDevelopment.pdf. Accessed April 2004.

8. American Society of Health-System Pharmacists. *ASHP Statement on Medication Use Policy Development.* Bethesda, MD: American Society of Health-System Pharmacists; draft.

Chapter 16

Development, Implementation, and Monitoring of Therapeutic Plans

John E. Murphy

Introduction

For every drug or other therapy a patient receives there should be a clearly planned purpose (therapeutic goal). The therapeutic goal should be determined based on the patient's needs and desires for treatment and the evaluation by clinicians caring for the patients of the benefits and risks compared to other treatment options or to no treatment at all. A monitoring plan should then be developed to evaluate whether the drug's potential positive effects are achieved and to prevent toxicity in individual patients. Routine recommendations for therapeutic goals and optimal monitoring can also be developed for populations of patients (e.g., evidence-based clinical guidelines).

Regrettably, not all patients respond equally to a certain dose or dosing schedule or even to target drug concentrations. Thus, the monitoring of therapeutic plans to assess response and side effects is necessary to enhance the potential for optimal patient outcome. The outcomes determined from monitoring should then lead to decisions on whether to continue or adapt the regimen.

A therapeutic plan begins with assessment of a patient's needs. For pharmacists the focus on the assessment relates to the need for drug therapy, either over-the-counter or prescription. Pharmacists can, of course, provide important triage functions for other types of therapy as well, but the focus of this chapter will be on a patient's need for drug therapy and the pharmacist's role in developing, implementing, and monitoring a chosen therapy.

Pharmacists and Drug Therapy Plans

Many studies have demonstrated the value that pharmacists can provide in the enhancement of patient outcomes. For example, Leape and colleagues showed that pharmacists decreased adverse drug reactions when working as a team member in intensive care units and Gattis and colleagues demonstrated the value of pharmacist monitoring by the decrease in negative heart failure outcomes in their patients.[1,2] Further, the economic impact of a variety of pharmacy services reported in the literature has been evaluated and found to be positive in a number of the studies.[3,4]

Pharmacists and other health care professionals do not always provide optimal plan implementation and monitoring for every patient, or the monitoring may be haphazard. Donald Francke once said "Today's drugs may be likened to ballistic missiles with atomic warheads, while we prescribe, dispense, and administer them as if they were bows and arrows" and Hepler wondered how pharmacists could provide "a drug, a poison, to a patient without knowing what effect the drug should produce?"[5,6] Hepler further questioned how pharmacists could know if a drug was working or not if the therapeutic plan is unknown. In order to avoid having these allegations be true and to enhance the potential for successful outcome in patients, it is important that pharmacists develop a therapeutic plan for each drug suggested for a patient, no matter how innocuous the drug may seem.

Conversely, the limits on available resources in the health care system suggest the need to determine the patients who would most benefit from time and effort spent on extensive development and monitoring of therapeutic plans. Studies have been conducted to better identify those patients who need a higher level of drug therapy monitoring. MacKinnon and Hepler examined indicators for preventable drug related morbidity in the aged.[7] They found that patients who had more diagnoses and prescribers (four or more of each), were on six or more prescription medications, were males, or were on antihypertensives were at greater risk and thus should be considered for targeted monitoring. Seeger and colleagues demonstrated that preventable adverse drug reactions in hospitalized patients tend to be dose related or to occur among patients with allergies to the drug.[8] Targeted and effective therapeutic plan development, implementation, and monitoring can have an important impact on preventing such events.

Pharmacists are extensively involved in the monitoring of drug therapy in the hospital setting. In their 1999 publication, Bond and colleagues reported that pharmacists participated in drug therapy monitoring in 42.9% of responding hospitals and that 56.0% of the patients in these institutions received these services.[9] However, the true total is even greater because pharmacokinetic consultations occurred in 52.9% and adverse drug reaction monitoring in 67.1% of the hospitals. These latter services could also be considered drug therapy monitoring.

Approaches

A standard approach to developing, implementing, and monitoring a drug therapy plan is to determine a patient's problem, define the goals of therapy, select a drug with known or suspected potential to affect the problem from among available therapeutic options, determine an initial empiric dose and schedule (often based on standard doses or less often on target drug concentrations), and begin therapy. The next step is to evaluate whether the patient is responding adequately and without toxicity through use of outcome monitoring. For those patients not responding optimally but who are not exhibiting signs of important drug toxicity and who are judged to be adherent to their treatment regimens, the dose may be increased or another drug or therapy added or substituted. In some cases it might also be possible to reduce the dose. For those responding well and without symptoms of toxicity, the regimen can remain as initially prescribed. For those responding but exhibiting signs and symptoms of important toxicity that is not of limited duration (e.g., drowsiness that dissipates over a fairly short time), the dose may be reduced or the drug therapy changed. Patients whose therapy is adjusted then cycle through the series again.

Purposes of a Therapeutic Plan

Therapeutic plans should take into account the patient's objectives as well as those of the various clinicians caring for that patient.[10,11] Issues for the patient may include their preferences for specific dosage forms and dosing schedules, as well as costs and social issues. The plans should be created as a partnership.

Four fundamentals assist in the development and monitoring of drug therapy plans.[12] These include the following:

1. Understanding the desired therapeutic outcome of the drug and a reasonable length of therapy for the individual patient

2. Assessing the potential efficacy of a selected drug versus other possible drug and nondrug therapies for the specific patient

3. Determining monitoring parameters (laboratory tests, symptom relief, etc.) that will indicate optimal therapeutic outcome

4. Determining monitoring parameters that will indicate toxicity or adverse reactions caused by the drug

Careful monitoring using the above four cornerstones or by what Strand and colleagues' called the pharmacist's workup of drug therapy (PWDT) can facilitate optimum outcome of the drug therapy.[13,14]

Drug therapy plans should be designed to "improve the patient's quality of life through (1) cure of a disease, (2) elimination or reduction of symptoms, (3) arresting or slowing of a disease process, or (4) prevention of a disease or symptoms."[15] Since drug-related problems (DRPs) can prevent achievement of optimal drug therapy outcomes, their avoidance should be considered for every patient receiving therapy with medications.[16] DRPs have been defined in terms of the patient:

1. Taking/receiving a drug for which there is no valid indication

2. Requiring drug therapy for an indication and not receiving/taking this therapy

3. Taking/receiving the wrong drug or drug product

4. Taking/receiving too little drug

5. Taking/receiving too much drug

6. Not taking/receiving the prescribed drug appropriately

7. Experiencing an adverse drug reaction (not dose related)

8. Experiencing a drug-drug, drug-food, or drug-laboratory interaction

In terms of developing, implementing, and monitoring drug therapy, clinicians can enter the evaluation of a patient's DRPs prospectively at point 2 above where therapy needs to be started in a patient or retrospectively as an assessment of current drug therapy at points 1 and 3 through 8. It might be assumed that if an appropriate plan were developed, implemented, and monitored for a patient's drug-related needs (number 2 above), then the risk of the rest of the remaining DRPs could be reduced.

Pharmacists have long advocated their professional role as providing the right drug, in the right dose, at the right time. Pharmaceutical care extends that mandate to require pharmacists to take responsibility for ensuring these outcomes so that a patient's quality of life improves. Developing, implementing, and monitoring therapeutic plans are a critical component of providing pharmaceutical care.

Therapeutic Plan Development and Documentation

Winslade and colleagues adapted Hepler and Strand's process for the provision of pharmaceutical care as follows[15,17]:

1. "Develop a covenantal relationship between the pharmacist and the patient.

2. Collect relevant drug, disease, and patient information.

3. Interpret this information to identify all of the patient's drug-related problems.

4. Prioritize the patient's drug-related problems.

5. Identify those drug-related problems for which the pharmacist will assume responsibility.

6. Identify patient-specific outcomes for each drug-related problem for which the pharmacist has assumed responsibility.

7. Develop a therapeutic plan to attain the desired patient-specific outcomes for each drug-related problem.

8. Develop a monitoring plan to assess whether predetermined outcomes have been attained.

9. Implement and follow the pharmacy care plan, which consists of desired outcomes, therapeutic plan, and monitoring plan."

Following each of these steps can help ensure the orderly development, implementation and monitoring (steps 7 to 9) of a therapeutic plan for individual patients.

Other traditional rubrics have been used to focus the thinking of clinicians as they examine patients and develop therapeutic plans. Two approaches used to collect information and write up an evaluation of patient needs in a chart are SOAP (Subjective findings, Objective findings, Assessments of the findings, and Plans for dealing with the patient's problems) and FARM (Findings, Assessments, Recommendations, and Monitoring). Each approach covers the same ground with regard to data gathering, assessment, and plans though they do have slightly different emphasis. Subjective and objective assessments are combined in the Findings of FARM while Recommendations and Monitoring should both exist under the Plan section of SOAP. Though either approach to writing in a chart can produce the desired results, the FARM rubric places greater apparent emphasis on monitoring the outcomes of recommended plans of action and may lead new pharmacist clinicians to better understand the importance of having a monitoring plan.

A number of forms and software have been created to assist in the data gathering, assessment, plan development, and monitoring of individual patients.[17,18] Winslade and colleagues developed a tool for the pharmacist's management of drug-related problems (PMDRP).[17] They use the tool in teaching pharmacists to provide pharmaceutical care services via collection of patient data and the writing of responses to questions about the data in order to interpret their significance. The tool was developed using two other pharmaceutical care monitoring tools, including the PWDT.[13] The PWDT allows pharmacists to assess a patients history, drug therapy, and signs and symptoms in order to identify drug-related needs. According to the authors, one of the valuable outcomes of the PMDRP project was to standardize the many different approaches used by the clinical pharmacists to monitor therapy. Using standardized approaches can facilitate the creation of similar outcomes for patients.

Appendices A, B, and C show forms for collecting, documenting, and evaluating data; for determining a patient's drug therapy problems; and for writing a therapeutic care plan. These were adapted from forms developed for the American Society of Health-System Pharmacists' (ASHP) Clinical Skills Program and those provided to students in ASHP's Clinical Skill Competition.[19,20]

Monitoring

Monitoring has been defined by Knowlton and Penna as "the process of obtaining and evaluating clinical indicators and other relevant information."[10] They further state that "In order for a pharmaceutical care system to work correctly, monitoring must be planned, intelligent, active, coordinated, and responsive."

Outcome monitoring ranges from simple approaches like asking the patient how they are feeling relative to a desired outcome or whether they are experiencing any problems, all the way through the ordering and interpretation of complex laboratory and diagnostic tests. Evaluating the results of outcome measurements is a critical component of decisions with regard to continuation or alteration in the current therapeutic plan. Regrettably, outcome measures do not always accurately represent what is going on with a patient. It is likely that almost every pharmacy student has heard the mantra from clinical faculty to "treat the patient and not the laboratory test result," and rightfully so since results that are contrary to other outcome measures should not automatically outweigh common sense. It is the interpretation of all monitoring parameters and not just laboratory tests that makes up the bulk of how a clinician should determine the outcome of therapy for a given patient. The unusual laboratory result or other unexpected diagnostic outcome represents an opportunity to evaluate whether the test or measurement is accurate. Laboratory tests and other outcome measurements can be inaccurate for a wide variety of reasons. Luckily, these are a rarity rather than the rule.

Outcomes

Desirable outcomes of drug therapy include the prevention of disease or the successful treatment of signs and symptoms of disease, while improving a patient's quality of life. There are, unfortunately, risks (positive and negative outcomes) along with the benefits for virtually every therapeutic option available. Prior to initiating therapy, the benefits and risks of available treatment options should be weighed by the clinicians involved in a patient's therapy in concert with the patient.

Many factors can alter a drug's efficacy and safety outcomes. Addition or deletion of other drug therapy, including over-the-counter and complementary medicines (and diet) that may interact with the drug being monitored, can alter outcomes and should be considered when evaluating benefit and risk. Other diseases and changes in the function of the primary organs of drug elimination (usually the liver and kidneys) or in cardiac function can also alter the benefit:risk relationships for a drug.

Monitoring the Therapeutic Plan Outcomes

The therapeutic plan outcomes should be monitored as a partnership with the various health care professionals caring for the patient and the patient/caregiver. Pharmacists can assist patients in becoming a partner in their therapy by helping them understand what should and should not happen from the drug that is being taken. While health professionals can add sophisticated diagnostic criteria to the evaluation mix, considering both simple and complex outcome measures is of value. The financial burden on the health care system could probably be reduced if the focus of monitoring was more routinely on what is easy and inexpensive to evaluate.

Far more often than not, monitoring provides data that is useful for the assessment of patient outcome. This data is then combined with subjective assessments of patient outcome and the therapeutic plan continued or revised.

When unexpected laboratory reports occur they can complicate monitoring and decision making. Several examples illustrate problems that can develop in the interpretation of drug concentration measurements (DCMs) and other diagnostic criteria.[12] Patients may be nonadherent with drug therapy, taking either more or less than was prescribed for them or their concentrations may not be at steady state. A patient who should have been fasting before a test may inadvertently be allowed to eat. In institutional settings administration errors can account for unexpected outcomes; a patient may be administered the wrong dose of a drug, may receive it at the wrong time, may not receive the scheduled drug at all, or may be given the wrong drug. Errors on medication administration records and laboratory documentation records also can occur. For example, it might be recorded that a drug was given at a time other than the actual time it was received by the patient. Incomplete drug delivery due to patient problems (e.g., infiltration of an intravenous fluid or clogging of a nasal cannula) can also influence DCM results and patient progress.

Problems in sample collection can also lead to unexpected laboratory results. A blood sample may be drawn at the wrong time or the collection time may be reported incorrectly. This is seen with too great a frequency with aminoglycoside concentration measurements for example. Samples can also be taken from the wrong patient or obtained incorrectly (e.g., through a drug administration line that was inadequately flushed prior to sample withdrawal). In addition, samples may be improperly stored or the test methods (e.g., instruments or assays) may be of poor quality.

Patient (or caregiver) adherence must be assessed whenever a decision to adjust therapy is based on the therapeutic plan monitoring parameters. Simply assuming appropriate adherence to the prescribed regimen can lead to grave errors in the worst case and a waste of resources in others. It is disturbing to consider how often patient drug therapy is altered due to lack of response, when the greatest potential reason for lack of response is usually lack of adherence. As former Surgeon General Everett Koop once said, "Drugs don't work in patients who don't take them."

Determining Need for Regimen Adjustments or Drug Therapy Changes

When unusual results are reported, the test or finding should likely be rechecked before the initially measured result is accepted as valid and the therapeutic plan altered. An example of this is the elevation in blood pressure that may be seen on the first measurement at an office visit. Repeating the measurement either confirms the elevation or the blood pressure may be decreased after the patient relaxes.

Determining whether a problem has occurred with a diagnostic test result can be done with careful detective work. A patient can be questioned about compliance or past outpatient pharmacy records can be checked to determine whether a lack of response is related to nonadherence, or the nurse who administered the drug or the phlebotomist drawing the blood sample can be interviewed to determine if dosing or timing errors occurred.

With poor or misleading information about response or toxicity, a clinician can make an erroneous decision about the drug therapy needs of the patient. Accurate monitoring information is essential to appropriately assess the therapeutic plan and its outcomes. Unfortunately, communication of problems and successful outcomes of a therapy can be compromised by patients as well as prescriber/clinicians. Gandhi and colleagues showed that patients often did not tell their physicians of side effects and physicians often did not ask patients about them.[21] Thus, both patients and clinicians should be encouraged to take time to discuss the successes and problems with therapy during care visits.

Results that appear normal may also be erroneous due to the above factors and the actual values may not actually be normal. When a patient is having problems, normal test results may not indicate that all is well and the possibility of error should be considered.

Once diagnostic outcome measures are found to be as accurate as possible and the patient has been determined to be adherent with therapy, the need for dosage adjustment or the removal or addition of drugs can be determined. This determination should be based on the diagnostic results, pharmacodynamic response, and overall patient outcome.

Monitoring Frequency

Monitoring must be accomplished at an acceptable and appropriate level. That is, excessive monitoring does not improve outcome, can be expensive and wasteful, and in some cases may even hamper success due to inordinate regimen changes from *chasing* results. This issue has been raised a number of times in the literature on both the positive and negative sides. For example, authors have questioned the value of always monitoring aminoglycosides, while others have proposed guidelines for ensuring appropriate monitoring of various agents.[22–25]

The frequency of monitoring for efficacy or side effects related to drug therapy varies with the drug used, the intensity of the disease process, the stability of body functions, and other factors. In general, more severely compromised patients should be monitored more frequently, while stable patients on long-term therapy may not need evaluation more often than once a year. Unstable patients with rapidly changing organ function, hydration status, drug therapy, or therapeutic response may need evaluation more than once a day.

Summary

Developing, implementing, and monitoring therapeutic plans provides a rational approach to drug therapy for individual patients and patient populations and can enhance positive outcomes while reducing negative ones. Use of standard rubrics, forms, or software can provide a framework to make these therapeutic plan processes easier to manage. In the end, rational approaches to the care of patients will help increase the chance that their quality of life is improved.

References

1. Leape LL, Cullen DJ, Clapp MD, et al. Pharmacist participation on physician rounds and adverse drug events in the intensive care unit. *JAMA*. 1999;282:267–70.

2. Gattis WA, Hasselblad V, Whellan DJ, et al. Reduction in heart failure events by the addition of a clinical pharmacist to the heart failure management team. *Arch Intern Med.* 1999;159:1939–45.

3. Shumock GT, Meek PD, Ploetz PA, et al. Economic evaluations of clinical pharmacy services: 1988–1995. *Pharmacotherapy.* 1996;16:1188–208.

4. Shumock GT, Butler MG, Meek PD, et al. Evidence of the economic benefit of clinical pharmacy services: 1996–2000. *Pharmacotherapy.* 2003;23:113–32.

5. Anon. The role of the pharmacist in comprehensive medication use management. APhA White Paper. American Pharmaceutical Association; 1992.

6. Hepler CD. The pharmacist's job is to provide total pharmaceutical care. *US Pharmacist.* 1991(Nov): 61–4, 68.

7. MacKinnon NJ, Hepler CD. Indicators of preventable drug-related morbidity in older adults 2. Use within a managed care organization. *J Managed Care Phar.* 2003;(9)2:134–41.

8. Seeger JD, Kong SX, Schumock GT. Characteristics associated with ability to prevent adverse drug reactions in hospitalized patients. *Pharmacotherapy.* 1998;18(6):1284–9.

9. Bond CA, Raehl CL, Franke T. Clinical pharmacy services and hospital mortality rates. *Pharmacotherapy.* 1999;19(5):556–64.

10. Knowlton CH, Penna RP. *Pharmaceutical Care.* 2nd ed. Bethesda, MD: American Society of Health-System Pharmacists; 2003.

11. Galt KA. *Developing Clinical Practice Skills for Pharmacists.* Bethesda, MD: American Society of Health-System Pharmacists; 2005.

12. Murphy JE. Monitoring drug therapy. In: Schumacher GE, ed. *Therapeutic Drug Monitoring.* Norwalk, CT: Appleton & Lange; 1995:105–18.

13. Strand LM, Cipolle RJ, Morley PC. Documenting the clinical pharmacist's activities: back to basics. *Drug Intell Clin Pharm.* 1988;22:63–7.

14. Cipolle RJ, Strand LM, Morley PC. *Pharmaceutical Care Practice: The Clinician's Guide.* 2nd ed. New York: The McGraw-Hill Companies; 2004.

15. Hepler CD, Strand LM. Opportunities and responsibilities in pharmaceutical care. *Am J Hosp Pharm.* 1990;47:533–43.

16. Johnson JA, Bootman JL. Drug-related morbidity and mortality—a cost-of-illness model. *Arch Intern Med.* 1995;155:1949–56.

17. Winslade NE, Bajcar JM, Bombassaro AM, et al. Pharmacist's management of drug-related problems: a tool for teaching and providing pharmaceutical care. *Pharmacotherapy.* 1997;17(4):801–9.

18. Bosinski TJ, Campbell L, Schwartz S. Using a personal digital assistant to document pharmacotherapeutic interventions. *Am J Health-Syst Pharm.* 2004;61:931–4.

19. Jones WN, Campbell S. *Clinical Skills Program Module 4: Designing and Recommending a Pharmacist's Care Plan.* Bethesda, MD: American Society of Hospital Pharmacists; 1994.

20. Clinical Skills Competition Forms. Bethesda, MD: American Society of Hospital Pharmacists.

21. Gandhi TK, Weingart SN, Borus J, et al. Adverse drug events in ambulatory care. *New Eng J Med.* 2003 Apr 17;348(16):1556-64.

22. Massey KL, Hendeles L, Neims A. Identification of children for whom routine monitoring of aminoglycoside serum concentrations is not cost effective. *J Pediatr.* 1986;109:897–901.

23. Averbuch M, Weintraub M, Nolte F. Gentamicin blood levels: ordered too soon and too often. *Hosp Formul.* 1989;24:598–612.

24. Pellock JM, Willmore LJ. A rational guide to routine blood monitoring in patients receiving antiepileptic drugs. *Neurology.* 1991;41:961–4.

25. Pippenger CE. The cost-effectiveness of therapeutic drug monitoring. *Ther Drug Monit.* 1990;12:418.

Appendix 16-1
Patient Database Form

Pharmacist _____

Patient name	Patient ID	Location
Address	Physician	
	Pharmacy	
Date of birth	Race	Sex
Height · · · · · Weight		
Date of admission/initial visit	Occupation	

Allergies/ADRs	**PRIORITIZED MEDICAL PROBLEM LIST** · · · · **MEDICATION PROFILE**
☐ **No Known Drug Allergies/ADRs**	
Drug · · · · · · · *Reaction*	
HPI, PMH, FH, SH, etc.	

Vital Signs, Laboratory Data, Diagnostic Test Results

Date											
Weight											
Temperature											
Blood pressure											
Pulse											
Respiratory rate											
Na											
K											
Cl											
CO_2 (HCO_3)											
BUN											
Creatinine											
Creat CL											
Glucose											
Hgb/Hct											
WBC											
Diff											
Platelets											
Ca											
Mg											
PO4											
Albumin											
AST											
ALT											
Alk phos											
T bili											
T chol											
LDL/HDL											
Triglyceride											
HgA1C											

NOTES

Appendix 16-2
Drug Therapy Problem Worksheet

TYPE OF PROBLEM	POSSIBLE CAUSES	PROBLEM LIST	NOTES
Correlation between drug therapy and medical problems	Drugs without obvious medical indications Medications unidentified Untreated medical conditions		
Need for additional drug therapy	New medical condition requiring new drug therapy Chronic disorder requiring continued drug therapy Condition best treated with combination drug therapy May develop new medical condition without prophylactic or preventative therapy or premedication		

Unnecessary drug therapy	Medication with no valid indication
	Condition caused by accidental or intentional ingestion
	  of toxic amount of drug or chemical
	Medical problem(s) associated with use of or withdrawal
	  from alcohol, drug, or tobacco
	Condition is better treated with nondrug therapy
	Taking multiple drugs when single agent as effective
	Taking drug(s) to treat an avoidable adverse reaction
	  from another medication		

Appropriate drug selection	Current regimen not usually as effective as other choices Current regimen not usually as safe as other choices Therapy not individualized to patient		
Wrong drug	Medical problem for which drug is not effective Patient has risk factors that contraindicate use of drug Patient has infection with organisms resistant to drug Patient refractory to current drug therapy Taking combination product when single agent appropriate Dosage form inappropriate		
Drug regimen	PRN use not appropriate for condition Route of administration/dosage form/mode of administration not appropriate for current condition Length or course of therapy not appropriate Drug therapy altered without adequate therapeutic trial Dose/interval flexibility not appropriate		
Dose too low	Dose/frequency too low to produce desired response in this patient Serum drug level below desired therapeutic range Timing of antimicrobial prophylaxis not appropriate Medication not stored properly		
Dose too high	Dose/frequency too high for this patient Serum drug level above the desired therapeutic range Dose escalated too quickly Dose/interval flexibility not appropriate for this patient		
Therapeutic duplication	Receiving multiple agents without added benefit		

TYPE OF PROBLEM	POSSIBLE CAUSES	PROBLEM LIST	NOTES
Drug allergy/adverse drug events	History of allergy or ADE to current (or chemically-related) agents Allergy/ADE history not in medical records Patient not using alert for severe allergy/ADE Symptoms or medical problems that may be drug-induced Drug administered too rapidly		
Interactions (drug-drug, drug-disease, drug-nutrient, drug-laboratory test)	Effect of drug altered due to enzyme induction/inhibition from another drug patient is taking Effect of drug altered due to protein binding alterations from another drug patient is taking Effect of drug altered due to pharmacodynamic change from another drug patient is taking Bioavailability of drug altered due to interaction with another drug or food Effect of drug altered due to substance in food Patient's laboratory test altered due to interference from a drug the patient is taking		
Failure to receive therapy	Patient did not adhere with the drug regimen Drug not given due to medication error Patient did not take due to high drug cost/lack of insurance Patient unable to take oral medication Patient has no IV access for IV medication Drug product not available		
Financial impact	The current regimen is not the most cost-effective Patient unable to purchase medications/no insurance		
Patient knowledge of drug therapy	Patient does not understand the purpose, directions or potential side effects of the drug regimen Current regimen not consistent with the patient's health beliefs		

Appendix 16-3
Therapeutic Care Plan

Patient _____   Pharmacist _____

Location/Room _____   Date _____

Health Care Need[a] (Medical and Drug Therapy Problems List)	Clinical Significance	Current Regimens Addressing Health Care Needs	Pharmacotherapeutic Goals and Desired Endpoints	Recommendations for Therapy	Therapeutic Alternatives (Drug and Nondrug)	Monitoring Parameter(s) and Frequency	Patient Education
	Most clinically significant problems Problems of major clinical significance Problems of lesser clinical significance						

[a]Health care needs include actual and potential medical problems and drug-related problems as well as any other health care services from which the patient may benefit.

Chapter 17

Leadership

Karol G. Wollenburg, Paul W. Bush

Introduction

Like most industries in the 21st century, health systems operate within a rapidly changing, highly regulated, and competitive environment. In turn, pharmacists and pharmacy departments in health systems are confronted with ongoing significant challenges. We are expected to provide the highest level of safe and effective care with excellent customer service and, in addition, are asked to closely manage our budgets. We are faced with staff shortages, drug diversion, medication errors, prescribers who do not practice evidence based medicine, patients who speak languages that are foreign to us, and many other problems, large and small.

At the same time, opportunities for health-system pharmacists in today's world are vast. Studies show that pharmacists on patient care teams improve outcomes.[1-3] Regulatory bodies that understand the value pharmacists bring to patient care are requiring pharmacists to be part of the medication use process in more comprehensive ways. The demand for pharmacists in many settings across the continuum of care is increasing. Pharmacists in many parts of the country continue to inch closer to provider status. This is an exciting time for pharmacists. We have many opportunities to expand our roles in patient care and meet our professional responsibility and mission to help people make the best use of medications. For this to be a reality, we need strong leadership to help us seize the opportunities amidst the challenges.

People are the most important asset in an organization. Their ability to work creatively, collaboratively and effectively toward a challenging, yet worthy goal is the magic that enables an organization to be successful. Leadership is the art of mobilizing people to want to struggle for shared aspirations.[4] It is the ability to inspire ordinary people to accomplish things they would not have thought possible.[5] Leadership is encouraging people to take risks in order to find better ways of doing things; to make a significant difference. Leadership is not a place or position, it is a process.[4] True leadership cannot be assigned. It comes from influence and must be earned.[6]

Consistently successful organizations encourage leadership at all levels. Many members of these organizations lead through influence, not assigned authority.[6] Individuals who exhibit credible attributes and competencies and have developed solid relationships can be informal leaders, inspiring a group, over whom they have no formal authority, to see a vision and work passionately toward that end. The complexity of leadership may be greater the higher one goes in an organization, but many of the principles that enable success are the same.

High performing pharmacy services develop when strong pharmacy leadership is found throughout the department. Although it is essential that directors are able to successfully lead staff as well as get support from senior leadership, it is also important for strong pharmacy leadership to be present within many other settings and levels of the organization. It is critical that leadership roles be assumed by all practitioners including pharmacy clinicians with their patient care teams, pharmacists on interdisciplinary information technology projects teams, medication safety pharmacists with their quality improvement or nursing peers, or supervisors in pharmacy distribution areas. For pharmacists to help patients make the best use of medications, strong pharmacy leadership is important at all levels of our organizations. Many people need to help with the leadership role.[7]

In this chapter we will examine the leadership process, the essentials for the leadership journey, and describe how ordinary people with core attributes and competencies can influence their spheres of activity and improve care to patients. In the process, they become leaders.

Attributes of a Leader

What makes people want to follow a leader? What characteristics are necessary for leaders to be credible, to earn the trust of others? Why is it that some leaders are more effective than others? The key to successful leadership begins with critical core attributes that provide a foundation for the development of leadership skills. Without these core attributes, strategies, tactics, and plans are empty. Leaders will not be able to garner the commitment from others needed to meet the challenges ahead.

There are many core attributes that researchers and authors have used to characterize effective leaders.[4,8–12] The foundation for credibility begins when leaders are competent and knowledgeable. Being trustworthy contributes to credibility and is generally earned through honesty, sound judgement, integrity, and consistency. Characteristics that help to build relationships also build credibility and include effective listening, respect, compassion, fairness, openness, and generosity. People must truly believe that their leader cares about them. People want their leaders to be forward looking with a true sense of concern for the future of the organization. And finally, to inspire others to move toward a common vision, leaders must be positive and passionate about the journey. In summary, people must believe that leaders' words can be trusted, that they will do what they say, that they are personally excited and enthusiastic about the direction in which they are headed, and that they have the knowledge and skill to lead.[4]

It is worthwhile noting that most of the characteristics listed above are centered on others. True leaders are not focused on their own well-being or personal gain. They are focused on the benefits to their team, their organization, their patients, or other stakeholders. If we take seriously our professional responsibilities as pharmacists, the characteristics of a professional align with many of those expected of leaders. A true profession is based first on service to others. Professionals must also possess a specialized body of knowledge and remain competent in that knowledge. Professionals are expected to use their knowledge ethically and compassionately in their responsibility to serve society.[8,10] There are leadership overtones in our daily responsibilities as pharmacists. And there are many places in our organizations where leadership is needed to ensure that patients receive the safest and most efficacious care within the constraints of good stewardship of our resources.

Attributes are qualities that develop daily. Our ability to exhibit them grows and matures, and the discovery of these attributes by other people also unfolds over time. And so it is that we return to the premise that true leadership cannot be assigned. It must be earned as others come to experience an individual's words and deeds.

Practices of Effective Leaders

"No matter what leaders set out to do—whether it's creating strategy or mobilizing teams to action—their success depends on *how* they do it."[13]

Take Risks—Drive Change

To lead implies that there will be change. Change that leads to improvement is vital on several fronts. First, in a rapidly changing world, we cannot maintain our status in our environment without also changing. Information about drugs changes daily. Likewise, the standard of care for our patients changes continuously. Technology that enables us to distribute drugs more safely, efficiently, and effectively is expanding rapidly. To advance beyond the ever-changing norm or pursue excellence requires an even greater focus on change. An additional, compelling reason for change is to provide motivation and fulfillment to our staff. The most talented and high performing individuals in our workforce thrive on challenge and innovation. If we want to engage them and retain them, we must create an environment where they are inspired by the opportunity to push toward a goal they feel is meaningful and worthy of their time and talent. Our most talented pharmacists want to work in an environment where the standard of care is high and their input to improve care is valued and acted on.

Encourage Innovation

Strong leaders have a good sense of the current state of their organization and search for opportunities to grow, innovate, and improve.[11] They are constantly on the outlook for new and innovative ideas. Leaders and staff in high performance groups are well-connected to information sources outside their organizations. They invest time and resources in keeping informed and developing relationships beyond their organization. To foster creative and forward looking thinking, leaders and their team members should be encouraged to attend professional meetings, read professional journals, and visit other closely and marginally related organizations. (Table 17-1).

Effective leaders value intellectual curiosity; the ability to see better ways of doing things. Some leaders are robust innovators themselves, generating creative ideas that drive the organization forward. Other leaders may not be strong innovators themselves but are good listeners with skills that draw out new ideas from others. They make an effort to talk to staff at all levels

Table 17-1
Information Sources

Journals and Newsletters

American Journal of Health-System Pharmacists
Annals of Internal Medicine
Annals of Pharmacotherapy
Harvard Business Review
Hospital Pharmacy
Hospitals and Health Networks
JAMA
Lancet
Managed Health Care
Modern Healthcare
New England Journal of Medicine
Pharmacotherapy

Websites

The Advisory Board Company. www.advisoryboardcompany.com
Agency for Healthcare Research and Quality. http://www.ahrq.gov/
ASHP Section of Pharmacy Practice Managers.
    http://ashp.org/practicemanager/
Harvard Business School Working Knowledge. http://hbswk.hbs.edu/
Institute for Safe Medication Practices. http://www.ismp.org/
Joint Commission on Accreditation of Healthcare Organizations.
    http://www.jcaho.org/
The LeapFrog Group for Patient Safety. http://www.leapfroggroup.org/
Modern Healthcare. www.modernhealthcare.com

about challenges and opportunities in the workplace and how to change and pursue them. They seek input from customers. Leaders value good ideas and reward staff for their innovation. No matter the source, strong leaders recognize good ideas, value them, and pursue them.

Take Risks

In outstanding and innovative organizations, one will generally find leaders who are willing to take risks and staff who feel safe taking risks. Using strategies that minimize risk and the presence of a culture that accepts failures as part of the road to success are characteristics found in innovative organizations. Risk might be minimized by beginning a new project with a pilot program. The smaller scope can minimize the risk of the entire project by enabling the team to identify and fix problems while the program is still small. If the problems cannot be solved, the project can be aborted

while it is still small in scope and other opportunities pursued. Careful communication with individuals affected by the change during the planning stages is another way to minimize risk. Accepting that some projects will fail and not placing blame on individuals is essential in creating an environment where people are willing to take risks. When projects are not successful, leaders and their teams should reflect on what went wrong and apply that knowledge to future endeavors.

The rate of change that an organization can endure is dependent on many factors. The sheer volume of concurrent change efforts and the maturity or cohesiveness of the team are just two factors to consider. Likewise, the timing of a particular change is important.

The same project could fail or be successful depending on other issues ensuing in the organization at the time the project is planned or implemented. For example, justification for the addition of a pharmacist to provide pharmaceutical care within the Emergency Department may be easier to accomplish if the health system has identified improvements in the ED as a strategic goal that year. Conversely, in the middle of a downsizing effort, the request for a new position may not be wise. Strategic leaders often hold many good ideas in abeyance until the climate and timing are favorable.

Invest in Opportunities

Strategic leaders invest heavily in opportunities. Drucker provides good insight when he advises, "Good executives focus on opportunities rather than problems. Problems have to be taken care of, of course; they must not be swept under the rug. But problem solving, however necessary, does not produce results. It prevents damage. Exploiting opportunities produces results."[14] Collins has similar advice, "Put your best people on your biggest opportunities, not your biggest problems."[15]

Almost every scientific breakthrough involves a break with tradition or old ways of thinking. For significant change to occur, we must first change our paradigm; the way we see and interpret the world.[16] Strong leaders value intellectual curiosity, seek out opportunities, and embrace change with optimism and hope. This ability to see a better way of doing things contributes to a new vision.

Inspire Excellence and Provide Clarity through a Vision

Covey recommends that we begin with the end in mind.[16] Effective leaders invest time in working with others to develop and clarify what their purpose is, where they are headed, and how they will get there. In this planning process, teams analyze current and anticipated factors and trends in their environment that could enhance or inhibit their future success. For departments of pharmacy this might include reviewing current and anticipated changes in factors such as technology, the workforce supply, regulations, or reimbursement. Teams also consider the strengths and weaknesses of their organization. Pharmacists can use practice standards such as ASHP's *Best Practices for Hospital & Health-System Pharmacy* standards to help assess strengths and weaknesses.[17] They can review resources available from other professional organizations, goals established by quality and patient safety organizations, and other local or national benchmarking structures. Most importantly, successful teams look for conditions that present opportunities. Effective strategic planning considers the needs of all the key stakeholders affected by their work. For a pharmacy team this might include stakeholders in the medication use process such as patients, physicians, nurses, hospital administrators, employees, third party payors, and others.

Define the Mission

The foundation of the strategic planning process is to first understand the mission of the team: why we are doing what we are doing. For most pharmacists and departments of pharmacy in health systems, their mission likely resembles the mission statement adopted by the American Society of Health-System Pharmacists— "To Help People Make the Best Use of Medications."[18] For members of a Medication Safety Team, the mission might be to ensure the safe use of medications or to "first, do not harm." Whatever the mission for the group, it must provide a clear sense of purpose, be inspiring, and be for the common good.

Create a Vision

With a clear understanding of their purpose in place, leaders then help their group develop a dream of how to best realize that mission. A vision describes what the group wants to be and where it wants to go. A compelling vision provides a unique and uplifting view of the future and fosters hope. It expresses a standard of excellence. Effective visions require a stretch, yet are attainable. They are specific enough to guide decision making, yet general enough to generate a broad appeal and to allow for conditions that may change.[7] The vision for a department of pharmacy may be to provide pharmacy services across the continuum of care that are safe, efficacious, and cost conscious. For an interdisciplinary task force, it might be to ensure that the medication history for every patient leaving the hospital is effectively communicated to the next health-care setting where care is provided for that patient. The mission and vision for a department or team in a larger organization must support the mission and vision of the larger organization.

Develop a Plan

Once a team has come to consensus on a vision, they must review the gap between the present and the desired future and develop a strategy and operational plan that will enable the team to achieve the vision. Specific strategies or goals must be defined, which when fulfilled will enable the team to achieve the vision. One strategy that might be identified for the department dreaming of expanding pharmacy services across the continuum of care could be to establish pharmacy managed anticoagulation clinics. As strategies are developed to pursue the vision, the team must also consider and define the capital and operational costs needed to accomplish the strategic goals, as well as the human resource needs. If there are new capital or operational costs, a business plan might be developed defining the goals, anticipated benefits, estimated costs, and projected revenue. If the new functions require expertise that does not currently exist, there must be a plan to acquire or develop that talent. Finally, the master plan must be broken down into manageable tasks. Operational plans must be developed that clearly outline what steps must be taken to accomplish the strategic goals, who is responsible for them, when specific steps in the process will be accomplished, and what metrics will be used to measure progress. Leaders may need to guide the process by clarifying priorities in order to help focus all the energy and talent on the work that will support the strategic plan.

Include Others

Although the complexity and scale of the team or vision will affect the amount of time required to develop a strategic plan, the process can not generally be accomplished in several meetings. Often the basic content for a mission statement is discussed by the team and a draft crafted by one individual. The team then responds to and further develops that idea. The idea is then tweaked and discussed until consensus is reached. Input from people at all levels of the organization and stakeholder groups is essential to ensure the vision will be supported by all the groups affected by it. If staff or individuals who will be counted on to carry out the mission and vision are involved in the development process, they will be more likely to feel ownership of the plan. True leaders take responsibility for beginning the process to create and refine a vision and strategic plan but capitalize on the synergies of the team in the development of the plan.[19]

Many departments find it helpful to hold retreats, removed from daily distractions, to allow a vision and strategic plan to emerge in a more focused setting. Once established, the mission and vision do not change for a long period of time (years). Operational planning, however, requires more frequent review and revision. Annual retreats can be used to reassess mission and vision, update strategic goals, and develop action plans for the year that will enable the department to continue the pursuit of their vision.

The strategy and planning that flow after the development of a mission and vision are essential for an organization to be successful. Even more important is the community, enthusiasm, and clarity that grows in the development process around that common purpose and shared vision. When led carefully, the process itself can create a community where people believe what they are doing is worthwhile and understand their role in making that worthwhile thing happen. Leaders cannot effectively build or pursue a dream on their own. They need a team to develop and passionately pursue that vision.

Build and Empower Teams

Grand dreams do not become realities through the actions of a single leader. Leadership is a team effort.[4] Leaders must build a team that feels a sense of ownership for the vision. With effective leadership, great teams can have synergy—where the group effort is greater than the sum of the parts.

Choose the Right Team Members

In emphasizing the importance of people decisions in building an effective team, Collins suggests that a leader must first "get the right people on the bus (and the wrong people off the bus) *before* you figure out where to drive it."[15] The input from a strong team when the mission and vision and operational plans are nurtured and developed enables a journey where there will be greater ownership of the work to be done.

The attitudes and character traits of individuals are key attributes that should be considered when putting together a strong team. The values of the individuals should be compared with the values desired for the team when selections are made. Would the individual respect and trust other team members? Would he work collaboratively with others on the team? Would she fulfill commitments? Would he be excited about taking on major challenges? Once basic characteristics such as these are confirmed, other areas of expertise needed to support the mission and vision such as education, specialized knowledge, and other skill sets, can be reviewed.

The right mix of people on a team is also important. Diversity can bring expanded dimensions of thought and opinion to dreaming and decision making. Diverse skill sets and areas of expertise broaden the knowledge base. Depending on the purpose of a team, a mix of talents such as creativity, organizational skills, people skills, or aptitude with numbers could provide depth to the team. It may be helpful to bring in "new blood" to provide fresh ideas and perspectives. Finally, in addition to a range of talents and skill sets, diverse life and work experiences and cultural differences can enable a more open, creative, and comprehensive approach to issues a team may face. Diverse teams may be more challenging for leaders to manage, but they will bring more innovative solutions to the organization.[20]

An additional consideration for team selection is to match individuals with a project or responsibilities. The background, skill sets, or passion of an individual may make that particular individual an important member of a particular team. A systematic and well-organized individual may be a good choice for setting up a 340B program. A creative staff member may be well-suited for devising new training programs for staff. The converse may also be appropriate; a leader may select an inexperienced individual for a team in order to provide an opportunity for that individual to grow and develop new skill sets.

Perhaps the most difficult responsibility for a leader is to take action when team members are not contributing to their team. This deficiency may be evident through their work, their attitude, or their unwillingness to support the team effort. Leaders should provide feedback to these individuals, in private, about specifics they have done or not done that have hindered the progress of the team, listen to their issues, and offer suggestions about what they can do to improve their performance. If sufficient progress is not noted after progressive discussions, the leader should remove the individual from the team. This is important not only because of the lack of contribution or output from one individual, but also because carrying the burden of poorly performing team members can be demotivating to others on the team.

Foster Collaboration and Synergy in Teams

Teams who are equipped with a solid understanding of their mission and vision have a solid foundation for their work. Teams who were involved with the development of the mission and vision have even greater ownership of the vision since they helped to develop it. The role of the leader is then to provide continued focus on the vision and action plans and to set clear expectations for teams and individuals. By ensuring a realistic understanding of the current state, defining the gap between the present and the future, and making clear the consequences of not moving quickly toward the vision, a sense of urgency is developed.

Outstanding teams are passionate about their work. This passion is most evident when teams and individuals feel their work is of value; the mission and vision they are contributing to is meaningful to them and connects with their personal values and mission. Members must also believe that their daily work truly contributes to that mission. Pharmacy leaders may help their staff understand the importance of their work by providing staff in distribution areas, opportunities to get closer to patients. Telling stories of near misses that were prevented by pharmacy staff at staff meetings is another example of actions leaders can take to help staff feel the value of their daily work.

Teams are more effective when there exists a sense of community and collaboration. Effective leaders value and work to build a sense of community in their team or workplace. Strong communities care about and support one another; they communicate effectively; they are honest; they coach and mentor one another; they share; they encourage one another; they are accountable to one another; and they laugh and play together.[10] Teams embedded with trust have the courage to question and challenge one another. They are especially powerful when they have a unified drive for excellence and when they realize that their success is determined by the collective effort of everyone in the community. When teams become trusting communities, the contributions of the group become greater than the sum of the parts.

Empower and Support Teams

For a team to be successful, the leader must create an empowering environment that enables the team to innovate and make decisions within defined parameters. Leaders and teams should carefully review their organizational structure to ensure that it supports their strategy and action plans. For example, if medication safety is a priority for a pharmacy department, is there an individual that can help the team infiltrate aspects of safety into all their initiatives? Leaders must also ensure that members have sufficient education and training for the new tasks that are essential to their success. For pharmacy teams, it should not be forgotten that the development of interpersonal skills such as communication or conflict management skills, can be equally important as technical skills or knowledge about drugs. Other resource needs should be considered as projects are initiated. Would wireless computers provide pharmacy staff working in patient care areas more timely and efficient access to drug information?

An important gift that leaders can provide to teams is the ability to work with an appropriate degree of autonomy. Granting teams and individuals the authority to make decisions that affect their daily work enables them to do their jobs more efficiently and effectively, and more importantly, gives them greater ownership of the results.

At the same time it is important for leaders to give teams autonomy, it is important for leaders to stay connected. Most teams will maintain metrics that define their progress, or information on how well they are sticking to their timeline. Leaders must review these and other signs of progress and provide feedback on a regular basis, related to how the leader views the progress of the team. To inspire and encourage the team, leaders should try to provide more positive than negative feedback. Teams may need help in maintaining their focus. Individuals on the team may benefit from coaching. There may be barriers that only the leader can remove. Leaders must learn the delicate art of when to help and when to keep a distance.

Leaders must select and retain the right people, establish a culture where individuals work collaboratively, and empower them to do their work. They must build a team who trust and respect one another and feel ownership for the vision and the tasks at hand. In the end, success depends on what an organization's people care about, what they do, and how they work together.[13] The role of a leader is to help them do their best.

Foster Development of Talents

In an environment of constant change, competitive organizations must continue to expand learning opportunities to develop teams of leaders who can create and communicate visions and strategies. Leaders that continue to methodically learn tend to exhibit habits that lead to success. Lifelong learners take risks, humbly reflect on successes and failures, actively seek opinions from others, listen carefully, and are open to new ideas. These habits are associated with leaders with high standards, ambitious goals, and a real sense of mission.[7]

As a learning organization, the key to success is the organization's capacity to create a social architecture capable of generating new knowledge and sustaining this intellectual capital. By setting an example as a learner, the leader sets the pace of learning and is key to realizing the full potential of intellectual capital.[21] It is important for the leader to continually improve his or her knowledge, while identifying those learning opportunities that will be helpful to staff. Learning opportunities and obligations arise continually and in several formats. An organization's leaders may encourage an informal process or implement a formalized approach, such as continuing professional development (CPD), which is a frame work for lifelong learning and is an individualized, ongoing learning and personal improvement approach.[22]

Successful leaders are people who understand the dynamics and value of group interaction and can use that understanding to effectively motivate members of their work group to achieve important goals. To accomplish this, a leader will develop a team of assigned leaders who have the authority over the people they are leading, as well as a group of influence leaders who lead people over whom they have no authority.[6] The role of the leader is to add value to other people so that they can be their best, and inspire them to succeed. To accomplish this, the leader will support, direct, empower, encourage, coach, and facilitate others to make the right choices.

In addition to developing the assigned leadership team, the leader will establish many workgroups, both short and long-term in duration and often with an interdisciplinary membership. Selecting the chair and complementary team members, defining the charge of the workgroup, timeline, and expectations are important tasks for the leader. Once the workgroup is underway, the leader will monitor progress and provide guidance and support through to the conclusion of the group's work. Leaders must not only provide opportunities for people to develop their talents and skills, they must also lead the organization to understand that continuous learning is valued and expected.

Communicate Effectively

Helping people to do their best requires extraordinary communication. The power of a vision is unleashed only when people involved have a common understanding of its goals and direction.[7] People need to be convinced that the mission and vision are worthy of their time and talents. They need to believe that the vision is achievable. They need to have confidence that their leadership has the ability to help them achieve the vision.

Explain Why Change is Necessary

When communicating the strategic plan, leaders should first lay the groundwork for why the strategic plan (i.e., change) is necessary; explaining their view of how the environment is changing and why their organization needs to change. People who understand the underlying issues necessitating the urgent need for change are more likely to be motivated to change and support the vision.[13] With this contextual perspective, a confirmation of the mission and a description of the vision should then be described and discussed. In some settings, the discussion should get down to the detail of specific actions plans and timelines. The goal of these global or detailed discussions is for staff to come to understand exactly what is expected of them and how their work contributes to the vision.

Tell Everyone

All groups affected by the vision should hear some version of the strategic plan. For pharmacy teams this could be pharmacy staff, patients, physicians, nurses, administration, finance, information systems, human resources, and potentially others. The message could be tailored to the specific group. For instance, physicians might hear a version focusing on quality when they are informed of a plan to establish a pharmacist managed ambulatory anticoagulation clinic. The presentation to the finance department might focus more on expense and revenue. In addition to communicating *to* many people, the vision must be effectively communicated *by* all the leaders in the organization, not just the leader at the top.

Communicate through Varied Means

Communication is most effective when it is continuous and consistent. Leaders should find as many ways as possible to weave the vision and strategic plan into ordinary events as well as special meetings. The vision and operational plans for the year can be communicated at a kick off meeting for the department. Specific responsibilities and their relationship to the vision can be discussed during weekly "walkarounds" or one-on-one meetings. Goals supporting the vision can be included in individual performance reviews. Posters can be placed in pharmacy areas to remind staff of the big picture. Pens can be distributed with symbols reminding the owner of the mission or vision. Stories can be told about actions by ordinary people that supported the vision. In these different venues, the message can be expressed with urgency, passion, humor, encouragement, or gratitude. But the message must be positive and sincere. When it consistently comes from different voices in different settings and in ways people can connect with, it has a better chance of being heard and remembered.[7]

Listen

Listening is a powerful part of communication that is often overlooked. Listening and answering questions can help to clarify the vision. It may enable a leader to learn about flaws in a plan. It helps the leader to find common ground; what matters to people. Through this process the leader has greater opportunity to understand diverse groups and individuals and to help bring the vision to life for them. Kouzes and Posner advise that leadership is a dialogue, not a monologue.[4]

Provide Feedback

As the vision is pursued, leaders must share information about progress. Feedback not only updates people, it serves as a reminder that the vision and action plan are still important to the organization. This communication can occur in various settings and mediums as mentioned above. Progress expressed in metrics is essential; charts and graphs can provide a clear picture. An annual report is one example of how a pharmacy department can share its accomplishments and plans

with a wide audience.[11] Anecdotal stories can also be powerful. If the CEO pays a complement about a new program that supports the vision, this feedback should be shared with the team. The leader should be honest and share good news as well as bad news. Whether the news is good or bad, the leader should offer encouragement and support. Whatever the means, the leader should find ways to tie the results back to the contributions of groups and individuals that have made a difference.

An old saying offers wise advice about effective communication: "Tell me and I'll forget, show me and I'll remember, involve me and I'll understand." Effective leaders will communicate often and actively engage others in many aspects of how the vision is to be acted out.

Listen and Keep Informed

A successful leader will continually listen, read, and observe to stay informed of institutional and departmental progress, issues, and concerns. This is accomplished by interacting with staff formally (staff meetings) and informally (walking around), monitoring outcomes, critical metrics, and progress toward the vision. Being accessible, actively listening, and sharing with others creates an atmosphere that promotes the free exchange of ideas and perpetuates learning and commitment within the organization. It also encourages a healthy breeding ground for the innovative ideas needed to keep the organization at the cutting edge.

Effective leaders develop broad-based knowledge and employ a method to stay informed and continually expand their knowledge and capabilities. Clinical competency and knowledge of contemporary pharmacy practice are basic requirements for leadership success and credibility within a pharmacy organization. This knowledge becomes obsolete and must be continually updated for the leader's continued success. To accomplish this, leaders develop a personal process for continual learning such as a four-step cycle of learning, analyzing, questioning, and acting.[8] The leader must maintain broad knowledge of current issues in business, health care, pharmacy practice, and drug therapy. This is accomplished through active listening, reading, attending courses, conferences, and involvement in organizations. Learning communities and email list serves have enhanced communication and networking by efficiently transferring information of relevance to targeted audiences. When the leader follows the four-step cycle, he or she will stay informed of institutional and departmental situations, issues and trends, analyze the information, instinctively and intuitively question the conclusions drawn, and then take action.[8]

Develop Relationships

Relationships lead to trust and influence and, ultimately, define a leader's effectiveness.[11] For many, building enduring relationships is not easy. It requires time, energy, and commitment, while at the same time there are multitudes of concrete tasks that need attention.[23] Relationships, however, can reap huge benefits both in terms of the ability to get things done as well as the personal satisfaction that results from working collaboratively with others. The capacity to develop connected relationships is perhaps the most important quality of true leadership and is essential to leadership without authority.

Cultivate Relationships throughout the Organization

When a leader sincerely cares about others, many important relationships develop through natural means. Astute leaders realize that they must also strategically seek out relationships with individuals that can help their team pursue their goals. For pharmacists this may mean cultivating positive relationships with the medical staff, leaders in the finance department, key people in the quality or human resource departments, and other areas depending on the strategic plan and power bases within the health system. Relationships with the front lines can be as helpful as those in the administrative suite. Accordingly, relationships at all levels in the organization should be fostered. Since much of the effectiveness of an organization can be reliant on people caring about one another, leaders must also cultivate relationships between individuals and groups in their organization. Team building exercises outside of the workspace can often provide a foundation for the growth of these relationships. Even with well-established groups, it is important for leaders to periodically provide opportunities for staff to intermingle outside of their daily work routines.

Pharmacists should cultivate professional relationships outside of their place of work. These friends can serve as a source of new ideas and suggestions. They can also provide objective advice and encouragement.

Be Sincere

Relationships must be based on sincerity. For relationships to flourish, leaders must be respectful of the ideas, needs, and concerns of others. Asking a staff member about their children or sending a note after the loss of a loved one can be powerful gestures, if sincere. Relationships often begin when one individual helps or supports another, without expecting something in return. They are strengthened when there is a track record of being fair and honest. People are more inclined to trust leaders who show trust in others.[4]

Volunteer

There are many opportunities for pharmacists in health systems to assume a proactive role in developing relationships. They can request to serve on committees. They might volunteer at community events or participate in fund raising events. They can stop to chat with people from other departments in the cafeteria. They can set up one-on-one meetings with individuals or departments to clarify issues or convey that they value and care about the others' input. Most pharmacists have valuable skill sets they can offer in their quest to develop reciprocal relationships such as their ability to compile and analyze data, effectively research a topic, apply an evidence-based approach to decision making, or complete a failure mode analysis. The key to these offerings is that they must be genuine, not manipulative.

Relationships with members at all levels of an organization are critical to engendering commitment and meeting goals. Time spent in meaningful conversations and supportive efforts can be an investment that will produce far-reaching dividends.[24] In successful organizations, people not only care about *what* they are doing (i.e., the mission and the vision); they also care about one another.

Lead by Example

The actions of leaders are the most powerful form of communication. Actions provide evidence of what leaders truly are and believe in. Leaders' actions demonstrate their level of commitment to the vision and the people in the organization. The credibility of leaders is dependent on the congruity of their words and their deeds.

Peoples' belief that a leader truly cares about them is strongly influenced by what a leader does, not just by what a leader says. Leaders show they value others when they seek out and listen to others. They visit staff in the workplace. They may ask about their progress in school. They listen to and, when possible, respond to comments about challenges in the workplace. They make decisions that are for the common good of the organization; not just good for themselves.

Caring leaders share credit and recognize the contributions of others. They become more human to others when they demonstrate that they are honest, caring, and compassionate.

Model Values

A leader's behavior not only determines the credibility of the leader, it also models the way for *how* things are done in an organization. A leader who treats others with respect can expect that others will be respectful of one another. A leader who believes that collaborative working relationships are important must invest time in listening to and helping others. A leader who admits mistakes sets the tone for honesty in an organization. Meeting deadlines and being punctual for meetings sends a signal that self-discipline is important. Credible leaders will not compromise when their principles are tested.[20] The end result is that when leaders consistently meet or exceed the standards they ask of others, people are not only more likely to believe in the leader, they are also more likely to exude these characteristics themselves.

Demonstrate Commitment to the Vision

Leaders must prove that they are committed to the vision they articulate. When leaders use the vision and goals as the basis for decisions, they fortify their commitment to the vision. When they frame a discussion around the vision, they illustrate their focus on the vision. If a COO wants all hospital staff to feel responsible for a clean environment, he or she will pick up litter from a hallway. If a pharmacy manager is compassionate about medication safety, he or she will begin every staff meeting by asking staff what they have done during the week to enhance medication safety. What a leader *does* leads people to believe that their leader is sincerely and passionately dedicated to the vision they articulate. The demonstration of this commitment must be constant, even in difficult times.

In effective organizations, people believe in their leaders. Leaders gain credibility when they enact the values they expect from others and demonstrate commitment to the vision and the people in the organization. Effective leaders lead by example.

Celebrate Success

The change required to achieve a mission or even to complete a project can be difficult and take a long time. Leaders can help sustain the energy and enthusiasm for the journey by creating opportunities to recognize the contributions of individuals and groups. It is also important to periodically take time as a group to reflect on progress and celebrate success.

Recognize People

Recognition is most powerful when it is related to actions or behaviors that contribute to the vision or the values of the organization. Recognition provides positive feedback for people whose actions and energies have contributed to the goals of the team. Recognition or rewards can be spontaneous or planned, can take on many forms, and are not always monetary in nature. Meaningful rewards can include a simple "thank you" in the workplace, a basket of candy in a pharmacy satellite, a lunch with the Director, a plaque, or a trip to a national pharmacy meeting. Stories that are told at the time appreciation is shown can be very powerful, especially when the actions being recognized are tied back to the vision or values of the organization. Honoring people who support the vision or values reinforce that the leader is serious about the vision and values. Genuine expressions of gratitude can encourage people and fuel their passion to support the vision and goals.

Celebrate Group Accomplishments

It is important for the organization or team to periodically celebrate the accomplishments of the entire group. Special milestones, such as the implementation of a new service, a successful JCAHO survey, reducing the incidence of a targeted adverse drug reaction, or sustaining a target for turnaround time could be celebrated. Pharmacy leaders can use pharmacy week to plan a celebration of pharmacy contributions to the health system. Other departments in the institution might be invited to enhance their understanding and appreciation for the goals and contributions made by pharmacy staff. A patient who has been touched by compassionate care provided by a pharmacist or a physician whose prescribing error was caught by a pharmacist might provide powerful messages of gratitude for all the pharmacy staff present. These types of messages can help staff realize that their work is meaningful and worthwhile. The injection of humor through skits, gag gifts, or having leaders dress in silly costumes is another vehicle for celebration. Humor can help to create positive attitudes and team spirit that will remain after the formal celebration is over. Whatever means are used, celebrating team accomplishments recognizes that extraordinary performance is the result of many people's efforts and reinforces the sense that the efforts of the team are greater than the sum of the individual efforts.

Recognition and celebrations are often underutilized by leaders. These events provide an opportunity for teams to take a break from the day to day grind and reflect on the progress that has been made. They provide a means to refocus on the vision and values of the organization. For pharmacy staff, they provide an opportunity to remember the value of their individual and collective work in helping people make the best use of medications. Acts of recognition and celebrations serve as reinforcement and give people the courage to continue to struggle with the challenges ahead of them.

Summary

Our health systems and patients need and deserve pharmaceutical care that is safe, effective, cost conscious, and compassionate. To meet these needs, departments of pharmacy must have effective leaders. In pharmacy departments where there is strong leadership, the work is innovative and challenging, the focus is clear, and people are informed and empowered. There are numerous leaders throughout the department, not just at the top. Leaders care about the people and the people care about and support one another. Pharmacy leadership is evident within the department and outside the department, in pharmacy satellites and on patient care teams, in community outreach programs, and in patient safety initiatives. Pharmacists are passionate about their responsibility to help people make the best use of medications. Leaders enable pharmacy staff to make a difference.

References

1. Boyko WL, Yurkowski PJ, Ivey MF, et al. Pharmacist influence on economic and morbidity outcomes in a tertiary care teaching hospital. *Am J Health Syst Pharm.* 1997 Jul 15; 54(14):1591–5.

2. Leape LL, Cullen DJ, Dempsey CM, et al. Pharmacists' participation on physicians rounds and adverse drug events in the intensive care unit. *JAMA.* 1999;282:267–70.

3. Gattis WA, Hasselblad V, Whellan DJ, et al. Reduction in heart failure events by the addition of a clinical pharmacist to the heart failure management team. *Arch Intern Med.* 1999;159:1939–45.

4. Kouzes JM, Posner BZ. *The Leadership Challenge.* New York: Wiley Johns and Sons; 2002.

5. Holdford DA. Leadership theories and their lessons for pharmacists. *Am J Health Syst Pharm.* 2003;60:1780–6.

6. American Society of Health-System Pharmacists. 2003 ASHP leadership conference on pharmacy practice management executive summary. Looking to the future: leading and managing change. *Am J Health Syst Pharm.* 2004;61:1052–8.

7. Kotter JP. *Leading Change.* Boston: Harvard Business School Publishing; 1996.

8. Woodward BW. The journey to professional excellence: a matter of priorities. *Am J Health Syst Pharm.* 1998;55:782–9.

9. Williams RB. Achieving excellence. *Am J Hosp Pharm.* 1986;43:617–24.

10. Wollenburg KG. Leadership with conscience, compassion, and commitment. *Am J Hosp Pharm.* 2004;61:1785–91.

11. Zilz DA, Woodward BW, Thielke TS, et al. Leadership skills for high-performance pharmacy practice. *Am J Health Syst Pharm.* 2004;61:2562–74.

12. Maxwell JC. *The 21 Irrefutable Laws of Leadership: Follow Them and People Will Follow You.* Nashville, TN: Nelson; 1988.

13. Goleman D, Boyatzis R, McKee A. *Primal Leadership.* Boston: Harvard Business School Publishing; 2002.

14. Drucker PF. What makes an effective executive? *Har Bus Rev.* 2004;82:58–63, 136.

15. Collins J. *Good to Great: Why Some Companies Make the Leap...and Others Don't.* New York: Harper Collins; 2001.

16. Covey SR. *The 7 Habits of Highly Effective People.* New York: Simon & Schuster; 1990.

17. American Society of Health-System Pharmacists. ASHP policy positions, statements and guidelines. Available at: http://www.ashp.org/bestpractices. Accessed February 24, 2005.

18. American Society of Health Systems Pharmacists. Mission statement of the American Society of Health-System Pharmacists, approved by the ASHP House of Delegates, June 4, 2001. Available at: http://www.ashp.org/AboutASHP/ASHPMission.cfm. Accessed February 24, 2005.

19. Gebelein SH, Stevens LA, Skube CJ, et al. *Successful Manager's Handbook: Development Suggestions for Today's Managers.* Minneapolis: Personnel Decisions International; 2000.

20. George B. *Authentic Leadership.* San Francisco: Jossey-Bass; 2003.

21. Bennis W. The Leadership advantage. *Leader to Leader.* 12(Spring 1999):18–23.

22. Rouse MJ. Continuing professional development in pharmacy. *Am J Health Syst Pharm.* 2004;61:2069–76.

23. Levine SL. *The Six Fundamentals of Success: The Rules for Getting It Right for Yourself and Your Organization.* New York: Doubleday & Company; 2004.

24. Abramowitz PW. Nurturing relationships: an ingredient of leadership. *Am J Health Syst Pharm.* 2001;58:479–84.

Chapter 18

Medication Safety

Scott M. Mark, Michelle C. Mercado

Introduction and Background

The goal of drug therapy is the achievement of defined therapeutic outcomes that improve a patient's quality of life while minimizing patient risk.[1] There are inherent risks, both known and unknown, associated with the therapeutic use of drugs (prescription and nonprescription) and drug administration devices.[2] The incidents or hazards that result from such risk have been defined as drug misadventuring, which includes both adverse reactions (ADRs) and medication errors.[3]

The release of the Institute of Medicine (IOM) report, *To Err Is Human: Building a Safer Health System,* in 1999 irrevocably changed the way medication errors were viewed in health systems. In many ways, this was the fist comprehensive report that quantified the problem of medical errors in health systems.

Selected information from the 1999 Institute of Medicine report on medical safety revealed[4]:

- Medical errors kill 44,000 to 98,000 patients annually.

- Errors cause more deaths each year than breast cancer, motor vehicle accidents, and AIDS.

- It is estimated that each year in our nation's hospitals, 6.7% of all admitted patients will experience a medical accident.

- Of those accidents, 3.1% will be adverse events and 13% of those adverse events will be fatal.

- Of these accidents, in total, 72% of them are recurring and, therefore, are predictable and preventable.

- Two out of every 100 admissions experienced a preventable adverse drug event, resulting in average increased hospital costs of $4,700 per admission.

- Medication errors alone, occurring either in or out of the hospital, are estimated to account for over 7,000 deaths annually.

Medication errors compromise patient confidence in the health care system and increase health care costs. Research conducted for the ASHP revealed that 61% of respondents stated that they were "very concerned" about being given the wrong medicine during a hospital stay.[5] The problems and sources of medication errors are multidisciplinary and multifactorial. They can be committed by both experienced and inexperienced staff, including pharmacists, physicians, nurses, supportive personnel (e.g., pharmacy technicians), students, clerical staff (e.g., unit clerks), administrators, pharmaceutical manufacturers, patients and their caregivers, and others.[2]

Many medication errors are probably undetected. According to the fourth annual report on medication errors by the United States Pharmacopeia (USP), 49% of medication errors never reached the patient.[6] The outcome(s) or clinical significance of many medication errors may be minimal, with few or no consequences that adversely affect a patient. According to the USP study, which was based on errors reported voluntarily through its MEDMARx™ database in 2002 using 190,000 errors, more than 98% of medication errors result in no harm to the patient. Tragically, however, some medication errors result in serious patient morbidity and mortality. The pharmacist's mission is to help ensure that patients make the best use of medications.[7] This applies to all drugs used by inpatient or ambulatory patients, including oral or injectable products, radiopharmaceuticals, radiopaque contrast media, anesthetic gases, blood-fraction drugs, dialysis fluids, respiratory therapy agents, investigational drugs, drug samples, drugs brought into the hospital setting by patients, and other chemical or biological substances administered to patients to evoke a pharmacological response.[8]

Definitions and Classification of Medication Errors

It is important that health practitioners within a given institution have a common set of definitions. The IOM defines an adverse drug event (ADE) as an injury resulting from medical intervention related to a drug, which can be attributable to preventable and nonpreventable causes.

The National Coordinating Council for Medication Error Reporting and Prevention (NCCMERP) defines a medication error as "Any preventable event that may cause or lead to inappropriate medication use or patient harm while the medication is in the control of the health care professional, patient, or consumer."

The July 1999 Health Care Financing Administration (HCFA) guidelines define a significant medication error as one that creates discomfort for the patient or compromises the patient's health and safety, based on the patient's condition, the drug's category, and the frequency with which the error occurs. Often medication errors are categorized by the segment of the medication use process that has failed. Therefore, they can be categorized as prescribing errors, dispensing errors, medication administration errors, monitoring errors, and patient compliance errors. The Joint Commission on Accreditation of Healthcare Organizations (JCAHO) has also adopted a similar approach in the revised 2004 medication management chapter standards. For the purpose of safe medication management, JCAHO divides the medication use process into six critical processes shown in Figure 18-1.

Studies indicate that 49% of medication errors occur during the ordering phase, 26% during the delivery (transcribing) phase, and 25% during the processing (preparing and dispensing) phase.[9]

Medication errors are also classified by type of technical error that occurred. The American Society of Health-System Pharmacists (ASHP) Guidelines on Preventing Medication Errors in Hospitals classifies these types of error as listed in Table 18-1.

An analysis has shown that the most common errors were those of omission (25.6%), in which the prescribed medication was not administered; dosage or quantity (25.5%); and prescription (18.5%), in which a medication was incorrectly prescribed.[6] Medication errors that are most likely to cause harm to the patient included wrong administration of medication (such as inappropriately crushing tablets); delivering drugs through the wrong route (such as intravenous vs. intramuscular); and issuing the wrong medications. Insulin, morphine, and heparin were cited as being most involved in errors resulting in harm to patients.

Another common way to classify medication errors is by patient harm (if any) that resulted due to the error. To understand this manner of classification, it is necessary to understand these terms:

- *Harm*—Impairment of the physical, emotional, or psychological function or structure of the body and/or pain resulting there from.

- *Monitoring*—To observe or record relevant physiological or psychological signs.

- *Intervention*—May include change in therapy or active medical/surgical treatment.

- *Intervention Necessary to Sustain Life*—Includes cardiovascular and respiratory support (e.g., CPR, defibrillation, intubation, etc.).

Simple classifications group the errors into clinically significant and minor.[10] Later, a more elaborate classification was developed by Hartwig, Denger and Schneider.[11] NCCMERP has developed the following classification system which has now gained widespread acceptance, shown in Figure 18-2.

Figure 18-1
Medication Use Process

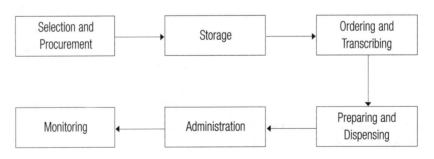

Table 18-1

Types of Medication Errors[12-24,a]

Type	Definition
Prescribing error	Incorrect drug selection (based on indication, contraindications, known allergies, existing drug therapy, and other factors), dose, dosage form, quantity, route, concentration, rate of administration, or instructions for use of a drug product ordered or authorized by physician (or other legitimate prescriber); illegible prescriptions or medication orders that lead to errors that reach the patient
Omission error[b]	The failure to administer an ordered dose to a patient before the next scheduled dose, if any
Wrong time error	The failure to administer a medication within a predefined time interval from its scheduled administration time (this interval should be established by each individual health care facility)
Unauthorized drug error[c]	Administration to the patient of a medication not authorized by a legitimate prescriber for the patient
Improper dose error[d]	Administration to the patient of a dose that is greater than or less than the amount ordered by the prescriber or administration of duplicate doses to the patient, i.e., one or more dosage units in addition to those that were ordered
Wrong dosage-form error[e]	Administration to the patient of a drug product in a different dosage form than ordered by he prescriber
Wrong drug-preparation error[f]	Drug product incorrectly formulated or manipulated before administration
Wrong administration-technique error[g]	Inappropriate procedure or improper technique in the administration of a drug
Deteriorated drug error[h]	Administration of a drug that has expired or for which the physical or chemical dose-form integrity has been compromised
Monitoring error	Failure to review a prescribed regimen for appropriateness and detection of problems, or failure to use appropriate clinical or laboratory data for adequate assessment of patient response to prescribed therapy
Compliance error	Inappropriate patient behavior regarding adherence to a prescribed medication regimen
Other medication error	Any medication error that does not fall into one of the above predefined categories

a The categories may not be mutually exclusive because of the multidisciplinary and multifactorial nature of medication errors.

b Assumes no prescribing error. Excluded would be (1) a patient's refusal to take the medication or (2) a decision not to administer the dose because of recognized contraindications. If an explanation for the omission is apparent (e.g., patient was away from nursing unit for tests or medication was not available), that reason should be documented in the appropriate records.

c This would include, for example, a wrong drug, a dose given to the wrong patient, unordered drugs, and doses given outside a stated set of clinical guidelines or protocols.

d Excluded would be (1) allowable deviations based on preset ranges established by individual health care organizations in consideration of measuring devices routinely provided to those who administer drugs to patients (e.g., not administered a dose based on a patient's measure temperature or blood glucose level) or other factors such as conversion of doses expressed in the apothecary system to the metric system and (2) topical dosage forms for which medication orders are not expressed quantitatively.

e Excluded would be accepted protocols (established by the pharmacy and therapeutics committee or its equivalent) that authorize pharmacists to dispense alternate dosage forms for patients with special needs (e.g., liquid formulations for patients with nasogastric tubes or those who have difficulty swallowing), as allowed by state regulations.

f This would include, for example, incorrect dilution or reconstitution, mixing drugs that are physically or chemically incompatible, and inadequate product packaging.

g This would include doses administered (1) via the wrong route (different from the route prescribed), (2) via the correct route but at the wrong site (e.g., left eye instead of right), and (3) at the wrong route of administration.

h This would include, for example, administration of expired drugs and improperly stored drugs.

Figure 18-2

NCC MERP Index for Categorizing Medication Errors[27]

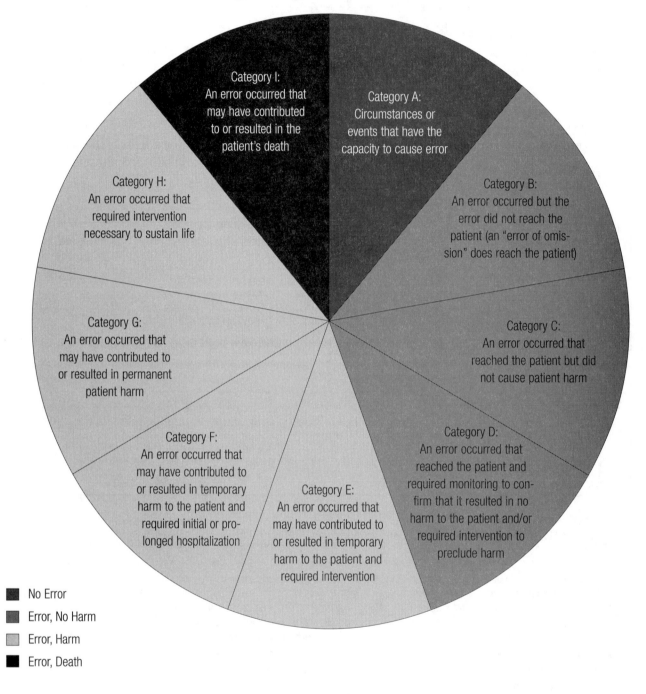

Category I:
An error occurred that may have contributed to or resulted in the patient's death

Category A:
Circumstances or events that have the capacity to cause error

Category H:
An error occurred that required intervention necessary to sustain life

Category B:
An error occurred but the error did not reach the patient (an "error of omission" does reach the patient)

Category G:
An error occurred that may have contributed to or resulted in permanent patient harm

Category C:
An error occurred that reached the patient but did not cause patient harm

Category F:
An error occurred that may have contributed to or resulted in temporary harm to the patient and required initial or prolonged hospitalization

Category E:
An error occurred that may have contributed to or resulted in temporary harm to the patient and required intervention

Category D:
An error occurred that reached the patient and required monitoring to confirm that it resulted in no harm to the patient and/or required intervention to preclude harm

■ No Error
■ Error, No Harm
■ Error, Harm
■ Error, Death

Source: National Coordinating Council for Medication Error Reporting and Prevention.

Preventing Medication Errors

Medication errors occur for a number of reasons. Some common reasons include the following:

- Ambiguous strength designation on labels or in packaging
- Drug product nomenclature (look-alike or sound-alike names, use of lettered or numbered prefixes and suffixes in drug names)
- Equipment failure or malfunction
- Illegible handwriting
- Improper transcription Inaccurate dosage calculation
- Inadequately trained personnel
- Inappropriate abbreviations used in prescribing
- Labeling errors
- Excessive workload
- Lapses in individual performance
- Medication unavailable

It is important to understand that it is human nature to make mistakes, and that no person is error-free. Further, medication use systems are extremely complex. Therefore, it becomes vital to create systems in which safeguards are built in order to reduce risk and promote safe use of medications. Systems for ordering, dispensing, and administering medications should be designed to minimize error. Medication errors may involve process breakdowns in more than one aspect of a system. For this reason, it is essential that each organization use a systematic approach to analyzing their medication use systems. The data collected will help drive decisions regarding system changes.

Error Reporting and Use of Data

In order to design safer medication delivery systems, medication data must be collected, analyzed and trended. System failures teach us a tremendous amount about the weaknesses inherent in our complex medical delivery processes. Ongoing quality improvement programs for monitoring medication errors are needed in each institution. While it is essential that data be collected and trended for analysis, the difficulty in detecting errors has long been recognized as a barrier to studying the problem effectively.[12] Medication errors should be identified and documented and their causes studied in order to develop systems that minimize recurrence.[13,14] Most health systems have a process for voluntary reporting of medication errors. Some are computerized, but most are paper systems that are designed to collect necessary information. The process can be laborious and as a result, reporting rates can be low. It is estimated that reported rates represent less than 10% of actual errors. Several error monitoring techniques exist and may be applied as appropriate to determine error rates.[11,14] There are differences in the validity of the data obtained by the various error monitoring techniques or combined techniques. Monitoring programs for medication errors should consider the following risk factors:[8,11,13,14]

- Work shift (higher error rates typically occur during the day shift)
- Inexperienced and inadequately trained staff
- Medical service (e.g., special needs for certain patient populations, including geriatrics, pediatrics, and oncology)
- Increased number of quantity of medications per patient
- Environmental factors (lighting, noise, and frequent interruptions
- Staff workload and fatigue
- Poor communication among health care providers
- Dosage form (e.g., injectable drugs are associated with more serious errors)
- Type of distribution system (unit dose distribution is preferred; floor stock should be minimized)
- Improper drug storage
- Extent of measurements or calculations required
- Confusing drug product nomenclature, packaging, or labeling
- Drug category (e.g., antimicrobials)
- Poor handwriting
- Verbal (orally communicated orders)
- Lack of effective policies and procedures
- Poorly functioning oversight committees

It is important to note that several items listed have a common denominator, the limitation of human performance. Studies on the negative effects of stress have shown that the human performance degrades in the face of significant stress. In a relaxed environment, clinicians can choose the correct medication off the shelf 99.9% of the time, but during periods of high stress the error rate can be as high as 25%.[38]

Fatigue can also have a tremendous influence on performance. Although being oncall all night and working double shifts is commonplace, fatigue impairs the ability to process complex information and care for patients. After 24 hours without sleep, cognitive performance is equivalent to a blood alcohol level of 0.10%.[15] Data published from Shindul-Rothschild et al. demonstrated that the root causes of medication errors could be stratified into six groups. Fifty-seven percent were attributable to stress, 45% to understaffing, 38% to lack of experience, 33% to unclear orders, 26% to fatigue, and 15% to illegible handwriting.[16]

Determination of the causes of medication errors should be coupled with assessment of the severity of the error. While quality management processes should include programs to decrease the incidence of all medication errors, effort should be concentrated on eliminating the causes of errors associated with greater levels of severity. There should be established mechanisms for tracking drugs or drug classes that are involved in medication errors. Correlations between errors and the method of drug distribution should also be reviewed (e.g., unit dose, floor stock, injectable etc.). Certain medications tend to be more problematic than others.

Listed below are drugs that are commonly associated with errors.[17]

1. Insulin
2. Albuterol
3. Morphine sulfate
4. Potassium chloride
5. Heparin
6. Cefazolin
7. Warfarin
8. Furosemide
9. Levofloxacin
10. Vancomycin

Currently, most medication error reporting systems are internal and health-system specific. Most states now have specific legislation in place which allows health systems to collect and review medication error data without the risk that it will be used against the organization in court cases. These peer-review statues, however, provide clear boundaries regarding how the information is communicated and used. In the most

general of terms, the information can only be used for the purpose of reviewing and improving systems and can only be communicated to those individuals deemed as a necessary part of the process. It is essential that individuals reviewing medication error information be familiar with the laws in their jurisdiction to ensure that they, their organization, and their data remain protected.

For those states under which it is permissible, there are several national reporting agencies available that will partner to collect and trend data. These national programs allow health care professionals to anonymously report concerns regarding the quality, safety, performance, or design of drug products. The information is collected nationally, and the aggregate information is shared for the purpose of identifying national trends.

There are currently three national reporting programs.[18]

- The FDA's MedWATCH program is mainly focused on postmarketing surveillance received from events reported by health professionals.

- The USP Medication Error Reporting (MER) Program allows individual practitioners to anonymously report actual or potential medication errors. If desired, professionals can provide contact information to USP, ISMP, FDA and/or pharmaceutical manufacturers so that they can be contacted for additional information.

- MEDMARx is also an anonymous program by which information can be reported. It is unique in that individual health systems can internally monitor their own progress and track the success of their improvement strategies against national trends.

For many health care professionals, there still remains a fear associated with reporting and an unwillingness to identify the errors of coworkers. For this reason, anonymous reporting systems offer an alternative. Concerns remain, however, over the security of the information and the legal risks incurred by sharing data with a third party. Many feel that a mandatory reporting system would force change in the health care system by highlighting competitive weaknesses. Payors have begun to ask for quality data and some have even developed incentive programs intended to improve quality which have predefined safety metrics. A well-informed public has also begun to question quality and use available quality reports from regulatory agencies such as JCAHO to guide their health care selections. Failures can be very traumatic events for both the families and all of the health care workers involved.

Organization Recommendations to Improve Medication Safety[2,19]

There are many strategies that can be employed to reduce medication errors. Regardless of the specific initiative, certain approaches have proven to be more effective. Figure 18-3 lists a rank order of error reduction strategies from most effective to least effective.[20]

Forcing functions—methods implemented that make it difficult to proceed erroneously with a process—are the most effective strategies because individuals only have the ability to do the right thing. Examples would include stocking oral syringes that will not fit IV sites, therefore making it impossible for oral medications to be administered intravenously. Another such example of a forcing function is limiting the stock of drug to one concentration or strength; if only one concentration of a drug is available then the wrong concentration cannot be selected. Preprinted order forms or computer options that *force* selection from a limited number of medications, available dosages, and routes of administration are also examples.

Using the principles of the formulary system, the P&T Committee (or its equivalent)—composed of

Figure 18-3
Methods Used to Minimize Medication Errors

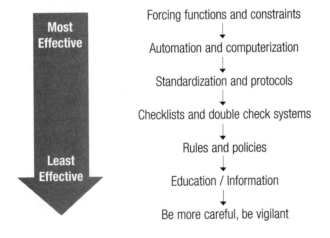

Source: Adopted from the Institute for Safe Medication Practices.

pharmacists, physicians, nurses, and other health professionals— should be responsible for formulating policies regarding the evaluation, selection, and therapeutic use of drugs in organized health care settings. JCAHO now requires that all medications on the formulary or to be added to the formulary be reviewed annually and that medication safety be considered. Institutions should develop a systematic method developed to assess a medication's risk profile based on potential side effects, approved uses, look-alike/sound-alike potential, difficulty in dose preparation, etc.

A review of the formulary should be conducted to identify any products that look-alike. Every attempt should be made to purchase products from alternative manufacturers to minimize potential confusion. When alternate products are not available, look-alike products should be physically separated in the pharmacy and automated dispensing cabinets and additional signage added when necessary. USP MER Program maintains a list of medication names which look-alike and sound-alike (Table 18-2). Remember that these names may not sound-alike as they are read or look-alike in print, but when handwritten or communicated verbally these names have caused or could cause a mix-up.

The use of a patient's own or *home* medications should be avoided to the fullest extent possible. Use of such medications should be allowed only if there is a need for the patient to receive the therapy, the drug product is not obtainable by the pharmacy, and no alternative therapy can be prescribed. If such medications are used, the prescribing physician must write and appropriate order in the patient's medical record. Before use, a pharmacist should inspect and identify the medication. If there are any unresolved questions with respect to product integrity, the medication must not be used.

Except in emergency situations, all sterile and non-sterile drug products should be dispensed from the pharmacy department for individual patients. The storage of nonemergency floor stock medications on the nursing units or in patient care areas should be minimized. Particular caution should be exercised with respect to drug products that have commonly been involved in serious medication errors or whose margin of safety is narrow, such as concentrated forms of drug products that are intended to be diluted into larger volumes (e.g., concentrated lidocaine and potassium chloride for injection concentrate). All drug storage areas should be routinely inspected by pharmacy personnel to ensure adequate product integrity and appro-

Table 18-2
Look-Alike, Sound-Alike Medications[a]

Accupril	*Accutane*
Acetohexamide	Acetazolamide
Doxepin	Doxycycline
DepoMedrol	*Solu-Medrol*
Cytovene	*Cytosar*
Coumadin	*Compazine*
Doxorubicin	Idarubicin
Depo-Estradiol	*Depo-Testadiol*
Cytoxan	*Cytotec*
Cyclobenzaprine	Cyproheptadine
DynaCirc	*Dynacin*
DiaBeta	*Zebeta*
Cytoxan	*Cytosar* (Cytarabine)
Cyclophosphamide	Cyclosporine
Feldene	*Seldane*
DynaCirc	*Dynacin*
Dolobid	*Slobid*
Dilaudid	*Demerol*
Flumadine	Fludarabine
Echogen	*Epogen*
Dopamine	Dobutamine
Diphenatol	Diphenidol
Fluorouracil	Flucytosine
Efudex	*Eurax*
Doxepin	Doxycycline
Diupres	*Daypro*
Folinic Acid	Folic Acid
Eldepryl	Enalapril
Doxorubicin	Idarubicin
Dobutrex	*Diamox*
Gamimune Nestraderm	*CytoGam*
DynaCirc	*Dynacin*
Dolobid	*Slobid*
Gamulin	*MICRhoGAM*
RhEstratest	*Estratab*
Echogen	*Epogen*
Dopamine	Dobutamine
Imipenem	*Omnipen*

Hydroxyzine	Hydralazine
Hemoccult	*Seracult*
K-Phos Neutral	*Neutra-Phos-K*
Inderal	*Isordil*
Lamictal	*Lomotil*
Lanoxin	*Lasix, Lomotil*
Interleukin 2	Interferon 2
K-Phos Neutral	*Neutra-Phos-K*
Klonopin	Clonidine
Lamictal	*Lomotil*
Lanoxin	*Lasix, Lomotil*
Klonopin	Clonidine
Inderal	*Adderall*
Lenoxin	*Levoxine, Lanoxin*
Leucovorin	*Leukine, Leukeran*
Propranolol	*Propulsid*
Prinivil	*Proventil*
Premarin	*Primaxin*
Provera	*Premarin*
Prinivil	*Prilosec*
Prepidil	Bepridil
Provera	*Provir*
Proctocream HC	*Proctocort*
Prilosec	*Prozac*
Soma	*Soma Compound*
Rimantadine	Amantadine, Ranitidine
Reglan	*Megace*
Stadol	*Haldol*
Reserpine	*Risperdal*, Risperidone
Reno-M-60	*Renografin-60*
Sulfasalazine	Sulfisoxazole
Roxanol	*Roxicet*
Ridaura	*Cardura*
Zonalon	*Zone A Forte*
Vincristine	Vinblastine
Tussi-Organidin DM	*Tussi-Organidin*
Zofran	*Zantac*
Zonalon	*Zone A Forte*
Zosyn	*Zofran*

[a] Brand names are italicized.

Source: Adopted from United States Pharmacopeia.

priate packaging, labeling, and storage. It is important that drug products and other products for external use be stored separately from drug products for internal use.

All discontinued or unused drugs should be returned to the department of pharmacy immediately on discontinuation or at patient discharge. Discharged patients must not be given unlabeled drug products to take home, unless they are labeled for outpatient use by the pharmacy in accordance with state and federal regulations. Discharged patients should be counseled about use of any medications to be used after discharge.

An effort should be made to reduce the number of concentrations that are available. Multiple concentrations lead to selecting the wrong drug and miscalculations. For example, multiple formulations of insulin are available, and product packaging can look similar in appearance.

The pharmacy director and staff must ensure that all drug products used in the organizational setting are of high quality and integrity. This would include, for example, (1) selecting multisource products supported by adequate bioavailability data and adequate product packaging and labeling, (2) maintaining an unexpired product inventory, and (3) keeping abreast of compendial requirements.

The pharmacy department must be responsible for the procurement, distribution, and control of all drugs used within the organization. Adequate hours for the provision of pharmaceutical services must be maintained; 24-hour pharmaceutical service is strongly recommended in hospital settings. In the absence of 24-hour pharmaceutical service, access to a limited supply of medications should be available to authorized nonpharmacists for use in initiating urgent medication orders. The list of medications to be supplied and the policies and procedures to be used (including subsequent review of all activity by a pharmacist) should be developed by the P&T Committee (or its equivalent). Items should be chosen with safety in mind, limiting wherever possible medications, quantities, dosage forms, and container sizes that might endanger patients. The use of well-designed night cabinets, after-hours drug carts, and other methods would preclude the need for nonpharmacists to enter the pharmacy. Access to the pharmacy by nonpharmacists (e.g., nurses) for removal of doses is strongly discouraged; this practice should be minimized and eliminated to the fullest extent possible. When 24-hour pharmacy service is not feasible, a pharmacist must be available on an oncall basis. Given that JCAHO now requires a pharmacist review of all nonemergent orders, many pharmacies have outsourced off-hours review of orders. Orders are either scanned to alternate locations, processed centrally for several hospitals, or processed through virtual private networks from remote locations.

Special labeling of medication storage bins can help avoid errors. For example tallman lettering—using capital letters to distinguish look-alike or sound-alike medications—avoid errors by drawing attention to small differences in drug names to ensure that the correct product is selected. Examples include DOButamine vs. DOPamine or HydrALazine vs. HydrOXyzine.

Studies indicate prescribing continues to represent the highest area of risk in the medication use process. Forty-nine percent of medication errors occur during the ordering phase.[22] For this reason hospitals nationwide have invested significant resources into implementing computerized prescriber order entry (CPOE) systems. Several advocacy groups such as the Leap Frog Group and the Institute for Safe Medication Practices (ISMP) have also endorsed this trend. Caution should be exercised though as these systems reduce risk in some areas of the medication use process and increase or transfer risk to other areas. In addition, these systems are challenging to implement. Without proper support and coordination, they can fail to provide a safer environment and may even introduce new risk.[23]

Functions important to the *ideal* computer order entry system include the following[24]:

- Prescriber order entry for verification by nurse and pharmacist

- Computer-generated medication administration records from a common data base shared with the pharmacy and the prescriber

- For each patient, lists of current medications that are readily accessible by caregivers

- Two-way interface between the pharmacy and other institutional systems (e.g., laboratory, admission and discharge, clinical records)

- Access to historical patient data (i.e., archived information)

- Ability to calculate and verify appropriate height-weight range and dosage for patient

- Access to vital patient and drug information directly from order entry, medication profile, and medication administration screens

- Ability of system to use patient and drug information to provide unsolicited information during order entry to reduce potential for adverse drug events (e.g., drug interactions, contraindications, excessive doses, allergies). This should be part of a comprehensive decision support program. These programs would include checking for laboratory results and advising the prescriber of the need for dosing modifications for specified medications. Automatic checking should also include drug-drug interactions, drug-nutrient interactions, drug duplication, therapeutic duplication, contraindicated medications, and weight-based dosage checking.

- Provide forced function by limiting the route and frequency by which a drug is ordered

To further promote safe medication use, consider the following:

1. To determine appropriate drug therapy, prescribers should stay abreast of the current state of knowledge through literature review, consultation with pharmacists, consultation with other physicians, participation in continuing professional education programs, and other means. It is especially crucial to seek information with prescribing for conditions and diseases not typically experienced in the prescriber's practice.

2. Prescribers should evaluate the patient's total status and review all existing drug therapy before prescribing new or additional medications to ascertain possible antagonistic or complementary drug interactions. To evaluate and optimize patient response to prescribed drug therapy, appropriate monitoring of clinical signs and symptoms and of relevant laboratory data is necessary.

3. In hospitals, prescribers should be familiar with the medication ordering system (e.g., the formulary system), participation in DUE programs, allowable delegation of authority, procedures to alert nurses and others to new drug orders that need to be processed, standard medication administration times, and approved abbreviations.

4. Drug orders should be complete. They should include the patient's name, generic drug name, trademarked name (if a specific product is required), route and site of administration,

dosage form, dose, strength, quantity, frequency of administration, and prescriber's name. In some cases, a dilution, rate, and time of administration should be specified. The desired therapeutic outcome for each drug should be expressed when the drug is prescribed. Prescribers should review all drug orders for accuracy and legibility immediately after they have prescribed them.

5. Care should be taken to ensure that the intent of medication orders is clear and unambiguous. Prescribers should adhere to the following:

   a. Write out instructions rather than using non-standard or ambiguous abbreviations. For example, write *daily* rather than *q.d.*, which could be misinterpreted as *q.i.d.* (causing a drug to be given four times a day instead of once) or as *o.d.* (for right eye).

   b. Do not use vague instructions, such as *take as directed*, because specific instructions can help differentiate among intended drugs.

   c. Specify exact dosage strengths (such as milligrams) rather than dosage form units (such as one tablet or one vial). An exception would be combination drug products, for which the number of dosage form units should be specified.

   d. Prescribe by standard nomenclature, using the drug's generic name (United States Adopted Name or USAN), official name, or trademarked name (if deemed medically necessary). Avoid the following: locally coined names (e.g., Dr. Doe's syrup); chemical names (e.g., 6-mercaptopurine [instead of mercaptopurine] could result in a sixfold overdose if misinterpreted); nonestablished, abbreviated drug names (e.g., *AZT* could stand for zidovudine, azathioprine, or aztreonam); acronyms; and apothecary or chemical symbols.

   e. Always use a leading zero before a decimal expression of less than one (e.g., 0.5 mL). Conversely, a terminal zero should never be used (e.g., 5.0 mL), since failure to see the decimal could result in a tenfold overdose. When possible, avoid the use of decimals (e.g., prescribe 500 m instead of 0.5 g).

Data published on tenfold errors show that overdoses are prescribed in 61% of the cases.[25] As a class, antimicrobials, cardiovascular agents, and central nervous system agents each accounted for ≥15% of errors.

Table 18-3

ISMP Error-Prone Abbreviations

Abbreviation	Potential Problem	Preferred Term
U (for unit)	Mistaken as zero, four, or cc	Write *unit*
IU (for international unit)	Mistaken as IV (intravenous) or 10 (ten)	Write *international unit*
Q.D., Q.O.D. (Latin abbreviation for once daily and every other day)	Mistaken for each other. The period after the *Q* can be mistaken for an *I* and the *O* can be mistaken for *I*.	Write *daily* and *every other day*
Trailing zero (X.0 mg) [Note: Prohibited only for medication-related notations]; Lack of leading zero (.X mg)	Decimal point is missed	Never write a zero by itself after a decimal point (X mg), and always use a zero before a decimal point (0.X mg)
MS MSO$_4$ MgSO$_4$	Confused for one another. Can mean morphine sulfate or magnesium sulfate.	Write *morphine sulfate* or *magnesium sulfate*
mg (for microgram)	Mistaken for mg (milligrams) resulting in one thousand-fold dosing overdose	Write *mcg*
H.S. (for half-strength or Latin abbreviation for bedtime)	Mistaken for either half-strength or hour of sleep (at bedtime). q.H.S. mistaken for every hour. All can result in a dosing error.	Write out *half-strength* or *at bedtime*
T.I.W. (for three times a week)	Mistaken for three times a day or twice weekly resulting in an overdose	Write *3 times weekly* or *three times weekly*
S.C. or S.Q. (for subcutaneous)	Mistaken as SL for sublingual or *5 every*	Write *Sub-Q, subQ,* or *subcutaneously*
D/C (for discharge)	Interpreted as discontinue whatever medications follow (typically discharge meds)	Write *discharge*
c.c. (for cubic centimeter)	Mistaken for U (units) when poorly written	Write *mL* for milliliters
A.S., A.D., A.U. (Latin abbreviation for left, right, or both ears)	Mistaken for OS, OD, and OU, etc.	Write *left ear, right ear,* or *both ears*

The tenfold errors were produced by a misplaced decimal point in 43.5% of cases and by adding an extra zero in 31.5% of cases.

    f. Spell out the work *units* (e.g., 10 units regular insulin) rather than writing *u*, which could be misinterpreted as a zero.

    g. Use the metric system.

In 2004, JCAHO developed a list of prohibited abbreviations based on recommendations made by ISMP. The list is expected to expand each year with regular additions. The 2004 list included abbreviations listed in Table 18-3.[26] These items may not be used in *any* form of handwritten documentation (orders, progress notes, nursing notes, etc.).

One very successful strategy for reducing prescribing errors has been to target violations in order writing. This process generates immediate feedback to the physician writing the order and serves to reinforce desired behavior. Children's National Medical Center in Washington, DC developed a top 10 list of critical elements required for all physician orders (see Box 18-1). Creating a system for providing feedback to individual prescribers can drastically reduce prescribing errors and improve safety.

6. Written drug or prescription orders (including signatures) should be legible. Prescribers with poor handwriting should print or type medication or prescription orders if direct order entry capabilities for computerized systems are unavailable. A handwritten order should be completely readable (not merely recognizable through familiarity). An illegible handwritten order should be regarded as a potential error. If it leads to an error of occurrence (that is, the error actually reaches the patient), it should be regarded as a prescribing error.

7. Verbal drug or prescription orders (that is, orders that are orally communicated) should be reserved only for those situations in which it is

---

Box 18-1
Children's National Medical Center Top 10 Critical Prescribing Practices

All orders must adhere to the following top 10 critical guidelines:

1. Weight must be included.

2. Parenteral narcotics require a mg/kg/dose (or mcg/kg/dose) in addition to the prescribed dose.

3. If the dosage is in units, *units* must be spelled out and not abbreviated as *U.*

4. One or more of the following is not included on the order: drug, route, frequency, or dosage.

5. Date must be included.

6. No leading decimal points (write 0.2 mg not .2 mg) are allowed.

7. No trailing zeros (write 2 mg not 2.0 mg) are allowed.

8. All digoxin orders must have two physician signatures.

9. Prescriber's signature and either printed name or pager must be included.

10. All orders must be legible.

Source: Adopted from Children's National Medical Center, Pharmacy & Therapeutics Committee, Washington, DC.

---

impossible or impractical for the prescriber to write the order or enter it in the computer. The prescriber should dictate verbal orders slowly, clearly, and articulately to avoid confusion. Special caution is urged in the prescribing of drug dosages in the teens (e.g., a 15-mEq dose of potassium chloride could be misheard as a 50-mEq dose). The order should be read back to the prescriber by the recipient (i.e., the nurse or pharmacist, according to institutional policies). When read back, the drug name should be spelled to the prescriber and, when directions are repeated, no abbreviations should be used (e.g., say "three times daily" rather than "t.i.d."). A written copy of the verbal order should be placed in the patient's medical record and later confirmed by the prescriber in accordance with applicable state regulations and hospital policies.

In 2004, JCAHO incorporated verbal order readback (VORB) into the National Patient Safety Goals (Goal #2). The goal requires each institution to implement a process for taking verbal or telephone orders or critical test results that requires a verification *read-back* of the complete order/results by the person receiving the order/result. RNs, respiratory therapists, and pharmacists must write down the telephone/verbal order or test result and read back to ensure correctness. It is important to note that this is a readback, not a repeat back. Orders should signify compliance by documenting *V.O.R.B.* with name when writing order in medical record.

8. When possible, drugs should be prescribed for administration by the oral route rather than by injection.

9. When possible, the prescriber should talk with the patient or caregiver to explain the medication prescribed and any special precautions or observations that might be indicated, including any allergic or hypersensitivity reactions that might occur.

10. Prescribers should follow-up and periodically evaluate the need for continued drug therapy for individual patients.

11. Instructions with respect to *hold* orders for medications should be clear.

12. Pharmacists should preview and provide advice on the content and design of preprinted medication order forms or sheets if they are used.

Preprinted order forms can reduce prescribing errors by clarifying complicated regimens and reminding prescribers to order concominent therapy or standardize doses.

Pharmacists should participate in drug therapy monitoring (including the following, when indicated: the assessment of therapeutic appropriateness, medication administration appropriateness, and possible duplicate therapies; review for possible interactions; and evaluation of pertinent clinical and laboratory data) and DUE activities to help achieve safe, effective, and rational use of drugs.

When appropriate, the patient should be observed after administration of the drug products to ensure that the doses were administered as prescribed and have the intended effect.

Establishing a Culture of Safety

Successful patient safety work has to address and incorporate factors related to the culture of medicine, the systems supporting care, and the human factor—how highly trained clinicians work in a highly complex environment.[40] A basic tenet of medical culture is that well-trained individuals will deliver error-free performance if they are paying attention and trying hard. So deeply rooted is this belief that clinicians link their sense of clinical competence and personal self-image with the absence of error.[41]

Everyone in the medication use process plays a vital role in preventing errors.[42] Each step in the process contains safety checks designed to failures from earlier points in the process. Each person depends on each other. Even the most knowledgeable and diligent professional will, in all probability, make a number of medication errors over the course of a career. Most will be intercepted by another heath care professional. For this reason, each person needs to take their role seriously.

It is also critical that patients and their families understand that they too can serve as a safety check in the process. Patients should be encouraged to ask questions, be informed, and challenge activities that appear inconsistent or unusual. If their medication is suddenly a different color they should determine why.

Creating a culture of safety is difficult. Errors are traumatic events and the natural tendency is to hold someone responsible. Cultures of fear and blame, however, tend to drive reporting and disclosure underground. The culture itself can be the very impediment to the learning and improvement needed to create a safer system. When people feel that they can share information without fear from reprisal, then the organization can learn from past mistakes. There are several ways in which this can be achieved.

One key cultural paradigm centers around blameless reporting. When people feel that they can communicate openly about medication errors without fear of punishment or disciplinary action then it is likely that they will share information about the actual contributing factors. The language used itself can send an unintended message. The words used can imply vastly different meanings. To some, investigating an event implies a punitive direction as opposed to studying an event, which implies learning. As a result, some hospitals have adopted standardized words for use when discussing medication related events in an attempt to minimize any negative connotations. Conversations need to stay depersonalized and nonjudgmental.

Hospital executives need to be personally involved if a culture of safety is going to be established. This means educating the board of trustees on the issue and making a significant place for patient safety initiatives in the budget. Creating an economic analysis of the cost of an error can help to justify expense allocation.

It is also essential that it be culturally acceptable to question other health care professionals, orders, or situations. Too often, a root cause analysis conducted after a major error reveals that one or more health care professionals thought there was a problem but that they didn't feel comfortable questioning it or they were scolded for questioning and, therefore, did not escalate their concern. A well-established process for questioning a medication order needs to be outlined (Figure 18-4).

Disclosure Policy

One key element of an open culture surrounds how the hospital communicated with patients and families when an accident has occurred. Some hospitals are reluctant to disclose information for fear of litigation. Ironically it can be this very behavior that can precipitate litigation as the family fears the unknown and seeks full disclosure in a lawsuit. Open and ongoing dialogue with families can often prevent escalation. Many organizations have now adopted a policy of full disclosure under the advice of legal counsel. Among the items included in the policy is the communication plan. Who will be serving as the primary source of

Figure 18-4
Process for Questioning Medication Order

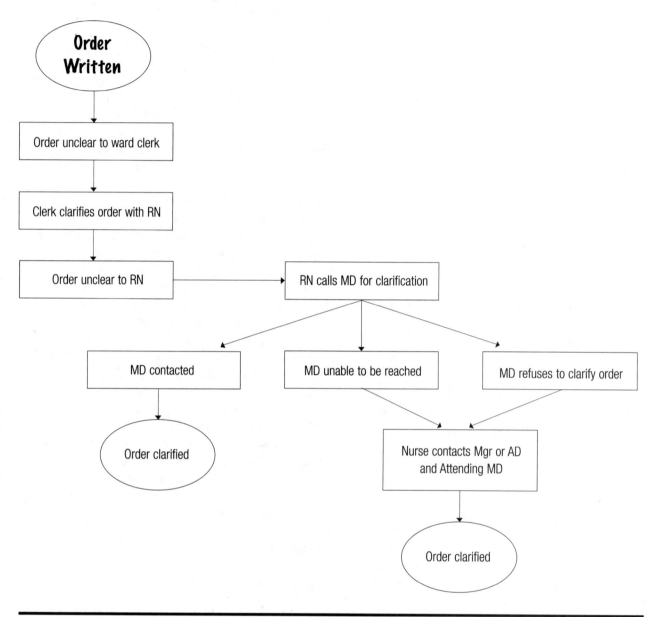

information for the family to ensure consistency of accurate information.

Infrastructure

A unified hospital vision for medication safety is critical to the institution's success. To drive change, senior leadership must create an organizational structure that demonstrates the support of top executives as well as the necessary leverage. Quality Councils or Patient Safety Steering Committees are a examples of the type of governing body created to evaluate medication safety concerns. Often such entities report directly to the hospital board to ensure that they can function autonomously and avoid conflicts of interest.

Many organizations have formed multidisciplinary groups designed to talk about frontline medication safety concerns. These Unit-Based Medication Safety Teams or Safety Action Teams then hold patient safety dialogues, which serve to bubble up issues. Approaching the issues from the bottom up generally promotes an increased level of support. This serves to engage the expertise of the people doing the work. It is important that these groups develop a common goal or desired state. Examples of goals are below:

- To conduct an ongoing assessment of the internal horizon of medication practice across the institution for inpatients and outpatients. This includes assessment of the following:
  - The education and tools for clinicians in order to deliver medications safely
  - The practices and policies of safe medication practice
  - Opportunities for improvement
  - Current state of the Medication Strategic Plan
- To assess the external horizon in order to remain ahead of the changing medical environment
  - External benchmarking with comparative hospitals
- To plan for a fundamental redesign of medication practice
  - Integration of the multiple medication teams

Establishing clear lines of medication safety accountability is necessary to ensure that issues can progress up the organizational structure if needed. Figure 18-5 is a diagram of how accountability could be structured within an organization.

Error Reduction Methodologies

Health care has begun to utilize techniques adopted from other industries to proactively analyze systems and identify areas of weakness. Three such processes include the following:

- Failure Mode and Effects Analysis (FMEA) commonly used in the aerospace and automotive industries.[43–45] It is a systematic method of identifying and preventing product, equipment, and process problems before they occur. Interdisciplinary teams are assembled to evaluate complicated systems and identify areas of concern. Proactive changes are then taken to strengthen these areas. Applied to health care, FMEA provides a safety tool for risk managers to improve the patient care environment.[46]
- Probabilistic Risk Assessment (PRAs) are a similar process that utilize error probabilities. Systems are mapped and failure probability is assigned to each process point. Pathways deemed to have a high risk of failure then become a point of focus for process redesign.

- Healthcare Failure Mode Effects Analysis (HFMEA) uses a simplified tool, the Hazard Scoring Martix, to assess risk. The matrix applies hazard analysis principles that factor in the severity and probability of the potential failure mode occurring. The matrix defines degrees of severity as catastrophic, major, moderate, and minor. Degrees of probability are defined as frequent, occasional, uncommon, and remote.[47]

JCAHO requires all institutions to develop a process for managing high-risk medications. Institutions should conduct an analysis across the medication use process (procuring, prescribing, transcribing, dispensing, administering, and monitoring) to determine where risk potential exists with these medications and take steps where possible to minimize risk.

It is also necessary to establish a baseline from which to evaluate the safety of the current system as well as the impact that changes or interventions may have. There are several ways to achieve this end. One commonly used method is to complete the comprehensive questionnaire developed by the ISMP. The ISMP Medication Safety Self-Assessment™ evaluates the current status of a health system at a particular point in time. It forces an institution to evaluate how well safety is incorporated into its medication processes, from how technology is used to how medications are securely stored to how well-lit drug-preparation areas are. It is recommended that the survey be completed by a multidisciplinary team as honestly as possible. Individual questions are weighted and scored directly by ISMP. Once a baseline is established, it can be used as an internal comparison from year to year. This process allows the individual hospital to determine areas of comparative weakness as well as receive guidance from best practice hospitals.

Evaluating Risk In Medication Use Process

To fully understand the complexity of a given medication use system, it must be flowed out. JCAHO standard MM 8.10 now requires all institutions to evaluate their medication use process. Once completed, the institution's medication-use strengths and risk points are identified as shown in Figure 18-6.

Flow diagrams are also useful for assessing changes that will occur with process redesigns. Minimizing steps, overlap, and rework is important when building safe systems. This process can then be repeated for selected high-risk processes.

Figure 18-5
Medication Safety Accountability

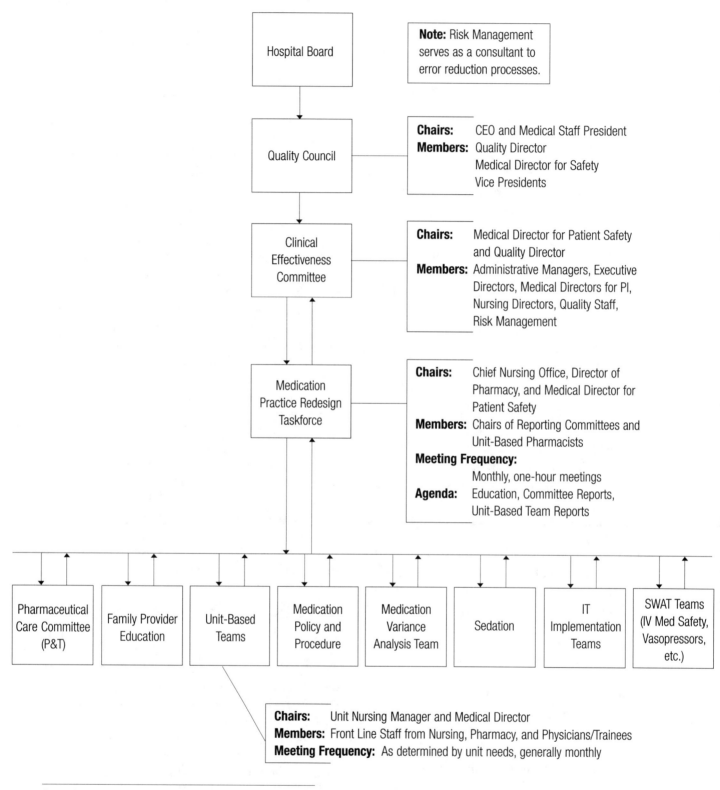

Source: Adopted from Children's National Medical Center, Washington, DC.

Figure 18-6
Identifying Risk in the Medication Use Process

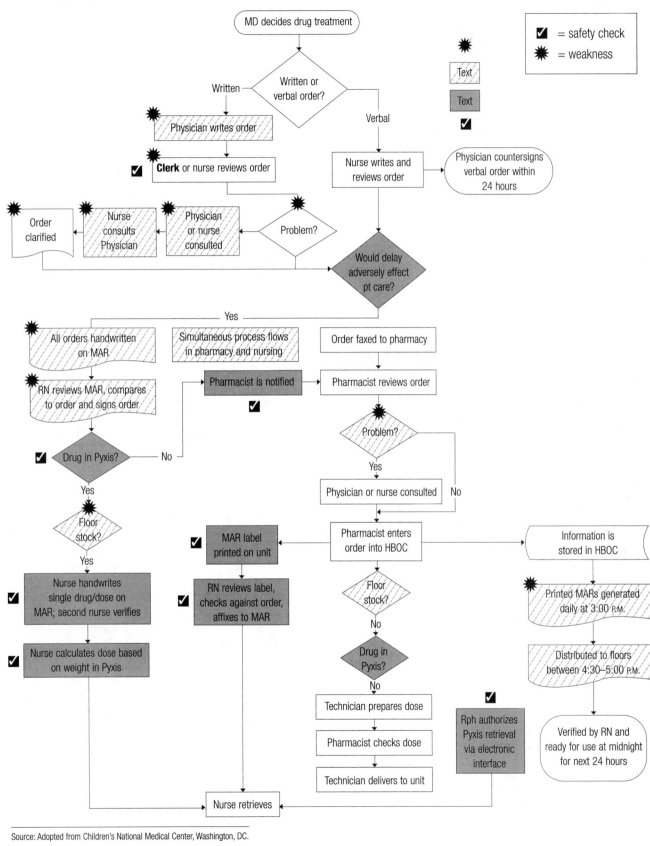

Source: Adopted from Children's National Medical Center, Washington, DC.

Creating an Institution-Wide Medication Safety Strategic Plan

Using the benchmark data received from the ISMP survey, internal data from variance reports, and information gathered from the flow diagrams, it should be possible to get sense of the safety needs and the prioritization of the risk associated with each. Using a multidisciplinary team, solutions should be identified to reduce or minimize the identified risks. These proposals are then consolidated and mapped along a timeline to create a Medication Safety Strategic Plan. This safety plan then serves is the guide for decisions and sets the vision for upcoming years. Note how it integrates the many ways to improve medication safety, including incorporation of automation and technology, expansion of clinical pharmacy services, policy development, and formation of unit-based teams. An example of a Medication Safety Strategic Plan is shown in Appendix 18-1.

Managing Medication Errors

Quality improvement programs should provide guidance for patient support, staff counseling and education, and risk management processes when a medication error is detected. The first priority is always the patient. As discussed, it is important to have a disclosure policy that is forthright and timely. Patients have a right to know when an error has occurred and be informed of all decisions that will need to be made as a result of the error.

Risk management processes for medication errors should be multidisciplinary and include pharmacists, physicians, and nurses, in addition to risk management specialists, legal counsel, and others as appropriate. The following actions are recommended upon error detection[4,8,26]:

1. Any necessary corrective and supportive therapy should be provided to the patient.

2. The error should be documented and reported immediately after discovery, in accordance with written procedures. For clinically significant errors, an immediate oral notice should be provided to physicians, nurses, and pharmacy managers. A written medication error report should follow promptly.

3. For clinically significant errors, fact gathering and investigation should be initiated immedi-

ately. Facts that should be determined and documented include what happened, where the incident occurred, why the incident occurred, and who was involved. Appropriate product evidence (e.g., packaging and labeling) should be retrieved and retained for future reference until causative factors are eliminated or resolved.

4. Reports of clinically significant errors and the associated corrective activities should be reviewed by the supervisor and department head of the area(s) involved, the appropriate organizational administrator, the organizational safety committee (or its equivalent), and legal counsel (as appropriate).

5. When appropriate, the supervisor and the staff members who were involved in the error should confer on how the error occurred and how its recurrence can be prevented. Medication errors often result from problems in systems rather than exclusively from staff performance or environmental factors.[3,49]

6. Information gained from medication error reports and other means that demonstrates continued failure of individual professionals to avoid preventable medication errors should serve as an effective management and educational tool in staff development or, if necessary, modification of job functions or staff disciplinary action.

7. Supervisors, department managers, and appropriate committees should periodically review error reports and determine causes of errors and develop actions to prevent their recurrence (e.g., conduct organizational staff education, alter staff levels, revise policies and procedures, or change facilities, equipment, or supplies).

8. Medication errors should be reported to a national monitoring program so that shared experiences of pharmacists, nurses, physicians, and patients can contribute to improved patient safety and to the development of valuable educational services for the prevention of future errors.

JCAHO now requires all institutions to perform a root cause analyses on all sentinel events. Root cause analyses are multidisciplinary reviews of serious errors, which help to identify all underlying causes or factors

Appendix 18-1
Medication Safety Strategic Plan

<u>INTERVENTION:</u> **Place a Clinical Pharmacist in the PICU**
<u>RATIONALE:</u> Pharmacist participation in patient care at the unit level has been shown to reduce drug cost, reduce errors, and improve overall service for drugs and related products. The PICU was chosen as the first unit because of the intensity and complexity of drug therapy in the area and because of the greatest opportunities for systems improvement.

<u>INTERVENTION:</u> **Assess all High-Risk Drugs and Related Procedures**
<u>RATIONALE:</u> Numerous groups (ASHP, IHI, ISMP, AHA, etc.) have identified several groups of drugs that are considered to be at high risk for patients, usually because of their toxicity and related negative outcome in the event of errors. Examples include concentrated potassium and other electrolytes such as calcium, chemotherapy, insulin, heparin, and opiates.

<u>INTERVENTION:</u> **Develop a Preprinted Electrolyte Order Form**
<u>RATIONALE:</u> Consistent with the continuing assessment of high-risk drugs, electrolyte ordering, dispensing, and administration continues to be an area for improvement. The development of an electrolyte ordering form would standardize dosing, prescribing, labeling, terminology, dosage forms, and units of measure and would provide concurrent education for all of those involved in the process.

<u>INTERVENTION:</u> **Establish a Hospitalwide Policy on Medication Errors**
<u>RATIONALE:</u> There is currently a hospital medication policy that is very thorough on procedures and policies related to medications. It has become clear that a policy is needed that specifically defines errors, severity ranking of errors, the nonpunitive nature of our reporting system, and the flow of how errors should be reported.

<u>INTERVENTION:</u> **Assign Palm Pilots to Housestaff with Prescribing Information**
<u>RATIONALE:</u> One of the highest reasons for prescribing errors is lack of information. By putting information at the fingertips of housestaff, they will have greater access to basic information and should use the resource as a means to write better orders.

<u>INTERVENTION:</u> **Implementation of Unit-Based Medication Error Reduction PI Effort**
<u>RATIONALE:</u> While this overall plan will help in restructuring the medication use process, there needs to be a front line ownership and participation in error reduction efforts. Each unit will be required to have a medication error reduction team that is multidisciplinary in makeup and focused on a problem specific to their area.

<u>INTERVENTION:</u> **Reformat Medication Labels**
<u>RATIONALE:</u> The labels for medications prepared in the pharmacy are difficult to read and have resulted in errors. A thermal printer label would have more of a laser type of print (big, bold fonts for the patient name, drug name, and dose with a smaller font for less important information).

Source: Adopted from Children's National Medical Center, Washington, DC.

that may have contributed to the event. They are particularly useful ways to determine both the causative factors but also the more subtle contributory elements that may not be immediately apparent. Trending the findings of root cause analysis can also uncover patterns that thread through many errors.

Participants generally find the process particularly enlightening as they learn to see the medication use process from the perspective of other professionals. The very nature of the discussion provides a point and counterpoint that reveal hidden defenses in the system and help to understand its complexity. Learning to evaluate the medication use process from a systematic perspective helps to reduce overall risk and understand how the actions of one professional influence those of another. For this reason, many organizations conduct mock-root cause analysis or focused event studies on nonsentinel events. These less serious, near misses can reveal a tremendous amount of information that can be used to prevent the next sentinel event. Often these studies are conducted with more than one facilitator to ensure that nonverbal behavior is observed. Even though there is a stated openness to the process, some may still be uncomfortable sharing, and a perceptive facilitator can recognize nonverbal clues and ensure that points are fully explored. According to JCAHO, communication is now the leading root cause of all types of sentinel events.[50]

Summary

Medication error prevention is an essential requirement for pharmaceutical care and must be a core mission of every pharmacy.[51] The medication use process is extremely complex and as a result, error-prone. It is the responsibility of everyone in the process to work to improve communication and clarity and take responsibility for their value in the system. Patient safety should always be the primary goal.

References

1. Hepler CD, Strand LM. Opportunities and responsibilities in pharmaceutical care. *Am J Hosp Pharm.* 1990;47:533–43.

2. ASHP Guidelines on Preventing Medication Errors in Hospitals. *Am J Hosp Pharm.* 1993;50(2):305–14.

3. Manasse HR Jr. Medication use in an imperfect world: drug misadventuring as an issue of public policy. Part 1. *Am J Hosp Pharm.* 1989;46:929–44.

4. Kohn, L Corrigan J, Donaldson M. *To Err Is Human: Building a Safer Health System.* Washington, DC: Institute of Medicine; 1999.

5. Telephone survey conducted for ASHP by International Communications Research (ICR). July 9–13, 1999.

6. *AHA News Now.* November 18, 2003.

7. Zellmer WA. ASHP plans for the future. *Am J Hosp Pharm.* 1986;43:1921. Editorial.

8. American Society of Hospital Pharmacists. ASHP statement on the pharmacist's responsibility for distribution and control of drugs. *Am J Hosp Pharm.* 1991;48:1782.

9. Bates DW, et al. Incidence of adverse drug events and potential adverse drug events: implications for prevention. ADE Prevention Study Group. *JAMA.* 1995;274(1):29–34.

10. Blum KV, Abel SA, Urbanski CJ, et al. Medication error prevention by pharmacists. *Am J Hosp Pharm.* 1988;45:1902–3.

11. Hartwig SC, Denger SD, Schneider PJ. A severity-indexed, incident-report based medication-error reporting program. *Am J Hosp Pharm.* 1991;48:2611–6.

12. Barker KN, McConnell WE. The problems of detecting medication errors in hospitals. *Am J Hosp Pharm.* 1962;19:361–9.

13. Barker KN, Pearson RE. Medication distribution systems. In: Brown TR, Smith MC, eds. *Handbook of Institutional Pharmacy Practice.* 2nd ed. Baltimore, MD: Williams & Wilkins; 1986:325–51.

14. McClure ML. Human error—a professional dilemma. *J Prof Nurs.* 1991;7:207.

15. Dawson D, Reid K. Fatigue, alcohol and performance impairment. *Nature.* 1997;388:235.

16. Shindul-Rothschild J, et al. *Am J Nurs.* 1996. Unpublished data. Wakefield B, et al. Nurses' perceptions of why medication administrations occur. *MedSurg Nursing.* 1998;7:39–44.

17. *Incorporating Safe Medication Principles into Daily Practice: Teaching Tool for Healthcare Practitioners.* Bethesda, MD: ASHP Research and Education Foundation; 2004.

18. ISMP Medication Safety Alert. USP launches MedMARx as the third major national reporting program for adverse drug events. June 17, 1998. Available at: http://ismp.org/MSAarticles/MedMARx.html.

19. American Society of Hospital Pharmacists. *Medication Errors: A Closer Look.* Videocassette. Bethesda, MD: ASHP; 1988. 20 min.

20. Cohen MR, Levine SR, Mandrack MM. *Confronting the Challenges of Neonatal and Pediatric Medication Safety.* Huntingdon Valley, PA: ISMP; 2003.

21. American Society of Hospital Pharmacists. Medication errors; a closer look. Videocassette. Bethesda, MD: ASHP; 1988. 20 min.

22. Bates DW, et al. Incidence of adverse drug events and potential adverse drug events: implications for prevention. ADE Prevention Study Group. *JAMA.* 1995;274(1):29–34.

23. Chin T. Doctors pull plug on paperless system. *Am Med News.* Feb 17, 2003.

24. Levine SR, Cohen MR, et al. Guidelines for preventing medication errors in pediatrics. *J Pediatr Pharmacol Ther.* 2001;6:426–42.

25. Lesar TS. Tenfold medication dose prescribing errors. *Ann Pharmacother.* 2002;36:1833–9.

26. Joint Commission on Accreditation of Healthcare Organizations. *2004 Accreditation Manual for Hospitals.* Oakbrook Terrace, IL: JCAHO; 2003.

27. Zellmer WA. Preventing medication errors. *Am J Hosp Pharm.* 1990;47:1755-6. Editorial.

28. American Society of Hospital Pharmacists. ASHP guidelines on the pharmacist's role in drug-use evaluation. *Am J Hosp Pharm.* 1988;45:3865–6.

29. American Society of Hospital Pharmacists. ASHP guidelines: minimum standard for pharmacies in institutions. *Am J Hosp Pharm.* 1985;42:372–5.

30. American Society of Hospital Pharmacists. ASHP guidelines on pharmacist-conducted patient counseling. *Am J Hosp Pharm.* 1984;41:331.

31. American Society of Hospital Pharmacist. ASHP statement on unit dose drug distribution. *Am J Hosp Pharm.* 1989;46:2346.

32. Folli HL, Poole RL, Benitz WE et al. Medication error prevention by clinical pharmacists in two children's hospitals. *Pediatrics* 1987;79:718–22.

33. Montazeri M, Cook DJ. Impact of a clinical pharmacist in a multidisciplinary intensive care unit. *Crit Care Med.* 1994;22:1044–8.

34. Broyles JE, Brown RO, Vehe KL, et al. Pharmacist interventions improve fluid balance in fluid restricted patients requiring parenteral nutrition. *Ann Pharmacother.* 1991;25:119–22.

35. Leape, LL, Cullen DJ, Clapp MD, et al. Pharmacist participation on physician rounds and adverse drug events in the intensive care unit. *JAMA.* 1999;282(3):267–70.

36. McMullin ST, Hennenfent JA, Ritchie DJ, et al. A prospective, randomized trial to assess the cost impact of pharmacist-initiated interventions. *Arch Intern Med.* 1999;159(19):2306–9.

37. ISMP Medication Safety Alert. Feb 10, 1999.

38. Salvendy G, ed. *Handbook of Human Factors and Ergonomics.* New York: John Wiley & Sons; 1997.

39. American Society of Hospital Pharmacists and American Nurses Association. ASHP and ANA guidelines for collaboration f pharmacists and nurses in institutional care settings. *Am J Hosp Pharm.* 1980; 45:1660.

40. Leonard M. Lessons from the sharp end: critical components of successful patient safety work. Focus on Patient Safety. *NPSF Newsletter.* 2003;6(2).

41. Rasmussen J, Jensen A. Mental procedure in real-life tasks: a case study of electronic trouble shooting. *Ergonomics.* 1974;17:293–307.

42. Cohen MR, ed. *Medication Errors.* Washington, DC: American Pharmaceutical Association; 1999.

43. McDermott R, Mikulak R, Beauregard M. The Basics of FMEA. 1996:3.

44. Cohen MR, Senders J, Davis NM. Failure mode and effects analysis: a novel approach to avoiding dangerous medication errors and accidents. *Hosp Pharm.* 1994; 29:319–30.

45. Williams E, Talley T. The use of failure mode effect and criticality analysis in a medication error subcommittee. *Hosp Pharm.* 1994;29:331–8.

46. Summy EA, et al. Strategies and tips for maximizing failure mode effects analysis in your organizations. *ASHRM.* July 2002;1–12.

47. *JCAHO Journal on Quality Improvement.* 2002;28(5):254.

48. Miwa LJ, Fandall RJ. Adverse drug reaction program using pharmacist and nurse monitors. *Hosp Formul.* 1986:1140–6.

49. Anderson ER Jr. Disciplinary action after a serious medication error. *Am J Hosp Pharm.* 1987;44:2690, 2692.

50. *JC Perspectives on Patient Safety.* 2002;2(9).

51. Walsh CS, Grissinger M. Medication error prevention guidelines. *Pharmacy Practice News.* November 2002.

Chapter 19

Reimbursement for Clinical Services

Michael D. Hogue

Introduction

Regardless of whether you practice in a traditional inpatient pharmacy, an ambulatory care clinic, or some other more specialized practice area within your health system, few topics bring about as much discussion and debate as reimbursement for nondispensing, clinical pharmacy services. The literature contains examples dating back to the mid- to late 1960s when pharmacists were struggling with a way to charge patients for professional services above and beyond the cost of the drug product.[1,2] This early debate led to what we now term the *dispensing fee,* which many would argue is hardly enough to cover the overhead associated with dispensing a prescription. In the fall of 1983, changes to Medicare created Diagnosis Related Groups, or DRGs, which no longer allowed hospitals and health systems to bill in the traditional fee-for-service format of prior years.[3] When DRGs were instituted, the role of the pharmacy department began to take a dramatic turn. No longer was the pharmacy department seen as a revenue source but a source of significant and escalating expense. Pharmacists began to realize that if they were to continue to be of value in the system, their practice must evolve beyond provision of drug orders. It was at this point that pharmacists began to emphasize their role as *cost containment guru,* carefully scrutinizing drug therapies for appropriateness and cost effectiveness. Many pharmacists since that time have successfully documented and demonstrated their value to the health system, with manuscripts providing such documentation appearing in prominent nonpharmacy journals, including *Journal of the American Medical Association* and *Archives of Internal Medicine,* in addition to the pharmacy literature.[4–6]

In 2006, pharmacists are presented with yet another new opportunity. The Medicare Modernization Act of 2003 created Medicare Part D. This new act demands that prescription drug plan (PDP) sponsors pay for Medication Therapy Management Services (MTMS), which may be provided by a pharmacist.[7] For the first time ever, Congress had recognized pharmacists as providers under Medicare. MTMS can be provided in any practice setting, and it is anticipated that opportunities for new revenue will be realized for health systems over the coming months and years as this new provision is implemented and as other insurers likely follow Medicare's lead. Therefore, it is imperative that pharmacists in all practice settings be familiar with basic reimbursement principles so as to capitalize on new and emerging professional opportunities.

Definitions

While Medicare Part A is largely hospitalization insurance in which DRGs apply, and Medicare Part B is outpatient insurance under which pharmacists may bill for certain immunizations and diabetes self-management services, Medicare Part D, prescription drug coverage, created new terminology previously undefined in pharmacy practice. The term *medication therapy management services* had not been used before the creation of Part D, and the Centers for Medicare and Medicaid Services (CMS) grappled with its definition. In an effort to assist CMS in defining MTMS and to create a preferred future for the profession of pharmacy, 11 national pharmacy organizations convened in Washington, DC and created a consensus definition for MTMS (Appendix 19-1). While CMS did not completely adopt the profession's language into final public regulation, the definition will serve as the basis for future advocacy on behalf of pharmacy.

The issue of reimbursement versus compensation is another interesting play on terminology. This author contends in previous works that reimbursement refers to payment for an item that has been purchased by one individual and resold to another, sometimes for little or no profit. Compensation may or may not involve a product but refers to a service or to some value that one adds to a product.[9] In reality, therefore, this chapter is more appropriately titled *Compensation for Clinical Services.* The difference in terminology may appear subtle, but to some payers the difference in meaning is tremendous.

Medical billing terminology can be sometimes complex and confusing. An entire industry flourishes around medical billing, including a special certification for billing and coding professionals.[10] While it is not necessary for every pharmacist to know specific billing codes, it is important for pharmacists to at least speak some of the basic *language* of billing. *CPT codes* refer to Current Procedural Terminology codes, which are used to provide a standardized mechanism for classifying medical procedures and interventions and were developed and are maintained by The American Medical Association (AMA).[11] *HCPCS codes*, Health Care Procedure Coding System, are very similar to CPT codes, except they are primarily focused on providing a standardized numerical code for products (i.e., drugs, medical devices) and certain procedures. HCPCS codes were developed and are maintained by CMS.[12] There are instances in which a CPT code and a HCPCS code both exist for the same product, procedure, or intervention. In this case, the insurer will issue guidance on which set of codes is preferred for the given intervention. Generally, Medicare and Medicaid prefer HCPCS codes when they exist, and defaults to CPT coding when a HCPCS code is not available. Private insurers, including Blue Cross and Blue Shield plans, almost exclusively utilize CPT coding.[9] In July 2005, the AMA CPT Advisory Panel

released a new coding set for use by pharmacists in billing for medication therapy management services. Table 19-1 lists the new codes along with their approved definitions.

ICD-9 refers to the International Classification of Diseases, 9th edition. ICD-9 is a standardized classification system for identifying the precise diagnosis of a patient for the current billing encounter. The World Health Organization (WHO) is responsible for maintaining the ICD, as these codes are used globally for reporting disease incidence and prevalence. In the United States, the Centers for Disease Control and Prevention (CDC) adapts ICD codes for more specific use in this country and refers to this adaptation as a Clinical Modification. Hence, one may see ICD codes in the U.S. referred to as ICD-9-CM. A new edition, ICD-10, is also now available, and some medical specialty disciplines have already transitioned to ICD-10.[9,12]

Pharmacists may also be familiar with a group of codes known as *PPS*, or Professional Pharmacy Services' codes. The creation of these codes, developed by The National Council for Prescription Drug Programs, was an attempt to standardize the electronic transmission of pharmacy service claims.[9] However, because pharmacy benefit management companies (PBMs) have largely refused to pay for nondispensing services

---

Table 19-1

CPT Codes for MTM Services[a]

Medication Therapy Management

Medication Therapy Management Service(s) (MTMS) describe face-to-face patient assessment, and intervention as appropriate, by a pharmacist. MTMS is provided to optimize the response to medications or to manage treatment-related medication interactions or complications.

    MTMS includes the following documented elements: review of the pertinent patient history, medication profile (prescription and nonprescription), and recommendations for improving health outcomes and treatment compliance. These codes are not to be used to describe the provision of product-specific information at the point of dispensing or any other routine dispensing-related activities.

● 0115T Medication therapy management service(s) provided by a pharmacist, individual, face-to-face with patient, initial 15 minutes, with assessment, and intervention if provided; initial encounter

Released July 1, 2005.
Implemented January 1, 2006.

● 0116T subsequent encounter

Released July 1, 2005.
Implemented January 1, 2006.

+● 0117T each additional 15 minutes

(List separately in addition to code for the primary service)

(Use 0117T in conjunction with 0115T, 0116T)

a CPT Codes and their descriptions are copyrighted by the American Medical Association, Chicago, Illinois. Used herein under fair use provisions.

except related to formulary compliance, and because PPS codes have not received adoption by major medical insurers, these codes are used only in a few instances in the outpatient or community pharmacy setting. They have little current applicability to clinical pharmacy services billing, although with the passage of the Health Insurance Portability and Accountability Act (HIPAA) it was hoped that they might become the electronic claims standard for pharmacy. While this remains a possibility with recent changes to Medicare, influential pharmacy advocacy groups' comments sent to CMS in anticipation of final regulations for billing of professional services under part D were advocating the use of CPT codes preferentially.[13-15]

The Pharmacist as Caregiver

It seems strange in a text designed for pharmacists that a discussion of the pharmacist as a giver of care would be necessary. However, it is important to recognize that not all patients, physicians, nurses, and others outside the esteemed profession of pharmacy view pharmacists as caregivers, but rather as dispensers of a commodity (drugs). Unfortunately, our profession has struggled with this image problem for a number of years, if not decades. This is in large part born out of the necessity to secure a facility's drug supply. Because the drug supply in any institution must be kept secure, the area in which pharmacists have traditionally found themselves providing service has often been out of view of patients and medical staff. Clinical pharmacy specialists and directors of pharmacy who have moved to more decentralized models of delivery of pharmacy services have discovered that this approach is more effective in creating a visualization of the activities of pharmacists. Arguably, *every* pharmacist in a health system is providing patient care at some level, not just the designated *clinical pharmacists*. The effort to make these individuals' work more visible within the facility is not only professionally important to the pharmacists but vitally necessary for continued recognition among administrators and medical staff of the value of the pharmacy department.

As mentioned earlier, the battle to justify the value of highly paid pharmacists to the health system continues. Table 19-2 summarizes selected literature documenting the value of pharmaceutical services in institutions. In addition, Bond and colleagues investigated whether there was a difference in death rate, length of stay, Medicare charges, bleeding transfusions, and

transfusions in hospitals that had pharmacist-run anticoagulation management services versus those that did not. In all cases the rate of occurrence of the negative health outcome investigated was significantly higher in hospitals that did not have a pharmacist-run service versus those that did. In the 758 hospitals studied that did not have pharmacist-provided heparin management, Medicare charges were an average of $1,145 per patient more than in the 197 hospitals that did provide the service.[16] Complete examination of the findings of this study makes a strong case that the pharmacist is certainly a valuable care giver.

Other works by the same research team examining four National Clinical Pharmacy Services database surveys found that if the core clinical pharmacy services of drug information, adverse drug reaction management, drug protocol management, medical rounds, and admission drug histories were implemented at every hospital across the nation for 100% of inpatients, a net requirement of 14,508 additional full-time pharmacists would be needed.[17] While the authors did not assess patient opinions in their research, it might be hypothesized that if one were to survey patients of their expectations of whether they should be receiving these services as inpatients, most would reply favorably that they should be receiving these services. Research of the patient population is needed to bolster pharmacy's position in this arena. The studies by Bond and colleagues illustrate in a very real way the value a caring pharmacist provides to a health system, and that more needs to be done to focus attention to the care of patients.

Once again, why bring up the pharmacist as caregiver? Because academia and the profession, at least on the surface, seem to have become so focused on training to the pharmaceutical portion of pharmaceutical care, the caring portion is perhaps being neglected. In fairness, the American Pharmacists Association-Academy of Students of Pharmacy (APhA-ASP) and the American Association of Colleges of Pharmacy (AACP) have formed their second task force to address issues of professionalism, which by nature will place greater emphasis on the care of and interaction with patients.[18]

A further illustration of the importance of pharmacists seeing themselves as caregivers was evidenced by a presentation from Dr. Rachel Remen, MD, at the 2004 AACP annual meeting. Dr. Remen's presentation focused on the importance of pharmacists finding meaning in their work. AACP's newsletter reported:

Table 19-2
Studies Documenting the Value of Pharmacist Services in Institutions[9,a,b]

Study	Purpose	Selected Results
Gattis et al. *Arch Intern Med.* 1999;159:1939–45	Evaluate the addition of a clinical pharmacist to heart failure management	All cause mortality and heart failure events significantly lowered in intervention group; higher dose ACE inhibition in intervention group; outcomes in heart failure improved after addition of a pharmacist
Halley *Am J Health-Syst Pharm.* 2000;57(suppl 3):S17–21	Evaluate implementation of a community-acquired pneumonia (CAP) pathway driven by pharmacist interventions	LOS reduced 1.2 days and readmissions for CAP lower in intervention group; cost savings of at least $22,000 annually projected
Chisholm et al. *Clin Transplant.* 2000;14 (Part 1):304–7	Evaluate pharmacist-managed immunosuppressant medication assistance program	61 patients enrolled with a net cost avoidance of $124,793; over the year of the program, for every dollar spent on pharmacist time, the institution received $4 in return
Dager et al. *Ann Pharmacother.* 2000;34:567–72	Evaluate the effect of daily consultation by hospital pharmacists on accuracy and rapidity of warfarin optimization	Significant reduction in hospital LOS; INR values above 3.5 reduced by more than half; readmissions for complication significantly reduced as well
Condron and Mann *Can J Hosp Pharm.* 1994;47(5):203–8	Evaluate the status of pharmacy-directed, drug-related patient-care programs by survey responses	Each pharmacist intervention resulted in cost savings of $49.24; for DUE, cost savings was $29.99 for every dollar invested in pharmacist time
Mutnick et al. *Am J Health-Syst Pharm.* 1997;54:392–6	Collect and analyze pharmacist intervention data at an 894-bed institution	Net therapy cost savings of $487,833 and further cost avoidance of $158,563 per annum; 87% of the pharmacist's recommendations were accepted
Janning et al. *Am J Health-Syst Pharm.* 1996;53:542–7	Describe the implementation of comprehensive pharmaceutical services	A fivefold increase in interventions, and cost savings and avoidance rose to a projected $562,402 over 4 years; however, major change was necessary to implement comprehensive pharmaceutical services
Hunter and Dormaier *Clin Ther.* 1995;17:534–40	Describe development and implementation of pharmacist-managed intravenous-to-oral step-down program	Expected annualized cost savings was $37,000
Phillips and Carr-Lopez *Am J Hosp Pharm.* 1990;47:1075–9	Evaluate the effect of a pharmacist on drug prescribing in a hospital-based geriatric clinic	32% reduction in total prescriptions, and a 42% reduction in prescriptions for medications associated with ADRs in the elderly; a direct cost savings of $53.75 per patient was realized
Bertch et al. *Drug Intell Clin Pharm.* 1988;22:906–11	Evaluate novel approach to cost-justifying clinical pharmacy services	Interventions had perceived impact on cost, quality, or both; a 1.9-day increase in therapeutic control was achieved, with physicians accepting 82% of recommendations

[a] Adapted from Albrant, D. Generating new revenue streams for institutions. In: *The Pharmacist's Guide to Compensation for Patient Care Services.* Washington, DC: American Pharmacists Association; 2002;74. Copyright 2002, American Pharmacists Association. Used with permission of APhA.

[b] LOS = length of stay; DUE = drug use evaluation; and ADRs = adverse drug reactions.

Remen described how increasingly health care professionals are experiencing disillusionment, depression, and apathy because of a loss of control over standards of care. Students are asked to practice in a way that compromises values and to function below a level of excellence, she said. It is harder to find satisfaction and this makes students and health care professionals vulnerable to burnout. She described her father as a pharmacist 'who compounded medicines, answered questions and eased fears. He would say, it's not about the medicines, it's about the people. He would ask his patients, 'Is there anything about taking this medicine that worries you?'

The title of her presentation, *Being a Blessing*, is from a card sent to her mother by a patient of her father's after he had died. The card, which her mother carried around in her wallet, contained this one sentence: "Your husband was a blessing." Later when Remen shared this story with her UCSF class, a medical student told her he wanted to learn not only how to be a physician but how to be a blessing."[19]

The realization that pharmacists must come to in the meaning of their work is core to the ability to assign a value to that work. Unless pharmacists return to their roots of giving care in a very conscious way, it will be difficult for others to view the services provided by pharmacists as valuable and worthy of direct compensation.

Documentation Requirements

There is an adage that has been repeated extensively, particularly directed toward pharmacists' novice to the concept: If you didn't document it, then you didn't do it. Unfortunately, computerized dispensing and patient profiling systems utilized in central hospital and ambulatory care pharmacies until very recently allowed only limited free text data input from the pharmacist. Additionally, particularly in ambulatory care pharmacies, data is often purged from the computer system after some specified length of time. Inpatient pharmacists who perhaps identified and resolved a drug-related problem in the pharmacy department had no real way to document that intervention, short of walking from central pharmacy to the floor, locating the patient's chart, and documenting the intervention—a time-consuming proposition at best for the centralized phar-

macist. The advent of electronic medical records and hand-held clinical intervention devices in which pharmacists have more direct access in the health system to medical documentation systems has allowed for simplified, less time-consuming documentation of patient interventions to occur. However, documentation skill relative to interventions is not to be assumed, and some baseline training may be necessary for staff unfamiliar with basic clinical documentation methods.

The SOAP note (Subjective, Objective, Assessment, and Plan) is the standard documentation format used by most clinicians. This universally recognized, problem-oriented documentation format systematically classifies types of information gleaned from patient interview and assessment, along with the clinician's evaluation notes and plans for action (both current and future). Table 19-3 contains a detailed description of the elements of a SOAP note. Following a standard documentation formation such as the SOAP format allows multiple caregivers within the institution to communicate patient intervention and care plans to each other. In order to ensure appropriate outcomes, each provider must be meticulous in following the institution's documentation standard, and detailed in the description of interventions. A variety of clinical practice guidelines and reports have been issued that emphasize the importance of documentation on patient outcomes.[20,21]

In some cases, a complete SOAP note is unnecessary, because the nature of the intervention is such that a complete patient assessment was not required. For example, a pharmacist that determines a drug to be incompatible with other drugs in the patient's profile and calls or emails the physician with a change in drug therapy would not have a subjective component. In this case, a simple notation in the patient record that details the nature of the intervention will suffice in most cases. Regardless, the most important payment-related consideration one must take into account is documentation requirements of the third-party insurer. Most insurers, including Medicare and Medicaid, have very specific documentation requirements.[22] At a minimum, a problem must be identified in writing, along with recommended and/or instituted changes with appropriate follow-up plans. Specific documentation requirements have been established for billing of MTM Services (see Table 19-1). Failure to adhere to at least minimum documentation requirements could result in the insurer recouping any funds paid, and in

Table 19-3

Elements of the Problem-Oriented Medical Record[a]

Problem name: Each "problem" is listed separately and given an identifying number. Problems may be a patient complaint (e.g., headache), a laboratory abnormality (e.g., hypokalemia), or a specific disease name if prior diagnosis is known. When monitoring previously described drug therapy, more than one drug-related problem may be considered (e.g., noncompliance, a suspected adverse drug reaction or drug interaction, or an inappropriate dose). Under each problem name, the following information is identified:

Subjective	Information that explains or delineates the reason for the encounter. Information that the patient reports concerning symptoms, treatments tried, medications used, and adverse effects encountered. These are considered nonreproducible data because the information is based on the patient's interpretation and recall of past events.
Objective	Information from physical examination, laboratory results, diagnostic tests, pill counts, and pharmacy patient profile information. Objective data are measurable and reproducible.
Assessment	A brief, but complete, description of the problem, including a conclusion or diagnosis that is supported logically by the above subjective and objective data. The assessment should not include a problem/diagnosis that is not defined above.
Plan	A detailed description of recommendation or intended further workup (laboratory, radiology, consultation), treatment (e.g., continued observation, physiotherapy, diet, medications, surgery), patient education (self-care, goals of therapy, medication use and monitoring), monitoring and follow-up relative to the above assessment.

[a] Sometimes referred to as the *SOAP* (subjective, objective, assessment, plan) note.
Source: Reprinted with permission from *Applied Therapeutics: The Clinical Use of Drugs.* Baltimore, MD: Lippincott Williams & Wilkins; 2001.

a worse case scenario, charges of fraudulent activity.

Documentation serves a legal purpose as well. In a litigious society, it is imperative that providers accurately document interventions. Failure to do so could result in adverse legal ramifications in the future if a patient were to file charges or make allegations against you or your facility. If an error in documentation occurs, for handwritten documentation a single line should be drawn through the error and the word error should be written, along with the documenting clinician's initials, above the error. If an error in documentation occurs in the electronic record, a new notation should be entered explaining the error in documentation and signed by the documenting clinician. Under no circumstance should erasures, deletions, or blotted markings (such as those made by Wite-Out®) be used to write over or correct a documentation error once it has been entered or saved to the patient profile.

Payers of Health Care Services

Health care has a variety of customers. Of course, the most important customer is the patient. However, the purchaser of health care may or may not be the patient. In some cases it is the patient's employer, in others the government (e.g., Veteran's Administration, Medicare, Medicaid, Ryan White Program, U.S. Military), in others the patient's family, and in still others charitable organizations or trusts. In many of these situations, the ultimate purchaser of health care has contracted with an organization to manage the limited amount of dollars designated for health care for a defined group of individuals (i.e., employees or beneficiaries). Health Maintenance Organizations (HMOs) and Preferred Provider Organizations (PPOs) have rapidly become a major payment source for most health systems. While the subtle differences are not necessarily important for the pharmacist to understand, the way in which HMOs and PPOs generally cover services is important. These organizations make money based upon how well they *manage* a given amount of money for the purchaser (employer), hence the term *managed care*. Because HMOs and PPOs are largely for-profit organizations, they tend to tightly control a variety of factors related to health care utilizations. For example, they might contract with physician groups, hospitals, or pharmacies for negotiated discounts on health care. They might arrange out-of-pocket copayment structures to incentivize the use of preferred providers that have agreed to these discounts. Some require preauthorization, second opinions, and other activities to ensure the necessity of a recommended procedure or medical equipment purchase. It is these organizations with whom pharmacy has had the greatest struggle as a profession for payment for nondispensing services. The reasons for this struggle are multifaceted but may include short-term contracts (typically 1 to 2 years) between the HMO and employer that do not focus on long-term benefits but short-term savings. It could also be that because pharmacists have not typically been recognized by agencies issuing provider identification numbers (such as the Drug Enforcement Administration or CMS), that creating a compensation mechanism for pharmacists is too cumbersome. More likely though, is a lack of understanding on the part of the payer as to the ability of the pharmacist to provide short- and long-term savings to the plan.

Fortunately, many of the challenges faced by pharmacists with regards to payers are being minimized or eliminated. As discussed previously, a mounting body of evidence documenting the value of the pharmacist to the health system continues to grow. Additionally, as a direct result of HIPAA, the Department of Health and Human Services (DHHS) has begun issuing a National Provider Identification (NPI) to health care professionals and health care entities in 2005.[23] These numbers will replace Universal Provider Identification numbers (UPIN) and DEA numbers so far as billing for health care services is concerned. (Note: DEA numbers will still be issued for drug control purposes just as they have in the past. It is unclear as to whether UPIN numbers will continue to be issued.) DHHS regulations will allow pharmacists, as well as pharmacies, to apply for these new 10-digit numbers and will require their use for any electronic claims.

Medicare is a source of nondispensing payment for certain pharmacist services, and has been for a number of years. Pharmacists and pharmacies qualify under Medicare Part B as mass immunizers. As a result, a pharmacist can apply for a Part B provider number using CMS form 855I (individual applicants) and be paid for administering inactivated influenza vaccine and pneumococcal vaccine to Medicare beneficiaries. Hepatitis B vaccine is also covered for those beneficiaries undergoing dialysis. Pharmacies may also bill for these immunizations; however, CMS form 855B (business or group applicants) should be used to obtain a Part B provider number. It is very important to note that this is one of the very few services for which hospital inpatient providers may bill Medicare Part B. The agency allows any qualified entity to bill for influenza, pneumococcal, and hepatitis B vaccines because of the tremendous health benefit they provide and to maximize the number of providers available to patients for receipt of the vaccines. Table 19-4 summarizes key billing information for pharmacists and health systems desiring to bill Medicare Part B for immunizations. One other note: the Medicare Part B provider number

for immunizations is not the same as the durable medical equipment (DME) provider number for Part B that many ambulatory care centers and pharmacies have utilized for billing home oxygen therapy, home infusion products and services, and durable medical equipment. DME suppliers bill through a regional carrier (DMERC), while immunization providers bill through a state-specific carrier, thus requiring separate identification numbers.[9,25]

Another service for which pharmacists may receive compensation is as part of a formal education program under Medicare Part B's diabetes self-management education (DSME) provisions. Under Medicare regulation, a program that wishes to receive payment for provision of DSME must first be recognized by the American Diabetes Association's (ADA) quality assurance recognition process. National Standards for DSME have been developed by a multidisciplinary task force and ensure quality DSME criteria "that can be implemented in diverse settings and will facilitate improvement in health care outcomes."[26] To date, dozens of programs representing every state have obtained ADA recognition for DSME programs. Most of these programs are in hospitals or health systems.[27] The precise requirements for becoming ADA recognized and for qualifying for Medicare Part B reimbursement are quite detailed. Interested providers should consult the ADA website at www.diabetes.org or a more comprehensive compensation textbook for specific information on these complex billing procedures.

Medicare Part D

Medicare Part D was created in December 2003 with the enactment of the Medicare Prescription Drug, Improvement, and Modernization Act of 2003. The Act contains an historic provision that mandates payment by prescription drug program (PDP) sponsors for medication therapy management services (MTMS). The Act states that MTMS may be provided by pharmacists. In further clarifying language giving legislative intent, lawmakers wrote that pharmacists are the most logical providers of MTMS.[7] This is the first time within the Social Security Act (the broader law which MMA 2003 amended) that pharmacists have specifically been identified as providers.

MTM is a term used for the first time in MMA 2003. The literature did not define MTM prior to MMA, nor did the specific provisions in the MMA. As a result, the profession of pharmacy took the initiative

Table 19-4
Considerations for Billing Medicare Part B for Immunization Services[11,24]

Application Process	Apply as a mass immunizer; pharmacists apply for provider status using CMS Form 855I; Pharmacies/Health Systems apply for provider status using CMS Form 855B
Eligible Vaccines	Inactivated influenza vaccine and pneumococcal vaccine for any Medicare Part B recipient; Hepatitis B vaccine for those beneficiaries undergoing dialysis; a beneficiary is only eligible for one influenza vaccine per influenza season, and a maximum of two pneumococcal vaccines per lifetime based upon current CDC recommendations *Note: Live-attenuated, intranasal influenza vaccine is currently not covered by Medicare.*
Billing Procedure	Mass immunizers can bill via one of two ways; first, using paper-based CMS Form 1500; the preferred method for billing, however, is electronically using software provided by your state's Medicare carrier; roster billing (billing of multiple patient claims utilizing only one form and a roster) is the quickest way to bill through either paper or electronic means; you can not bill both influenza and pneumococcal vaccine on the same roster
Billing Codes	Mass immunizers receive compensation for both the vaccine and for the act of administering the vaccine; the current billing codes should be used to bill Medicare Part B for covered vaccines

Vaccine	ICD-9 Code	CPT Code
Influenza (≥3 yrs)	V04.81	90658
Pneumococcal	V03.82	90732
Hepatitis B	V05.3	90747*

Administration Codes (HCPCS Codes)**	
Influenza	G0008
Pneumococcal	G0009
Hepatitis B	G0010

Compensation Rates	Reimbursement rates for covered vaccines, as well as compensation rates for vaccine administration, are updated annually; rates vary by state and, in some cases, by region within a given state; current rates are posted on the provider page of the CMS website at www.cms.gov.

* The CPT Code for Hepatitis B vaccine listed here is for dialysis or immunosuppressed patient dosage since the vaccine is only covered for Medicare Part B beneficiaries undergoing dialysis. Current Procedural Terminology (CPT) codes are copyright, American Medical Association, Chicago, Illinois. Consult the most recent edition of CPT for updates and a more expansive listing of codes.

**Healthcare Common Procedure Coding System (HCPCS) codes are maintained by the Centers for Medicare and Medicaid Services and, in general, not used by private insurers.

to define the term since MMA specifically identified pharmacists as the potential providers for this service. In July 2004, eleven national pharmacy associations representing the broad professional interests of practitioners and pharmacist employers convened a consensus conference, which resulted in the creation of a definition for MTM. Additionally, the consensus conference spelled out specific criteria, which programs that offer MTM as a covered benefit should meet as

minimum standards. The consensus document is reprinted in Appendix 19-1 and will be utilized by all national and state pharmacy advocacy groups moving forward.

PDP sponsors are newly defined fiscal intermediaries for the Medicare Part D prescription drug benefit. PDP sponsors may offer drug-only programs, or offer prescription drug programs as part of existing Medicare Advantage (Medicare Managed Care, Part C) plans.

The Act calls for a minimum of two PDP sponsors per Medicare Part D region, one of which must be a drug-only program. CMS has announced a total of 34 PDP regions and 26 Medicare Advantage regions. Many of these regions consist of a single state, while others combine two or more states to form a region.[28] A listing of the PDP and MA regions appears in Table 19-5. It is anticipated that most regions will have more than the minimum of two PDP sponsors per Part D region, as CMS documents state, the agency is encouraging competition and a choice.[29]

As this publication goes to press, CMS has decided not to specify the types of services provided by a pharmacist that will be specifically compensable under the MTM services provision. The MMA states that MTM services is designed to ensure that "covered part D drugs under the prescription drug plan are appropriately used to optimize therapeutic outcomes through improved medication use, and to reduce the risk of adverse events, including adverse drug interactions. Such a program may distinguish between services in ambulatory and institutional settings." Furthermore, the Act specifically mentions that MTM service programs may include elements designed to (a) enhance enrollee understanding of appropriate medication use (i.e., education and counseling); (b) increase adherence with medication regimens (i.e., compliance packaging and monitoring); and (c) detect adverse events and patterns of over- and under-utilization of medications.[7] It is yet unclear whether further, more specific guidance will be given to PDP sponsors and providers as to those services that will qualify for remuneration. It is also unclear if a standard billing procedure (such as that using Current Procedural Terminology [CPT] codes) or if a standard compensation formula that considers the time, clinical intensity, and resources required for provision of the services will be adopted by CMS as it has done with other services billable to the agency.

Principles of Billing

Four basic principles should be followed by pharmacists seeking remuneration from a third-party insurer.

Bill in an Acceptable Format with Acceptable Codes

The fact that a CPT code exists for a given service does not necessarily mean that it will be compensable by the particular third party to which you are submitting a claim. For example, CPT code 99371 is for "a tele-

phone call specifically by a physician to a patient or for consultation or medical management with other health care professionals."[8] Neither Medicare, Medicaid, nor any known Blue Cross entity will pay for this code at this time. Codes 99372 and 99373 are also for telephone consults. Will these codes ever be compensable for pharmacists? Perhaps, but the main issue here is to be familiar with the third party's acceptable billing practices *before* you submit your claim. Doing so will reduce the time associated with being paid due to rejected claims that result from billing errors.

Also related to coding is the issue of bundling or unbundling of services. This refers to instances when multiple services are provided at the same health care encounter. If a single code can be utilized to describe the services that were provided at the particular encounter, generally speaking, most insurers would prefer one code be utilized. Some providers attempt to bill for several codes for the same visit when one code would have sufficed. This attempt to increase reimbursement through unbundling is rarely successful, and often forbidden by the insurer. Again, consult the insurer to whom you are submitting a claim anytime you are uncertain of the correct procedure for billing multiple services provided during a single encounter.

The CMS Form 1500 has become the recognized claim form used by virtually all public and private insurers in the United States (Figure 19-1). However, electronic billing standards mandated by HIPAA will eventually require all health claims to be submitted online, eliminating the use of the CMS Form 1500 for the vast majority of health care billing.[9] For the time being, the most crucial factor associated with the billing form is ensuring that all necessary fields of the form are completed to the satisfaction of the third-party payer. Certain third-party payers require some fields to be completed in full, while other fields should be left blank. Other payers require any blank field to contain the marking *N/A* for any field not applicable to the particular claim. While it is beyond the scope of this text to detail the instructions for completion of CMS Form 1500, a copy of the form is provided at the end of this chapter and one can seek guidance for completion of the form from the third-party entity to which you desire to send a claim.

Charge All Necessary Copayments and Collect all Deductibles

Pharmacist services are generally covered by the major medical benefit, not the pharmacy benefit, if they are

Table 19-5
Prescription Drug Plan (PDP) and Medicare Advantage (MA) Regions[28]

PDP Regions

PDP Region 1—Northern New England (New Hampshire and Maine)

PDP Region 2—Central New England (Connecticut, Massachusetts, Rhode Island, and Vermont)

PDP Region 3—New York

PDP Region 4—New Jersey

PDP Region 5—Mid-Atlantic (Delaware, District of Columbia, and Maryland)

PDP Region 6—Pennsylvania, West Virginia

PDP Region 7—Virginia

PDP Region 8—North Carolina

PDP Region 9—South Carolina

PDP Region 10—Georgia

PDP Region 11—Florida

PDP Region 12—Alabama, Tennessee

PDP Region 13—Michigan

PDP Region 14—Ohio

PDP Region 15—Indiana, Kentucky

PDP Region 16—Wisconsin

PDP Region 17—Illinois

PDP Region 18—Missouri

PDP Region 19—Arkansas

PDP Region 20—Mississippi

PDP Region 21—Louisiana

PDP Region 22—Texas

PDP Region 23—Oklahoma

PDP Region 24—Kansas

PDP Region 25—Upper Midwest and Northern Plains (Iowa, Minnesota, Montana, Nebraska, North Dakota, South Dakota, and Wyoming)

PDP Region 26—New Mexico

PDP Region 27—Colorado

PDP Region 28—Arizona

PDP Region 29—Nevada

PDP Region 30—Oregon, Washington

PDP Region 31—Idaho, Utah

PDP Region 32—California

PDP Region 33—Hawaii

PDP Region 34—Alaska

MA Regions

MA Region 1—Northern New England (New Hampshire and Maine)

MA Region 2—Central New England (Connecticut, Massachusetts, Rhode Island, and Vermont)

MA Region 3—New York

MA Region 4—New Jersey

MA Region 5—Mid-Atlantic (Delaware, District of Columbia, and Maryland)

MA Region 6—Pennsylvania and West Virginia

MA Region 7—North Carolina and Virginia

MA Region 8—Georgia and South Carolina

MA Region 9—Florida

MA Region 10—Alabama and Tennessee

MA Region 11—Michigan

MA Region 12—Ohio

MA Region 13—Indiana and Kentucky

MA Region 14—Illinois and Wisconsin

MA Region 15—Arkansas and Missouri

MA Region 16—Louisiana and Mississippi

MA Region 17—Texas

MA Region 18—Kansas and Oklahoma

MA Region 19—Upper Midwest and Northern Plains (Iowa, Minnesota, Montana, Nebraska, North Dakota, South Dakota, and Wyoming)

MA Region 20—Colorado and New Mexico

MA Region 21—Arizona

MA Region 22—Nevada

MA Region 23—Northwest (Idaho, Oregon, Utah, and Washington)

MA Region 24—California

MA Region 25—Hawaii

MA Region 26—Alaska

Figure 19-1
CMS Form 1500, front

PLEASE DO NOT STAPLE IN THIS AREA

HEALTH INSURANCE CLAIM FORM

PICA   PICA

1. MEDICARE   MEDICAID   CHAMPUS   CHAMPVA   GROUP HEALTH PLAN   FECA BLK LUNG   OTHER   1a. INSURED'S I.D. NUMBER   (FOR PROGRAM IN ITEM 1)
☐ (Medicare #) ☐ (Medicaid #) ☐ (Sponsor's SSN) ☐ (VA File #) ☐ (SSN or ID) ☐ (SSN) ☐ (ID)

2. PATIENT'S NAME (Last Name, First Name, Middle Initial)
3. PATIENT'S BIRTH DATE   MM DD YY   SEX   M ☐ F ☐
4. INSURED'S NAME (Last Name, First Name, Middle Initial)

5. PATIENT'S ADDRESS (No., Street)
6. PATIENT RELATIONSHIP TO INSURED   Self ☐ Spouse ☐ Child ☐ Other ☐
7. INSURED'S ADDRESS (No., Street)

CITY   STATE
8. PATIENT STATUS   Single ☐ Married ☐ Other ☐   Employed ☐ Full-Time Student ☐ Part-Time Student ☐
CITY   STATE

ZIP CODE   TELEPHONE (Include Area Code) (   )
ZIP CODE   TELEPHONE (INCLUDE AREA CODE) (   )

9. OTHER INSURED'S NAME (Last Name, First Name, Middle Initial)
10. IS PATIENT'S CONDITION RELATED TO:
11. INSURED'S POLICY GROUP OR FECA NUMBER

a. OTHER INSURED'S POLICY OR GROUP NUMBER
a. EMPLOYMENT? (CURRENT OR PREVIOUS)   ☐ YES ☐ NO
a. INSURED'S DATE OF BIRTH   MM DD YY   SEX   M ☐ F ☐

b. OTHER INSURED'S DATE OF BIRTH   MM DD YY   SEX   M ☐ F ☐
b. AUTO ACCIDENT?   PLACE (State)   ☐ YES ☐ NO
b. EMPLOYER'S NAME OR SCHOOL NAME

c. EMPLOYER'S NAME OR SCHOOL NAME
c. OTHER ACCIDENT?   ☐ YES ☐ NO
c. INSURANCE PLAN NAME OR PROGRAM NAME

d. INSURANCE PLAN NAME OR PROGRAM NAME
10d. RESERVED FOR LOCAL USE
d. IS THERE ANOTHER HEALTH BENEFIT PLAN?   ☐ YES ☐ NO   If yes, return to and complete item 9 a-d.

READ BACK OF FORM BEFORE COMPLETING & SIGNING THIS FORM.
12. PATIENT'S OR AUTHORIZED PERSON'S SIGNATURE I authorize the release of any medical or other information necessary to process this claim. I also request payment of government benefits either to myself or to the party who accepts assignment below.
SIGNED _____   DATE _____
13. INSURED'S OR AUTHORIZED PERSON'S SIGNATURE I authorize payment of medical benefits to the undersigned physician or supplier for services described below.
SIGNED _____

14. DATE OF CURRENT: ILLNESS (First symptom) OR INJURY (Accident) OR PREGNANCY(LMP)   MM DD YY
15. IF PATIENT HAS HAD SAME OR SIMILAR ILLNESS. GIVE FIRST DATE   MM DD YY
16. DATES PATIENT UNABLE TO WORK IN CURRENT OCCUPATION   FROM MM DD YY TO MM DD YY

17. NAME OF REFERRING PHYSICIAN OR OTHER SOURCE
17a. I.D. NUMBER OF REFERRING PHYSICIAN
18. HOSPITALIZATION DATES RELATED TO CURRENT SERVICES   FROM MM DD YY TO MM DD YY

19. RESERVED FOR LOCAL USE
20. OUTSIDE LAB?   ☐ YES ☐ NO $ CHARGES

21. DIAGNOSIS OR NATURE OF ILLNESS OR INJURY. (RELATE ITEMS 1,2,3 OR 4 TO ITEM 24E BY LINE)
1. |__.__| 3. |__.__|
2. |__.__| 4. |__.__|
22. MEDICAID RESUBMISSION CODE   ORIGINAL REF. NO.
23. PRIOR AUTHORIZATION NUMBER

24.
A DATE(S) OF SERVICE From MM DD YY To MM DD YY	B Place of Service	C Type of Service	D PROCEDURES, SERVICES, OR SUPPLIES (Explain Unusual Circumstances) CPT/HCPCS MODIFIER	E DIAGNOSIS CODE	F $ CHARGES	G DAYS OR UNITS	H EPSDT Family Plan	I EMG	J COB	K RESERVED FOR LOCAL USE
1										
2										
3										
4										
5										
6										

25. FEDERAL TAX I.D. NUMBER   SSN EIN ☐ ☐
26. PATIENT'S ACCOUNT NO.
27. ACCEPT ASSIGNMENT? (For govt. claims, see back)   ☐ YES ☐ NO
28. TOTAL CHARGE $
29. AMOUNT PAID $
30. BALANCE DUE $

31. SIGNATURE OF PHYSICIAN OR SUPPLIER INCLUDING DEGREES OR CREDENTIALS (I certify that the statements on the reverse apply to this bill and are made a part thereof.)
SIGNED _____   DATE _____
32. NAME AND ADDRESS OF FACILITY WHERE SERVICES WERE RENDERED (If other than home or office)
33. PHYSICIAN'S, SUPPLIER'S BILLING NAME, ADDRESS, ZIP CODE & PHONE #
PIN# _____   GRP# _____

(APPROVED BY AMA COUNCIL ON MEDICAL SERVICE 8/88)   PLEASE PRINT OR TYPE
APPROVED OMB-0938-0008 FORM CMS-1500 (12/90),   FORM RRB-1500,
APPROVED OMB-1215-0055 FORM OWCP-1500,   APPROVED OMB-0720-0001 (CHAMPUS)

CARRIER
PATIENT AND INSURED INFORMATION
PHYSICIAN OR SUPPLIER INFORMATION

Figure 19-1, continued
CMS Form 1500, *back*

BECAUSE THIS FORM IS USED BY VARIOUS GOVERNMENT AND PRIVATE HEALTH PROGRAMS, SEE SEPARATE INSTRUCTIONS ISSUED BY APPLICABLE PROGRAMS.

NOTICE: Any person who knowingly files a statement of claim containing any misrepresentation or any false, incomplete or misleading information may be guilty of a criminal act punishable under law and may be subject to civil penalties.

REFERS TO GOVERNMENT PROGRAMS ONLY

MEDICARE AND CHAMPUS PAYMENTS: A patient's signature requests that payment be made and authorizes release of any information necessary to process the claim and certifies that the information provided in Blocks 1 through 12 is true, accurate and complete. In the case of a Medicare claim, the patient's signature authorizes any entity to release to Medicare medical and nonmedical information, including employment status, and whether the person has employer group health insurance, liability, no-fault, worker's compensation or other insurance which is responsible to pay for the services for which the Medicare claim is made. See 42 CFR 411.24(a). If item 9 is completed, the patient's signature authorizes release of the information to the health plan or agency shown. In Medicare assigned or CHAMPUS participation cases, the physician agrees to accept the charge determination of the Medicare carrier or CHAMPUS fiscal intermediary as the full charge, and the patient is responsible only for the deductible, coinsurance and noncovered services. Coinsurance and the deductible are based upon the charge determination of the Medicare carrier or CHAMPUS fiscal intermediary if this is less than the charge submitted. CHAMPUS is not a health insurance program but makes payment for health benefits provided through certain affiliations with the Uniformed Services. Information on the patient's sponsor should be provided in those items captioned in "Insured"; i.e., items 1a, 4, 6, 7, 9, and 11.

BLACK LUNG AND FECA CLAIMS

The provider agrees to accept the amount paid by the Government as payment in full. See Black Lung and FECA instructions regarding required procedure and diagnosis coding systems.

SIGNATURE OF PHYSICIAN OR SUPPLIER (MEDICARE, CHAMPUS, FECA AND BLACK LUNG)

I certify that the services shown on this form were medically indicated and necessary for the health of the patient and were personally furnished by me or were furnished incident to my professional service by my employee under my immediate personal supervision, except as otherwise expressly permitted by Medicare or CHAMPUS regulations.

For services to be considered as "incident" to a physician's professional service, 1) they must be rendered under the physician's immediate personal supervision by his/her employee, 2) they must be an integral, although incidental part of a covered physician's service, 3) they must be of kinds commonly furnished in physician's offices, and 4) the services of nonphysicians must be included on the physician's bills.

For CHAMPUS claims, I further certify that I (or any employee) who rendered services am not an active duty member of the Uniformed Services or a civilian employee of the United States Government or a contract employee of the United States Government, either civilian or military (refer to 5 USC 5536). For Black-Lung claims, I further certify that the services performed were for a Black Lung-related disorder.

No Part B Medicare benefits may be paid unless this form is received as required by existing law and regulations (42 CFR 424.32).

NOTICE: Any one who misrepresents or falsifies essential information to receive payment from Federal funds requested by this form may upon conviction be subject to fine and imprisonment under applicable Federal laws.

NOTICE TO PATIENT ABOUT THE COLLECTION AND USE OF MEDICARE, CHAMPUS, FECA, AND BLACK LUNG INFORMATION
(PRIVACY ACT STATEMENT)

We are authorized by CMS, CHAMPUS and OWCP to ask you for information needed in the administration of the Medicare, CHAMPUS, FECA, and Black Lung programs. Authority to collect information is in section 205(a), 1862, 1872 and 1874 of the Social Security Act as amended, 42 CFR 411.24(a) and 424.5(a)(6), and 44 USC 3101;41 CFR 101 et seq and 10 USC 1079 and 1086; 5 USC 8101 et seq; and 30 USC 901 et seq; 38 USC 613; E.O. 9397.

The information we obtain to complete claims under these programs is used to identify you and to determine your eligibility. It is also used to decide if the services and supplies you received are covered by these programs and to insure that proper payment is made.

The information may also be given to other providers of services, carriers, intermediaries, medical review boards, health plans, and other organizations or Federal agencies, for the effective administration of Federal provisions that require other third parties payers to pay primary to Federal program, and as otherwise necessary to administer these programs. For example, it may be necessary to disclose information about the benefits you have used to a hospital or doctor. Additional disclosures are made through routine uses for information contained in systems of records.

FOR MEDICARE CLAIMS: See the notice modifying system No. 09-70-0501, titled, 'Carrier Medicare Claims Record,' published in the <u>Federal Register</u>, Vol. 55 No. 177, page 37549, Wed. Sept. 12, 1990, or as updated and republished.

FOR OWCP CLAIMS: Department of Labor, Privacy Act of 1974, "Republication of Notice of Systems of Records," <u>Federal Register</u> Vol. 55 No. 40, Wed Feb. 28, 1990, See ESA-5, ESA-6, ESA-12, ESA-13, ESA-30, or as updated and republished.

FOR CHAMPUS CLAIMS: <u>PRINCIPLE PURPOSE(S):</u> To evaluate eligibility for medical care provided by civilian sources and to issue payment upon establishment of eligibility and determination that the services/supplies received are authorized by law.

<u>ROUTINE USE(S):</u> Information from claims and related documents may be given to the Dept. of Veterans Affairs, the Dept. of Health and Human Services and/or the Dept. of Transportation consistent with their statutory administrative responsibilities under CHAMPUS/CHAMPVA; to the Dept. of Justice for representation of the Secretary of Defense in civil actions; to the Internal Revenue Service, private collection agencies, and consumer reporting agencies in connection with recoupment claims; and to Congressional Offices in response to inquiries made at the request of the person to whom a record pertains. Appropriate disclosures may be made to other federal, state, local, foreign government agencies, private business entities, and individual providers of care, on matters relating to entitlement, claims adjudication, fraud, program abuse, utilization review, quality assurance, peer review, program integrity, third-party liability, coordination of benefits, and civil and criminal litigation related to the operation of CHAMPUS.

<u>DISCLOSURES:</u> Voluntary; however, failure to provide information will result in delay in payment or may result in denial of claim. With the one exception discussed below, there are no penalties under these programs for refusing to supply information. However, failure to furnish information regarding the medical services rendered or the amount charged would prevent payment of claims under these programs. Failure to furnish any other information, such as name or claim number, would delay payment of the claim. Failure to provide medical information under FECA could be deemed an obstruction.

It is mandatory that you tell us if you know that another party is responsible for paying for your treatment. Section 1128B of the Social Security Act and 31 USC 3801-3812 provide penalties for withholding this information.

You should be aware that P.L. 100-503, the "Computer Matching and Privacy Protection Act of 1988", permits the government to verify information by way of computer matches.

MEDICAID PAYMENTS (PROVIDER CERTIFICATION)

I hereby agree to keep such records as are necessary to disclose fully the extent of services provided to individuals under the State's Title XIX plan and to furnish information regarding any payments claimed for providing such services as the State Agency or Dept. of Health and Human Services may request.

I further agree to accept, as payment in full, the amount paid by the Medicaid program for those claims submitted for payment under that program, with the exception of authorized deductible, coinsurance, co-payment or similar cost-sharing charge.

SIGNATURE OF PHYSICIAN (OR SUPPLIER): I certify that the services listed above were medically indicated and necessary to the health of this patient and were personally furnished by me or my employee under my personal direction.

NOTICE: This is to certify that the foregoing information is true, accurate and complete. I understand that payment and satisfaction of this claim will be from Federal and State funds, and that any false claims, statements, or documents, or concealment of a material fact, may be prosecuted under applicable Federal or State laws.

According to the Paperwork Reduction Act of 1995, no persons are required to respond to a collection of information unless it displays a valid OMB control number. The valid OMB control number for this information collection is 0938-0008. The time required to complete this information collection is estimated to average 10 minutes per response, including the time to review instructions, search existing data resources, gather the data needed, and complete and review the information collection. If you have any comments concerning the accuracy of the time estimate(s) or suggestions for improving this form, please write to: CMS, Attn: PRA Reports Clearance Officer, 7500 Security Boulevard, Baltimore, Maryland 21244-1850.

covered at all. The exception to this, of course, is Medicare Part D. Nearly all major medical plans in place today have either a coinsurance or a deductible or both in place for their beneficiaries. Failure to collect any coinsurance or deductible from a patient could result in automatic rejectionof your claim. Additionally, it is considered insurance fraud to waive deductibles and coinsurance when providing service. Deliberate waiving of these out-of-pocket fees could result in a fine or, in some states, imprisonment.

Make Sure Your Documentation Matches Your Billing Code

CPT evaluation and management codes and MTM services codes have very specific documentation requirements that must accompany their use. It is critical to ensure you have documented your services appropriately and only bill for a code for which you have firm clinical documentation.

Be Persistent and Consistent

Anyone who wishes to bill for his or her professional services will only be successful if they are both persistent and consistent. Particularly in the early going, persistence is necessary with many third-party insurers as they may not be accustomed to paying for pharmacist-directed services. Don't give up with the first rejected claim! Bill the patient, and encourage the patient to advocate with their insurer for payment as well. It has been reported elsewhere that some pharmacists simply choose not to bill most third parties for their services, choosing rather to bill the patient directly. This mechanism of billing utilizes the value the patient sees in the relationship with their pharmacist to get the ultimate payer (patient or employer) to demand reimbursement from their insurer.[9]

While persistence is certainly important, perhaps even more important is consistency. It is absolutely imperative that what you choose to charge one patient you charge to all. Many would consider it unethical, and some consider it illegal, to charge a third-party payer for something one is unwilling to charge a patient paying fully out-of-pocket. It is always best to set professional fees, post them or publish them, and be consistent in seeking remuneration from all parties.

Summary

Compensation for professional services is a topic that has received significant attention in the pharmacy literature over the past three decades. Documentation of the value of the pharmacist and the pharmacist's role as a caregiver in the health system has been ongoing since the establishment of DRGs. The efforts of those clinicians who have taken a leadership role in substantiating their value to the health care system have long reaped professional rewards but have often not seen significant financial incentives for their hard work.

Passage of MMA 2003 may well represent the first significant opportunity for pharmacists practicing in diverse health systems to be paid for their nondispensing services. Only time will tell if the changes enabled by this law will be of positive, negative, or neutral impact on the profession of pharmacy. It is also yet to be seen if private insurers will follow the lead of Medicare and begin payment for MTM services. One thing is for certain—the profession is at a critical juncture for which it has long been advocating, and the failure of the profession to step up and provide the services that are compensable could be one of monumental proportions. Health-system pharmacy directors must actively engage themselves, their institutions, and their pharmacists in laying the framework to meet or exceed MTM services provisions under Medicare and beyond. The opportunity for new revenue streams has never been better for the health-system pharmacy.

References

1. Apple WS. Pharmacy's new Rx evolution. *J Am Pharm Assoc.* 1967; NS7(9):474–7, 484.

2. Myers MJ. Professional fee: renaissance or innovation? *J Am Pharm Assoc.* 1968;NS8(12):628–31.

3. 42 C.F.R. § 405.1804.

4. Gattis WA, Hasselblad V, Whellan DJ, et al. Reduction in heart failure events by the addition of a clinical pharmacist to the heart failure management team. *Arch Intern Med.* 1999;159:1939–45.

5. Leape LL, Cullen DJ, Clapp MD, et al. Pharmacist participation on physician rounds and adverse drug events in the intensive care unit. *JAMA.* 1999;282:267–70.

6. McMullin ST, Hennenfent JA, Ritchie DJ, et al. A prospective, randomized trial to assess the cost impact of pharmacist-initiated interventions. *Arch Intern Med.* 1999;159:2306–9.

7. Medicare Prescription Drug, Improvement, and Modernization Act of 2003. 42 CFR Part 423.

8. MTM services definition finalized. *Pharmacy Today.* Aug 2004;10(8):15.

9. Hogue MD. *The Pharmacist's Guide to Compensation for Patient Care Services.* Washington, DC: American Pharmacists Association; 2002.

10. National Healthcareer Association. Medical coding and billing homepage. Available at: http://www.medical codingandbilling.com/. Accessed December 13, 2004.

11. American Medical Association. *Current Procedural Terminolog: 2005*. Chicago, Illinois: American Medical Association; 2004.

12. National Center for Health Statistics, Centers for Disease Control and Prevention. Classification of diseases. International classification of diseases. 10th revision. Clinical modification. Available at: www.cdc.gov/nchs/about/otheract/icd9/abticd10.htm. Accessed November 30, 2004.

13. ASHP urges CMS to take stronger hand in assuring appropriate medication therapy for Medicare patients. Available at: http://www.ashp.org/news/ShowArticle. cfm?cfid=3603233&CFToken=41348908&id=7954. Accessed November 30, 2004.

14. APhA letter to CMS on the Medicare prescription drug benefit proposed regulation. Available at: www.aphanet.org. Accessed November 30, 2004.

15. ASCP Final Comments to CMS on Proposed Rules for Medicare Drug Benefit Available at: www.ascp.com/ medicarerx/docs/ASCP_CMS_MMA_Comments.pdf. Accessed November 30, 2004.

16. Bond CA, Raehl CL. Pharmacist-provided anticoagulation management in United States hospitals: death rates, length of stay, Medicare charges, bleeding complications, and transfusions. *Pharmacotherapy*. 2004;24(8):953–63.

17. Bond CA, Raehl CL, Patry R. Evidence-based core clinical pharmacy services in United States Hospitals in 2020: services and staffing. *Pharmacotherapy*. 2004;24(4):427–40.

18. Pharmacy professionalism toolkit for students and faculty. Available at: http://www.aacp.org/Docs/Main Navigation/ForDeans/6428_PharmacyProfessionalism Toolkitv.1.pdf. Accessed December 2, 2004.

19. Zoeller JL, ed. Finding meaning in our work. *AACP News*. August 2004;35(8):3.

20. Quality of care and outcomes research in CVD and stroke working groups. Measuring and improving quality of care: a report from the American Heart Association/ American College of Cardiology First Scientific Forum on assessment of healthcare quality in cardiovascular disease and stroke. *Circulation*. 2000;101:1483–93.

21. Soto CM, Kleinman KP, Simon SR. Quality and correlates of medical record documentation in the ambulatory care setting. *BMC Health Services Research*. (serial online). 2002;2:22.

22. 1997 documentation guidelines for evaluation and management services. Available at: http://www.cms.hhs. gov/medlearn/master1.pdf. Accessed December 2, 2004.

23. Office of the Secretary, Department of Health and Human Services. HIPAA administrative simplification: standard unique health identifier for health care providers, final rule. *Federal Register*. January 23, 2004; 69(15).

24. How to bill Medicare for influenza and pneumococcal immunizations. Available at: http://www.cms.hhs.gov/ preventiveservices/2f.pdf. Accessed December 13, 2004.

25. Hogue MD, Foster S, eds. *Pharmacy-Based Immunization Delivery: A National Certificate Program for Pharmacists Self-Study*. Washington, DC: The American Pharmacists Association; 2004.

26. Task Force to Review and Revise the National Standards for Diabetes Self-Management Education Programs. National standards for diabetes self-management education. *Diabetes Care*. 2000;23(5):682–89.

27. Education recognition program. Available at: http://www.diabetes.org/education/eduprogram.asp. Accessed December 6, 2004.

28. MA and PDP region specific fact sheets. Available at: http://www.cms.hhs.gov/medicarereform/mmaregions/ pdpmaorsfs.asp. Accessed December 13, 2004.

29. Medicare prescription drug benefit program application and contracting process summary. Available at: http://www.cms.hhs.gov/pdps/PartD%20white%20paper. pdf. Accessed December 13, 2004.

Appendix 1
Medication Therapy Management Services Definition and Program Criteria

Medication Therapy Management is a distinct service or group of services that optimize therapeutic outcomes for individual patients. Medication Therapy Management Services are independent of, but can occur in conjunction with, the provision of a medication product.

Medication Therapy Management encompasses a broad range of professional activities and responsibilities within the licensed pharmacist's, or other qualified health care provider's, scope of practice. These services include but are not limited to the following, according to the individual needs of the patient:

a. Performing or obtaining necessary assessments of the patient's health status;

b. Formulating a medication treatment plan;

c. Selecting, initiating, modifying, or administering medication therapy;

d. Monitoring and evaluating the patient's response to therapy, including safety and effectiveness;

e. Performing a comprehensive medication review to identify, resolve, and prevent medication-related problems, including adverse drug events;

f. Documenting the care delivered and communicating essential information to the patient's other primary care providers;

g. Providing verbal education and training designed to enhance patient understanding and appropriate use of his/her medications;

h. Providing information, support services, and resources designed to enhance patient adherence with his/her therapeutic regimens;

i. Coordinating and integrating medication therapy management services within the broader health care-management services being provided to the patient.

A program that provides coverage for Medication Therapy Management Services shall include:

a. Patient-specific and individualized services or sets of services provided directly by a pharmacist to the patient*. These services are distinct from formulary development and use, generalized patient education and information activities, and other population-focused quality assurance measures for medication use.

b. Face-to-face interaction between the patient* and the pharmacist as the preferred method of delivery. When patient-specific barriers to face-to-face communication exist, patients shall have equal access to appropriate alternative delivery methods. Medication Therapy Management programs shall include structures supporting the establishment and maintenance of the patient*-pharmacist relationship.

c. Opportunities for pharmacists and other qualified health care providers to identify patients who should receive medication therapy management services.

d. Payment for Medication Therapy Management Services consistent with contemporary provider payment rates that are based on the time, clinical intensity, and resources required to provide services (e.g., Medicare Part A and/or Part B for CPT & RBRVS).

e. Processes to improve continuity of care, outcomes, and outcome measures.

---

* In some situations, Medication Therapy Management Services may be provided to the caregiver or other persons involved in the care of the patient. Approved July 27, 2004 by the Academy of Managed Care Pharmacy, the American Association of Colleges of Pharmacy, the American College of Apothecaries, the American College of Clinical Pharmacy, the American Society of Consultant Pharmacists, the American Pharmacists Association, the American Society of Health-System Pharmacists, the National Association of Boards of Pharmacy,** the National Association of Chain Drug Stores, the National Community Pharmacists Association, and the National Council of State Pharmacy Association Executives.

**Organization policy does not allow NABP to take a position on payment issues.

Chapter 20

Financial Management and Cost Control

Andrew L. Wilson

Introduction

Financial management and cost control are key activities for pharmacists in leadership roles in institutional practice. The high cost of pharmaceuticals, growing salaries for pharmacists, combined with the compelling need for pharmacy services and medication therapy require thoughtful, cost-conscious management to ensure success. The growth of support systems and technology to manage the safety and effectiveness of the medication use process, including automation and information systems also add to the scope of financial management and cost control responsibilities of pharmacists. Pharmacy directors and managers encounter conflicts between their patient care leadership and their management roles as they work to balance costs, benefits and outcomes in delivering patient care. A working knowledge of financial management is essential to ensure that high quality services are effectively delivered, and that the patient care mission of the pharmacy is carried out optimally.

As pharmacists, we are charged with developing and maintaining a medication use system that provides the highest quality of care and one that serves the medical and pharmaceutical needs of the patient to their fullest. However, in a health care delivery system where resources are finite, the pharmacy leadership role requires monitoring, allocating, and actively managing pharmaceutical and professional resources to use them to their greatest advantage. Building working relationships with administration, physicians, nurses and others is based on an understanding of the key relationships in cost management and finance. In some instances, the resource limitations and the balance between cost and benefit for pharmacy services and medication therapy may not be well-defined by senior management, adding the burden and opportunity of developing a broader, financially responsible plan for the hospital or health system to pharmacy leadership.

An active, engaged pharmacy leader is well-versed in clinical and professional disciplines surrounding medication use and pharmaceutical care. The leader also possesses a keen understanding of the financial and productivity performance for his or her areas of responsibility and works to understand the role of the pharmacy service in the context of the institution. A knowledgeable pharmacy manager works to communicate the impact of pharmacy services and medication therapy, and secure the necessary resources to accomplish these goals. Audiences and forums for these discussions include the medical staff, in Pharmacy and Therapeutics Committee meetings, and other discussions and Senior Administrative leadership in budget review and other administrative meetings. Because of the scope, magnitude, costs and outcomes associated with medication therapy, health-system boards of trustees and corporate leaders rely on pharmacists to contribute to the understanding the impact of medication costs. Increasingly, a key role of pharmacy leadership is to articulate a coherent plan for clinical pharmacists and other pharmacy staff to understand the balance of cost, benefit, and outcome in their daily professional decision-making.

Thoughtful financial management and cost control strategies allow institutional pharmacy directors to ensure that their department receives resources appropriate to meet patient care needs and organizational mission. The controls and reporting mechanisms that the institutional and pharmacy leadership put in place and maintain, ensure that these goals are met and that patient care quality and outcomes are optimized.

Practice Standards

ASHP Practice standards and guidelines refer to the leadership responsibilities of pharmacists and identify key roles and responsibilities related to financial management of a pharmacy service[1,2]:

- *Budget Management*—The pharmacy should have a budget consistent with the organization's financial management process that supports the scope of and demand for pharmaceutical services.

- *Workload and Productivity Management*— Oversight of workload and financial performance should be managed in accordance with the organization's requirements.

- *Analysis and Control Methods*—Management should provide for (1) determination and analysis of pharmaceutical service costs, (2) analysis of budgetary variances, (3) capital equipment acquisition, (4) patient revenue projections, and (5) justification of personnel commensurate with workload productivity.

- Processes should enable the analysis of pharmaceutical services by unit-of-service and other parameters appropriate to the organization (e.g., organization-wide costs by medication therapy, clinical service, specific disease management categories, and patient health plan enrollment). The director should have an integral part in the organization's financial management process.

- *Drug Expenditures*—Specific policies and procedures for managing drug expenditures should address such methods as competitive bidding, group purchasing, utilization review programs, inventory management, and cost-effective patient services.

- *Revenue, Reimbursement, and Compensation*—The director should be knowledgeable about revenues for pharmaceutical services including reimbursement for the provision of drug products and related supplies and compensation for pharmacists' cognitive services.

- Processes should exist for routine verification of patient benefits and for counseling patients about their anticipated financial responsibility for planned medication therapies. A process should also exist for responding to services requests from medically indigent patients.

Financial Terms

Medical terminology is precise, and so is financial terminology. Pharmacists are trained to value thoughtful, direct, and evidence-based evaluations of medications, procedures, policies and programs. They work to communicate professional assessments and directions in a precise manner to ensure that appropriate actions are undertaken. Leadership colleagues including the institution's Chief Executive Officer (CEO) and Chief Financial Officer (CFO) expect similar precision in descriptions of the financial and operational performance of the pharmacy service.

Financial terms and expectations must be learned within the context and goals of each institution. For-profit hospitals; not-for-profit hospitals; HMOs; integrated health systems; state, federal and other types of institutions each have different reporting needs and management structures. Pharmacists must learn the full meaning and implications of each of these terms in the context of their organization. The use and importance of each term will vary with the goals of the institution and with the financial status of the organization. Key terms to understand in all types of organizations include the following:

Expense

An *expense* is a payment made by the health system to others for value received. Pharmacy expenses fall into several categories. Direct expenses are those expenses that are incurred by the pharmacy to deliver services and products. Supplies are the largest category of direct expense; predominately pharmaceuticals. Other categories of supplies managed by pharmacy include blood products, intravenous fluids, syringes and needles, administration sets, and other *nonpatient care* supplies such as packaging materials, paper, labels, and other office supplies. Human resources are generally the second largest category of direct expense. Human resource expenses consist of the salary and benefit costs for pharmacists, pharmacy technicians, pharmacy managers, and others.

Other direct expenses incurred by the pharmacy include the following:

- Leases for hardware and software to manage medication delivery, including automated medication cabinets, dispensing robots, pharmacy computer systems, and intravenous pumps

- Services including hood certification, service agreements for technology and equipment, and maintenance and repairs for pharmacy facilities

- Professional education and development expenses including meetings, travel, and competency programs

- Licenses, taxes, and other fees associated with accreditation, including pharmacy residency program accreditation

Direct expenses can also be classified as fixed or variable. Fixed expenses are defined as costs that do not vary significantly in the short-term with the volume of activity. Property and equipment are examples. *Variable expenses* are costs that vary in the short-term with the level of activity. Purchase costs for pharmaceuticals are an example; costs rise and fall as the number of patients and prescriptions change. Pharmacy activity volume may be expressed based on the number of patient days, prescriptions or orders processed, or as the number of doses dispensed. Most health-system budgets base variable costs for pharmacy supply and manpower on a combination of inpatient days, emergency department visits, and clinic or other ambulatory volumes.

Indirect expenses are payments for services that support the pharmacy but are not directly paid by the pharmacy. These include housekeeping, heat and air-conditioning, electricity, hospital administration, hospital purchasing, information systems support, human resources, hospital finance, and others. The cost of these indirect services may also be referred to as overhead. In the modern health system the magnitude of these costs is substantial. Because the costs are beyond the control of the pharmacy manager, they are not generally a part of regular financial reports. However, indirect costs are considered when business plans and profitability of a service or program are reviewed, including pharmacy services.

An additional expense category in which a pharmacy service is involved is capital expenses. *Capital expenses* are defined as the cost of an improvement or a piece of equipment that will provide benefit over a number of years. Health systems budget and manage capital expense separately from regular operating expenses. Accounting methods can report capital expenses spread across several years. Capital expenditures are typically significant in size and scope. Pharmacy examples of capital expenses might include new IV admixture hoods, remodeling of a pharmacy, or building a new pharmacy satellite. Health systems typically specify a financial test (e.g., an expense >$5,000) and a duration of useful life of the purchase (e.g., >5 years) to identify an item or project as a capital expense.

Revenue

Revenue is defined as money received for products or services provided to customers. Pharmacy revenues consist primarily of patient charges. Patient charges may arise from doses administered in an inpatient setting or from prescriptions dispensed in an outpatient setting. Pharmacies may also generate revenue by providing professional services, including consultation, management of research studies, providing education and other support services, and for medication therapy management.

Inpatient pharmacy revenues appear on patients' hospital bills as charges. A total of all charges posted by the pharmacy to all bills for an accounting period (e.g., a month), are reported as the pharmacy's gross revenue.

Although charges for medications and for pharmacy services are a focus for pharmacy managers, they are typically not the payments received by the hospital. Most inpatient care is paid at a case rate. A case rate is a payment that is negotiated based on a diagnosis-related group (DRG), a per diem (daily) amount, or other benchmark method to determine the hospital's payment. The hospital receives the case rate payment for the patient's care, irrespective of the individual charges posted to the patient's account. Some hospital contracts pay a discounted percentage of billed charges, and most payers provide supplemental payments for patients whose care substantially exceeds the negotiated amount. However, almost no payer, including the federal government pays full charge. Patients without insurance often are unable to pay their hospital bill, requiring the hospital to "write off" their bill, considering the cost of care as a charitable loss.

The case rate payment method is designed to encourage hospitals to provide care economically. It also allows the hospital to be the beneficiary of savings and efficiencies or to incur the cost of inefficient care. Although this approach works well in theory, it creates challenges for pharmacy managers in understanding the impact and goals of therapy selection and management of the medication use process. Because case rates are diagnosis-specific, diagnoses where medications are a significant expense are of the greatest financial and cost control interest to pharmacists. Formulary decisions, practice guideline development, and therapeutic decisions at the bedside may have a significant impact on the health system's ability to meet financial objectives treating these patients. This is discussed later in this chapter.

When the hospital receives payment for services, the case-rate based payment is matched to the charge-based patient bill, and the "discount" is calculated and subtracted; the resulting payment is the net revenue. The net revenue consists of the gross revenue minus the discounts resulting from case rate-based payment. The hospital's accounting system allows the deductions from the gross revenue to be applied to the charges posted by the pharmacy and other departments. The resulting adjustment determines the net revenue to each department. The pharmacy's overall net revenue is calculated by subtracting the pharmacy's share of discounts, contractual allowances, and nonpayments for all patient bills to the hospital from the pharmacy gross revenue.

Outpatient prescriptions are typically charged in the same fashion. The pharmacy contracts with a third party (insurance provider, state Medicaid program, or Pharmacy Benefits Manager (PBM)) to fill prescriptions at a fixed rate based on medication costs and service fees. Rate structures are typically based on a percentage of average wholesale prices for the medication plus a filling fee. Outpatient prescription payment methods are typically handled electronically at the time of dispensing; generally referred to as adjudication at the point of service. Each prescription claim is electronically verified and payment posted through access to a centralized information system. These systems provide recordkeeping and revenue tracking systems for outpatient pharmacy in real time.

Assets

Assets are the real, intangible and financial items that are owned by the health system. These include land, buildings, equipment, and the value of inventory. Assets also include cash, accounts receivable (unpaid bills owed by patients, insurance companies and others) for services delivered but not yet paid. In the case of pharmacy, the majority of assets of interest are equipment and the inventory of drugs and supplies. Assets are offset by liabilities, the debts (unpaid bills the hospital owes to creditors, loans, bonds issued) owed against them. The net of assets and liabilities is equal to the equity held by the institution. In a for-profit organization, equity is a form of liability representing what the corporation owes to the stockholders.

Work Volumes

Work volumes for pharmacy consist of work units and paid hours. Workload volume for a hospital is generally reported as adjusted discharges or patient days. Health-system pharmacy workload calculations may be based on patient counts such as inpatient admissions or discharges, prescriptions filled, orders processed, or doses dispensed and combinations of these components. Typical indicators for pharmacy workload are adjusted using case-mix-index (CMI) or another indicator of acuity to recognize the additional cost and resources required to care for sicker patients. Outpatient workload is generally reported as prescriptions filled and may include patient counseling and other direct patient care activities in some settings. Institutional pharmacy workload should also be adjusted to reflect the significant amount of effort and cost required to support outpatient surgery, emergency department activity, outpatient infusion services, and other areas that are not reflected in patient day or inpatient discharge count.

As pharmacy has evolved from a primary focus on medication dispensing to include more substantial clinical and cognitive services, workload models based on doses charged, or doses dispensed have fallen out of favor. Workload models based solely on medication doses handled do not reflect the full range of pharmacy service activities, and their use is discouraged.

Health Care Institution Accounting Methods

Accounting is a standard method for reporting the expenses, revenues, and accumulation of assets, and other financial results. An institution maintains a balance sheet that lists the assets, liabilities, and equity. The balance sheet is a financial statement which lists the wealth of the institution at a specific point of time. Traditionally, assets appear on the left and liabilities on the right and the two must be in balance. The balance sheet is described by the equation:

$$\text{Assets} = \text{Liabilities} + \text{Equity}$$

Double entry bookkeeping ensures that both sides of the equation remain balanced at all times. Double entry bookkeeping enters any transaction on both sides of the balance sheet (as a debit on one side and a credit on the other) to keep the equation balanced. As an example, a purchase of an IV hood creates a liability but creates and asset of equal value. Table 20-1 is a simplified example of a balance sheet for a health system.

The second part of an organization's periodic financial review is the income statement. The income statement lists the Revenue, Expense, and Profit (or loss) of the institution over a period of time. Traditionally, revenue appears on the right and expenses on the left. The income statement and balance sheet together comprise the financial statement. Hospitals prepare financial statements monthly and generally report results to a Board or other oversight body on a monthly, quarterly, and annual basis.

The balance sheet and income statement are fed by data maintained in the hospital's general ledger. The general ledger is a record of each transaction of the hospital. Balances on the general ledger are referred to as trial or unaudited balances, as corrections and changes may be made through an audit process. Reports generated from the general ledger provide significant detail about the institution's activities and finances. A monthly report comparing the actual expenses and activities to the budget for the same period provides pharmacy managers and administrators with information to understand the financial status of

Table 20-1
Hospital Balance Sheet

Balance Sheet Community Hospital June 30, 2005			
Assets		**Liabilities and Equity**	
Cash	$1,000,000	Accounts Payable	$250,000
Accounts Receivable	$3,000,000	Long-Term Debt	$12,000,000
Inventory	$200,000	Equity	$5,950,000
Land	$1,000,000		
Buildings	$10,000,000	**Total**	**$18,200,000**
Equipment	$3,000,000		
Total	**$18,200,000**		

the department. These monthly activity reports or responsibility summaries are a key to understanding the financial performance of the pharmacy. Table 20-2 is an example of a monthly operations report.

Financial Planning

The annual budget is an important part of the pharmacy manager's financial responsibility. A budget is a plan for future expenses and revenue, typically over a 12-month period. A budget does not represent the actual amount of money available to be spent. The pharmacy budget is a thoughtful forecast of future expenses and revenue and a benchmark for measuring financial performance.

The Budget Process

Each year the institution develops an annual plan. The institutions CEO, CFO, and Board of trustees develop goals for services, activity levels, expenditures, and revenues. This is typically done 6–9 months before the fiscal year begins. Forecasts are developed for admissions, service activity, growth, expansion, or other program changes. The director of pharmacy receives these forecasts and begins the process of developing the pharmacy budget. Each institution's budget process varies slightly. However, the CFO provides a budget manual or other instructions, including a calendar format for budgeting and required approvals and reviews. Instructions may also specify the projections for forecasting inflation and other price increases to be used in budget development. As discussed earlier in the chapter, parts of the budget represent fixed costs that will not vary with activity while others are variable

costs, requiring the manager to carefully review forecasts for admissions, patient days and other volume indicators.

Capital Budget

The budget cycle typically begins with the development of a capital budget. The *capital budget* is typically comprised of items that cost more than a fixed threshold (e.g., an expense >$5,000) and a useful life greater than 5 years. These thresholds are set by the institution's Board. Capital expense budgets are generally set several years in advance because many capital expenses can be forecast. The need to replace equipment, renovate or build facilities, or to incur expenses for a new program lends themselves to forward planning.

Capital budget needs are typically larger than the institution can afford, so some prioritization of need may be undertaken, normally a focused review of the expense (Is it required by a new regulation or standard? Is the current equipment broken or nonfunctioning? Is the equipment necessary to support a new patient care program?). A review of the return on investment (ROI) is also generally used to prioritize or determine the wisdom of the capital expense. ROI is a structured calculation of the operating cost and revenue changes that the institution with incur with the new capital expense (Will fewer employees be needed due to increased productivity? Will additional patient volume be available due to increased capacity? Will more revenue be collected?). ROI calculations are generally stated in terms of the number of months or years that a capital purchase takes to pay back its purchase cost. Shorter payback periods are generally more favorable, and capital expenses that do not result in payback of

Table 20-2
Example Monthly Operating Statement—Inpatient Pharmacy

Current Month Actual	Current Month Budget	Difference	0415 INPATIENT PHARMACY PATIENT SERVICES REVENUE	Fiscal Year to Date Actual	Fiscal Year to Date Budget	Difference
			INPATIENT SERVICES			
$8,485,475	$8,315,766	$169,710	3010102 ANCILLARY SERVICES	$25,456,425	$24,947,297	$509,129
$8,485,475	*$8,315,766*	*$169,710*	*TOTAL INPATIENT REVENUE*	*$25,456,425*	*$24,947,297*	*$509,129*
			OUTPATIENT SERVICES			
$1,274,799	$1,249,303	$25,496	3010202 SPECIAL MEDICAL SERVICES	$3,824,397	$3,747,909	$76,488
$110,852	$108,635	$2,217	3010203 EMERGENCY SERVICES	$332,556	$325,905	$6,651
$1,385,651	*$1,357,938*	*$27,713*	*TOTAL OUTPATIENT REVENUE*	*$4,156,953*	*$4,073,814*	*$83,139*
$9,871,126	**$9,673,703**	**$197,423**	**PATIENT SERVICES REVENUE**	**$29,613,378**	**$29,021,110**	**$592,268**
$(5,653,838)	$(5,540,761)	$(113,077)	3020399 DEDUCTION FOR CONTRACTUAL	$(16,961,514)	$(16,622,284)	$(339,230)
$(5,653,838)	*$(5,540,761)*	*$(113,077)*	*TOTAL CONTRACTUAL ADJUSTMENT*	*$(16,961,514)*	*$(16,622,284)*	*$(339,230)*
$4,217,288	**$4,132,942**	**$84,346**	**NET PATIENT REVENUE**	**$12,651,864**	**$12,398,827**	**$253,037**
$16,916	$16,578	$338	3040204 SALES–NP DRUG SALES	$50,748	$49,733	$1,015
$16,916	*$16,578*	*$338*	*TOTAL OTHER OPERATING REVENUE*	*$50,748*	*$49,733*	*$1,015*
$4,234,204	**$4,149,520**	**$84,684**	**TOTAL REVENUE**	**$12,702,612**	**$12,448,560**	**$254,052**
$32,485	$31,835	$650	4010101 SALARY–MGMT & SUPERVISION	$97,455	$95,506	$1,949
$360,198	$352,994	$7,204	4010102 SALARY–TECHNICIAN	$1,080,594	$1,058,982	$21,612
$10,043	$9,842	$201	4010106 SALARY–SUPPORT STAFF	$30,129	$29,526	$603
$2,057	$2,016	$41	4010107 SALARY–OTHER	$6,171	$6,048	$123
$404,783	*$396,687*	*$8,096*	*TOTAL SALARIES*	*$1,214,349*	*$1,190,062*	*$24,287*
$33,180	$32,516	$664	4010202 WAGES–TECHNICIAN	$99,540	$97,549	$1,991
$4,664	$4,571	$93	4010205 WAGES–AIDES & ORDERLIES	$13,992	$13,712	$280
$37,844	*$37,087*	*$757*	*TOTAL WAGES*	*$113,532*	*$111,261*	*$2,271*
$9,818	$9,622	$196	4010302 OVERTIME–TECHNICIAN	$29,454	$28,865	$589
$370	$363	$7	4010306 OVERTIME–SUPPORT STAFF	$1,110	$1,088	$22
$10,188	*$9,984*	*$204*	*TOTAL SALARIES OVERTIME*	*$30,564*	*$29,953*	*$611*
$172	$169	$3	4010406 OVERTIME–SUPPORT STAFF	$516	$506	$10
$172	*$169*	*$3*	*TOTAL WAGE OVERTIME*	*$516*	*$506*	*$10*
$9,146	$8,963	$183	4010502 SHIFT–DIFFERENTIAL TECHNICIAN	$27,438	$26,889	$549
$9,146	*$8,963*	*$183*	*TOTAL SHIFT DIFFERENTIAL*	*$27,438*	*$26,889*	*$549*
$262	$257	$5	4010602 ON CALL–TECHNICIAN	$786	$770	$16
$262	*$257*	*$5*	*TOTAL ON CALL*	*$786*	*$770*	*$16*
$(6,439)	$(6,310)	$(129)	4010909 VACANCY REDUCTION–SALARY	$(19,317)	$(18,931)	$(386)
$(6,439)	*$(6,310)*	*$(129)*	*TOTAL OTHER PERSONNEL*	*$(19,317)*	*$(18,931)*	*$(386)*
$36,278	$35,552	$726	4020101 FICA	$108,834	$106,657	$2,177
$43,626	$42,753	$873	4020104 GROUP HEALTH INSURANCE	$130,878	$128,260	$2,618
$29,026	$28,445	$581	4020105 RETIREMENT BENEFITS	$87,078	$85,336	$1,742
$2,501	$2,451	$50	4020106 WORKER'S COMP INSURANCE	$7,503	$7,353	$150
$1,927	$1,888	$39	4020107 GROUP LIFE INSURANCE	$5,781	$5,665	$116
$1,577	$1,545	$32	4020109 DISABILITY INSURANCE	$4,731	$4,636	$95
$114,935	*$112,636*	*$2,299*	*TOTAL EMPLOYEE BENEFITS*	*$344,805*	*$337,909*	*$6,896*
$570,891	**$559,473**	**$11,418**	**TOTAL PERSONNEL EXPENSE**	**$1,712,673**	**$1,678,420**	**$34,253**

Table 20-2, continued

Current Month Actual	Current Month Budget	Difference	0415 INPATIENT PHARMACY PATIENT SERVICES REVENUE	Fiscal Year to Date Actual	Fiscal Year to Date Budget	Difference
$1,573,726	$1,542,251	$31,475	4050201 DRUGS	$4,721,178	$4,626,754	$94,424
$32,401	$31,753	$648	4050202 INTRAVENOUS SUPPLIES	$97,203	$95,259	$1,944
$458,717	$449,543	$9,174	4050203 BLOOD & BLOOD PRODUCTS	$1,376,151	$1,348,628	$27,523
$9,761	$9,566	$195	4050206 REAGENT & CHEMICALS	$29,283	$28,697	$586
$13,512	$13,242	$270	4050503 GENERAL MED/SURG SUPPLY	$40,536	$39,725	$811
$2,088,117	*$2,046,355*	*$41,762*	*TOTAL SPECIAL SUPPLIES*	*$6,264,351*	*$6,139,064*	*$125,287*
$527	$516	$11	4060101 OFFICE SUPPLIES	$1,581	$1,549	$32
$61	$60	$1	4060301 OFFICE EQUIPMENT	$183	$179	$4
$159	$156	$3	4060305 COMMUNICATION EQUIPMENT	$477	$467	$10
$45	$44	$1	4060405 COMPUTER SUPPLIES	$135	$132	$3
$792	*$776*	*$16*	*TOTAL GENERAL SUPPLIES*	*$2,376*	*$2,328*	*$48*
$247	$242	$5	4080201 REPAIR OF MEDICAL EQUIP	$741	$726	$15
$99	$97	$2	4080202 REPAIR NON-MEDICAL EQUIP	$297	$291	$6
$8	$8	$0	4080401 FREIGHT	$24	$24	$0
$4,987	$4,887	$100	4080405 PRINTING	$14,961	$14,662	$299
$41,539	$40,708	$831	4080601 PHARMACY SCHOOL SERVICE CONTRACT	$124,617	$122,125	$2,492
$30	$29	$1	4080801 GENERAL SERVICES	$90	$88	$2
$46,910	*$45,972*	*$938*	*TOTAL PURCHASED SERVICES*	*$140,730*	*$137,915*	*$2,815*
$527	$516	$11	4140203 TELEPHONE	$1,581	$1,549	$32
$527	*$516*	*$11*	*TOTAL OTHER EXPENSES*	*$1,581*	*$1,549*	*$32*
$2,136,346	**$2,093,619**	**$42,727**	**TOTAL NON-PERSONNEL EXPENSES**	**$6,409,038**	**$6,280,857**	**$128,181**
$2,707,237	**$2,653,092**	**$54,145**	**TOTAL OPERATING EXPENSES**	**$8,121,711**	**$7,959,277**	**$162,434**
$2,707,237	**$2,653,092**	**$54,145**	**TOTAL EXPENSES**	**$8,121,711**	**$7,959,277**	**$162,434**
$1,526,967	**$1,496,428**	**$30,539**	**NET EXCESS**	**$4,580,901**	**$4,489,283**	**$91,618**

their costs may not be easily approved and budgeted, unless they are required to meet a legal or accreditation standard.

Operating Budget

The *operating budget* represents a forecast of the daily expenses required to operate the pharmacy. Development of the health-system budget generally takes advantage of the fact that most expenses are similar in size and scope to prior years. In many organizations, the pharmacy director is presented with a preliminary budget based on the activity for the prior fiscal year. Even when this is not done, it is incumbent on the pharmacy director to review proposed expenses and revenues in light of the past 1–2 fiscal years and to

base changes on institutional and industry trends, news, and other information. The budget review and approval process generally uses this method to ensure continuity and prevent errors.

Volume Budget

The *volume budget* is prepared by the CFO and supplies the number of admissions, patient days, CMI, outpatient visits, emergency department visits, and other activities. The Pharmacy director should examine historical relationships between these volume statistics and pharmacy activity to develop a pharmacy volume budget. Table 20-3 is an example of a pharmacy volume budget developed based on the CFO's base statistics.

Table 20-3
Pharmacy Volume Budget

LOCATION	JUL	AUG	SEP	OCT	NOV	DEC	JAN	FEB	MAR	APR	MAY	JUN	TOTAL	Monthly Average
Inpatient Pharmacy	369,392	369,392	357,476	369,392	357,476	369,392	369,392	333,644	369,392	357,476	369,392	357,476	4,349,292	362,441
Inpatient Pharmacy Total	**369,392**	**369,392**	**357,476**	**369,392**	**357,476**	**369,392**	**369,392**	**333,644**	**369,392**	**357,476**	**369,392**	**357,476**	**4,349,292**	**362,441**
Orders/Day	11,915.87	11,915.87	11,915.87	11,915.87	11,915.87	11,915.87	11,915.87	11,915.86	11,915.87	11,915.87	11,915.87	11,915.87		11,915.87
Outpatient Pharmacy #1	16,557	15,869	16,180	16,197	15,716	15,997	16,197	14,768	16,213	15,656	16,213	15,656	191,220	15,935
Outpatient Pharmacy #2	9,617	9,885	9,916	9,446	9,898	10,064	9,446	10,063	9,953	9,631	9,953	9,631	117,503	9,792
Outpatient Pharmacies Total	**26,174**	**25,755**	**26,097**	**25,644**	**25,613**	**26,061**	**25,644**	**24,830**	**26,166**	**25,287**	**26,166**	**25,287**	**308,724**	**25,727**
Rx/Day	1,106	1,088	1,140	1,084	1,118	1,101	1,084	1,162	1,106	1,104	1,106	1,104		1,108.55
Home Infusion Pharmacy	11,935	11,935	11,550	11,935	11,550	11,935	11,935	10,780	11,935	11,550	11,935	11,550	140,525	11,710
Rx/Day	385.00	385.00	385.00	385.00	385.00	385.00	385.00	385.00	385.00	385.00	385.00	385.00		385.00
GRAND TOTAL:	**407,501**	**407,082**	**395,123**	**406,971**	**394,639**	**407,388**	**406,971**	**369,254**	**407,493**	**394,313**	**407,493**	**394,313**	**4,798,541**	**399,878**

Expense Budget

Pharmacy expenses can be divided into three categories: human resources, supplies, and other expenses.

Human Resource Expense

Human resource expense includes the salaries for all professional, technical, and support staff, and their benefits including insurance, workers compensation, disability, etc. The cost is typically stated as a percentage of the annual salary. Benefits costs can run as high as 25–30% in some markets. Benefit percentage for a budget calculation is typically provided by the CFO in the annual budget instructions. The pharmacy manager takes the number of approved positions in each job class (Pharmacist, Pharmacy Technician, Secretary, etc.) and multiplies them by the number of paid hours and the hourly rate for the year to arrive at the salary cost. Benefits are added as a percent of the final salary figure. A spreadsheet detailing the calculation for each incumbent employee and with vacant positions listed ensures a correct calculation. Projected raises and salary increases for the coming year should be included in this calculation. New positions added to the pharmacy service are typically added to this calculation during the budget review and approval process as they are approved.

Supply Expense

The vast majority of pharmacy supply expense is drugs, and the size and scope of drug expense have material impact on the hospital's overall budget. A thoughtful, well-supported supply budget for drugs is crucial for success. Forecasting drug and other supply expense is a combination of four factors: (1) price inflation, (2) drug utilization, (3) drug mix, and (4) a blend of utilization and mix representing expensive but innovative medications. The authors of a continuing series of articles examining trends in drug cost recommend a nine-step process to ensure success in forecasting this expense[3]:

- *Step 1*—Collect data. Historical purchase data can be gathered from wholesaler data systems and utilization data from hospital and pharmacy information systems. Group purchasing organizations provide reports on anticipated contract price changes and an annual forecast that serves as a resource for predictions of new drug approvals, adoption of recently approved drugs, generic drug introductions, and overall trends.

- *Step 2*—Review financial history. Evaluate the pharmacy's performance against budget for the most recent full fiscal year and for the current fiscal year (annualizing current fiscal year-to-date data). Compare actual fiscal year data to identify local inflationary trends by drug and, if possible, by disease, diagnosis, or service. Identify areas of exceptional variance for more detailed assessment. Review the performance of current cost containment efforts.

- *Step 3*—Build a high-priority drug budget. A relatively small number of drugs (50–60 products) represent 80–90% of total purchases and utilization in most health systems. Create a drug product-specific budget for these drugs based on historical utilization, and project changes in volume of use.

- *Step 4*—Build a new-product budget. Consider new drugs expected to be approved during the period covered by the budget. Work with prescribers to identify which new drugs will be used, how they will be used, and how often.

- *Step 5*—Build a nonformulary drug budget. Budget commonly used nonformulary products separately for financial monitoring purposes.

- *Step 6*—Build a low-priority drug budget. The low-priority drug budget represents a small portion of the total drug budget and can be safely budgeted as a lump sum. This component of the budget should be predicted on a volume-specific basis, taking into consideration any anticipated change in overall patient volume. Other medical supplies and general supplies can also be forecast using this method.

- *Step 7*—Establish a drug cost containment plan. Include drug-use-evaluation results indicating inappropriate prescribing, drug classes with multiple competing agents, and reports of successful cost-containment efforts published by other institutions. For each cost-containment target identified, produce a targeted prediction that includes the scope of the plan, what the intervention will entail (e.g., guideline implementation, formulary change), the timing of intervention implementation, and an estimate of the costs for a fully successful plan.

- *Step 8*—Finalize and present the total drug budget. The total drug budget is the sum of expected expenditures on the high priority list, new products, nonformulary agents, and low-priority products minus the total cost impact expected from the cost-containment plan. In many cases, the initial estimate of expenditures will be higher than hospital leadership is comfortable with. Using this budgeting model, requests for additional cuts can be met in a variety of ways.

- *Step 9*—Vigilance. Budgets established using the eight steps above provide a level of detail and a robust baseline for comparison with actual performance and variance reporting.

Other Fixed Expense

Other nonsupply expense generally varies only in response to inflation and price changes. Table 20-4 shows a full range of expenditures budgeted on this basis.

Revenue Budget

Although, as previously discussed, few payers actually pay full charge for pharmacy items, the development of a revenue budget remains an important component of the budget process. Charges offer an opportunity to track the operations of the pharmacy and serve as a proxy for net revenue after discounts and allowances.

Revenue can be predicted from workload volume and from supply expense. Because a detailed volume budget has been developed, the charges associated with this volume can be forecast. However, since most pharmacy charges are derived from the cost of service, including drug cost, it is important to account for the influence of changes in case mix and the influence if increased drug supply cost. Further, revenue targets set by the CFO may be set as an overall departmental gross revenue figure. It is incumbent on the pharmacy manager to develop a detailed plan that meets the big target using the expense budget.

Budgeting for a New Program

New pharmacy programs that involve operating expense should be considered carefully. New drug and supply expense, additional personnel, and other expenses merit careful consideration. The budget for a new pharmacy program is a smaller version of the process identified above. Rather than including these expenses "buried" in the entire budget, a spreadsheet identifying the costs by category as described above and as outlined in Tables 20-2 through 20-4 should be prepared. A narrative supporting the new program including objectives, program description, advantages, resources required, and a bottom line should be developed. Many organizations also consider indirect costs for new programs, although they are generally not a significant part of the annual budget process for the pharmacy.

Budget Negotiation, Review, and Approval

After all departments develop their budgets, they are returned to the CFO for a "roll-up" where they are all aggregated and a first version of a working health-system budget is created. Because the budget development process takes place at the department level, the resulting budget draft generally needs substantial work. The CFO works to balance the budget, to identify frank errors and problematic assumptions, and to develop a workable plan.

The institution's administration, led by the CEO and CFO set priorities for funding, ask departments to cut, reduce, or otherwise modify their budget requests. Some requests may be deferred to future years or denied outright. Budget development is both a rational and a political process; negations revolve around the organization's highest priorities and the quality of preparation and presentation made by the respective department leaders.

Pharmacy budgets developed as described above are evaluated against prior fiscal year experience to ensure that they are realistic and reasonable. The integrity of the development process and the level of support for key assumptions such as pharmacy volumes, drug price increases, and new drug adoption are also a factor in considering how the pharmacy budget is accepted. The track record of the pharmacy and pharmacy manager in meeting prior budgets often has significant influence on the outcome of the current budget review. A thoughtful, well-developed budget supported by data has the greatest chance of success and provides the health system with the best forecast of the future.

Monitoring the Budget

Volume, expense, and revenue data are collected in real time by the institution's data financial management systems. Monthly activity reports are provided to pharmacy managers. These reports should be reviewed and action taken to ensure that the pharmacy department meets targets set during the budget process. Alternatively, if changes occur, and the pharmacy will not meet the target set during the budget process, regular review will ensure that action is taken to resolve the problem or appropriately alter the budget to reflect the new reality.

Variance Analysis

Table 20-2 provides an example of a monthly operating statement for a pharmacy department. A *variance* is a difference between the budgeted amount and the actual amount spent for a period. Variances are typically evaluated monthly, and an assessment is made of the monthly variance and the variance from the start of the fiscal year to date. Variances can be described as positive (expenses lower than forecast; revenues higher than forecast) or negative (expenses higher than forecast; revenue lower than forecast). Variances can be absolute—the total actual amount is higher irrespective of volume—or volume-adjusted; the variance in cost cannot be explained solely by changes in activity volume.

Some variation in expense and revenue is expected. Pharmacy managers should consider the magnitude of variance based on their ability to control the associated cost or revenue. Human resource cost should be managed within 2% of forecast after volume adjustment. Drug expense is not as directly controlled by pharmacy; a 5–10% variance might be acceptable if explained by changes in CMI, prescribing practices or other variables. The absolute variation in expense may also be considered cause for review; typically a threshold is set by the CEO or CFO.

Determining the Cause of Variance

Table 20-5 is an example of a report designed to identify the nature of expense variance. To determine the sources of variance, the pharmacy manager must look at each category of expense that meets the threshold for investigation. Reasons for human resource expense variance might include an open position where expense was not incurred or the use of overtime to meet a specific patient care need. Supply expense might have a positive variance if a high-cost drug was released later than expected. Supply expense might show a negative variance if an outbreak of an infectious disease caused a higher than anticipated use of a costly antibiotic. Alternatively, supply expense might also increase if a shortage of medication caused the pharmacy to switch to a more costly drug or if prices rose faster than forecast. Both human resource and supply cost might be higher than anticipated if the hospital census was higher than budgeted.

Pharmacy leaders are expected to have a continuing, current understanding of the nature and source of expense variance. Their understanding should include both the business and clinical therapeutics understanding for which they are trained. The regular discipline of monthly analysis provides an opportunity to understand.

Integrating Cost and Revenue Analysis

As reimbursement for health care services has become more competitive, pharmacy managers have had to come to terms with profitability of services. Although it is tempting to examine the cost alone when working to determine the most appropriate course of action in management of drug use and pharmacy costs, the payment for a patient care service or DRG often creates the need to consider a more complex alternative. Does the hospital make or lose money on treating this type of case?

Most case rates are determined based on a standard practice or on a current norm. When a costly new drug or treatment is introduced or when treatment protocols or standards change, the cost of medications and the profitability of the case changes. Formulary additions, practice guidelines, and other decisions made by P&T committees and pharmacists should consider not only the cost and cost-benefit relationships associated with a particular drug therapy, but also the reimbursement received by the hospital. Revenues and costs are time-consuming to track in a health system. However, a thoughtful pharmacy leader must consider the implications of revenue and margin in choosing a course of action. This is a critical skill as high cost and high impact drugs are considered for use in a hospital.

Productivity Measurement and Benchmarking

Productivity measurement is a byproduct of the budgeting process. Productivity is defined using the following equation:

$$Productivity = Output/Input$$

Because the budget develops indicators of input (supply costs, hours worked, salary costs) and outputs (doses dispensed, patients treated, patients discharged) a baseline for productivity results. As discussed previously, the movement to a more knowledge and outcome based assessment of the impact of pharmacy has complicated the development and use of workload and productivity measures. Although we distinguished between fixed and variable costs earlier in the chapter, this distinction blurs when considered in a productivity

Table 20-4
Pharmacy Operating Budget

0415 INPATIENT PHARMACY	JUL	AUG	SEP	OCT	NOV	DEC	JAN	FEB	MAR	APR	MAY	JUN	TOTAL
PATIENT SERVICES REVENUE													
INPATIENT SERVICES													
3010102 ANCILLARY SERVICES	7,880,727	8,485,475	8,822,211	8,714,977	7,949,128	8,363,443	7,568,410	8,069,571	7,671,084	7,646,254	7,621,188	8,239,793	97,032,261
TOTAL INPATIENT REVENUE	7,880,727	8,485,475	8,822,211	8,714,977	7,949,128	8,363,443	7,568,410	8,069,571	7,671,084	7,646,254	7,621,188	8,239,793	97,032,261
OUTPATIENT SERVICES													
3010202 SPECIAL MEDICAL SERVICES	1,183,946	1,274,799	1,325,387	1,309,278	1,194,222	1,256,466	1,137,025	1,212,317	1,152,451	1,148,720	1,144,955	1,237,889	14,577,455
3010203 EMERGENCY SERVICES	102,952	110,852	115,251	113,850	103,845	109,258	98,872	105,419	100,213	99,889	99,561	107,643	1,267,605
TOTAL OUTPATIENT REVENUE	1,286,898	1,385,651	1,440,638	1,423,128	1,298,067	1,365,724	1,235,897	1,317,736	1,252,664	1,248,609	1,244,516	1,345,532	15,845,060
PATIENT SERVICES REVENUE	9,167,625	9,871,126	10,262,849	10,138,105	9,247,195	9,729,167	8,804,307	9,387,307	8,923,748	8,894,863	8,865,704	9,585,325	112,877,321
3020399 DEDUCTION FOR CONTRACTUAL	(5,075,959)	(5,653,838)	(5,900,828)	(5,803,603)	(5,292,160)	(5,449,855)	(4,905,266)	(5,130,224)	(4,890,408)	(4,876,444)	(4,935,855)	(5,233,475)	(63,147,915)
TOTAL CONTRACTUAL ADJUSTMENT	(5,075,959)	(5,653,838)	(5,900,828)	(5,803,603)	(5,292,160)	(5,449,855)	(4,905,266)	(5,130,224)	(4,890,408)	(4,876,444)	(4,935,855)	(5,233,475)	(63,147,915)
	1	1	1	1	1	1	1	1	1	1	1	1	12
NET PATIENT REVENUE	4,091,666	4,217,288	4,362,021	4,334,502	3,955,035	4,279,312	3,899,041	4,257,083	4,033,340	4,018,419	3,929,849	4,351,850	49,729,406
3040204 SALES–NP DRUG SALES	15,711	16,916	17,588	17,374	15,847	16,673	15,088	16,087	15,293	15,243	15,193	16,426	193,439
TOTAL OTHER OPERATING REVENUE	15,711	16,916	17,588	17,374	15,847	16,673	15,088	16,087	15,293	15,243	15,193	16,426	193,439
TOTAL REVENUE	4,107,377	4,234,204	4,379,609	4,351,876	3,970,882	4,295,985	3,914,129	4,273,170	4,048,633	4,033,662	3,945,042	4,368,276	49,922,845
4010101 SALARY–MGMT & SUPERVISION	32,243	32,485	32,485	31,216	32,703	34,388	31,700	30,191	34,720	31,700	33,210	33,210	390,251
4010102 SALARY–TECHNICIAN	359,852	360,198	361,293	344,871	364,614	382,704	350,186	333,908	384,153	351,847	369,005	371,322	4,333,953
4010106 SALARY–SUPPORT STAFF	9,957	10,043	10,043	9,586	10,043	10,650	9,723	9,261	10,724	9,791	10,257	10,257	120,335
4010107 SALARY–OTHER	2,057	2,057	2,057	1,964	2,057	2,151	1,964	1,870	2,151	1,964	2,057	2,119	24,468
TOTAL SALARIES	404,109	404,783	405,878	387,637	409,417	429,893	393,573	375,230	431,748	395,302	414,529	416,908	4,869,007
4010202 WAGES–TECHNICIAN	32,930	33,180	33,391	32,068	33,695	35,227	32,163	30,638	35,234	32,212	33,781	33,880	398,399
4010205 WAGES–AIDES & ORDERLIES	4,651	4,664	4,664	4,452	4,669	4,881	4,457	4,245	4,887	4,462	4,725	4,791	55,548
TOTAL WAGES	37,581	37,844	38,055	36,520	38,364	40,108	36,620	34,883	40,121	36,674	38,506	38,671	453,947
4010302 OVERTIME–TECHNICIAN	9,805	9,818	9,845	9,845	9,880	9,900	9,923	9,941	9,947	9,991	10,007	10,072	118,974
4010306 OVERTIME–SUPPORT STAFF	367	370	370	370	370	376	376	376	378	378	378	382	4,491
TOTAL SALARIES OVERTIME	10,172	10,188	10,215	10,215	10,250	10,276	10,299	10,317	10,325	10,369	10,385	10,454	123,465
4010406 OVERTIME–SUPPORT STAFF	171	172	172	172	172	172	172	172	172	172	174	176	2,069
TOTAL WAGE OVERTIME	171	172	172	172	172	172	172	172	172	172	174	176	2,069
4010502 SHIFT–DIFFERENTIAL TECHNICIAN	9,146	9,146	9,146	9,146	9,146	9,146	9,146	9,146	9,146	9,146	9,146	9,146	109,752
TOTAL SHIFT DIFFERENTIAL	9,146	9,146	9,146	9,146	9,146	9,146	9,146	9,146	9,146	9,146	9,146	9,146	109,752

Account	Total												
4010602 ON CALL—TECHNICIAN	3,144	262	262	262	262	262	262	262	262	262	262	262	262
TOTAL ON CALL		*262*	*262*	*262*	*262*	*262*	*262*	*262*	*262*	*262*	*262*	*262*	*262*
4010909 VACANCY REDUCTION—SALARY	(77,686)	(6,675)	(6,634)	(6,322)	(6,895)	(5,989)	(6,278)	(6,860)	(6,545)	(6,163)	(6,458)	(6,439)	(6,428)
TOTAL OTHER PERSONNEL	*(77,686)*	*(6,675)*	*(6,634)*	*(6,322)*	*(6,895)*	*(5,989)*	*(6,278)*	*(6,860)*	*(6,545)*	*(6,163)*	*(6,458)*	*(6,439)*	*(6,428)*
4020101 FICA	414,841	35,227	32,583	32,690	32,796	34,500	32,357	35,756	33,985	37,259	37,718	36,278	33,692
4020104 GROUP HEALTH INSURANCE	498,869	42,363	39,183	39,312	39,439	41,488	38,912	42,999	40,869	44,806	45,355	43,626	40,517
4020105 RETIREMENT BENEFITS	331,910	28,185	26,069	26,154	26,240	27,603	25,889	28,608	27,191	29,810	30,178	29,026	26,957
4020106 WORKER'S COMP INSURANCE	28,604	2,429	2,247	2,254	2,261	2,379	2,231	2,465	2,343	2,569	2,602	2,501	2,323
4020107 GROUP LIFE INSURANCE	22,032	1,871	1,730	1,736	1,742	1,832	1,718	1,899	1,805	1,979	2,004	1,927	1,789
4020109 DISABILITY INSURANCE	18,029	1,531	1,416	1,421	1,425	1,499	1,406	1,554	1,477	1,619	1,640	1,577	1,464
TOTAL EMPLOYEE BENEFITS	*1,314,285*	*111,606*	*103,228*	*103,567*	*103,903*	*109,301*	*102,513*	*113,281*	*107,670*	*118,042*	*119,497*	*114,935*	*106,742*
TOTAL PERSONNEL EXPENSE	**6,797,983**	**580,548**	**569,596**	**549,170**	**588,782**	**533,322**	**546,307**	**596,278**	**568,736**	**555,831**	**576,767**	**570,891**	**561,755**
4050201 DRUGS	18,157,177	1,519,980	1,384,655	1,402,981	1,382,728	1,508,429	1,385,952	1,534,187	1,456,395	1,636,774	1,647,390	1,573,726	1,723,980
4050202 INTRAVENOUS SUPPLIES	370,514	31,463	29,101	29,197	29,292	30,813	28,900	31,935	30,353	33,278	33,689	32,401	30,092
4050203 BLOOD & BLOOD PRODUCTS	5,084,006	453,616	440,773	428,451	454,651	424,396	426,834	469,026	447,582	450,639	465,707	458,717	163,614
4050206 REAGENT & CHEMICALS	111,623	9,479	8,767	8,796	8,825	9,283	8,706	9,621	9,144	10,025	10,150	9,761	9,066
4050503 GENERAL MED/SURG SUPPLY	154,514	13,121	12,136	12,176	12,215	12,850	12,052	13,318	12,658	13,878	14,049	13,512	12,549
TOTAL SPECIAL SUPPLIES	*23,877,834*	*2,027,659*	*1,875,432*	*1,881,601*	*1,887,711*	*1,985,771*	*1,862,444*	*2,058,087*	*1,956,132*	*2,144,594*	*2,170,985*	*2,088,117*	*1,939,301*
4060101 OFFICE SUPPLIES	6,023	511	473	475	476	501	470	519	493	541	548	527	489
4060301 OFFICE EQUIPMENT	699	59	55	55	55	58	55	60	57	63	64	61	57
4060305 COMMUNICATION EQUIPMENT	1,818	154	143	143	144	151	142	157	149	163	165	159	148
4060405 COMPUTER SUPPLIES	520	44	41	41	41	43	41	45	43	47	47	45	42
TOTAL GENERAL SUPPLIES	*9,060*	*768*	*712*	*714*	*716*	*753*	*708*	*781*	*742*	*814*	*824*	*792*	*736*
4080201 REPAIR OF MEDICAL EQUIP	2,826	240	222	223	223	235	220	244	231	254	258	247	229
4080202 REPAIR NON-MEDICAL EQUIP	1,137	97	89	90	90	95	89	98	93	102	103	99	92
4080401 FREIGHT	93	9	7	7	7	8	7	8	8	8	8	8	8
4080405 PRINTING	57,027	4,843	4,479	4,494	4,508	4,743	4,448	4,915	4,672	5,122	5,184	4,987	4,632
4080601 PHARMACY SCHOOL SERVICE CONTRACT	498,471	41,542	41,539	41,539	41,539	41,539	41,539	41,539	41,539	41,539	41,539	41,539	41,539
4080801 GENERAL SERVICES	348	30	27	27	28	29	27	30	29	31	32	30	28
TOTAL PURCHASED SERVICES	*559,902*	*46,761*	*46,363*	*46,380*	*46,395*	*46,649*	*46,330*	*46,834*	*46,572*	*47,056*	*47,124*	*46,910*	*46,528*
4140203 TELEPHONE	6,022	511	473	475	476	501	470	519	493	541	547	527	489
TOTAL OTHER EXPENSES	*6,022*	*511*	*473*	*475*	*476*	*501*	*470*	*519*	*493*	*541*	*547*	*527*	*489*
TOTAL NON-PERSONNEL EXPENSES	**24,452,818**	**2,075,699**	**1,922,980**	**1,929,170**	**1,935,298**	**2,033,674**	**1,909,952**	**2,106,221**	**2,003,939**	**2,193,005**	**2,219,480**	**2,136,346**	**1,987,054**
TOTAL OPERATING EXPENSES	**31,250,801**	**2,656,247**	**2,492,576**	**2,478,340**	**2,524,080**	**2,566,996**	**2,456,259**	**2,702,499**	**2,572,675**	**2,748,836**	**2,796,247**	**2,707,237**	**2,548,809**
TOTAL EXPENSES	**31,250,801**	**2,656,247**	**2,492,576**	**2,478,340**	**2,524,080**	**2,566,996**	**2,456,259**	**2,702,499**	**2,572,675**	**2,748,836**	**2,796,247**	**2,707,237**	**2,548,809**
NET EXCESS	**18,672,044**	**1,712,029**	**1,452,466**	**1,555,322**	**1,524,553**	**1,706,174**	**1,457,870**	**1,593,486**	**1,398,207**	**1,603,040**	**1,583,362**	**1,526,967**	**1,558,568**

measurement context. Although human resource costs and drug costs are variable over a typical operating variance, larger changes may not provide a direct unitary change.

Productivity measures can also be designed using detailed time and motion studies or through the use of external benchmarking. Time and motion studies determine the resources necessary to complete a task or set of tasks and set goals for improvement or change. External benchmarking uses data collected from peer institutions to set standards for performance. All three methods (budget, time and motion, benchmarking) seek to develop a ratio of input to output expressed as $ cost/unit of output or hours worked/unit of output. Table 20-6 lists examples of productivity measures that are in use in evaluating pharmacy services and medication therapy. Productivity measures based on doses charged or doses dispensed have significant negatives, because they do not measure the full range of pharmacy service activities and their related patient care outcomes.

External benchmarking is a process of measuring costs, services, and practices against the organization's peers or against industry leaders. The goal of external benchmarking is to find and implement the best practices of peer organizations. External benchmarking presents a significant challenge. The idea behind benchmarking is attractive, but because there is limited information about peer institutions, there is a chance that incorrect or inappropriate comparisons may be made. The real cause of differences shown in key ratios may result from factors outside the scope of the data being collected and compared. External benchmarking does offer an opportunity to identify variation in performance across a group of industry peers and to target opportunities for investigation. Excessively rigid or overly casual use of external cost and labor benchmarks can create significant problems. Internal benchmarking against prior department and health-system performance offers nearly the same improvement opportunities and achieves them in a more data-rich fashion. A full understanding of quality and safety issues, combined with a broad assessment of changes in case mix, programs, and other variables make internal benchmarking a more robust methodology. Because productivity and operational benchmarking lack a quality of care and outcome dimension, they are being displaced by *dashboard* and *scorecard* methodologies that incorporate indicators of quality and outcome into efficiency and effectiveness review.

Table 20-5
Pharmacy Expense Variance Report

Month	IP Revenue Actual	IP Revenue Budget	OP Revenue Actual	OP Revenue Budget	Total Revenue Actual	Total Revenue Budget	Revenue Difference	Difference %	Revenue: Expense Ratio Actual	Revenue: Expense Ratio Budget	Units of Service (UOS) Actual	Units of Service (UOS) Budget	Difference	Difference %
July	$8,527,162	$8,245,371	$4,646,435	$3,695,395	$13,173,597	$11,940,766	$1,232,831	10.3%	2.74	2.51	336,472	329,921	6,551	2.0%
August	$8,628,643	$8,533,718	$3,807,882	$3,865,367	$12,436,525	$12,399,085	$37,440	0.3%	2.53	2.61	404,417	349,201	55,216	15.8%
September	$8,829,684	$8,874,755	$4,983,629	$4,033,035	$13,813,313	$12,907,790	$905,523	7.0%	2.67	2.63	389,297	362,517	26,780	7.4%
October	$9,277,092	$8,768,942	$4,718,853	$4,199,857	$13,995,945	$12,968,799	$1,027,146	7.9%	2.89	2.60	394,874	361,667	33,207	9.2%
November	$9,768,914	$7,997,775	$3,896,291	$3,505,613	$13,665,205	$11,503,388	$2,161,817	18.8%	2.61	2.60	395,055	327,999	67,056	20.4%
December	$9,746,353	$8,416,325	$5,645,850	$4,143,021	$15,392,203	$12,559,346	$2,832,857	22.6%	2.90	2.53	373,987	348,401	25,586	7.3%
January														
February														
March														
April														
May														
June														
Total	$54,777,848	$50,836,886	$27,698,940	$23,442,288	$82,476,788	$74,279,174	$8,197,614	11.0%	2.72	2.58	2,294,102	2,079,706	214,396	10.3%
Projected Year End	$109,555,696	$101,673,772	$55,397,880	$46,884,576	$164,953,576	$74,279,174	$90,674,402	122.1%	2.72	1.29	4,588,204	4,159,412	428,792	10.3%

	Personnel Expenses Actual	Personnel Expenses Budget	Personnel Expenses Difference	Difference %	Drug Actual	Drug Budget	Drug Expense Difference	Difference %	Other Actual	Other Budget	Total Non-Personnel Expenses Actual	Total Non-Personnel Expenses Budget	Total Non-Personnel Expenses Difference	Difference %	Total Actual	Total Budget	Total Expense Difference	Difference %
Total																		
July	$1,008,779	$841,344	$167,435	19.9%	$3,251,167	$3,485,893	$(234,726)	-6.7%	$552,816	$428,391	$3,803,983	$3,914,284	$(110,301)	-2.8%	$4,812,762	$4,755,628	$57,134	1.2%
August	$890,164	$847,009	$43,155	5.1%	$3,351,488	$3,127,174	$224,314	7.2%	$673,339	$782,551	$4,024,827	$3,909,725	$115,102	2.9%	$4,914,991	$4,756,734	$158,257	3.3%
September	$833,353	$851,714	$(18,361)	-2.2%	$3,217,945	$3,317,227	$(99,282)	-3.0%	$1,116,671	$742,442	$4,334,616	$4,059,669	$274,947	6.8%	$5,167,969	$4,911,383	$256,586	5.2%
October	$857,321	$826,092	$31,229	3.8%	$3,249,268	$3,386,318	$(137,050)	-4.0%	$739,677	$774,846	$3,988,945	$4,161,164	$(172,219)	-4.1%	$4,846,266	$4,987,256	$(140,990)	-2.8%
November	$837,757	$789,400	$48,357	6.1%	$3,491,771	$2,952,081	$539,690	18.3%	$910,479	$686,702	$4,402,250	$3,638,783	$763,467	21.0%	$5,240,007	$4,428,183	$811,824	18.3%
December	$881,493	$905,202	$(23,709)	-2.6%	$3,539,117	$3,287,121	$251,996	7.7%	$895,089	$778,942	$4,434,206	$4,066,063	$368,143	9.1%	$5,315,699	$4,971,265	$344,434	6.9%
January																		
February																		
March																		
April																		
May																		
June																		
Total	$5,308,867	$5,060,761	$248,106	4.9%	$20,100,756	$19,555,814	$544,942	2.8%	$4,888,071	$4,193,874	$24,988,827	$23,749,688	$1,239,139	5.2%	$30,297,694	$28,810,449	$1,487,245	5.2%
Projected Year End	$10,617,734	$10,121,522	$496,212	4.9%	$40,201,512	$39,111,628	$1,089,884	2.8%	$9,776,142	$8,387,748	$49,977,654	$47,499,376	$2,478,278	5.2%	$60,595,388	$57,620,898	$2,974,490	5.2%

Month	Drug Cost per UOS Actual	Drug Cost per UOS Budget	Difference	Difference %	Salary Cost per UOS Actual	Salary Cost per UOS Budget	Difference	Difference %	Total Cost per UOS Actual	Total Cost per UOS Budget	Difference	Difference %	Revenue per UOS Actual	Revenue per UOS Budget	Difference	Difference %
July	$9.66	$10.57	$(0.90)	-8.5%	$2.55	$3.00	$0.45	17.6%	$14.30	$14.41	$(0.11)	-0.8%	$39.15	$36.19	$2.96	8.2%
August	$8.29	$8.96	$(0.67)	-7.5%	$2.43	$2.20	$(0.22)	-9.3%	$12.15	$13.62	$(1.47)	-10.8%	$30.75	$35.51	$(4.76)	-13.4%
September	$8.27	$9.15	$(0.88)	-9.7%	$2.35	$2.14	$(0.21)	-8.9%	$13.28	$13.55	$(0.27)	-2.0%	$35.48	$35.61	$(0.12)	-0.3%
October	$8.23	$9.36	$(1.13)	-12.1%	$2.28	$2.17	$(0.11)	-4.9%	$12.27	$13.79	$(1.52)	-11.0%	$35.44	$35.86	$(0.41)	-1.2%
November	$8.84	$9.00	$(0.16)	-1.8%	$2.41	$2.12	$(0.29)	-11.9%	$13.26	$13.50	$(0.24)	-1.8%	$34.59	$35.07	$(0.48)	-1.4%
December	$9.46	$9.43	$0.03	0.3%	$2.60	$2.36	$(0.24)	-9.3%	$14.21	$14.27	$(0.06)	-0.4%	$41.16	$36.05	$5.11	14.2%
January																
February																
March																
April																
May																
June																
Total	$8.76	$9.40	$(0.64)	-6.8%	$2.43	$2.31	$(0.12)	-4.9%	$13.21	$13.85	$(0.65)	-4.7%	$35.95	$35.72	$0.24	0.7%
Projected Year End	$8.76	$9.40	$(0.64)	-6.8%	$2.43	$2.31	$(0.12)	-4.9%	$13.21	$13.85	$(0.65)	-4.7%	$35.95	$35.72	$0.24	0.7%

Table 20-6

Example Pharmacy Productivity Ratios

Labor Productivity Ratios

Hours worked per adjusted patient day

Hours worked per adjusted discharge

Hours worked per 100 orders processed

Hours paid per adjusted patient day

Hours paid per adjusted discharge

Hours paid per 100 orders processed

Cost-Base Productivity Ratios

Drug cost per 100 orders processed

Supply cost per 100 orders processed

Labor cost per 100 orders processed

Total cost per 100 orders processed

Drug cost per adjusted patient day

Supply cost per adjusted patient day

Labor cost per adjusted patient day

Total cost per adjusted patient day

Drug cost per adjusted discharge

Supply cost per adjusted discharge

Labor cost per adjusted discharge

Total cost per adjusted discharge

Summary

Thoughtful financial management by pharmacy leadership is critical to the success of the organization's pharmaceutical care plan. Development of an organized data-based budget, monitoring of variance, and the assessment and management of costs and revenues supports the modern pharmacy department.

References

1. American Society of Health-System Pharmacists. ASHP guidelines: minimum standard for pharmaceutical services in ambulatory care. *Am J Health-Syst Pharm.* 1999;56:1744–53.

2. American Society of Health-System Pharmacists. ASHP guidelines: minimum standard for pharmacies in hospitals. *Am J Health-Syst Pharm.* 1995;52:2711–7.

3. Hoffman JM, Shah ND, Vermeulen LC, et al. Projecting future drug expenditures—2005. *Am J Health-Syst Pharm.* 2005;62:149–67

4. Murphy JE. Using benchmarking data to evaluate and support pharmacy programs in health systems. *Am J Health-Syst Pharm.* 2000;57(suppl 2):S28–31.

5. Knoer SJ, Could RJ, Folker T. Evaluating a benchmarking database and identifying cost reduction opportunities by diagnosis-related group. *Am J Health-Syst Pharm.* 1999;56(11):1102–7.

Chapter 21

Purchasing and Inventory Control

Jerrod Milton

Introduction

An effective purchasing and inventory control system requires the understanding and active participation of all pharmacy staff.

This chapter describes the basic principles of pharmaceutical purchasing and inventory control. It applies to all types of pharmacy settings including decentralized, centralized, home infusion, and ambulatory care pharmacy operations.

The Formulary System

Most hospitals and health care systems develop a list of medications that may be prescribed for patients in the institution or health care system. This list is usually called a formulary and serves as the cornerstone of the purchasing and inventory control system.[1-3] The formulary is developed and maintained by a committee of medical and allied health staff called the Pharmacy and Therapeutics (P&T) committee. This group generally comprises physicians, pharmacists, nurses, and administrators, although other disciplines may be present, including dieticians, risk managers, and case managers. They collaborate to ensure that the safest, most efficacious, and least costly medications are included on the formulary. The products on the hospital formulary dictate what the hospital pharmacy should keep in inventory. Third-party prescription drug benefit providers will also establish plan-specific formularies for their ambulatory patients. Ambulatory (retail) pharmacy staff frequently encounter insurance plan-specific drug formularies in serving their patients and adjust their inventory accordingly. Most retail pharmacies do not rigidly restrict items in their inventory, because in this setting, inventories are largely dependent on the dynamic needs of their patient population and, to some degree, their patients' respective insurance plans. Therefore, the concept of formulary management differs greatly depending on the perspective taken (e.g., that of the hospital compared with that of the retail pharmacy).

The hospital formulary is usually available in print form and may also be maintained in an online format. The formulary is produced exclusively for all health practitioners involved in prescribing, dispensing, and monitoring medications, and this tool is formatted generally to inform users of product availability, the appropriate therapeutic uses, and recommended dosing of medications. Most formularies are organized alphabetically by the generic drug's name, which is typically cross-referenced with the trade name products. In most cases, the drug storage areas in the pharmacy are arranged alphabetically by either the generic or trade name of the drug. Therefore, the formulary can help the pharmacy technician determine if a product is stocked in the pharmacy and where it would be.

Drugs are added and deleted from the formulary on a regular basis, but the frequency with which drugs are added or deleted varies among organizations. Formularies typically are updated every 12 to 18 months. Loose-leaf formularies and those maintained online can be updated continuously in a timelier manner, whereas bound formulary handbooks rely on supplementary updates or publication of serial editions.

Other important information that may be available in the formulary, specified under each listing, is the dosage form, strength, and concentration; package size(s); common side effects; and administration instructions. Some institutions also indicate the actual or relative cost of a given item. When selecting a drug product from inventory, the technician must consider all product characteristics, such as name, dosage form, strength, concentration, and package size (see Figure 21-1). Detailed review and consideration of each listing helps minimize errors in product selection.

Ordering Pharmaceuticals

Some pharmacies employ a dedicated purchasing agent to manage the procurement and inventory of pharmaceuticals; others employ a more general approach, whereby a variety of staff are involved in ordering pharmaceuticals.[4] The state-of-the-art practice involves

Figure 21-1
Formulary Listing

CEFTAZIDIME[1]   8:12.06[2]
   (Antibiotic)[3] (Fortaz®)[4]

Note: This product is restricted to Pulmonary Medicine, Hematology/Oncology or
Infectious Disease Service Approval.[5]

DOSAGE[6]

Neonates:
   Postnatal age less than 7 days: 100
      mg/kg divided q 12h
   Postnatal age greater than 7 days:
      Less than 1200 g: 100 mg/kg per day
         divided q 12h
      Greater than 1200 g: 150 mg/kg per
         day divided q 8h
   Infants & children 1 month to 12 yr.:
      100–150 mg/kg per day divided
      every 8 hours; Maximum = 6 g/day

Adjust dosage with creatinine clearance

INJECTION, 500 mg, 1 g & 2 g vials[7]

Formulary book listings usually include:
   [1] generic name, [2] numeric cross
   reference to the American Hospital
   Formulary Service, [3] class of drug,
   [4] proprietary/trade name,
   [5] restricted uses within the institution,
   [6] dosing information, and [7] dosage
   form and package sizes

the use of computer and Internet technology to manage the process of purchasing and receiving pharmaceuticals from a drug wholesaler.[5] This technology
includes using bar codes and hand-held computer
devices for online procurement and purchase order
generation and for electronic receiving processes. Using
computer technology for these purposes has many
benefits, including up-to-the-minute product availability information, comprehensive reporting capabilities,
accuracy, and efficiency. It also encourages compliance
with various pharmaceutical purchasing contracts.

Receiving and Storing Pharmaceuticals

Receiving is one of the most important parts of the
pharmacy operation. A poorly organized and executed
receiving system can put patients at risk and elevate
health care costs. For example, if the wrong concentration of a product were received in error, it could lead
to a dosing error or a delay in therapy. Misplaced products or out-of-stock products also jeopardize patient
care as well as the efficiency of the department—both
are undesirable and costly outcomes.

The Receiving Process

Some pharmacies create processes whereby, as much
as possible, the person receiving pharmaceuticals is
different from the person ordering them. This process
is especially important for controlled substances
because it effectively establishes a check in the system
to minimize potential drug-diversion opportunities.

   In a reliable and efficient receiving system, the
receiving personnel verify that the shipment is complete
and intact (i.e., they check for missing or damaged
items) before putting items into circulation or inventory.[2] The receiving process begins with the verification
of the boxes containing pharmaceuticals delivered by
the shipper. The person receiving the shipment begins
the process by verifying that the name and address on
the boxes is correct and that the number of boxes
matches the shipping manifest. Many drug wholesalers
use rigid plastic crates because they protect the contents of each shipment better than foam or cardboard
boxes. These crates are also environmentally friendly
because they are returned to the wholesaler for cleaning and reuse. Regardless, each box should be inspected for gross damage.

   Products with a cold storage requirement (i.e.,
refrigeration or freezing) should be processed first. The
shipper is responsible for taking measures to ensure
the cold storage environment is maintained during the
shipment process and will generally package these
items in a shippable foam cooler that includes frozen
cold packs to keep products at the correct storage temperature during shipment.

   Receiving personnel play a critical role in protecting
the pharmacy from financial responsibility for products
damaged in shipment, products not ordered, and products not received. Any obvious damage or other discrepancies with the shipment, such as a breach in the
cold storage environment or an incorrect product,
should be noted on the shipping manifest, and, if warranted, that part of the shipment should be refused.
Ideally, identifying gross shipment damage or incorrect
box-counts should be performed in the presence of the
delivery person and should be well-documented when
signing for the order. Other problems identified after
delivery personnel have left, such as mispicks, product
dating, or internally damaged goods, must be resolved
according to the vendor's policies. Most vendors have
specific procedures to follow in reporting and resolving
these sorts of discrepancies.

   The next step of the receiving process entails checking the newly delivered products against the receiving

copy of the purchase order. This generally occurs after the delivery person has left. A purchase order, created when the order is placed, is a complete list of the items that were ordered. Traditionally, a purchase order will be executed in multiple copies, including an original file copy, a copy used in the receiving process, and a copy for the supplier (see Figure 21-2).

Figure 21-2
Documenting Receipt on a Purchase Order

PURCHASE ORDER
Department of Pharmacy Services
Community Hospital
1 Valley Road
Suburbia, MD 20777
(333) 555-1010

Purchase Order
No. 0849
THIS NUMBER MUST APPEAR ON ALL INVOICES, PACKING SLIPS, BILLS, PACKAGES AND CARTONS

Vendor: Pharmaceutical Labs
185 Commerce Ave.
Ft. Washington, PA
1-800-555-3753
Acc# 123-12345

BY_____DIRECTOR
PHARMACY SERVICES/DESIGNEE

ORDER DATE	FOB		DATE REQUIRED IN HOSPITAL	TERMS	DEPARTMENT	SHIP VIA
4/1/97	☐ HOSPITAL	☐ SHIPPING POINT	ASAP	N/A	Pharmacy	Standard

QUANTITY RECEIVED	ORDERED	DESCRIPTION	UNIT PRICE	AMOUNT
4	5	Orimune 50 × 1	$450.00	$2,250.00
50	50	Haemophilus B Vaccine Via 4s	$ 52.92	
13	12	Piperacillin 40 g Vial each	$110.00	$2,646.00
30	30	DPT Vaccine Vial 7.5 ml each	$ 56.50	
		Quantity received as indicated / one vial of piperacillin broken in shipment.		$1,320.00
				$1,695.00
		Joe Johnson, Pharmacy Technician 4/15/97		

1. Goods not in accordance with specifications will be rejected and held at vendor's risk awaiting disposal. Vendor must pay transportation both ways on all rejected material.
2. The right is reserved to cancel all or part of this order if not delivered within the time specified.
3. No price change allowed unless authorized by this office.
4. Packing slips must accompany all shipments.
5. All shipments must be prepaid.
6. Equipment supplied under this purchase order must meet all applicable O.S.H.A. Standards.

The quantity received is recorded in the "received" column by the person receiving the order. Damaged merchandise is noted on the purchase order, and the receiver signs and dates the receipt. This information enables the purchasing agent to confirm back orders, address mechanisms for retaining or returning overages, and determine financial accountability for damaged merchandise.

The person responsible for checking products into inventory uses the receiving copy. This ensures that the products ordered have been received. The name, brand, dosage form, size of the package, concentration strength, and quantity of product must match the purchase order. Once the accuracy of the shipment is confirmed, the purchase order copy is generally signed and dated by the person receiving the shipment (Figure 21-2). At this point, the product's expiration date should be checked to ensure that it meets the department's minimum expiration date requirement.

Frequently, departments will require that products received have a minimum shelf life of 6 months remaining before they expire. It is noteworthy to mention that on occasion, the manufacturer/wholesaler inadvertently may ship an excess quantity of an ordered product to the pharmacy. The ethical response is to notify the manufacturer or wholesaler of this situation immediately and subsequently arrange for the return of any excess quantity.

Controlled substances require additional processing on receipt.[2,6] Regulations specific to Schedule II controlled substances require Drug Enforcement Administration (DEA) form 222 to be completed on receipt of these products and filed separately with a copy of the invoice and packing slip accompanying each shipment. If a pharmacist or pharmacy technician other than the receiving technician removes a product from a shipment before it has been properly received and cannot locate the receiving copy of the purchase order, then a written record of receipt should be created. This is done by listing the product, dosage form, concentration/strength, package size, and quantity on a blank piece of paper (see Figure 21-3) or the supplier's packing slip/invoice and checking off the line item received (see Figure 21-4). In both cases, the name of the person receiving the product should be included, and the document should be given to the receiving technician to avoid confusion and an unnecessary call to the wholesaler or manufacturer.

The Storing Process

Once the product has been received properly, it must be stored properly.[7] Depending on the size and type of the pharmacy operation, the product may be placed in a bulk, central storage area or into the active dispensing areas of the pharmacy. In any case, the expiration date of the product should be compared with the products currently in stock. Products already in stock that have expired should be removed. Products that will expire in the near future should be highlighted and placed in the front of the shelf or bin. This is a common practice known as stock rotation. The newly acquired products will generally have longer shelf lives and should be placed behind packages that will expire before them. Stock rotation is an important inventory management principle that encourages the use of products before they expire and helps prevent the use of expired products and waste. Table 21-1 identifies the optimum storage temperatures and humidity.

Figure 21-3
Receipt of Pharmaceutical on Blank Piece of Paper

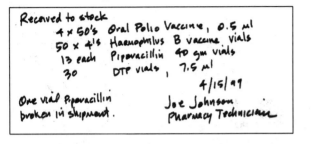

Received to stock
  4 x 50's   Oral Polio Vaccine, 0.5 ml
 50 x 4's   Haemophilus B vaccine vials
 13 each   Pipavacillin 40 gm vials
   30   DTP vials, 7.5 ml
                              4/15/99

One vial Pipavacillin
broken in shipment.   Joe Johnson
                             Pharmacy Technician

Figure 21-4
Receipt of Pharmaceutical on Packing Slip/Invoice

Invoice

Shipper	Buyer
Pharmaceutical Labs	Community Hospital
185 Commerce Avenue	1 Valley Road
Ft. Washington, PA	Suburbia, MD 20777

Invoice # 12346
Invoice Date 4/01/97

Quantity		Product #	Product Description	Unit Price	Amount
5	4 rec.	6190	Orimune 50 × 1	$450.00	$2,250.00
4	✓	7183	Haemophilus B Vaccine	$ 52.92	$2,646.00
13	12 rec.	4391	Piperacillin 40 g Vial	$110.00	$1,320.00
30	✓	2727	DPT Vaccine 7.5ml Vial	$ 56.50	$1,695.00

Quantity received as indicated
one vial Pipavacillin broken in shipment.
Received 4 x 50's Orimune
          50   Haemophilus B Vaccine
          13   Piperacillin 40 gm vial
          30   DTP Vaccine 7.5 ml
                        4/15/99
                   Joe Johnson
                   Pharmacy Technician

Product Handling Considerations

The Role of the Pharmacy Technician

Pharmacy technicians usually spend more time handling and preparing medications than do pharmacists. This presents pharmacy technicians with the critical responsibility of assessing and evaluating each product from both a content and a labeling standpoint. It also provides the technician with an opportunity to confirm that the receiving process was performed properly.

Just as checking the product label carefully at the time a prescription or medication order is filled is important, taking the same care when receiving pharmaceuticals and accurately placing them in their storage location is essential. The pharmacy technician should read product packaging carefully, rather than rely on the general appearance of the product (e.g., packaging type, size or shape, color, logo), because a product's appearance may change frequently and may be similar to other products. Technicians play a vital role in minimizing dispensing errors that may occur because of human fallibility. They are generally the first in a series of checks involved in an accurate dispensing process.

When performing purchasing or inventory management roles, the technician must pay close attention to the product's expiration date. For liquids or injectable products, the color and clarity of the items should also be checked for consistency with the product standard. Products with visible particles, an unusual appearance, or a broken seal should be reported to the pharmacist.

Because pharmacy technicians handle so many products each day, they are in a perfect position to identify packaging and storage issues that could lead to errors. The technician should pay close attention to these three main issues:

1. *Look-Alike/Sound-Alike Products*—Stocking products of similar color, shape, and size could result in error if someone fails to read the label carefully. All staff members should be alerted to look-alike or sound-alike products (see Figure 21-5).[9]

2. *Misleading Labels*—Sometimes the company name or logo is emphasized on the label instead of the drug name, concentration, or strength (see Figure 21-6).[10]

3. *Product Storage*—Storing products that are similar in appearance adjacent to one another can result in error if someone fails to read the label (see Figure 21-7).[11]

Alerting other staff members to products that fall into one of these categories is essential. Some pharmacies routinely discuss product-handling considerations at staff meetings or in departmental newsletters—dispensing errors may be averted by simply relocating a look-alike/sound-alike product or by placing warning notes (i.e., auxiliary labeling or highlights) on the shelf or directly on the product itself. Pharmacy technicians should also discuss their concerns with coworkers and advocate changes to products with poor labeling.

Table 21-1
Defined Storage Temperatures and Humidity[8]

Freezer	(-)25° to (-)10°C	(-)13° to 14°F
Cold (Refrigerated)	2° to 8°C	36° to 46°F
Cool	8° to 15°C	46° to 59°F
Room Temperature	The temperature prevailing in a working area	
Controlled Room Temperature	20° to 25°C	68° to 77°F
Warm	30° to 40°C	86° to 104°F
Excessive Heat	Any temperature above 40°C (104°F)	
Dry Place	A place that does not exceed 40% average relative humidity at controlled room temperature or the equivalent water vapor pressure at other temperatures. Storage in a container validated to protect the article from moisture vapor, including storage in bulk, is considered a dry place.	

Maintaining and Managing Inventory

An inventory management system is an organized approach designed to maintain just the right amount of pharmaceutical products in the pharmacy at all times. A variety of inventory management systems are used, ranging from simple to complex. They include the order book, the minimum/maximum (par) level, the Pareto (ABC) Analysis, the economic order quantity (EOQ), product storage and, finally, the fully automated, computerized system.[3]

Economic Models

The Pareto ABC analysis is also known as the 80/20 rule, and it essentially groups inventory products by aggregate value and volume of use into three groupings (A, B, and C). This analysis is useful in determining where inventory control efforts are best directed. For example, group A may include 10% of all items that make up 70% of the inventory cost. Tight control over these items would be sensible. Group B may include 20% of items and 15% of the inventory cost. An automatic order cycle might be useful here based on well-established par levels. Group C may include 70% of items and 10% of the inventory cost. Less aggressive monitoring of these items may be justifiable.

The EOQ is a model for calculating inventory order quantities and is also known as the Minimum Cost Quantity approach. In essence, this approach is an accounting formula used to determine the point at which the combination of order costs and inventory holding costs are minimized. One variation of the EOQ formula is as follows:

EOQ relies heavily on the accuracy of various data inputs, such as annual product usage, fixed costs associated with each order (including processing the purchase order, receiving, inspection, processing the invoice, vendor payment, and inbound freight costs), and the annual cost per average on-hand inventory unit. If calculated accurately, it results in the most cost-efficient order quantity. Economists would argue that anytime one has repetitive purchasing tasks, EOQ should be considered. Some organizations may find EOQ useful in aspects of their operation; applying it universally is relatively difficult in pharmacy practice because of the wide variability of the individual patient's pharmaceutical needs. Therefore, some pharmacies may find it useful to use a combination of the systems mentioned here.

Automation

The ideal system for inventory management is an automated or computerized system that supports a just-in-time product inventory.[12] Just-in-time inventory management is a philosophy that simply means products are ordered and delivered at just the right time—when they are needed for patient care—with a goal of minimizing wasted steps, labor, and cost. Pharmaceuticals are neither overstocked nor understocked. In pharmacy, this business philosophy couples responsible financial

Figure 21-5
Look-Alike/Sound-Alike Products

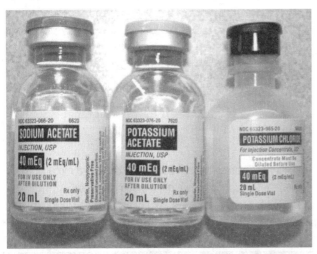

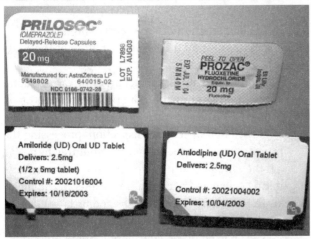

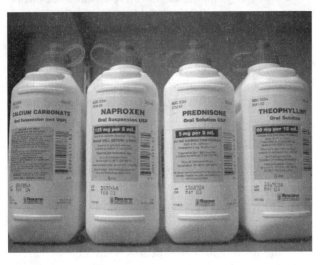

management of pharmaceutical purchasing with the clinical aspects of patient care. A related business philosophy is known as maximizing inventory turns, which means that because a product should not sit on the shelf, unused for long periods of time, specific drug inventory ideally is purchased and used many times throughout the course of a year. A simple means of calculating inventory turns in a given period is to divide the total purchases in that period by the value of physical inventory taken at one point in time. For example, if total pharmaceutical purchases for fiscal year (FY) 2004 were $10,243,590, and the physical inventory value on 12/31/2003 was $521,550, then the calculated inventory turns for FY2004 would be 19.6 times ($10,243,590/$521,550 = 19.6). This method assumes a relatively constant volume of pharmaceutical purchases and constant residual inventory over time.

The economic principle is simple: One does not want to buy pharmaceuticals that won't be used in a timely manner. Minimizing inventory carrying costs (or holding costs) is an important aspect of sound business administration. Carrying cost can be defined as all costs associated with inventory investment and storage costs, which might include interest, insurance, taxes, and storage expenses.

Although automated inventory management modalities are available, they are not the mainstay in practice today. Generally, today, a manual inventory management system is employed. Manual systems require the active oversight of pharmacy technicians and are usually based on a minimum/maximum, or par-level, system. Staff may create a pharmaceutical order using a hand-held bar-code scanning device or may enter product stock numbers directly into a personal computer. Manual systems typically involve a minimum/maximum, or par-level, shelf-sticker that corresponds to each product. The minimum and maximum inventory level is written on this label, and the information is used as a relative guide for pharmacy staff involved in purchasing. To that end, staff strive to maintain pharmaceutical inventories within the minimum to maximum range to avoid running short on a product or overstocking. Running short on a product may affect patient care, and overstocking adds unnecessary expense to the organization. This system requires pharmacy staff to routinely scan inventory levels and place orders accordingly. With either the electronic or manual system, pharmacy staff should realize that the diversity of their patients' specific needs may require modification in a particular product's par-level. In the fully

Figure 21-6
Product Labeling—Emphasis on Manufacturer Name

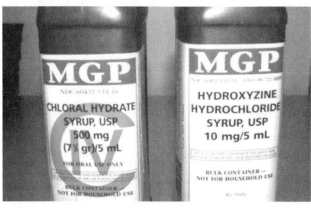

Figure 21-7
Product Inventory—Shelf Position

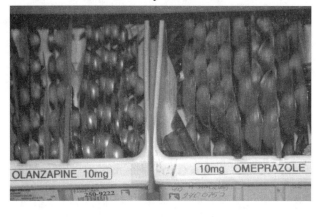

computerized inventory system, each dispensing transaction is subtracted from the perpetual inventory log that is maintained electronically in the computer; conversely, all products received are added to the inventory log. When the quantity of a pharmaceutical product in stock reaches a predetermined point (often called par or par-level), a purchase order is automatically generated to order more of the product. The system does not depend on any one employee to monitor the inventory or to reorder pharmaceuticals. The technology is available to have a computerized inventory in most pharmacies, but interfacing a computerized inventory system with existing pharmacy computer systems designed for dispensing and patient management systems is often difficult. In addition, other variables, such

as product availability, contract changes, and changing use patterns (either up or down), make relying on the fully computerized model challenging. Consequently, even the most sophisticated electronic or automated systems will require human oversight.

The use of automated dispensing devices in inpatient hospital nursing units, clinics, operating rooms, and emergency rooms has facilitated the use of computers for inventory management. Similar devices are evolving in retail pharmacy and hold promise for not only making the dispensing process safer and more efficient but also serving, possibly, to assist in inventory management. These devices are essentially repositories, or pharmaceutical vending machines, for medications that will be dispensed directly from a patient care area. A variety of manufacturers of automated dispensing devices are in the market today. The Pyxis Medstation, Meditrol, Omnicell, and SureMed are examples of products available to institutions today. These machines generally are networked via a dedicated computer file server within the facility, and they allow both unit-dose and bulk pharmaceuticals to be stocked securely on a given patient care unit location. Each unit's inventory is configurable and allows for variation and flexibility from device to device, depending on the unit's location. The machines are capable of tracking perpetual inventory at the product level. They also limit access to only authorized personnel, record the identities of those who access inventory, and record how much of a specific drug was removed for a given patient. A useful feature in many of these systems allows pharmacy personnel to automatically generate a fill-list of what needs to be replenished on the basis of a par-level system. In essence, the nursing and medical personnel who use these automated dispensing devices have a computerized inventory and billing system that the pharmacy staff manages. Medications used to restock these devices may be taken from the pharmacy's main inventory, or a separate purchase order may be executed for each device on a periodic basis.

The minimum/maximum, or par-level, inventory system relies on a predetermined order quantity and an order point. Shelf labels are placed on the storage bin or shelf to alert all staff to the minimum stock quantity (see Figure 21-8). The pharmacy technician should always determine if the minimum stock quantity has been reached when removing a product and inform the appropriate purchasing personnel or list the item on a designated order book as described below. An assigned staff member performs a periodic inventory of

Figure 21-8
Shelf Labels

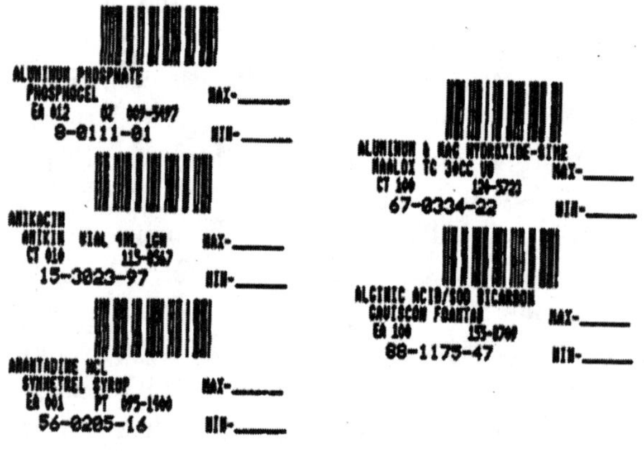

the stock to identify products that have a stock level at or below the reorder point. When the inventory is reduced to, or below, the order point, designated pharmacy personnel initiate a purchase order, or electronically transmit a purchase order, to a drug wholesaler.

Many pharmacies will use an order book system, also called a want list or want book. When pharmacists or pharmacy technicians determine that a product should be reordered, they write the item in the order book. Although this approach is simple, it provides the least amount of organized control over inventory. Its success is highly dependent on the participation of staff. Therefore, the order book system is usually not the sole method of inventory management and is often used in conjunction with one of the other systems mentioned previously.

Drug Recalls

A manufacturer, on its own or at the direction of the Food and Drug Administration (FDA), will occasionally recall pharmaceuticals for such reasons as mislabeling, contamination, lack of potency, lack of adherence to the acceptable Good Manufacturing Practices, or other situations that may present a significant risk to public health. A pharmacy must have a system for rapid removal of any recalled products.[2]

Role of the Food and Drug Administration

The FDA plays an active role in initiating the drug-recall process. It coordinates drug recall information, helps manufacturers and distributors develop specific recall plans, and performs health hazard evaluations to assess the risk facing the public by products being recalled. It also classifies recall actions in accordance with the level of risk and formulates recall strategies on the basis of the health hazard presented by the product in addition to other factors, including the extent of distribution of the product to be recalled. It decides on the need for public warnings and assists the recalling agency with public notification about the recall as needed. The following are the top 10 reasons for drug recalls in 2003[13]:

1. cGMP deviations
2. Subpotency
3. Stability data does not support expiration date
4. Generic drug or new drug application discrepancies
5. Dissolution failure
6. Label mix-ups
7. Content uniformity failure
8. Presence of foreign substance
9. pH Failures
10. Microbrial contamination of nonsterile products

Role of Manufacturer/Distributor

Because of their responsibility to protect the public consumer, manufacturers or distributors typically implement voluntary recalls when a marketed drug product needs to be removed from the market. This method of recall is more efficient and effective in ensuring timely consumer protection than an FDA-initiated court action or seizure of the product. Recall notices are sent in writing to pharmacies by the manufacturer of the product or by drug wholesalers. These notices indicate the reason for the recall, the name of the recalled product, the manufacturer, all affected lot numbers of the product, and instructions on how to return the product to the manufacturer. On receipt of the recall notice, a pharmacy staff member, usually a pharmacy technician, will check all pharmaceutical inventory stores to determine if any recalled products are in stock. If none of the recalled products are in stock, a note indicating "none in stock" is written on the recall notice and filed in a recall log to document that the recall was properly addressed. If a recalled product is in stock, all products should be gathered, packaged, and returned to the manufacturer according to the instructions on the recall notice. The package should be reviewed by the pharmacist in charge before returning it to the manufacturer. If patients have received a recalled product, the pharmacist in charge must take the recommended action. On completion of all activity regarding the product recall, a summary of actions taken should be documented on the recall letter and filed in the pharmaceutical recall log. The FDA has been known to request documentation of all recall activities to ensure compliance and, ultimately, patient safety. The technician should keep in mind that it may be necessary to order replacement stock to compensate for recalled items that were removed from stock. In some instances, the recall may encompass all products, and it will be impossible to order replacement stock.

The pharmacist in charge should be notified in this case because he or she will need to decide which, if any, alternative products may be required to place into inventory as therapeutic alternatives to the out-of-stock items.

Drug Shortages

Occasionally, manufacturers will be unable to supply a pharmaceutical because of various supply and demand situations. This may involve the inability to obtain raw materials, manufacturing difficulties related to equipment failure, or simply the inability to produce sufficient quantities to stay ahead of the market demand for the pharmaceutical. Although unfortunate, drug shortages are a reality that must be dealt with to avoid compromising patient care. As with drug recalls, the pharmacist in charge should be notified so he or she can communicate drug shortages and recommend alternative therapies effectively to prescribers.

Ordering and Borrowing Pharmaceuticals

Pharmaceutical Purchasing Groups

Most health-system pharmacies are members of a group purchasing organization (GPO).[4,14] Health systems and hospitals join together in a purchasing group to leverage buying power collectively and take advantage of any lower prices manufacturers offer to large groups that can guarantee a significant volume of orders over long periods of time (typically 1 to 2 years). Retail, chain pharmacies also are able to negotiate better pricing based on volume. Contracts may involve sole-source or multisource products. Sole-source products are products available from only one manufacturer, whereas multisource products (frequently termed

generic products) are available from numerous manufacturers. Sole-source products may be produced from only one manufacturer; however, the product may be included in what is known as a competitive market basket (i.e., proton-pump-inhibitors, such as omeprazole and lansoprazole), where competing brand-only products are on the market.

GPOs negotiate purchasing contracts that are mutually favorable to members of the group and to manufacturers. In addition to lower prices, pharmacies also benefit because this reduces the time staff spend establishing and managing purchasing contracts with product vendors. A GPO guarantees the price for pharmaceuticals over the established contract period, which may be 1 year or more. With the purchase price predetermined, the pharmacy can order the product directly from the manufacturer or from a wholesale supplier. Occasionally, manufacturers are unable to supply a given product that the pharmacy is buying on contract, which may require the pharmacy to buy or substitute a competing product not on contract at a higher cost. Most purchasing contracts will include language to protect the pharmacy from incurring additional expenses in the event this occurs. Generally, the manufacturer will be liable to rebate the difference in cost back to the pharmacy when this occurs. Therefore, it is important that the pharmacy technician documents any resulting off-contract purchases and shares these with the pharmacist in charge for reconciliation with the contracted product vendor.

Direct Purchasing

Direct purchasing from a manufacturer involves the execution of a purchase order from the pharmacy to the manufacturer of the drug. The advantages of direct purchasing include not having to pay handling fees to a third-party wholesaler, the ability to order on an infrequent basis (e.g., once a month), and a less demanding system for monitoring inventory. Some disadvantages include the following: a large storage capacity is needed; a large amount of cash is invested in inventory; the pharmacy's return/credit process becomes more complicated; and staff resources required in the pharmacy and accounts payable department to prepare, process, and pay purchase orders to more companies is increased. Other disadvantages have to do with the likelihood that the manufacturer's warehouse is not local in relation to the pharmacy, which creates a dependency on the shipping firms used by the manufacturers to ship products reliably. In addition, the delivery schedule is often unpredictable or not available on weekends, and there may be delays in delivery.

For most pharmacies, the disadvantages of direct ordering outweigh the advantages. As a result, most pharmacies primarily purchase through a drug wholesaler. Some drugs, however, can be purchased only directly from the manufacturers. These products generally require unique control or storage conditions. Consequently, most pharmacies will have a combination of direct purchases from manufacturers and drug wholesalers.

Drug Wholesaler Purchasing/Prime Vendor Purchasing

Purchasing from a drug wholesaler permits the acquisition of drug products from different manufacturers through a single vendor. When a health-system pharmacy agrees to purchase most (90–95%) of its pharmaceuticals from a single wholesale company, a prime vendor arrangement is established, and, customarily, a contract between the pharmacy and the drug wholesaler is developed. Usually, wholesalers agree to deliver 95–98% of the items on schedule and offer a 24-hour/ 7-day-per week emergency service. They also provide the pharmacy with electronic order entry/receiving devices, a computer system for ordering, bar-coded shelf stickers, and a printer for order confirmation printouts. They may also offer a highly competitive discount (minus 1–2%) below product cost/contract pricing and competitive alternate contract pricing. Some wholesalers will offer even larger discounts to pharmacies that may prefer a prepayment arrangement. In these situations, the wholesaler monitors the aggregate purchases of the pharmacy (e.g., a rolling 3-month average) and bills the pharmacy this amount in advance (prepayment). This may be attractive to both the wholesaler and the pharmacy because it creates larger cash flow and investment capital for the wholesaler while saving the organization money on its pharmaceutical purchases.

These wholesaler services make the establishment of a prime vendor contract appealing and result in the following advantages: more timely ordering and delivery, less time spent creating purchase orders, fewer inventory carrying costs, less documentation, computer-generated lists of pharmaceuticals purchased, and overall simplification of the credit and return process.

Purchasing through a prime vendor customarily allows for drugs to be received shortly before use, supporting the just-in-time ordering philosophy mentioned earlier in this chapter. Purchasing from a wholesaler is a highly efficient and cost-effective approach toward pharmaceutical purchasing and inventory management.

Borrowing Pharmaceuticals

No matter how effective a purchasing system is, there will be times when the pharmacy must borrow drugs from other pharmacies. Most pharmacies have policies and procedures addressing this situation. Borrowing or loaning drugs between pharmacies is usually restricted to emergency situations and limited to authorized staff.

Borrowing is also limited to products that are commercially available, thus eliminating items such as compounded products or investigational medications. Most pharmacies have developed forms to document and track merchandise that is borrowed or loaned (see Figure 21-9). These forms also help staff document the details imperative to error-free transactions.

The pharmacy department's borrow and loan policies and procedures should provide detailed directions on how to borrow and loan products, which products may be borrowed or loaned, sources for the products, and reconciliation of borrow-loan transactions (the pay-back process). Securing the borrowed item may require the use of a transport or courier service or may include the use of security staff or other designated personnel. This information is vital for pharmacy technicians to understand and fulfill their responsibility when borrowing and loaning products.

Products Requiring Special Handling

Most pharmaceuticals will be handled and processed in the inventorying and purchasing systems described above, with the exception of controlled substances, investigational drugs, compounded products, repackaged drugs, and drug samples.

Controlled Substances

Controlled substances have specific ordering, receiving, storage, dispensing, inventory, record-keeping, return, waste, and disposal requirements established under the law. The Pharmacist's Manual: An Informational Outline of the Controlled Substances Act of 1970 and the ASHP Technical Assistance Bulletin on Institutional Use of Controlled Substances provide detailed information on the specific handling requirements for controlled substances.[6]

Figure 21-9
Borrow/Loan Form

```
                    Community Pharmacy
                         555-3779
Borrowed                              Lent
   From: _____  To: _____
Drug: _____
Amount: _____
              (# of vials, tablets, etc. and bulk or unit dose packaging)
Date:_____  By: _____
◆◆◆◆◆◆◆◆◆◆◆◆◆◆◆◆◆◆◆◆◆◆◆◆◆◆◆◆◆◆◆◆◆◆◆◆◆◆◆◆◆◆◆◆◆◆◆◆◆◆◆◆◆◆◆◆◆◆◆◆◆◆◆◆
Date ordered:_____From: _____ By: _____
Date returned:_____By: _____
Date in Loan Book:_____By: _____
Value: $_____
```

In some pharmacies, pharmacy technicians work with pharmacists to manage inventory and order, dispense, store, and control narcotics and other controlled substances. The pharmacy technician should know two principles regarding controlled substances: (1) Ordering and receiving Schedule II controlled substances requires special order forms and additional time (1 to 3 days), and (2) these substances are inventoried and tracked continuously. This type of inventory method is referred to as a perpetual inventory process, whereby each dose or packaged unit, such as a tablet, vial, or mL of fluid volume, is accounted for at all times.

Investigational Drugs

Investigational drugs also require special ordering, inventorying, and handling procedures. Generally, the use of investigational drugs is categorized into two distinct areas: (1) in a formal protocol approved by the institution, and (2) for a single patient on a one-time basis that has been authorized by the manufacturer and the FDA. In both cases, the physician may be responsible for the ordering, and the pharmacy staff handles the inventory management of the investigational drug.

Some pharmacies associated with academic affiliations or institutions conducting clinical research may have formally organized investigational drug services managed by a pharmacist principally dedicated to pharmaceutical research activities. In these cases, the investigational drug service pharmacist may be responsible for the ordering, dispensing, and inventory management of investigational drugs according to the research protocol.

Compounded Products

Compounded pharmaceuticals are another type of product handled by pharmacy personnel, and, unlike drugs ordered from an outside source, compounded products are extemporaneously prepared in the pharmacy as indicated by scientific compounding formulas. These products may include oral liquids, topical preparations, solid dosage forms, or sterile products.

The use of these products requires that prescribing patterns and expiration dates be monitored closely. Compounded products typically have short expiration dates ranging from days to months. Because it is pharmacy technicians who likely will identify usage patterns and determine stock and product needs, procedures for monitoring patient use, product expiration dates, and additional stock needs must be well-known and adhered to by technicians to prevent stock shortages. Specific pharmacy technicians may initiate compounding activities, but this may vary according to departmental procedures.

Repackaged Pharmaceuticals

Although manufacturers supply many drugs in a prepackaged unit dose form, the pharmacy staff is responsible for packaging some products. These items are generally unit-dose tablets and capsules, unit-dose oral liquids, and some bulk packages of oral solids and liquids. Each pharmacy establishes stocking mechanisms for these products and relies on pharmacy technicians to identify and respond to production and stock needs. Generally, designated technicians coordinate repackaging activities, but some pharmacies may integrate repackaging with other pharmacy technician responsibilities. Knowledge of the department's procedures for repackaging is required to prevent disruptions in dispensing activities.

Nonformulary Items

Nonformulary items also require special handling. No matter how much planning is devoted to formulary management, some patients will still need medications not routinely stocked in the pharmacy. The pharmacist usually determines when a nonformulary medication should be ordered into stock. However, the pharmacy technician is often in the best position to monitor the supply and determine when and if additional quantities should be ordered. Nonformulary medications generally are not mixed into the shelving system of formulary products in the pharmacy; they fall outside normal inventorying mechanisms. Often, manual tracking mechanisms and computer system queries of active nonformulary orders are the two most common techniques used to monitor and order these products.

Medication Samples

The last products requiring special handling are medication samples. Traditional inventory management and handling practices do not work well with medication samples for two reasons. First, medication samples are not ordered by the pharmacy—they are usually provided to physicians on request by the drug manufacturer free of charge. This often occurs without the pharmacy's knowledge. Second, samples are not usually dispensed by the pharmacy. These factors make it difficult to know whom to contact if a medication sample is recalled and to ensure that medication samples are not sold. Because of difficulties in controlling samples, organizations may allow samples to be stored and dispensed in ambulatory clinics only after being registered with the pharmacy for tracking purposes. These difficult logistical and control factors have led many organizations to adopt policies that simply disallow medication samples altogether.

If an organization does allow samples, they will probably be stored outside the pharmacy and require that pharmacy personnel register and inspect the stock of medication samples. Pharmacy technicians are sometimes involved in inspecting medication sample storage units. These technicians are often responsible for determining if a sample is registered with the pharmacy, stored in acceptable quantities, labeled with an expiration date that has not been exceeded, and, generally, stored under acceptable conditions. Many hospitals strive to maintain compliance with the standards of the Joint Commission on Accreditation of Healthcare Organizations (JCAHO). Its standards on medication management are intended to promote consistently safe practices related to the procurement, storage, dispensing, and administration of pharmaceuticals and the use of sample drug products that fall into this standard.

Proper Disposal and Return of Pharmaceuticals

Expired Pharmaceuticals

The most common reason drugs are returned to the manufacturer is because they are expired. Each year, approximately 2% of all drugs shipped to pharmacies are returned to the manufacturer.[15] The process for returning drugs in the original manufacturer packaging is relatively simple and not particularly time-consuming when done routinely. Returning expired products to the manufacturer or wholesaler prevents the inadvertent use of these products while enabling the department to receive either full or partial credit for them. Some wholesalers limit credit given on returns of short-dated products. Generally, wholesalers will not give full credit on returns of products that will expire within 6 months. To return products, pharmacy personnel must complete the documentation required by the product's manufacturer or wholesaler and package the product so it can be shipped. Many wholesalers have implemented electronic documentation systems to further simplify the return process.

Technicians often perform these duties under the supervision of a pharmacist. Some pharmacies contract with an outside vendor that completes the documentation and coordinates the return of these products for an agreed on fee. In that case, the pharmacy technician need only assist the returned goods vendor with the location and packaging of expired pharmaceuticals.

Pharmaceuticals compounded or repackaged by the pharmacy department cannot be returned and, for safety reasons, must be disposed of after they have expired. Proper disposal prevents the use of subpotent products or products without guaranteed sterility. The precise procedure for disposal depends on the type and content of the product. Some products, such as expired repackaged solids, can be disposed of using the general trash removal system, whereas others, such as expired compounded cytotoxic products, must be disposed of according to hazardous waste removal procedures. Each pharmacy has detailed procedures for hazardous waste removal, and the pharmacy technician should be familiar with these procedures. Disposal of expired compounded or repackaged pharmaceuticals by the pharmacy technician should be completed under the supervision of the pharmacist.

Other products requiring disposal rather than return are chemicals used in the pharmacy laboratory. Most pharmacies will stock a supply of chemical-grade products used in extemporaneous pharmaceutical compounding. Examples of chemical products include sodium benzoate or sodium citrate (preservatives), lactose or talc (excipients), buffers, and active ingredients, such as hydrocortisone, triamcinolone, neomycin, or lidocaine powders. When such products expire, they should be disposed of in accordance with the pharmacy's hazardous waste procedures.

Figure 21-10
DEA Form 41 (Registrants Inventory of Drugs Surrendered)

OMB Approval No. 1117 - 0007	U. S. Department of Justice / Drug Enforcement Administration **REGISTRANTS INVENTORY OF DRUGS SURRENDERED**	PACKAGE NO.

The following schedule is an inventory of controlled substances which is hereby surrendered to you for proper disposition.

FROM: *(Include Name, Street, City, State and ZIP Code in space provided below.)*

Signature of applicant or authorized agent

Registrant's DEA Number

Registrant's Telephone Number

NOTE: CERTIFIED MAIL (Return Receipt Requested) IS REQUIRED FOR SHIPMENTS OF DRUGS VIA U.S. POSTAL SERVICE. See instructions on reverse (page 2) of form.

NAME OF DRUG OR PREPARATION	Number of Containers	CONTENTS (Number of grams, tablets, ounces or other units per container)	Controlled Substance Content, (Each Unit)	FOR DEA USE ONLY		
				DISPOSITION	QUANTITY	
					GMS.	MGS.
Registrants will fill in Columns 1,2,3, and 4 ONLY.						
1	*2*	*3*	*4*	*5*	*6*	*7*
1						
2						
3						
4						
5						
6						
7						
8						
9						
10						
11						
12						
13						
14						
15						
16						

FORM DEA-41 (9-01) Previous edition dated **6-86** is usable. *See instructions on reverse (page 2) of form.*

Source: Drug Enforcement Administration. Available at: http://www.deadiversion.usdoj.gov/21cfr_reports/surrend/41/41_blank.pdf

Expired controlled substances are disposed of uniquely. These products may not be returned to the manufacturer or wholesaler for credit. They must be destroyed, and the destruction must be documented to the satisfaction of the DEA.[6] The DEA provides a specific form, titled "Registrant's Inventory of Drugs Surrendered" (Form 41), for recording the disposal of expired controlled substances (see Figure 21-10). Ideally, the actual disposal of expired controlled substances should be completed by a company sanctioned by the DEA or by a representative of the state board of pharmacy. In other cases, the DEA may allow the destruction of controlled substances by a pharmacy, provided the appropriate witness process is followed and documented. The DEA disposal of controlled substances form should be completed properly and submitted to the DEA immediately after the disposal. A copy of the record of disposal form will be signed by a DEA representative and returned to the pharmacy, where it is kept on file. Previously, the DEA allowed .for shipment of expired controlled substances and the completed disposal form to the regional DEA office, but this practice is no longer permitted.

The usage and disposition of investigational drugs must also be documented carefully. Expired investigational drugs should be returned to the manufacturer or sponsor of an investigational drug study according to the instructions they provide. Investigational drug products that expire because of product instability or sterility issues should never be discarded. These doses should be retained with the investigational drug stock and be clearly marked as expired drug products because the investigational study sponsor will need to review and account for all expired investigational drug products.

Pharmaceuticals that need to be returned because of an ordering error require authorization from the original supplier and the appropriate forms. The Prescription Drug Marketing Act mandates that pharmacies authorize and retain records of returned pharmaceuticals to prevent potential diversion of pharmaceuticals. The pharmacy technician must be familiar with pharmacy department procedures for returning medications to a supplier. Typically, a pharmacy will have a process for returning misordered medications to the prime drug wholesaler on a routine basis, which prevents the need for storage in the pharmacy of overstocked or misordered products. The pharmacy technician may be responsible for relevant documentation, filing paperwork, and packaging returned products under the supervision of the pharmacist.

Summary

The movement of pharmaceuticals into and out of the pharmacy requires an organized, systematic, and cooperative approach. Each pharmacy staff member plays a role in the management of their pharmacy's system.

References

1. American Society of Hospital Pharmacists (ASHP). ASHP statement on the formulary system. *Am J Hosp Pharm.* 1983;40:1384–5.

2. Soares DP. Quality assurance standards for purchasing and inventory control. *Am J Hosp Pharm.* 1985;42: 610–20.

3. Bicket WJ, Gagnon JP. Purchasing and inventory control for hospital pharmacies. *Top Hosp Pharm Manage.* 1987;7(2):59–74.

4. Yost DR, Flowers DM. New roles for wholesalers in hospital drug distribution. *Top Hosp Pharm Manage.* 1987;7(2):84–90.

5. Roffe BD, Powell MF. Quality assurance aspects of purchasing and inventory control. *Top Hosp Pharm Manage.* 1983;3(3):62–74.

6. US Department of Justice Drug Enforcement Administration. Pharmacist's manual: an informational outline of the Controlled Substances Act of 1970. Washington, DC: DEA; April 2004. Available at: http://www.deadiversion.usdoj.gov/pubs/manuals/ pharm2/pharm_manual.htm. Accessed May, 2005.

7. Joint Commission on Accreditation of Healthcare Organizations (JCAHO). *Hospital Accreditation Standards 2005.* Oakbrook Terrace, IL: JCAHO; 2005. MM11–13.

8. United States Pharmacopeia (USP). *USP 28/The National Formulary 23.* Rockville, MD: USP; 2004:10.

9. Joint Commission on Accreditation of Healthcare Organizations (JCAHO). *Hospital Accreditation Standards 2005.* Oakbrook Terrace, IL: JCAHO; 2005. NPSG3.

10. Cohen MR. *Medication Errors.* Washington, DC: American Pharmaceutical Association; 1999. p13.1-13.22.

11. Cohen MR. *Medication Errors.* Washington, DC: American Pharmaceutical Association; 1999:9.1–9.9.

12. Hughes TW. Automating the purchasing and inventory control functions. *Am J Hosp Pharm.* 1985;42:1101–7.

13. US Food and Drug Administration/Center for Drug Evaluation and Research. Report to the nation— improving public health through human drugs. Washington, DC: FDA; 2003. Available at: http://www.fda.gov/cder/reports/rtn/2003/Rtn2003.pdf. Accessed May, 2005.

14. Wetrich JG. Group purchasing: an overview. *Am J Hosp Pharm.* 1987;44:1581–92.

15. Orey M. Cottage industry finds niche in expired drugs. *WSJ (Eastern Ed).* New York: Aug 29, 2001:B.1.

Chapter 22

The Policy and Procedure Manual

David J. Tomich, George J. Dydek

Introduction

Over the past couple of decades the practice of pharmacy has undergone many changes. The forces responsible for these changes have been numerous, including automation, computerization, new drug therapies, utilization of pharmacy technicians, advanced training for pharmacists, introduction of government regulation, growth of professional organizations, and society shifts. Change has fostered the revision of pharmacy practice standards and the creation of many new ones. Incorporating new standards into the operational dynamics of a department of pharmacy presents a challenge to the health-system pharmacy manager.

Development and implementation of practice standards in health-system pharmacy can be traced to the 1950s when the American Society of Hospital Pharmacists adopted the minimum standard for pharmacies in hospitals.[1] These standards charged the director of pharmacy with responsibility for development and implementation of rules and regulations to be utilized for the operation of the pharmacy department within the hospital.

Today, the minimum standard for pharmacies in hospitals as adopted by American Society of Health-System Pharmacists states, "An operations manual governing pharmacy functions (e.g., administrative, operational, and clinical) shall exist."[2] Beyond basic policies and procedures necessary for the appropriate conduct of business, the manual should include long-term goals for the pharmacy. The manual must be revised when necessary to reflect changes in policies, procedures, organizations, and objectives. All personnel should be familiar with the contents of their manual. Appropriate mechanisms to ensure compliance with the policies and procedures should be established." Guidance regarding pharmacy policies and procedures can also be found in the American Society of Health-System Pharmacists Technical Assistance Bulletin on Hospital Drug Distribution and Control.[3]

Development and maintenance of a policy and procedure manual can provide an efficient and systematic approach to manage change. The purpose of this chapter is to discuss the processes for writing policies and procedures and provide guidance on developing and maintaining a policy and procedure manual.

Definitions

Before discussing the development of the manual and how-to-write policies and procedures, it is important to understand the definition and purpose of policies and procedures. Webster defines *policy* as "a definite course or method of action selected from among alternatives and in light of given conditions to guide and determine present and future decisions" and *procedure* as "a particular way of accomplishing something or of acting; a step in a procedure or a series of steps followed in a regular definite order."[4] Policies are written statements that provide guidance on the position and values of an organization. They are often considered broad operating guidelines, but they should clearly define the direction and activities of an organization or department. An example of a policy for a Department of Pharmacy might be for Reporting Adverse Drug Reactions (ADR). The policy might sound something like, "To establish a systematic continuous process to monitor, assess, and improve ADR reporting and management at Generic Medical Center."

Procedures are written instructions that describe the recommended methods of sequential steps to follow to perform a task or activity. In short, procedures help define the process for completing a task. They might be considered the instruction manual that goes with each policy, which outlines how a policy is to be carried out or followed. For the example policy above on Reporting Adverse Drug Reactions, the procedure might look something like this "The ADR will be reported by any health care provider witnessing the

---

The opinions or assertions contained herein are the private views of the authors and are not to be construed as official or reflecting the views of the U.S. Department of Army or the Department of Defense.

reaction through any of the following ADR reporting options:

- Contacting the Clinical Pharmacist assigned to the ward or clinic
- Calling the ADR telephone reporting system 123-RASH (123-7274) and leaving the requested information on voicemail
- Sending an email using a hospital network computer system (HNCS) with patient information, description of the reaction, suspected medication and provider information
- Completing Hospital Form 1698 and sending a copy to the Department of Pharmacy

Benefits of the Policy and Procedure Manual

Aside from any requirements, many benefits can be derived from a well-developed and maintained policy and procedure manual including the following:

- *Improving Inter- and Intra-Departmental Communication*—The content of policies and procedures identifies and explains what is to be done by whom, when, where, and how. Having a policy and procedure manual that allows personnel in and outside of the department or organization to learn how daily operations and business practices are conducted. An example of this could be using the information in a policy to answer questions from nursing, medical staff, or patients. Standardization of the information minimizes communication breakdowns or process malfunction. Procedures that are well-defined and documented make it easier and more efficient to share information amongst staff to assure that a particular task is performed the same way. Medication errors may be minimized when all staff in the organization understand and operate from the same policies and procedures.

- *Creation of Standards of Care*—Creating and utilizing policies and procedures promotes standardization of services. Developing metrics based on content of the policy and procedure can be measured and tracked over time. Data can be benchmarked with comparisons and changes made to improve a service process, etc.

- *A Mechanism to Document Standards of Care and Other Important Activities*—Publishing the policy and procedure manual serves to formally identify standards of practice and care. This can be important for risk management cases and potential litigation that may occur. Or it could be used against you if not followed carefully.

- *Enhancement of Staff Orientation and Training*—The policy and procedure manual; because it is an organized collection of how to work or operate in the department becomes the conduit for standardized learning. It gives new employees the opportunity to "get up to speed" quickly with vital information necessary to function within the department and organization. Likewise, when policies or procedures are changed, staff can refer to the updated manual for new information.

- *Improvement and Maintenance of Staff Morale*—Recruiting staff in the process of revising or developing policies and procedures can create pride and satisfaction. It lets the staff know that management values their opinion and work.

- *Ability to Systematically, Objectively, and Efficiently Measure Staff and Departmental Performance*—Policies and procedures are standards for performing tasks and conducting business. Management can utilize the policy and procedure manual to direct and mentor staff by holding them accountable for performing according to standards. Performance of both individuals and the department can be measured and monitored.

- *A Source of Information*—The policy and procedure manual is the "go to" source for information pertaining to the operational aspects of the department. The content is designed by the department or organization and, therefore, is generally not available in other resources.

- *Quality Improvement Processes*—Standards in the manual can be measured and outcomes tracked and assessed over time. This provides the organization or department a mechanism to modify polices and/or procedures to improve performance and services. A complete review of the manual should be done at least annually.

- *Cost Effective Use of Resources*—The manual can save time and money. Policies and procedures provide rules and regulations for the staff. Adopting standards for operating procedures takes the guess work out of performing tasks. There is less chance of having to repeat processes and waste time and materials. Answers for many recurring questions can also be answered efficiently. Staff will not have to chase down a solution to problems or research answers to questions each time a situation presents itself.

- *Effective Administrative Tool for Planning, Developing, and Improving Pharmacy Services and Patient Care*—The process of developing policies and procedures promotes teamwork and camaraderie among staff in and outside the department. It provides the department a mechanism to review and evaluate all of the important aspects and correct inefficiencies.

- *Comprehensive Source*—The manual should be recognized by every individual in a department of pharmacy as *the* comprehensive source of information relevant to the daily operation of the entire department. It should contain all of the policies and procedures for the department. The contents must be current, accurate, and readily available.

Writing Policies and Procedures

Writing policies and procedures will usually take practice and time. There have been several books written on this process.[5,6] While there are some similarities, creating a policy requires a different approach than writing a procedure.

Format and Style

Policies and procedures can have many formats. The format and style of each policy and procedure document will vary depending on the organization and practice environment. Some organizations have adopted conventions for every department to follow when developing policies and procedures.

Many policies and procedures contain the following format:

- *The Purpose*—This section explains the objective of the policy and procedure. This is usually summarized in a few sentences. It should state the benefits of the policy to both staff and organization.

- *A History Section*—The history section provides the reader with the date when the policy and procedure was originally approved and any modifications, to include the date of the modifications. This information provides a snapshot of practice environment and philosophy over time.

- *Personnel Affected by the Policy and Procedure*—This section identifies who is impacted by the policy. This can vary widely from a few individuals to the entire organization or patient population.

- *The Policy Statement*—The policy statement should contain a statement of justification. The statement should be general but not too broad that it is meaningless.

- *References for the Policy*—This section should contain all pertinent references, which serve as the basis of the policy. This may include citations of regulation or law, journal articles, books, other manuals, etc.

6. *Policy Number*—Numbering policies and procedures provides a way to organize the manual and provide the reader with an easy convenient method to access the policies. Various numbering schemes have been developed, so choose one that best fits your pharmacy department's needs. Once a policy has been deleted the number assigned to that policy should either be retired or if used again, staff should be informed regarding its use. This will avoid any confusion.

7. *Use of Definitions, Terms, Acronyms, Words, or Abbreviations*—This section contains the explanation of words, terminology, and other syntax. Do not assume the reader will understand the terminology in the policy and procedure. If staff is expected to comply with policy they need to understand what it is they are reading. Do not take short cuts.

8. *Responsibilities for Personnel Involved with the Procedure*—The information in this section identifies who is responsible for what.

9. *The Procedure*—This is a key section. It should define how the policy is to be carried out. This should include step-by-step methods for completing a task. Action words should always be used. Language should be succinct and clear. An active voice should be used. Use of diagrams can be useful to help explain complex processes. The amount of detail to include or the number of steps required to describe a procedure depends on the policy, environment, skill level of staff, etc. Do not skip over important parts of the process. However, too much detail or complexity will make it difficult for staff to process the required information contained in the procedure. This will almost guarantee failure. When the procedure is in the draft stage, include a variety of staff in the

review process. This will save time and yield a better product. Do not work in a vacuum!

Other helpful hints when writing policies and procedures:

- Use clear concise writing
- Use positive statements
- Use present tense, active verbs
- If abbreviations are used, provide a definition of them

Consider the skills, education, and experience of the reader and the work culture and specific environment.

Examples of policies and procedures can be found on the worldwide web and in books. Never forget to network with colleagues to get help with development of policies and procedures. They may be able to share examples. Consult with the appropriate administrator in the organization for guidance as needed.

Several example formats of policies and procedures are located at the end of the chapter (Appendices 22-1, 22-2, and 22-3). Take some time and review the format and content of each. Refer back to the discussion on each section above to reinforce the purpose of each section.

Process for Drafting and Implementing Policies and Procedures

The process for writing meaningful policies and procedures can be time consuming. Table 22-1 provides an example outline for guiding the writer through the process. With experience, managers will develop a mechanism that works for their department. Do not be afraid to experiment.

Content and Format of the Policy and Procedure Manual

Like the individual policies and procedures contained in the manual, the format, content, and style of policy and procedure manuals will vary based on the organization and practice environment. An example content outline for a policy and procedure manual is located at the end of the chapter (Appendix 22-4). A pharmacy department policy and procedure manual often contains several common sections or divisions: (1) general information; (2) administrative information; and (3) professional practice. The general information section usually contains policies pertaining to the general operation of the organization and department. This

may include the mission statements, goals and objectives, scope of services, patients served, institutional philosophy, and organizational charts. It will often include a preamble or preface that introduces the reader to content of the manual, subject matter experts and authors of the manual, definitions or conventions used throughout the manual, processes of developing and approving the policies and procedures, and procedures for reviewing the manual. The administrative section may contain policies such as standards of operation, human resource management, resource and fiscal management, departmental and organizational relationships, safety, and security. The professional practice section usually contains the meat of the policy and procedure manual. It contains policies addressing topics such as medication use and management. This includes procurement, storage, preparation, and distribution of medications, investigational drugs, controlled substances, and clinical services.

A well-designed policy and procedure manual contains many cross-referenced policies, both inter- and intradepartmental. By design, this will provide the staff with a clear vision on how policies and procedures provide a common pathway for identifying and obtaining goals and objectives throughout the organization. It is important to remember that the format for each policy and procedure should be consistent and follow a logical sequence. This will make it easier for staff to become oriented to the content and format of the manual. If the format is not user friendly and the content pertinent, chances are the manual may be used as a doorstop instead of a "go to" reference.

Distribution of the Policy and Procedure Manual

Once the policy and procedure manual is approved it is ready for distribution. Distribution can be accomplished in a variety of methods. The electronic medium available today allows an organization to distribute policies to many locations. Desktop PCs, networks, laptops, and Personal Digital Assistants (PDAs) are now commonplace in the health care environment. The electronic medium offers many advantages over a paper medium including ease of access, graphic display, and ability to make quick edits or modifications, resulting in decreased costs to maintain and update the manual. Policies and procedures can be posted on websites for easy access. Web-based technology also allows links between pages for cross-referencing poli-

Table 22-1

Steps to Developing a Policy and Procedure Manual

1. Assign an individual to be accountable for oversight of the development, implementation, review, and maintenance of the policy.

2. Before writing, take the time to research the topic for which a policy and procedure are being written. Ask the following questions: What should the policy state and why? Whom will the policy affect? What data or information is needed to support the policy? What information is needed to define the procedure? What steps are necessary for the procedure?

3. Develop a policy team composed of staff and management with subject matter expertise. Include individuals from both in and outside the department. Having input from other departments within an organization can save time, minimize the number of revisions, and create a more robust policy.

4. Develop a draft of the policy and procedure. The draft should be written in the style and format defined by the department or organization (see above guidance).

5. Have the draft reviewed by staff, not part of the policy team. Getting the staff involved in the process of policy and procedure development can save time as stated above. Asking staff to review draft copies of proposed policy and procedure provides management a "reality check" to assure the policy is likely to achieve what it claims.

6. Modify draft to incorporate any recommended changes as appropriate.

7. Redistribute the draft for review by staff again.

8. Distribute modified draft to other outside departments, such as risk management, quality assurance department, or legal department for their review and approval as required or needed.

9. Modify draft to incorporate any recommended changes as appropriate.

10. Distribute the draft for final review to all in the review process.

11. Make any final changes to the draft prior to submission for approval by the approving authority.

12. Once approved, inform and educate all staff affected by the policy.

13. Update the Policy and Procedure manual with the revised or new policy and procedure.

15. Select a date to evaluate the impact of the policy and procedure.

16. Evaluate the effectiveness of the policy and procedure. This can be accomplished by designing outcome metrics to measure and evaluate.

17. Modify policy as necessary to improve effectiveness through the steps above.

18. Periodically review the policies and procedures, at least annually or when appropriate.

cies. If paper is the only medium that is used to distribute the manual, management needs to assure that enough copies are printed and available for staff in the work environment. Remember, the more copies distributed, the more diligent you must be in ensuring updates are distributed.

Revision of Policies and Procedures

Once the policies and procedures have been implemented, at some point an assessment should be made to determine if the policies are effective and the procedures are current and accurate. If the policies do not appear to be effective, reconvene a group and find out why they are not effective. All policies and procedures should be reviewed on a regular basis. They should reflect current practice, and policies that are obsolete should be deleted. Procedures change as practice changes so developing and maintaining a policy and procedure manual is a dynamic process. Applying the Deming Plan-Do-Check-Act (PDCA) Cycle[7] to develop and maintain policies and procedures can be helpful.

Summary

As the practice of institutional pharmacy has evolved, the operational dynamics of a department of pharmacy have become complex. The institutional pharmacy must adapt to constant change. Development and maintenance of a policy and procedure manual can provide the pharmacy manager a valuable tool to manage such change. The policy and procedure manual should be regarded as a living, breathing document. It should be maintained to reflect current standards of practice in the organization and department. Therefore, it is important to assure that all policies are routinely reviewed and updated on a regular basis and that the staff is properly oriented to the use of the policy and procedure manual.

References

1. *The Minimum Standard for Hospital Pharmacies.* Bethesda, MD: American Society of Hospital Pharmacists; 1950.

2. *Best Practices for Health-System Pharmacy: Positions and Guidance Documents of ASHP. 2002–2003 Edition.* Bethesda, MD: American Society of Health-System Pharmacists; 2003.

3. Drug distribution and control: distribution. ASHP technical assistance bulletin on hospital drug distribution and control. Bethesda, MD: American Society of Health-System Pharmacists.

4. Merriam-Webster Online Dictionary. Available at: http://www.m-w.com.

5. Page SB, ed. *Establishing a System of Policies and Procedures.* Westerville, OH: Process Improvement Publishing; 2002.

6. Page SB, ed. *7 Steps to Better Written Policies and Procedures.* Westerville, OH: Process Improvement Publishing; 2004.

7. Gitlow H, Gitlow S, Oppenheim A, et al. *Tools and Methods for the Improvement of Quality.* Homewood, IL: Irwin, Inc.; 1989.

Appendix 22-1
Administration Policies and Procedures—Introduction

Policy 1-1   **20 September 2005**

I. PURPOSE. To assign responsibility for the contents, establishment, and annual review of all policies and procedures for the operation of the Department of Pharmacy.

II. REFERENCES

    A. Hospital Policy (Regulation) 40-3, Chapter 11.

    B. *Accreditation Manual for Hospitals.*

    C. *Best Practices for Health-System Pharmacy: Positions and Guidance Documents of ASHP.* Bethesda, MD: American Society Health-System Pharmacists.

III. APPLICABILITY. The provisions of these policies and procedures are applicable to all personnel assigned to the Department of Pharmacy.

IV. RESPONSIBILITIES

    A. The Director, Department of Pharmacy is responsible for the establishment and contents of all policies and procedures.

    B. The Administrative Office of the Department of Pharmacy will ensure that all policies and procedures are reviewed annually.

    C. Service Directors and Section Supervisors will ensure that assigned personnel adhere to established policies and procedures and that service policies and procedures are updated as required.

    D. All assigned pharmacy personnel will conform to the provisions of published policies and procedures and are responsible for reviewing these policies and procedures on an annual basis.

V. PROCEDURES. All policies and procedures will be reviewed and updated as necessary and at least annually according to the following schedule:

Service	Review Date
Administration	Jan–Jul
Ambulatory Care	Mar–Jun
Inpatient Care	Mar–Jun
Specialty Pharmacies	May–Aug
Hematology/Oncology	Jul–Oct
Nuclear	Jul–Oct
Supply Support/Informatics	Sep–Dec

// Original Signed //
Name Here
Director, Department of Pharmacy

Appendix 22-2
Administration—Provision of Patient Care

Policy 1-2

I. PURPOSE. To describe how the care needs of patients and the patient population are assessed and met.

II. REFERENCES

A. Hospital Policy (Regulation) 40-3, Chapter 11, Pharmacy Management.

B. *Accreditation Manual for Hospitals.*

III. APPLICABILITY. This Policy and Procedure is applicable to all personnel assigned and/or attached to the Department of Pharmacy.

IV. RESPONSIBILITIES The Director, Department of Pharmacy is responsible for the establishment and contents of this policy and procedure.

V. PROCEDURES

A. Scope of Services

1. The Department of Pharmacy is a contemporary hospital pharmacy offering sound, well-balanced, and innovative pharmaceutical services. It is organized on a centralized basis with an inpatient pharmacy, a main ambulatory care pharmacy, and refill pharmacy. The major functions of the Department of Pharmacy's scope of care include preparation and dispensing of medications; distribution and control of medications; and provision of clinical pharmacy services.

2. Purchasing and administrative support for all pharmacy locations is provided by the main pharmacy. Additional pharmacy areas specializing in Hematology-Oncology, Nuclear Medicine, and Anticoagulation, Diabetes, and Lipids are located within the Medical Center.

3. The inpatient pharmacy offers unit dose, drug distribution, and complete sterile products services to all nursing units, several outpatient clinics, and the Emergency Room. Sterile products include all intravenous fluids with additives and such specialized fluids as total parenteral nutrition solutions, cardioplegia, and kidney perfusion solutions.

4. Clinical pharmacy programs are offered throughout the medical center. Specific programs are in Oncology, Nuclear Medicine, Internal Medicine, Critical Care Medicine, Family Practice, Clinical Investigations, Diabetes, and Cardiology. The Department of Pharmacy is also represented on the Nutrition Support team.

B. Patients Served. The patient population includes approximately 300,000 beneficiaries. The hospital serves as a referral center for the XYZ Healthcare Organization. This population encompasses all age groups.

C. Complexity of Patient Care Needs. Primary patient care needs are met by the Department of Pharmacy on both an inpatient and outpatient basis. Inpatient pharmacy offers unit-dose drug distribution and complete sterile products services to all nursing units, several outpatient clinics, and the Emergency Room. Ambulatory Care pharmacy processes and fills prescriptions written by in-house providers.

D. Meeting Patients' Needs

1. Patient needs are identified through periodic patient satisfaction surveys, Pharmacy Quality Assurance meetings, and through the Pharmacy & Therapeutics Committee (P&TC) and Subcommittees. These methods provide local control and evaluation procedures in order to ensure that only the most efficacious and economical therapeutic agents for our specific patient population are accepted for use in the medical facility.

2. The P&TC set local prescribing policies and selects the best agents based on sound clinical evidence without unnecessary duplication. An updated formulary is available in hardcopy from the Pharmacy, on the hospital web page under Department of Pharmacy, and this information posted on the Hospital Computer System accessible to all practitioners.

E. Support Services

1. *Purchasing Support Services*—The Department of Pharmacy is supported by several administrative services throughout

the Medical Center. The prime vendor provides the primary support service, which works jointly with pharmacy to ensure the availability of the highest quality of pharmaceuticals for our patients.

2. *Personnel Support Services*—Personnel support for the Department of Pharmacy is coordinated through the Human Resources Division.

3. *Equipment Support Services*—Some pharmacy equipment is leased and maintained by contracted companies. Other equipment upkeep is supported by medical maintenance.

4. *Pharmacy Support Services:*

a) The Department of Pharmacy provides a myriad of support services to the hospital, to include the inpatient and outpatient functions. The inpatient section stocks and checks the medication components of emergency (Crash) carts. The supply/support section maintains an adequate supply of emergency drugs as well as handling drug recalls, provision, and storage.

b) Other support services provide include clinical services, which provides drug information for patients, physicians, nurses, and other health care providers. The Pharmacy staff also develops drug monographs, participates in drug use review, publishes therapeutics newsletters, evaluates adverse drug reactions (ADRs), and provides educational in-services for physician, nursing, and pharmacy staff members. The clinical pharmacy staff provides pharmacokinetics counseling, patient counseling, patient care rounds, discharge counseling, and nutrition support consultations throughout the hospital.

c) The Hematology-Oncology Pharmacy and the Nuclear Pharmacy also provide numerous support services to their respective departments in addition to the support they provide by dispensing cytotoxic medications and radiopharmaceuticals.

d) The Investigational Drug Pharmacy is staffed by a pharmacist, which provides services related to investigational drug protocols approved by the facilities Investigational Review Board. Services provided include preparation of investigational protocol impact statements, drug information, investigational drug storage, preparation and dispensing.

F. Clinical Necessity and Timeliness. The support services the Department of Pharmacy provides are integrated into almost every facet of hospital operations. Pharmacy personnel provide this support in a timely and accurate fashion every day to ensure the highest quality and continuity of patient care.

G. Staff Availability. Pharmaceutical services are provided 24 hours a day, 7 days a week, by a staff consisting of pharmacists, research pharmacists, pharmacoeconomic pharmacists, technicians, supply technicians, a health systems specialist, and a pharmacy assistant. Specially trained staff members assigned to specific areas within the department may be utilized in other areas as needed due to staffing fluctuations.

H. Recognized Standards or Guidelines for Practice. The Department of Pharmacy follows state and federal laws, Joint Commission on Accreditation of Hospital Organization standards and current professional guidelines and standards for practice.

I. Methods Used to Assess and Meet Patient Care Needs

1. The Department of Pharmacy has a Quality Improvement (QI) program, which is reviewed and updated at least annually. It is a planned, systematic, ongoing, comprehensive, and integrated program. It utilizes a Total Quality Management approach to continually measure, assess, and improve important processes related to patient care and organizational functions.

2. The Pharmacy QI committee meets monthly to review indicators and data collection techniques, review data collected, analyze trends, and to implement corrective actions when necessary.

J. Customer Service. Patient satisfaction surveys are conducted periodically to assess patient needs and rectify real or perceived shortcomings. The Department of Pharmacy works with the Patient Representative office to improve customer service. Patient comments and complaints are stored in a database and reviewed periodically by supervisor and during the Department's QI meetings.

K. <u>Patient Confidentiality.</u> In support of HIPAA requirements, all pharmacy personnel will receive HIPAA training and will take measures to secure the confidentiality of patient information. Secure physical protective measures will be employed to store both active and inactive records. Access to storage space will be limited to assigned pharmacy personnel; all others must sign an access log and be escorted by a staff pharmacy member. Prescription labels and/or reports identifying patients will be disposed of according to hospital policy to protect patient confidentiality.

// Original Signed //
Name Here
Director, Department of Pharmacy

Appendix 22-3
Inpatient Care Unit Dose Section

Policy 4-2   **20 September 2005**

I.   PURPOSE. To describe in adequate detail, the standard methodology to be followed in conducting routine functions within the Unit Dose Section (UDS), Inpatient Activities Section, Department of Pharmacy.

II. REFERENCES

    A. Hospital Policy (Regulation) 40-3, Chapter 11, Pharmacy Management.

    B. Hospital Policy (Regulation) 40-114, Medication Use and Prescribing Policy.

    C. "ASHP Guidelines for Pharmacists on the Activities of Vendors' Representatives in Organized Health Care Systems."

III. APPLICIBILITY. The provisions of this policy and procedure are applicable to all pharmacy personnel.

IV. GENERAL

    A. The UDS objective: provision of a specific quantity of medication, for a specific patient or Unit to cover a specific length of time. A Pharmacist will have the responsibility for supervision and distribution.

    B. All changes from the posted work schedule will be cleared through the Director/Supervisor of the Section.

V.   RESPONSIBILITIES

    A. Pharmacists assigned to any shift in the UDS are professionally responsible for the quality of pharmaceutical dispensing that occurs during their shift. Such responsibility applies not only to their actions but also extends to the work performed by pharmacy technicians assigned to their shifts.

    B. Concerning matters not covered by this policy, the registered pharmacist assigned to the UDS on the evening or night shift (or weekends/holidays) will act in the best interest of the patient and the Pharmacy. The Branch/Section Director should be called for support in any circumstances that cannot be resolved by the pharmacist on duty.

    C. Pharmacists will use the Inpatient Pharmacy Service Communication Boards and the email system to alert subsequent shifts (and the Director) to problems experienced during the shift and to provide general information that will promote internal efficiency and responsibility.

VI. DEFINITIONS

    A. Terms

        1. *Unit Dose Section (UDS)*—Issue point for a 24-hour supply of unit dose medications in unit-of-use packaging.

        2. *Unit-of-Use*—A single medication dose, clearly identifiable as to drug, strength, commercial or Pharmacy Service lot number and expiration date.

        3. *Pharmacy Service Lot Number*—Seven-digit number given to repackaged drugs. The first number is always 6 (identifies U/D section). The next two numbers are the product number (from 01 to 99), and the last four digits are the last digit of the year plus the Julian date.

        4. *Medication Profile*—The patient record generated by the Hospital Computer System, which reflects the medication orders a patient receives during their stay in the hospital. The medication profile is maintained by the Pharmacy. The computer generated medication profile is used daily for filling unit dose (U/D) orders and for electronically compiling work counts.

        5. *Unit*—Term replacing ward. Refers to a separate nursing unit or floor (WICU, 6S etc.).

        6. *Patient Medication Drawer*—A sliding compartment used to hold the medications dispensed for administration to a specific patient during a 24 hour period. Duplicate sets of drawers exist for each patient; one set is in use on the Unit for administration to the patient; the other is in the Pharmacy being prepared for subsequent issue to the Unit for the next 24 hour period.

7. *Unit Cassette*—A holder containing drawers of a unit's individual patient medication drawers. Units may have up to four cassettes.

8. *Replenish on Request or On-Call*—Term for multidose medications, such as inhalers, ophthalmic, narcotic drips/PCA, selected IV fluids, and topical preparations, which are replenished or reissued to the unit upon verbal/telephonic request by the unit.

B. Forms

1. *Doctor's Orders (Form 42)*—This is a three-part form used for ordering a patient's medication when the hospital computer system is down or in special situations where the hospital computer system is not the primary order entry method. The first copy (white) is faxed to the pharmacy for input on the patient's medication profile and remains in the patient's record. The second copy (pink) is used by nurses for posting and may be sent to the pharmacy if the fax machine is not working on the unit. The third copy is not used by pharmacy.

2. *Packaging Control Log Sheet*—A quality control log sheet used to record lot numbers assigned to extemporaneous unit-dose packaging. One sheet will be used per drug.

3. *Unit Dose Pharmacy Cart List*—This is a list of all scheduled unit dose medications to be administered for a 24-hour-period of time and is sorted by unit and patient name. This list should not contain medications that are indicated in the hospital computer system as ward stock or replenish on request items. Pharmacy personnel should screen the list daily to look for replenish on request items and ensure they are not sent unless a need is verified with the unit.

4. *Unit Dose Pharmacy Cart List Update*—This is not a total cart list but only the new orders since the cart list was printed.

VII. REQUIREMENTS

A. Dispensing of Medications by the UDS of the Pharmacy Inpatient Activities Section Will Normally Follow These Sequential Events:

1. Receipt of Doctor's Orders by the Hospital Computer System or Fax

   a) Upon receipt, doctor's orders are to be reviewed by a pharmacist/technician. STAT orders are to be handled as priority.
   b) Orders will be checked for dosage change, drug addition/deletion, allergies, and interactions/incompatibilities by pharmacist/technician and entered into the hospital computer system medication profile.

2. Entering, Filling, and Delivering of Medications

   a) Patient Administration Division (PAD) is responsible for admitting and discharging patients in the hospital computer system. Patient profiles should be accessed through the unit dose pathway by their assigned units, patient name, or identification number.
   b) Name, actual strength stocked by the pharmacy, route of administration, and the daily dosage regimen of each drug ordered will be entered into the medication profile. Any clinical screens will be reviewed by a pharmacist with an appropriate comment recorded at the comment prompt. A pharmacist will review all orders entered into the hospital computer system medication profile.
   c) The delivery of medication to inpatients must support the Hospital Medication Automatic Stop Order Policy in accordance with Regulation 40-114.
   d) Medications sent to units, other than the once-a-day exchange of cassettes, will be placed in sealed disposable plastic bags and labeled with the hospital computer system patient specific unit dose label. Each plastic bag must contain medication for only one patient. All filled orders will be double-checked by another pharmacist/technician before delivering to the unit.
   e) Doctor's orders entered by technicians must be verified by a pharmacist. Doctor's orders are compared to the hospital computer system medication profile for accuracy of the patient's name, unit, allergies, drug nomenclature, dose, frequency quantity, and possible drug interactions or incompatibilities. The pharmacist will initial the verification block for the order in the hospital computer system.

f) The unit dose pharmacy cart list update will be printed and filled 1 hour before cart delivery to maintain the accuracy of the unit dose cassette fill.

3. *Filing of Completed Doctor's Orders*—Blue plastic bins for each day of the week are located in the UDS to file completed doctor's orders. Hospital computer system generated orders do not require filling and will be placed in the shedder box after they have been entered. Handwritten orders will be filed throughout the day in alphabetical order by last name. The day begins at 0700 for filing purposes. The orders will remain in the daily file bin until the same day of the following week at which time the old orders are discarded to the patient privacy destruction box for later shredding.

B. Filling of Unit Dose Cassettes

1. Cassettes are filled during the assigned shift of the UDS operation. The U/D drawers will be arranged alphabetically for filling. Patient-drawer name labels will have, when possible, hospital computer-system printed, patient-name labels that should be affixed to the patient's unit dose drawer.

a) Medication drawers are filled from the hospital computer system unit dose pharmacy cart list. The filler fills each drawer, recording on the cart list all doses dispensed and his/her initials for each unit.

b) All oral liquid medications will be prepared daily and as needed in the appropriate size oral syringe, cup, or bottle. Labels will be printed using the oral liquid computer program. Labels will contain the patient's name, ward, date, drug name and concentration, volume and strength, route, sig, lot number, expiration date, and the fillers and checkers initials. The expiration date will not exceed 72 hours and may be less depending on the expiration of the stock product and the stability of the item. The technician filling oral liquids each day must reconcile the active labels in the oral liquid computer program against the patient's CIS medication profile to determine if the order is still valid and accurate.

c) Oral liquid antibiotics or other liquid medications requiring refrigeration returned to the pharmacy will not be reused. These should be removed from the U/D drawer and replaced with fresh doses prepared when filling the cassettes.

d) The filler will initial all oral liquid labels filled and leave the used medication container next to the filled U/D oral liquid container for checking. The checking pharmacist will initial on the oral liquid label for all correctly filled U/D oral liquid containers.

e) Multiple-dose containers (e.g., creams, inhalers, etc.) that are not supplied in sealed containers will be sealed by placing tape over box ends or using a ziplock bag seal.

f) When a patient is discharged or a medication is discontinued, all unused medication must be removed from the patient's medication drawer and returned to stock if usable.

g) Returned medications that cannot be reused (e.g., ointments, ophthalmic or otic preparations, etc.) will be placed in an appropriate container for destruction.

2. The dispensing of investigational drugs will follow the hospital investigational medication policy.

C. Delivery of Unit Cassettes

1. Filled and checked cassettes are exchanged with duplicate used cassettes on a schedule determined by nursing and pharmacy.

2. During the delivery, all cassettes will be checked for bulk medications (e.g., creams, ointments, MDIs, etc.). These should be removed from the old cassettes and transferred to the new cassettes.

D. Unit Dose Work Units. Work units for the U/D section will be calculated using the hospital computer system work unit report. At the end of each month, the total unit dose work units will be calculated and reported to the Director, Pharmacy Service.

E. Packaging of Unit Dose Medications

1. All containers issued by the UDS will have uniform labeling to include the name of the drug (generic and trade if applicable), strength, a lot number, expiration date, and special instructions, if necessary.

2. In single-ingredient tablets or capsules, the strength of each drug will be in terms of intrinsic units (e.g., mg, units, mEq.). In oral liquids or injections, the strength will be indicated in terms of the number of milliliters and its equivalence as intrinsic units.

3. A hospital department of pharmacy lot number will be assigned to each extemporaneous unit dose (tablets, capsules, or liquid) packaging effort unless the automated packager automatically uses the manufactures lot number. This applies regardless of the number of doses prepared. A log is maintained to determine what the lot number should be for each medication packaged.

   a) Packaging control log sheet file (one sheet per drug) will be maintained for this purpose. The sheet will have the name and strength of the medication packaged, date of the packaging, the manufacturer's name, lot number and expiration date, the quantity packaged, the assigned hospital pharmacy lot number, the assigned expiration date, the initials of the technician packaging, and the initials of the pharmacist who released the packaged material.

   b) Repackaged U/D medication cannot be dispensed or returned to stock after the expiration date on the package has been reached. All repackaged U/D medication must be destroyed when expired.

   c) The maximum level of drugs packaged is a 3-month supply for fast movers.

4. Expiration dates will not exceed 6 months and will be dated for the last day of the appropriate month.

   a) If the expiration date from the manufacturer's container is less than 6 months, the manufacturer's expiration date will be used instead of 12-month dating. Round down the expiration date to the previous full month for any dates not at the end of the month.

   b) Expiration dates are calculated from the current month the product is packaged for a 6-month duration or manufacturer's expiration date, whichever is sooner. Start counting the months with the current month regardless of the number of days remaining in that month.

5. The prepack machine will be cleaned with 70% isopropyl alcohol between each drug packaged. Personnel prepacking drugs will wear disposable gloves during handling of all medications. All printed labels will be removed from the prepack machine after the last drug is packaged.

F. Packaging Half Tablets

1. Medication orders for half tablets will be evaluated by a pharmacist for the clinical indication of the half-tablet dose. The Inpatient Pharmacy should not prepare half-tablet doses when not clinically indicated or common sense would prohibit it (i.e., half-tablet vitamins or subtherapeutic doses). Below are options for half-tablet medication orders:

   a) Request a medication change to a clinically significant dose or an accurately measurable dose (whole tablet or half of a scored tablet).

   b) Change the medication to liquid if available.

   c) Prepare the half tablets from scored or unscored tablets ensuring the best cut or break for the half tablet.

G. Medication Brought to the Hospital by Patient.

1. It is policy at example hospital not to administer medications brought to the hospital by patients who are admitted. Health care personnel will attempt to have the patient's family member/significant other take home any medications and will inform patients and prescribers of this policy.

2. Patients admitted to the wards. All medications brought in by patients admitted to the wards will be collected by nursing personnel. Medications not given to a family member will be turned in to the pharmacy for disposition as follows:

   a) If the medication is not in stock at the inpatient pharmacy and the physician writes an order to continue the therapy in the hospital, then the pharmacy will identify the medication and take steps necessary to deliver the medication to the patient. The pharmacist must make a positive identification of the medication and prepare the medication to be delivered to the ward utilizing the unit dose system. The pharmacy will procure the medication as quickly as possible.

   b) If the medication is carried in stock, the pharmacy will either discard the medication or store the medication until the patient is discharged. If the patient has the same medication prescribed upon discharge and the retained medication is suitable for reissue, then it may be returned to the patient with appropriate labeling after coordination with the prescriber.

3. *Patients Not Admitted to Wards*—Patients who are not admitted to wards but are held in observational/ambulatory status (Observational Ward(s) for less than 23 hours, Sleep Clinic, etc.) may be allowed to utilize their personal medications as follows:

    a) The personal medications must be positively identified by pharmacy personnel and/or the patient's LIP, to ensure verification of labeled contents.

    b) The medication is documented in the hospital's medical information system (e.g., computer system's medication profile).

    c) The personal medication will be appropriately secured and will be administered and documented by the health care staff.

H. Discontinued Medications

1. Notification from the unit when a medication has been discontinued will be provided to the UDS verbally or via facsimile machine.

2. The medication will be discontinued in the computer system's medication profile and the medication removed from the patient's drawer.

I. Discharge and Inter-Unit Transfer of Patients

1. The Pharmacy is generally notified of discharge or transfer of patients via the hospital computer system.

2. The discharge of a patient requires pharmacy personnel to remove the drugs and patient name label from the patient's medication drawer. Drug orders will automatically be discontinued when PAD discharges patient in the hospital computer system. Pharmacy personnel should manually discontinue orders in the hospital computer system if there is a significant delay between the discharge order and the PAD initiated discharge in the hospital computer system.

3. When a patient is transferred, units are expected to forward medication with the patient to their new unit. Doctor's orders for medications must be reviewed and approved for the new unit by the transferring physician. The new unit is responsible for notifying PAD and transferring the patient in hospital computer system from the previous unit.

4. Patients on pass for more than 3 days will be considered discharged unless the Pharmacy has been otherwise notified.

J. Unit Stock Distribution

1. All Units have selected items maintained on the unit in their point-of-use cabinets.

2. Pharmacy personnel will restock the point-of-use cabinets twice a day.

3. These items will be reviewed yearly by unit nursing personnel and pharmacy personnel.

           // Original Signed //
           Name Here
           Director, Department of Pharmacy

Appendix 22-4
Department of Pharmacy
Policies and Procedures
Table of Contents

Chapter 23

Pharmacy Information Systems

Rowell Daniels

Introduction

Pharmacy information systems have regularly been used in the delivery of pharmacy services since the early 1980s.[1] Over the past decade, technology has advanced so dramatically that pharmacies would be lost without the aid and assistance of information systems. Pharmacy information systems provide the building blocks of the medication-use system. They are the repositories for medication usage information. Today's pharmacy information systems manage many basic tasks such as producing Medication Administration Records (MARs), managing inventories, and alerting users to drug-drug interactions, dose-range checking, and drug-allergy checking. More advanced systems have *rules engines* that are capable of combining several sets of data to proactively monitor complex combinations of events (e.g., high-potassium lab value when potassium supplementation has been ordered). Pharmacy systems track the dispensing history of patients' medications as well as information surrounding these events. This information includes the prescribers' name and other prescriber demographic information (DEA, License Number, place of practice, etc.), the date the medication was prescribed/ordered, the number of doses or days prescribed, drug name, strength, dose, route, pharmacy location, pharmacy technician responsible for entering, pharmacist responsible for review and approval, nursing unit (if acute care), and patient demographics (name, age, address, age, height, weight). This chapter will discuss the uses, selection, implementation and various other aspects of pharmacy information systems.

Background

Early pharmacy systems were primarily developed with operational, financial, and data management functions in mind.[2-4] "Some of the key features of early pharmacy information systems included pharmacy billing, inventory management, and report generation consisting of medication labels, fill lists, and patient profiles."[2,5-9] As recent as the mid-1990s, pharmacy information systems were still limited to distributive, managerial, and limited drug-use checks. Separate programs had to be used to perform pharmacokinetic dosing. With the advent of operating systems such as Microsoft® Windows, graphical user interfaces have improved the ease which computer technology has been incorporated into pharmacy practice. Other advances in technology including the evolution of the personal computer (PC), high-speed network connectivity (e.g., ethernet, fiber optic cables, local area networks) along with advances in processor technology have significantly pushed the capabilities of pharmacy information systems.[1] Even with these great advancements in technology, there is still significant room to maximize the use of pharmacy information systems and share data across systems. In a study of Florida hospitals, 100% of larger institutions had implemented pharmacy information systems, whereas only 69.6% of small hospitals had implemented the same technology.[10] Recent national data shows that "larger hospitals were most likely to have computer-accessible laboratory data available to pharmacists. For example, over 97% of hospitals with 400 or more, 300–399, and 200–299 beds had computerized laboratory data available to pharmacists, compared with 88.9% of hospitals with 100–199 beds, 58.2% of hospitals with 50–99 beds, and 59.1% of hospitals with fewer than 50 beds.[11] These great variations show the need for further expansion of the use of information technology and data.

System Selection

Changing from one pharmacy information system vendor to another is a significant and most often one of the largest decisions a Pharmacy Department will ever make. A significant amount of effort is required to select, purchase, and implement pharmacy information systems. Some institutions will allow pharmacy departments to make independent choices in the selection of information systems. However, due to the need for significant integration of practice area specific systems and, therefore, the level of complexity associated with this decision, many departments of pharmacy are not allowed to make independent choices in the selection of their own system. Regardless of the situation, pharmacists have a professional responsibility to ensure the proper selection of a pharmacy information system. Pharmacists are the most qualified individuals to perform a proper assessment of the clinical and operational functionalities within a potential system. Pharmacy departments should make every effort to participate in the selection process of their own information system. Efforts should be made to educate health system leadership on important topics such as medication error prevention, the ability to comply with laws and standards, and the significance of being able to report on drug usage. Since the consideration of a new pharmacy information system happens so infrequently in the life of an organization, lack of pharmacy participation in such a critical decision could have safety and financial ramifications for a decade or greater.

A multidisciplinary selection team of pharmacists, hospital information technology experts, nurses, and physicians, is often established to obtain an institution wide perspective. An executive team may also be established to "convey the institutional vision for future computerization, and strategic plans to the selection team; make important hardware, software, support, financial, and operating decisions for the selection team; participate in the executive managers' meeting; review the selection team's recommendation for a preferred vendor; and make the final decision as to the vendor and system of choice."[1]

The choice of "Best of Breed" versus "one size fits all" is being strongly influenced by many institutions that are now focusing on *enterprise-wide* or a *suite* of solutions from one single vendor. With the advent of health systems, the choice of one single information systems vendor for lab, radiology, pharmacy, finance, etc., is even more likely. Purchasing a group of information systems products from one vendor provides health systems the advantage of negotiating a lower purchase price than if all systems were purchased from separate vendors. It also allows an enterprise to leverage service and support for more than one product. The need for pharmacy system integration with other systems is essential as the sharing of data to improve patient safety and create positive outcomes (see Chapter 26). On the other hand, there are many positives for selecting a best of breed (i.e., industry leader). Most often, by selecting an industry-leading product,

pharmacy departments are able to buy the product that best matches their clinical and operational needs due to the quality and depth of features.[12] However, this may also mean a loss of functionality in areas such as interfaces, which are key to institutional success.

Several steps should be used in selecting a pharmacy information system. They include listing the strengths and weaknesses of the current pharmacy system, developing a wish list of functions and capabilities needed in a new system, developing a potential vendor list, developing a Request for Proposal (RFP), setting up demonstrations, and contract negotiation.[13] Use of all these steps will ensure a quality purchase that best meets the needs of a pharmacy department as well as the institution.

The development of a functionality wish list and a prospective vendor list can often be aided by performing on-site visits and phone surveys of other institutions. These types of interactions can often provide insight into vendor selection that the RFP is unable to illuminate. Institutions should have a standard list of questions they are interested in asking their peers (Table 23-1). Attending exhibitor showcases at local, state, or national pharmacy society meetings are also a valuable low cost method for identifying vendors.

After the research for system specifications is completed, the RFP is utilized to summarize the ideal pharmacy information system's specifications

Table 23-1
On-Site Visit and Phone Survey Questions[13]

What are the strengths and weaknesses of your system?
Do you feel the vendor responds to your requests in a timely manner?
Was the vendor efficient, thorough, and helpful during the installation process?
Did the contract negotiation process meet your expectations?
How flexible was the vendor during the contract negotiation process?
Once the contract was signed, was there a noticeable change in the vendor's response to requests or problems?
Does the vendor have a strong user committee?
Does the vendor listen to the user committee?
Who decides which upgrades and changes are made in the software?

(Table 23-2). The RFP is released to vendors interested in pursuing business with the institution. A time-limit for responding to the RFP should be placed on vendors pursuing the institution's business. Care should be given to the review of the RFP responses to ensure that questions are being clearly answered. Depending on responses, vendors may be invited to demonstrate the live functionality of their system.

Again, a multidisciplinary group should participate in the live demonstration. To provide continuity in the selection process, members of the selection team should be a part of the demonstrations. Taking notes and video taping demonstrations serve as useful reminders when the review group is completing the analysis. A standardized review form or script should be provided to all demonstrations participants so that the institution can quantify and qualify likes, dislikes, and concerns.[1,13] This introduces a more scientific approach to vendor selection and reduces the chance of a purely emotional decision.

The final step in a system's selection is contract negotiation. It is very helpful to include institutional experts in this endeavor. Subject experts in contract development such as purchasing agents, information services hardware and software experts, and the institution's attorneys should all participate in this process to ensure that the pharmacy department is well protected in such a large purchase. A checklist of items to be included in the contract should be developed to ensure that all aspects are adequately covered (Table 23-3). A sound contract is the basis for the ongoing relationship between the institution and the vendor. Up until the point at which the contract is signed, the customer has all the leverage with the vendor. After the contract is signed, all leverage over the vendor rests with the contract. Therefore, contract development is critical to the successful implementation of the vendor's system and the ongoing relationship with the vendor post implementation.

Table 23-2
Request for Proposal Elements

Element	Description
Introduction	Review of institutional goals and objectives for computerization and automation; instructions to vendors on how to respond, to the RFP and potential future steps in the selection process
Information Systems Overview	Review of hardware, software, operating, and interface requirements for the institution
Departmental Overview	Description of services, physical layout, and workload of the Department of Pharmacy, including future vision for automated and robotic systems, how services will be provided, and descriptions of the number of workstations and peripherals
Functional Specifications	Description of departmental needs subdivided by the following operational areas and functions: order entry, order verification, patient and medication profiles, formulary structure, clinical practice, labeling and other outputs, automation, reporting, investigational drugs, technical, inventory control, billing and financial, interface and connectivity, ambulatory care systems, home infusion, and required customizations
Contractual Information	Listing of warranties desired, performance criteria, payment schedules, support and maintenance requirements, contractual requirements, acceptance testing criteria, and so forth
Vendor Profile	Financial information, listing of institutions where their system is currently installed including the version of the software installed, contact names and telephone numbers, description of their training and support services, and the background and experience level of vendor executives and staff
System Pricing	Preformatted response sheet that the vendor completes and that describes the quantities, models, and unit costs for system hardware and software, as well as system maintenance, support, interface, enhancement, training, and implementation costs

Table 23-3
Contract Negotiation Checklist[13]

Critical functionality identified through site visits, multidisciplinary review, vendor demonstrations, or negotiated are documented
Vendor promises for current functionality are documented
Interfaces and interface functionality are documented
Customizations along with costs and programming time are documented
Additional modules purchased but not intended for immediate installation during system implementation are documented along with a clearly defined future implementation support structure
System development and implementation support structures and processes (on-site and remote) are documented
Vendor's service standards and response times to system breakdowns (e.g., urgent vs. nonurgent response times) are documented
Hardware and software specifications are documented
Warranties are documented

Interfaces and Standalone vs. Integrated Pharmacy Information Systems

Another concept issue with information technology is understanding the key differences between whether a system is interfaced or integrated. One-vendor solutions are often marketed as integrated solutions. Since one vendor may be offering a suite of products that includes a pharmacy product, health care institutions are left with the thought that the pharmacy system is integrated with all other products (e.g., lab, physician order entry, medication administration charting, etc.). "In the old days of mainframe-based product offerings this claim was more likely to be true because products such as pharmacy systems could reside on the same platform as the main hospital system, and actually read and write to databases of other systems, such as admitting and billing, without the need for interfaces."[12] Generally speaking, many of today's systems are completely separate or standalone systems and require interfaces to be effective. In many aspects, interfaces are the lifeblood of any information system. The robustness of an interface determines the quality, amount, and type of information received by a pharmacy system from various external sources. The most common type of interface is the Admission, Discharge, and Transfer (ADT) interface. This interface passes along informa-

tion such as name and address of the patient, sex, height, weight, allergies, medical record number, financial account number, admission date, unit, floor, room number, transfer location information, discharge date and time, etc. Other interfaces may include laboratory, drug formulary, orders, and pharmacy automation interfaces. Pharmacy automation is driven by the information created from the pharmacy information system. Depending on the vendor, automation interfaces may include formulary interfaces, patient profile (i.e., MAR) interfaces, inventory interfaces, and clinical alert interfaces (see Chapter 24). Integrated systems are constructed in such a way that all individual systems (Pharmacy, Nursing, Radiology, CPOE, Laboratory, etc.) all reside on top of one common database platform. As a result, no interfacing is required between these systems. This arrangement also avoids the complexities of matching numerous disparate database fields across interfaces. The future's most successful information systems vendors will develop their systems in this manner.

As Computerized Provider Order Entry (CPOE) continues to expand in usage, institutions are finding that there is a significant opportunity to unite these systems with pharmacy information systems. As mentioned previously, one inappropriate assumption made by organizations, is that if one vendor provides both the Pharmacy and CPOE systems, they will be integrated or interfaced in such a manner that information will easily flow between the two. However, in reality most of these one-vendor solutions may not communicate at all. As a result, health systems are forced to develop bidirectional orders interfaces, unidirectional orders interfaces, or manually transcribe printed information from the CPOE system to the pharmacy system.[2] The bidirectional orders interface represents one of the most complicated types of interfaces due to the complexity of the information being sent between both systems. Dose, route, frequency, administration time, special instructions, modified orders, discontinued orders, prescriber, patient, etc., must all cleanly match between both systems. Complicating this even further is the fact that many systems may use different vendors for their clinical decision support database (e.g., First Data Bank®, Multum®, etc.) This then requires even further manipulation of interface data as one system communicates information to another (e.g., clinical alert data).

Electronic Drug Information Knowledgebases

Several companies such as First DataBank and Multum provide electronic drug knowledgebase information for clinical decision support. The content provided by these companies supports such functions as electronic prescribing, patient education leaflets, pharmacy claims data, and clinical alerts (drug-drug, drug-allergy, etc.) within CPOE and pharmacy information systems. Standards for the use of this information is developed and maintained by the Federal Government (Centers for Medicare and Medicaid Services) and non-profit groups such as the National Council for Prescription Drug Programs (NCPDP). These standards promote the accurate transfer of data to and from the pharmacy services sector of the health care industry. When selecting a pharmacy information system, organizations should consider the source and reliability of the system's drug information vendor. Questions should be asked such as how often is this data updated (monthly, quarterly, annually), how much time does an update take, and is downtime required.

Telemedicine and Pharmacy Information Systems

With the advance of technology, the ability to share data and information across long distances instantaneously has now become a reality. New practice standards mandated by organizations such as the Joint Commission for Accreditation of Healthcare Organizations (JCAHO) require the availability of pharmacist review of medication orders prior to the administration of medications. Centralized after-hours remote pharmacy support is remarkably easy with the use of virtual private networks, secure (encrypted) Internet access, and peer-to-peer connections. Through these processes, a pharmacist may review physician orders and have access to patient profiles from any number of hospitals at one single location. For smaller hospitals that do not maintain 24-hour in-house pharmacist support, this technology has provided a very strong presence for the provision of pharmacist level knowledge without a physical presence. This technology may also be used along with a flexible workforce. As turnaround times increase for the review of medication orders, pharmacies may call in a flexible, part-time at home or otherwise distant workforce. Through the use of this technology, part-time workers can connect to the hospital or outpatient pharmacy's system to review, clarify, and approve medication orders or prescriptions. When the service is back within normal turnaround standards and/or back to manageable level, the pharmacists essentially sign off.

System Implementation

The planning for the implementation of an information system starts with the development of a project plan. The project plan should cover all aspects of the project such as resources, timeline, assigned roles, hardware installation, software development and testing, and staff education. "One of the biggest impediments to successful implementation of IT projects is 'scope creep.'"[14] Scope creep is the addition of unexpected and /or unplanned functionality resulting in the need for additional time, resources, or funding. A solid project plan enables the project team to successfully stay on track with the goals of the project and avoid the pitfalls of scope creep.

Human resources are incredibly important to the success of the implementation of a new information system. The project team should include pharmacists, the institution's information systems specialists, and representatives from the information system's vendor at a minimum. Nurses and physicians should be included if the system is being interfaced to nursing documentation systems and/or CPOE. Teams should be given specific tasks along with deadlines for the completion of these tasks to ensure success.

Database conversion or transfer is one of the most complex aspects of a new system's implementation. The ability to convert data relies on the format and availability of corresponding fields from one database to another. One would expect that with today's advanced systems, all fields from one system's databases could be simply copied to the new system's databases much the way that one can copy from Microsoft® Access to Excel or vice versa. This is simply not possible in all cases. Therefore, efforts should be made up front to establish how the critical fields from one database will be transferred to the new system. Critical fields may be determined in any number of ways. Relative value to the organization and complexity of the information are two important indicators of the need to transfer data. Unfortunately, when a vendor is unable to electronically convert a database, the organization is then left to decide if a manual entry of the data is worth the effort. Questions such as, has the vendor performed a similar conversion in the past, what has worked, and where have the failures been for previous installations are essential in this area. Care and consideration should also be given to the conversion of historical data from the current system. In many instances, conversion of historical data may be complicated, especially if you are changing vendors. If you are unable to convert your historical data, an effort should be made to determine how much will it cost or what amount of time and effort will be required to export this historical data to a separate database. In some instances, the previous vendor may allow the maintenance of their system purely for the purpose of historical data extraction.

System testing is one of the most critical steps in the development and implementation of a pharmacy information system. In this phase, extreme care should be given to fully explore all aspects of system functionality. Testing should include aspects such as operational, clinical, and volume testing. Operational testing includes reviewing such functions as medication batches, order entry flow, connectivity to automation, interfaces, and billing. Clinical testing includes reviewing dose-range checking, allergy checking, intervention checking, etc. Volume testing includes simulating a period of high volume activity on the system. This allows testing of processor speed. An example of volume testing might include having 10 or 12 pharmacists or technicians enter orders for 30 minutes to 1 hour and at the same time that the interfaces are open to stress the system. While this is occurring, special attention should be paid to size, disc space, and processor speed. Fiscal compatibility and compliance should be considered during the testing phase. Specific efforts should be made to validate billing from the new system all the way through to a patient's bill. This type of testing should include a direct comparison of outputs between the new system and old system.

One of the most important yet least planned for events in converting to a new information system is training. However, a successful training program will make the difference between a go-live fraught with confusion, desperation, and the thought of impending doom and a triumphant go-live where everyone knows their roles as well as the capabilities and limitations of the new system. One of the most challenging aspects of developing a training program early in the new system development process is actually knowing how the system functions. This may create conflict between the development team and the training team. The training team will need to have definitive answers as to system

functions and their impact on clinical and operational services. While the development team may know some of the answers, they may not be at the point of clearly understanding the system. Therefore, a lucid answer may not be possible. Providing required training time of all staff is also essential. Efforts should be made to accommodate all training needs, regardless of staffing conflicts or shift times. The more individuals that are familiar with system functionality, the more hands that are available to answer questions, trouble shoot, and provide services as per usual during the very difficult process of conversion.

Prior to go-live, time should be invested in the development of a conversion plan. This plan should include an assessment of human resource needs for the day of go-live. Human resource needs for go-live should be clearly identified and committed very early. Staff should know their roles, locations, and expectations.

If the new vendor is unable to convert historical data, then a critical conversion planning decision is necessary. How will data for patients currently being cared for be manually placed into the new vendor's system? This particular issue will have a significant impact on the number of people required on the day of go-live. In addition, assuming most conversions will require some amount of manual intervention, consideration should be given to the location of the conversion, preferably, a location that will accommodate all employees involved in the effort to promote ease of communication should issues be identified. This type of conversion will happen above and beyond the provision of normal services (which must go on regardless of the conversion). For this reason, preplanning should include the setup of additional computers if necessary to accommodate a larger than normal staffing load.

Depending on the size of the institution and, therefore, size and volume of the department's workload the time of the day and the day of the week should be carefully chosen. For outpatient services that traditionally are open and available during normal business hours and smaller acute care hospital pharmacies (not operational 24 hours a day, 7 days a week), this choice is much easier and can usually occur after business hours. However, for inpatient services at larger institutions, conversions must take place in a concurrent fashion with the provision of regular services. Days with the heaviest patient volumes and, therefore, most significant pharmacy workload should be avoided. At most institutions, this would be reflected in a Saturday or Sunday night conversion. Human resources might be scarce for a weekend conversion. However, with advanced planning limited staff availability will be avoided.

In order to determine the amount of time a conversion will take, several factors must be taken into account. How much time will be required to convert historical data, frequency tables, dosing algorithms, formulary tables, etc.? How much time is required for ADT and other interfaces to prepopulate the patient census? If not electronically converted, how much time will it take to back-enter live medication orders? These questions are necessary to develop a strong estimate of the number of personnel and the amount of time required to convert from the old to the new information system.

Communication is another crucial planning point. Determining in advance what methods you will use to communicate new findings to all staff (e.g., memos, email, intranet, staff meetings, etc.) will make the conversion much more successful.

In an effort to validate the conversion plan, one or more "dry runs" should be completed. The validation process should include an actual test conversion of data from the current system to the new pharmacy system. In fact this process should occur several times so that on the actual day of conversion this process is second nature.

In order to have a true sense of the human effort and or intervention required for any given conversion step, estimations should be made on the amount of time each step requires. A simple check of the watch to see how long database transfers require, how long it takes to enter different order types (IVs versus unit dose). Then multiply the amount of time required to perform the function by the number of occurrences. For example, if it takes 1 minute per unit dose order and you have estimated that there are 600 unit-dose orders to be entered then this part of the conversion will require 600 minutes or 10 work hours. Of course, one step in a conversion process may not be dependent on another and for that reason in the example of 10 work hours could be shared by five people to make that particular issue a 2-hour event.

For environments that operate 24-hours per day, coordinating the conversion with the functions of a work area is essential. For example, at what point will the new system generate MARs, billing, batches, first dose labels, etc. It is important that thought be given to this step to avoid confusion with nursing, prevent over and/or under billing, and avoid medication errors. At what point will all orders be converted over to the new system and how does this relate to the last time nurses performed a 24-hour MAR review? Or, if nursing is using an electronic MAR, how and when will the old information be electronically replaced by new information? Does the system bill in 24-hour batches on the day of dispense or the day of administration or does it bill at the time of dispense or administration? These are all significant considerations. If billing has already occurred for the previous 24 hours how and at what point will billing convert to the new system? As the orders are populated into the new system, attention should be paid to label generation. Labels should be diverted to a secure area or turned off so that extra doses are not inadvertently sent to nursing units. Likewise, with electronic MARs, the interface should only be started after an "all clear" is communicated to the nursing units.

There should be no limitations to the length that a pharmacy department can go to in order to test and train for the implementation of a new system. The strongest conversion plan includes the development of three distinct electronic environments. They include a testing and/or development environment, a training environment, and a live environment. The live environment is considered to be the final product and should be kept pristine and clear of all activity. It represents the final work product and should not be altered other than to update it to reflect final clinical and operational functional standards within the system. It should be kept under lock-and-key. The training environment should be a facsimile of the live account. This will allow pharmacists and technicians the ability to touch and feel the system prior to go-live. The training environment can continue to function after go-live for training new employees. The testing and development environment is the area in which staff working on the implementation can test alternative functionalities within the system without affecting the live environment. As final system design decisions are made, these settings should be also made in or copied to the live environment.

Interfaces should be started after interface development and testing is concluded but in sufficient time prior to go-live so that the system's census is adequately populated. For acute care environments, this would include some estimation of the average length of stay for patients. One can then make estimates over how many patients will be prepopulated if the interface is opened for the average length of stay or even two or three times the length of stay. The goal is to limit the number of times that pharmacists and technicians will have to manually admit patients. Manual admissions if not performed correctly may cause unexpected billing and dispensing problems. Manual admissions also delay the overall time it takes to convert to the new system. For these reasons prepopulation of the census becomes even more important.

The best go-live events are those that are seamless. The staff is able to come in and immediately pick up where they left off the shift before. Nurses are able to immediately utilize the new MAR and administer medications, billing works as designed. There are no major billing compliance issues or medication errors. On the day of go-live, all members of the go-live team should know their roles, the times that they should be present, and be prepared to take on additional tasks as necessary. Workload should be assigned in logical units and preferably with the most skilled participants scheduled accordingly. The conversion from one system to another offers invaluable training opportunities for all staff and should be promoted as such. All participants should also have an understanding of the overall plan and the timelines required for each step to occur. In those situations whereby manual entry of medication orders is necessary, thought should be given as to how staff will know what the current orders are in order to enter them. A printed version of the patient's profile, either from the MAR or from a report would be a couple of alternatives. The go-live team should include a clinical/ operational lead (pharmacy informatics specialist), technical lead (information systems specialist), and a vendor lead. It is important that the clinical/ operational Lead direct the go-live event. This individual will possess the knowledge required to determine if changes to the go-live plan are necessary and be able to assess their impact. Contingency planning and problem issue and resolution paths should also be developed. Undoubtedly, even the best-developed go-live plan will encounter unexpected twists. Some issues might be easily resolvable; however, others may require intensive research and troubleshooting. For these reasons, developing a plan for the documentation, prioritization, communication, and resolution of unexpected issues will be necessary. These issues can then be routed to the appropriate individual for resolution. For example, having someone available to make immediate changes to the formulary database in the case of an unexpected discovery of an incorrect dose, route, frequency, etc.

Post go-live monitoring and quality assurance testing and review should occur after the go-live event. How will you know if billing is in line with billing on the prior system? How will you know if the transfer of patient data (e.g., ADT, medication orders, allergies, etc.) occurred appropriately? From a medication safety point of view, double-checking the accuracy of medication orders in the new system is essential (e.g., comparing MARs between the old and new systems). From a fiscal point of view, comparing historical daily, weekly monthly charges to that coming from the new system are also incredibly important. In many cases the first true system performance (speed and response) is either at go-live (manual entry) or the day after go-live. It's at this point that all processes should be functioning. The system should be closely monitored to identify any delays in response and ensure that processing time is kept to a minimum.

High Availability and Disaster Planning

In the post-"911" world and with the advent of systems integration, disaster planning for computer systems has become a critical task. Historically speaking, many pharmacy departments may have kept, monitored, and administered their own servers. However, the standard of practice today includes having pharmacy system servers kept and maintained in secure, secluded environments. Many times these servers are not even within the same building and are often kept at a different site altogether. In addition, pharmacies have long since left the handwritten kardex world of maintaining patient profiles. Pharmacies now rely on information systems around the clock to drive clinical and operational functions. Zero pharmacy system downtime is now necessary to consistently provide the highest level of patient care. Regardless of the server location, designing a server configuration that provides never-failing uptime is essential. One level of precaution includes performing a daily back-up or copy of data (both live and historical). This information can then be retrieved if something should happen to the server or if the live data should become unexpectedly corrupted. The downside of this method is that depending on when the last back-up was performed, a certain amount of data will have to be manually rebuilt (e.g., if data were normally copied at 12:00 midnight and the system goes down at 8 A.M., 8 hours of data would have to be reentered into the system. A second level of precaution includes having a fully redundant server available. *High availability*, as it is called, keeps two servers in synchronization with each other at all times. As data is entered into one system, the data is copied and transferred to the mirror image second server. In the event that the primary server should fail, users and processes are seamlessly transferred to the secondary server. This type of server arrangement supports a zero downtime environment.

Clinical Practice/Medication Safety

The clinical practice of pharmacy has been dramatically advanced through the use and development of pharmacy information systems. Today's systems perform many clinical decision support functions such as dose-range checking, drug-drug interaction checking, food-drug interaction checking, and drug-laboratory results checking.

Functionality for dose-range checking involves comparing several patient parameters such as height, weight, and/or age against a prescribed dose. Most often individuals recognize the purpose of this functionality as a tool to prevent overdoses. In addition, this clinical functionality also supports the detection of supratherapeutic doses. The identification of doses above and below a recommended range allows pharmacists to maximize drug therapy. However, there are many other patient factors that basic dose-range checking may or may not take into account. These patient factors may include disease state, creatinine clearance, sex, disease state, etc. Therefore, the clinical disposition of the patient will always dictate the appropriateness of a dose. Dose-range checking does not replace the pharmacist's clinical practice experience.

Drug-drug interaction checking consists of electronically comparing a new drug that is being added to a patient's drug regimen to the drug(s) that the patient is currently receiving. Studies have shown that between 6.5% and 23% of adverse drug reactions are attributable to drug interactions.[15-19] Therefore, drug-drug interaction checking may produce an inordinate number of alerts depending on the number and type of medications a patient is taking. Many of these alerts may actually represent false-positives or insignificant interactions. Database companies (Multum®, First Databank®), therefore, have classified interactions into severity levels such as moderate, moderately severe, and severe. Information systems vendors use this classification scheme to give flexibility to the sensitivity of the alerts reviewed by pharmacists. Up until recently,

the option to set alerts for medication interactions was an all-or-none case. However, over the past decade, information systems have evolved to allow for global sensitivity settings as well as the capability to make exceptions to those settings. For example, users may downgrade or upgrade the sensitivity of a particular interaction based on the practice experience with a particular patient population.

While drug-drug interaction checking occurs in somewhat of a controlled fashion (e.g., checked prior to dispensing new medications whether that be in the acute care environment or ambulatory environment), food-drug interaction checking is different in that food is an unknown daily variable. Similar to drug-drug interaction checking, this clinical check compares food and drug combinations that are known to alter drug absorption (increase or decrease) or potentiate the effects of a drug (e.g., leafy green vegetables and warfarin). This may of course result in adverse outcomes. Institutional systems may include interfaces that pass food and/or drug information between pharmacy and dietary systems to alert pharmacists or dieticians when the potential for an interaction may occur. In the absence of any interface in institutional settings, alternative methods for communicating the potential for food drug interactions include the generation of a report to pharmacy, nursing, or dietary staff that is then used as a trigger to perform patient education. In the ambulatory environment, pharmacy information systems generate drug-drug and food-drug interaction warnings in the form of patient education monographs for counseling.

Combining pharmacy information with laboratory results can also prevent many errors. In one study, "adverse drug events occurred in 6.5 of 100 admissions; 28% of these adverse drug events were judged preventable. Errors were most often due to drug dosing and selection problems related to laboratory parameters."[20] Other studies have shown that 13.9% of 2,100 inappropriate medication dosing errors was due to patients having impaired renal and hepatic function and that 79% of pharmacy to lab related adverse drug events went without notice.[21,22] Therefore, combining these data sets may affect the selection, dosing, and monitoring of medications.[23]

Rules engines are perhaps the most exciting area of development with pharmacy information systems. Rules engines take disparate information from various sources and help identify complex scenarios. They may be used to significantly improve patient outcomes through the prevention of situations resulting in negative events. Examples of rules include: comparing microbiology culture and sensitivity data with a patient's antibiotic regimen and disease state, monitoring creatinine clearance in relation to drug therapy, or monitoring geriatric patients for combinations of drug therapies that may lead to hypotension, oversedation, etc. Such as system in one hospital generated 36,640 alerts on 14,740 patients resulting in 5,776 pharmacist interventions over the course of 1 year.[24]

The time from problem identification to intervention by pharmacists has been shown to vary widely. Without the aid of clinical decision support, pharmacists are left to review patients' data (e.g., medication profiles, laboratory information, progress notes and other pertinent information) and act on issues based on memory and ability to absorb great amounts of information.[24] One study showed that "only 27.5% of pharmacists' interventions are made within 12 hours of the prescription having been written, and even those with a potentially serious outcome have a mean lag time of 23.9 hours."[25,26] However, a few studies have reported on the use of computer-generated clinical alerts in an attempt to significantly reduce the time between the development of the critical event and resolution of the incident and thus also improve patient outcomes.[27–29] These *real-time* notifications can come in many forms. Critical alerts may come in the form of alpha-pages to personal beepers, alerts to handheld technologies such as Palm® devices, and notifications via other wireless technologies such as laptops or tablet devices, and email.[24,27] With real-time notification, many times this information can then be used to modify medication therapy hours or perhaps even days sooner than was previously possible. This type of clinical alert technology, most often comes in the form of pop-up screens to alert the pharmacist as he/she adds information to the patients' profile. Unfortunately, as the number of alerts increase, productivity and the ability to correctly respond to these alerts decreases. They may become more of a nuisance and hindrance than that of assistance. Care should be taken in activating these alerts so that only the most important and clinically relevant alerts are introduced to the care process.

The point in time in which clinical alerts are triggered may also have an impact on the clinical effectiveness of a pharmacy information system. If clinical checking only occurs when a patient profile is accessed, this will significantly impact the ability to proactively manage clinical pharmacy services. However, more advanced pharmacy information systems will have rules engines that function regardless of whether the patient profile is currently being accessed. This allows critical information to be communicated at any time of the day.

Alerts function in a binary fashion (yes or no). However, pharmacists must still utilize their knowledge of pharmacotherapy, disease states, and current literature to make the best patient care decisions. Ultimately, the pharmacist must choose to accept or reject these alerts. Pharmacy systems can now report on the acceptance rate for clinical alerts. This allows pharmacy departments to investigate and fine-tune the acuity of alerts.

Pharmacist intervention documentation is also an increasingly important function as pharmacists try to document their value. Processes to document pharmacist interventions have been paper-based (manual), bar-code scanner, notebook personal computer (PC), PC local area network, pharmacy information system, hospital information system, electronic medical record, personal organizer, personal digital assistants, and intranet websites.[30] Most often, the original methods of compiling and organizing intervention documentation were paper based. More advanced practices utilized electronic databases. However, for those institutions that did utilize electronic methods for documentation, most often these methods were physically separate from the pharmacy information system. Therefore, communication and coordination of pharmacist intervention information proved difficult. Pharmacy systems of today enhance this process by allowing the pharmacist to easily document information from within the information system's application. Intervention documentation can occur on multiple levels. Intervention documentation may occur at the patient demographic level, the medication order level, and the individual medication dose level. For instance, documentation that all medications for a patient have been adjusted for renal insufficiency would occur at the patient profile level. The discontinuation of an antibiotic based on a pharmacist's recommendation might occur at the medication order level. Whereas, the recommendation to withhold an evening dose of labetalol would be documented at the individual medication dose level. Regardless of the level at which documentation occurs, advanced pharmacy information systems, allow the easy review of this data from one location. Therefore, pharmacists do not have to hunt and search for intervention documentation. One of the most powerful benefits of having intervention documentation incorporated within the pharmacy system is the ability to report and trend intervention information in relationship to the cost of care. The use of this information has proven to be very beneficial to the cost-justification for the expansion of pharmacy services.

Many times clinical pharmacy also crosses over into ADR/ADE prevention. For example, when a pharmacist recommends a lower dose of warfarin to prevent excessive bleeding, this is not only a clinical intervention but also results in the prevention of patient harm. Pharmacies that utilize clinical intervention documentation tools can document and report how they have prevented numerous errors. Many studies have shown the value of pharmacists in reducing medication costs and preventing errors.[31–36] By utilizing technology to document interventions, pharmacists may easily promote their value to organizations.

Medication Administration Record

The Medication Administration Record (MAR) is the one document uniting nursing and pharmacy in the safe administration of medications. It commonly lists a patient's allergies, medications, and standardized medication administration times. Additionally, the MAR may include specific administration (e.g., infuse over 1hour). Historically speaking, the MAR was maintained by nursing. It represented the nurse's transcription of the physician's medication orders. Prior to the advent of computers, pharmacies would also maintain patient profiles in much the same manner manually handwriting new medications and discontinuing deleted medications. With the advent of the computer, it became increasingly easy for pharmacies to provide printed MARs to cover a specific period of time (e.g., 8 hr, 12 hr, 24 hr, 7 d). This reduced the amount of manual transcription by nursing and gave nursing a way to double-check the accuracy of the pharmacist as well as the nurse who transcribed the order in between printings. Today's most advanced systems utilize computer-based MARs in which the nurse electronically documents medication administration via touch screen technology or through the reading of a bar code on the patient's wrist and the medication packaging. This level of functionality allows for immediate feedback to the nurse if he or she tries to administer a medication inappropriately (e.g., attempt to administer a wrong medication, the wrong dose, at the wrong time, etc.)

Technician Order Entry

Technician order entry has been used as one method to improve the efficiency of order entry. However, this process has come into and out of favor numerous times. Several issues must be considered in determining if technician order entry is beneficial. Technician order entry has mostly been used to bridge the gap between the prescriber's order and the technical task of transcribing the order into the pharmacy information system. It includes all tasks up to but not including the final step of clinical review by the pharmacist. Training and length of technician experience along with the system's efficiency or ease of order review by pharmacists are all factors affecting the choice of using technician order entry. However, systems utilizing physician order entry that include a bidirectional interface or systems that are integrated obviate the need to utilize the technician for order entry. Utilizing technicians for order entry within these interfaced or integrated environments is nonvalue adding. Advanced pharmacy information systems will have tools such as an unverified orders queue that alerts the pharmacist as to which orders (technician or physician entered) are ready for review and final approval.

Inventory Management

Many pharmacy information systems have the capability to manage pharmaceutical inventories. However, there is variability in the success of using such functionality in inpatient versus outpatient pharmacy environments. Inventory management via these systems utilizes various methodologies. Outpatient or retail pharmacies have much more success in maintaining perpetual inventories due to their contained or limited access environments. Perpetual inventories account for the use of each and every tablet, bottle, tube, syringe, etc. Reordering in this perpetual environment is based on incremental utilization in relationship to "par" levels or order-points. The inventory system is triggered to reorder a medication when the inventory, based on actual usage, drops below the par level. When this occurs, an inventory order is then generated. The order may be automatically sent to the drug wholesaler, or the system may place the order into a queue for review by the pharmacist or technician before it is released. However, due to the numerous access points, large numbers of personnel involved, and continual transferring of medications (stocking pharmacy satellites, missing doses, pilferage) most inpatient pharmacies are not conducive to the support and use of inventory management software.

Reporting

The wealth of information available through pharmacy information systems has become well recognized within hospitals, health systems, retail pharmacy chains, pharmacy benefit management companies, and group purchasing organizations. Medication-use trending information may be utilized for such things as Medication Use Evaluations (MUE), ADR/ADE tracking and trending, drug budget forecasting, market share management, and bioterrorism detection and surveillance.[37]

Many tools are available for reporting information from pharmacy information systems. The most advanced systems are accessible and reportable via intranet websites and wireless portable or handheld devices. Reporting may also come in the form of clinical alerts. Advanced systems are capable of sending critical values and alerts to printers, email accounts, and even alpha-numeric pagers. Advanced systems allow for graphical representation of information. For example, one may look at trending information of one or more lab values such as potassium, creatinine clearance, hematocrit, etc., in relationship to the administration of specific medications. *Data mining* has also become easier with the advancement of pharmacy information systems. Reporting from early systems required extensive training and skills to master the extraction of data. Knowledge to perform these tasks was often limited to a small group of devoted pharmacists or information systems personnel when available. Over time, pharmacists have asked for easier front-end reporting tools. These tools allow pharmacists and others to essentially "drag-and-drop" categories or fields of information into a series of if-then statements. This allows the user to quickly develop reports for specific information. While this still has its limitations, it does allow for easier access to data.

Ease of Access

Access to pharmacy information systems has significantly evolved over time as well. Traditionally, client–server applications would have to be loaded onto each computer (client) that would be utilized to access the server. However, with today's web-based technologies such as Citrix®, pharmacy applications may be securely accessed from anywhere (patient care units, pharmacies, home, and abroad) via web browsers. Portable electronic technology has also allowed incredible flexibility to pharmacists' practice. Wireless laptops, tablet PCs, and Palm® devices are all becoming standards of practice. These technologies allow the pharmacist to access a patient's profile while attending rounds or interviewing a patient.

However, even with the advancement of technology and ease of electronic access to medication-use information, many pharmacists are still most comfortable with the traditional printed format. Perhaps this reluctance is mostly related to the size, weight, and awkwardness of carrying around electronic devices. While Palm® devices are easy to carry, their screen size limits the amount of viewable data while their memory limits the amount of storable information. In addition, Palm® devices may or may not provide wireless access to data and may require physical synchronization with another computer to rely on the most up-to-date patient information. Wireless laptops overcome these limitations, yet they are bulky and weigh significantly more. Many times, laptops are attached to mobile stands in a locked fashion to overcome weight issues and prevent the loss of technology. Most recently, tablet PCs have come into the market. They usually consist of a single 15–17" screen and may come with and without a keyboard. They allow the user to reorient the screen such that it can be held much like a pad of paper. Much like the smaller handheld devices, tablet PCs also utilize handwriting recognition technology along with touch–screen technologies to eliminate the need for a keyboard. As with any new technologies, tablet PCs are rapidly evolving. Early complaints of this technology related to length of battery life along with limitations of the handwriting recognition technology. However, battery life has been a complaint of all of these technologies. Due to expense, many of these technologies are shared by groups of clinicians. Preventative maintenance, remembering to recharge batteries, and care in use often get overlooked ultimately leading to poorly maintained devices. Technical support and servicing of these technologies take shape in several forms. In some cases pharmacies choose to maintain equipment themselves; however, it's rare that this task can be completely supported by a pharmacy department alone. In most cases, these types of technologies are supported by internal information systems departments or it is outsourced to vendors or companies specializing in hardware support.

System Security/HIPAA

Security and confidentiality of patient specific health care information have always been a concern of pharmacists. As information systems have evolved, so too has the requirement to have a user ID and a password when logging onto a pharmacy system. By having pharmacists and technicians sign-on to a system, pharmacies may track who has reviewed, approved, and dispensed medications. This is very helpful when errors occur and there is a need to provide educational follow-up to the individual pharmacist or technician. It is also helpful in the prevention of malicious acts by ill-doing individuals. Pharmacy systems require unique user identifications and passwords. Advanced systems require the user to change his/her password after a given interval of time to further ensure the privacy of the user's access. The Health Insurance Portability Accountability Act (HIPAA) of 1996 has also strongly influenced the usage of system security. This law was originally developed to decrease health care costs through the computerization of health care records. However, this lead to privacy concerns and additional laws were developed under the HIPAA umbrella to further protect patient confidentiality. HIPAA describes who may access health information. It also describes the circumstances when health information may be utilized and reported against. Today's pharmacy information systems provide significant user access auditing tools. These tools enable pharmacies to determine who accessed a patient profile on what date and time. They are also able to report any actions performed by an individual.

The Future of Pharmacy Information Systems

The future of pharmacy information systems promises to be very exciting. System integration resulting from the consolidation of disparate databases will be the standard offering from information services vendors. All clinicians (pharmacists, nurses, physicians, etc.) will, therefore, have the same picture of the care given to a particular patient. Clinicians will access patient care information through a common web-based portal or hub. Even though all disciplines will have access to the same information, the clinician will have the ability to self-arrange the patient data contained within the website in a manner that best suits his or her practice needs. User ids and passwords will give way to bio-identification (e.g., fingerprint, voice, retina, etc.) as

the common method to protect access to patient data. Medication profile data will be seamlessly shared electronically between retail pharmacies and acute care settings. As a result, the risk of medication related continuity of care errors as patients transition across inpatient and outpatient environments will be eliminated. Information systems will allow clinicians to easily select medications they wish to continue from the outpatient environment to the inpatient environment and vice versa. Many new clinical roles will open for pharmacists. Instead of only being at the receiving end of a prescriber's order, pharmacists will design electronic care pathways to include the proper use of drugs. Through this process, one pharmacist will be able to impact the clinical practice of numerous prescribers. With integrated systems, there will no longer be the need to have technicians enter handwritten or printed orders into the pharmacy system for a pharmacist's verification. Technicians will, therefore, focus, on the management of pharmacy automation, and the preparation and dispensing of products. Handheld, wireless technologies such as personal digital assistants and tablet PCs will further evolve and decrease in price. Pharmacy systems will be integrated with these technologies in such a way that voice recognition may be used to navigate all patient data or assist with the entry, approval, modification, or discontinuation of medication orders. All pharmacists will be mobile with constant access to patient care data. These advances and many others will allow all pharmacists to find themselves where they should have been all along— out of the pharmacy and at the patients bedside or interacting face to face with other caregivers.

Summary

Pharmacy information systems have had a dramatic impact on the practice of pharmacy. From the basics of inventory management and billing to the most recent real-time, mobile clinical alerts, pharmacy information systems have catapulted the expansion of clinical pharmacy services and improved the overall safety of patients. However, many questions remain around the best and most effective ways to utilize pharmacy information technology. It is also unclear as to how information technology may impact manpower needs in the pharmacy profession. Nevertheless, with the rapid evolution of computer technology, new and exciting advancements in pharmacy practice are sure to be enabled. Those pharmacists and technicians that embrace the use and understanding of pharmacy technologies will be the most sought after and valued pharmacy professionals of the future. Likewise, pharmacies that quickly employ the use of new technologies will easily attract the most talented practitioners.

References

1. Ryan ML, Rinke R, de Leon RF. Selecting a pharmacy computer system for the future. *Pharm Pract Manage Q.* 1995;15(3):1–14.

2. Chaffee BW, Bonasso J. Strategies for pharmacy integration and pharmacy information system interfaces, part 1: history and pharmacy integration options. *Am J Health-Syst Pharm.* 2004;61:502–6.

3. Evans SJ, Howe DJ. A computerized unit dose pharmacy system. *Am J Hosp Pharm.* 1971;28:500–6

4. Derewicz HJ, Zellers DD. The computer-based unit dose system in The Johns Hopkins Hospital. *Am J Hosp Pharm.* 1973;30:206–12.

5. Fish KH. Charging for hospital pharmaceutical services: computerized system using a markup and a dose fee. *Am J Hosp Pharm.* 1979;36:360–3.

6. Winters BH, Hernandez L. A computerized drug inventory control system. *Am J Hosp Pharm.* 1972;29:780–5.

7. Souder DE, Gouveia WA, Sheretz D, et al. A computer-assisted intravenous admixture system. *Am J Hosp Pharm.* 1973;30:1015–20.

8. Freund RG. Evolution of a computerized drug profile. *Am J Hosp Pharm.* 1973;30:160–4.

9. McGovern D. Print, prepare, check, and deliver a 24-hour supply of unit dose medication for 600 patients in one hour. *Hosp Pharm.* 1981;16:193–4 199–200, 203–6.

10. Warner A, Menachemi N, Brooks RG. Information technologies relevant to pharmacy practice in hospitals: results of a statewide survey. *Hosp Pharm.* 2005;20:233–9

11. Pedersen CA, Schneider PJ, Scheckelhoff DJ. ASHP national survey of pharmacy practice in hospital settings: monitoring and patient education—2003. *Am J Health-Syst Pharm.* 2004;61:457–71.

12. Barcia SM. Pharmacy computer systems—best-of-breed or one-vendor solutions? *Health Manag Technol.* 1999 Jul;20(6):16–8.

13. Saya FG, Shane R. A stepwise approach to the evaluation and selection of a hospital pharmacy information system. *Pharm Pract Manage Q.* 1995;15(3):15–22.

14. Ambrose JA, Hummel J. Developing an information technology plan. *Health System Fellowship Reports.* 1999;1(2):11–4.

15. Boston Collaborative Drug Surveillance Program. Adverse drug interactions. *JAMA.* 1972;220:1238–9.

16. Durrence CW, DiPiro JT, May JR, et al. Potential drug interactions in surgical patients. *Am J Hosp Pharm.* 1985;42:1553–5.

17. Blaschke TF, Cohen SN, Tatro DS. Drug-drug interactions and aging. In: Jarvik LF, Greenblatt DJ, Harman D (eds). *Clinical Pharmacology in the Aged Patient.* New York: Raven; 1981.

18. Borda IT, Slone D, Hick H. Assessment of adverse reactions within a drug surveillance program. *JAMA.* 1968;205:645–7.

19. Stanaszek WF, Franklin CE. Survey of potential drug interaction incidence in an outpatient clinic population. *Hosp Pharm.* 1978;13:255–63.

20. Bates DW, Cullen D, Laird N, et al. Incidence of adverse drug events and potential adverse drug events: implications for prevention. *JAMA.* 1995;274:29–34.

21. Lesar TS, Briceland L, Stein DS. Factors related to errors in medication prescribing. *JAMA.* 1997;277:312–7.

22. Tegeder I, Levy M, Muth-Selbach U, et al. Retrospective analysis of the frequency and recognition of adverse drug reactions by means of automatically recorded laboratory signals. *Br J Clin Pharmacol.* 1999;47:557–64.

23. Schiff GD, Klass D, Peterson J, et al. Linking laboratory and pharmacy: Opportunities for reducing errors and improving care. *Arch Intern Med.* 2003;163:893–900.

24. Amsden D. Push technology in the pharmacy. *Health Manag Technol.* 2003 Jan;24(1):28–31.

25. Tully M. The impact of information technology on the performance of clinical pharmacy services. *J of Clin Pharm Ther.* 2000;25(4):243–9.

26. Farrar KT, Stoddart MJ, Slee AJ. Clinical pharmacy and reactive prescription review—time for a change? *Pharmaceutical Journal.* 1998;260:759–61.

27. Degnan D, Merryfield D, Hultgren S. Reaching out to clinicians: implementation of a computerized alert system. *J Healthc Qual.* 2004 Nov–Dec;26(6):26–30.

28. Raschke RA, Gollihare B, Wunderlich TA, et al. A computer alert system to prevent injury from adverse drug events: development and evaluation in a community teaching hospital. *JAMA.* 1998;280:1317–20.

29. Kuperman GJ, Teich JM, Tanasijevic MJ, et al. Improving response to critical laboratory results with automation: results of a randomized controlled trial. *J Am Med Inform Assoc.* 1999;6:512–22.

30. Simonian AI. Documenting pharmacist interventions on an intranet. *Am J Health-Syst Pharm.* 2003;60:151–5.

31. Lee AJ, Boro MS, Knapp KK, et al. Clinical and economic outcomes of pharmacist recommendations in a Veterans Affairs medical center. *Am J Health-Syst Pharm.* 2002;59:2070–7.

32. Carter BL, Malone DC, Billups SJ, et al. Interpreting the findings of the IMPROVE study: impact of managed pharmaceutical care on resource utilization and outcomes in Veterans Affairs medical centers. *Am J Health-Syst Pharm.* 2001 Jul 15;58(14):1330–7.

33. Nesbit TW, Shermock KM, Bobek MB, et al. Implementation and pharmacoeconomic analysis of a clinical staff pharmacy practice model. *Am J Health-Syst Pharm.* 2001;58:784–90

34. Yanchick JK. Implementation of a drug therapy-monitoring clinic in a primary care setting. *Am J Health-Syst Pharm.* 2000;57(suppl 4):S30–34.

35. McMullin ST, Hennenfent JA, Ritchie DJ, et al. A prospective, randomized trial to assess the cost impact of pharmacist-initiated interventions. *Arch Intern Med.* 1999 Oct 25;159(19):2306–9.

36. Leape LL, Cullen DJ, Dempsey CM, et al. Pharmacists' participation on physicians rounds and adverse drug events in the intensive care unit. *JAMA.* 1999;282:267–70.

37. Lober WB, Karras BT, Wagner MM, et al. Roundtable on bioterrorism detection: Information system-based surveillance. *J Am Med Inform Assoc.* 2002;9:105–15.

Chapter 24

Automation in Practice

Steve Rough, Jack Temple

Introduction

In today's health care marketplace, payers and patients demand high quality, efficient, and cost-effective service. Technological advancements are a constant, which pharmacy departments must successfully implement to provide quality service. Efficient use of technology and automation is a prerequisite to the survival of the profession and the advancement of pharmacist patient care services. Automation is designed to streamline and improve the accuracy and efficiency of the medication-use process. All automation is technology, but the inverse is not necessarily true. The purpose of this chapter is to provide some background on the use of automation in inpatient pharmacy practice, to identify best practices for maximizing the safe and efficient use of automation, and to provide a predictive model for the impact automation will have on the future of pharmacy practice. This chapter is not a comprehensive review of all available automated devices and technologies. While this chapter briefly mentions components of pharmacy informatics, CPOE, and clinical decision support systems as they relate to pharmacy automation and rank order of implementation, a detailed review of these topics is provided in other chapters.

Definitions

Adverse Drug Event (ADE)—An injury from a medication or lack of intended medication.

Automation—Any technology, machine or device linked to or controlled by a computer and used to do work.

BCMA—Bar Code Medication Administration

Carousel Automation—A medication storage cabinet with rotating shelves used to automate medication dispensing.

CPOE—Computerized Prescriber Order Entry.

Medication Error—Any preventable event that may cause or lead to inappropriate medication use or patient harm while the medication is in the control of the health care professional, patient, or consumer.

Smart Pumps—Infusion devices with clinical decision support software and drug libraries that perform a test of reasonableness at the point of medication administration.

Technology—For the purposes of this chapter, this refers to anything that is used to replace routine or repetitive tasks previously performed by people, or which extends the capability of people.

Unit-Based Dispensing Cabinets—Secure storage cabinets capable of handling most unit-dose and some bulk (multiple-dose) medications.

History

The application of automated dispensing systems within the practice of pharmacy began in the early 1960s. However, changes in the health care system and the profession's transition to pharmaceutical care have dramatically increased the demand for incorporating automation into pharmacy practice over the past 15 years. Corporate and organizational goals of reducing costs, improving operating efficiencies, growing revenues, enhancing safety and quality, integrating and managing data, and providing outstanding customer service are primary drivers of this trend. Pharmacy managers are expected to improve efficiency (i.e., reduce pharmacy staff, reduce nursing workload) and quality (i.e., reduce medication delivery time, improve patient safety and clinical programs), both of which can be accomplished through appropriate use of automation. As the profession has accepted increased responsibility for improving patient outcomes through implementation of pharmacist patient care services, automation has been relied upon to free the pharmacist from technical tasks. Shortages of qualified pharmacists and technicians, coupled with shrinking operating budgets, are leading managers to explore technologies that can perform tasks traditionally performed by pharmacists and technicians.

Strategic partnerships between health systems and pharmaceutical wholesalers are increasing the rate of availability and deployment of new automation and technologies. Wholesalers are middlemen businesses that purchase pharmaceuticals from most drug manufacturers for resale to pharmacy customers. Rising complexities and costs of running day to day pharmacy operations, shrinking personnel resources, and limited technology expertise have led pharmacy directors to seek partnerships with vendors possessing a broad line of automated products. This trend, coupled with traditionally strong pharmacy/wholesaler business relationships and declining wholesaling drug distribution business margins, has created incentives for wholesalers to develop more profitable (automation-related) business ventures. Thus, since the mid-1990s wholesalers have acquired pharmacy technology and automation companies. Such mergers with automation companies have been a key component to drug wholesaler survival. Traditional automated distribution and information system technologies used by wholesalers to provide services to their pharmacy customers are now being sought after by these same customers to improve pharmacy purchasing and inventory management efficiency. Today's largest pharmaceutical wholesalers (AmerisourceBergen, Cardinal Health, and McKesson) offer similar suites of pharmacy automation dispensing products.

Medication Errors Versus Adverse Drug Events

According to a consensus definition reached by the National Coordinating Council for Medication Error Reporting and Prevention (NCCMERP), a medication error is "any preventable event that may cause or lead to inappropriate medication use or patient harm while the medication is in the control of the health care professional, patient or consumer." A medication error may also be defined as "the failure of a planned action to be completed as intended or the use of a wrong plan to achieve an aim."[1] The key elements of these definitions are that medication errors are preventable, do not always cause patient harm, and that they may be caused by errors in planning (e.g., prescribing), not just errors in execution (e.g., dispensing the wrong drug for a patient). The majority of medication errors do not result in adverse drug events (ADEs). An ADE is an injury from a medication or lack of intended medication. Reported medication error rates in the literature reach up to 19%.[2] Reported ADE rates vary in the literature depending on the detection method ranging from 0.2% using a voluntary, self-reporting system to 10%

when a system of chart review and computerized screening was used.[3–6] Medication errors resulting in ADEs (preventable ADEs) result in significant consumption of resources in the form of increased lengths of stay, increased cost of care, rework time, malpractice claims, and patient costs (suffering and lost productivity). Prospective, case-control studies estimate that preventable ADEs may result in an additional length of stay of 4.66 days and a $5,857 increase in hospitalization costs.[7,8]

The Medication-Use Process

The medication-use process encompasses all areas of medication use and is a highly complex, multidisciplinary process. In its simplest form, the medication-use process consists of five domains: (1) purchasing/inventory management; (2) prescribing/medication determination; (3) medication preparation, dispensing, and counseling; (4) medication administration; and (5) patient monitoring/assessment. Thinking of medication use in terms of a multistep process or system is critical to being able to understand and develop strategies to improve medication safety. Bates et al. used a four-phase medication-use model to categorize the potential and preventable ADEs that were detected using an intensive surveillance process.[5] These four phases include: (1) ordering, (2) transcription, (3) dispensing, and (4) administration. In this study, the majority of preventable and potential ADEs occurred in the ordering and administration phases (49% and 26%, respectively). The dispensing and transcription phase were associated with 14% and 11% of the preventable and potential ADEs. When only medication errors that caused patient harm were considered (i.e., preventable ADEs), 56% occurred during the ordering phase, 34% during administration, 6% during transcription, and 4% during dispensing.

These data suggest that system changes aimed at improving the ordering and administration phases of the medication-use process are likely to have the greatest impact on reducing medication errors and preventable ADEs. The high incidence of preventable ADEs in the ordering phase is one of the major reasons why a well-designed, CPOE system is touted as being so critical to improving the safety of the medication-use process. The study by Bates and colleagues also confirmed that errors are more likely to be intercepted if they occur early in the process.[5] If errors occur later in the medication-use process, they are far less likely to be detected as evidenced by the fact that no administration errors were intercepted in this study. This, coupled with the fact that the administration phase had the second highest incidence of preventable ADEs, reinforces the need for appropriate double checks in the administration process and, if possible, the use of bar code medication administration (BCMA) technology to build in another layer of protection into the medication-use system.

Although only a macro-level view of the medication-use process has been presented thus far, the medication-use system in hospitals is inherently complex often containing more than 100 steps with multiple hand-offs. Flowcharting the existing medication-use process lays the foundation for a system approach for reducing medication errors and preventable ADEs. Flowcharting the process also helps to illustrate weaknesses and unnecessary steps in the existing system and can help identify the multiple points in the system where breakdowns could occur and cause errors.

Strategies for Automation

A wide array of automation is currently in use in many health systems within all phases of the medication-use process. Automated tasks include counting, inventory control, packaging, compounding, labeling, distribution, dispensing, and verification of accurate medication administration, while electronically documenting all transactions. Goals for the use of automation include improving patient care, customer services, and resource utilization. This section describes several inpatient pharmacy automated dispensing systems and technologies, their advantages and disadvantages, and their intended roles in various aspects of the medication-use process. Table 24-1 provides a comprehensive list of technology and automation that can be applied throughout the medication-use process. It is important to note that intended benefits are not always actualized within organizations. Pharmacists must understand both the positive effects and limitations for automated systems and the areas for improvement they present. Several opportunities exist for further development of all technologies discussed in this section.

Drug Purchasing and Supply Chain Management Systems

Pharmacy asset management (order to pay process) can be improved by linking supply reordering channels to

Table 24-1

Technologies and Automated Devices Applied throughout the Medication-Use Process

Prescribing

> Clinical decision support software
> Computerized prescriber order entry

Dispensing

> Carousel technology
> Centralized robotic dispensing technology
> Centralized narcotic dispensing and inventory tracking devices
> Decentralized automated dispensing devices
> Intravenous and total parenteral nutrition compounding devices
> Pneumatic tube delivery systems
> Unit dose medication repacking systems

Administration

> Bar code medication administration technology
> Clinical decision support-based infusion pumps

Monitoring

> Electronic clinical documentation systems
> Web-based compliance and disease management tracking systems

the medication distribution system.[9,10] Goals include centralizing and automating supply chain management to reduce on-hand drug product inventory, improving accuracy and labor efficiency, paying invoices in a timely manner to optimize wholesaler discounts, and reducing product acquisition costs. Supply chain management essentially means the distribution of medication supplies throughout the medication-use process. For years, many pharmacies have been using bar coded product shelf labels and hand-held product reordering devices for physical product inventory and value documentation and for reordering pharmaceuticals. Historically, complete and accurate automation of inventory tracking and product reordering has been primarily limited to large chain store pharmacies, which have invested millions of dollars into developing systems to remove human error and labor costs from this process. Many hospital pharmacies continue to experience inefficiencies in this area. However, this gap is closing. Inefficient processes on front-end product ordering and inventory procedures can hamper a pharmacist's ability to provide direct patient care. Poor product procurement systems can result in pharmacists spending excessive time trying to locate products. Several technologies are available that can improve the supply chain management process.

In order for a pharmacy to develop an efficient supply chain management program, it is a requirement to partner with a pharmaceutical wholesaler. Some wholesalers use state-of-the-art inventory management technology within their distribution centers, which use bar codes and radio frequency signals to track and assure accurate product filling for customers. Since many wholesalers also own automated dispensing technologies and have extensive interface capabilities, they are able to electronically connect with pharmacy automated dispensing software, prescription processing computer systems, and point-of-sale cash register systems. Accomplishing such integration is a major hurdle in accurately and efficiently automating the procurement process. For example, if a pharmacy's computer order processing system is capable of maintaining an accurate perpetual inventory of products on the shelf and account for all dispensing and crediting transactions, that system may be able to electronically communicate real-time inventory levels to the wholesaler's order management system and automatically place an order to the wholesaler when inventory levels fall below a predetermined quantity. Such a system works best with robotic dispensing technology that maintains a closed perpetual inventory record of drug products. When products are received in the pharmacy from the wholesaler, the same interface permits new inventory quantities received to be added to the pharmacy computer system's or automated dispensing system's perpetual inventory. Health systems have been slow to implement such systems, largely due to dispensing system complexities and multiple drug inventory locations within the hospital. Some hospitals have implemented automated procurement systems for a limited supply of medications such as those maintained in a centralized robotic dispensing system or in a pharmacy stockroom, but not for the majority of their inventory. Automated inventory management systems, when properly managed, have the potential to result in dramatic one-time cost savings via reducing drug inventory (assets) on hand and result in long-term savings and efficiency via maximizing drug inventory turn rates, avoiding expired inventory, and reducing labor required for the drug procurement process.

Some wholesalers are beginning to provide handheld scanning devices with integrated bar code readers to pharmacies in order to automate the pharmaceutical receiving process at the product (or even the tote) level. This provides the pharmacy with an automated receiving and invoice reconciliation process, thus automating the labor-intensive and error-prone product check-in process. This process begins with a pharmacy technician scanning a bar code on a delivery tote containing products from the wholesaler, which in turn generates an electronic invoice. Each product bar code is then scanned as it is removed from the tote and the products received are automatically reconciled versus the invoice. The system will automatically credit product invoicing discrepancies, arrange for mispicks (shipping errors) to be returned, and updates the pharmacy's perpetual inventory for products received. This same scanner may be used to generate return requests for damaged or unused products the pharmacy wishes to return to the wholesaler and can be used for order generation. After products are received, the next step is to generate payment to the wholesaler. It is now possible for accounts payable information for all products received to be securely available as a billing statement via the Internet immediately following the automated electronic product receiving process. Thus, pharmacies may confirm via real-time Internet access exactly what products were received on specific invoices, as well as which invoices have been paid and which are outstanding. The combination of the ordering, receiving, and reconciliation technologies described above may help to improve efficiency of the pharmacy supply chain management process and dramatically reduce inventory carrying costs.

Drug Distribution and Dispensing Systems

This section briefly describes the advantages, disadvantages, and issues surrounding the use of several existing technologies, which, if appropriately deployed, may help improve the safety of the medication-use process. This section describes only those technologies thought to have the greatest potential impact on patient safety and is not designed to be all-inclusive. Comprehensive reviews of pharmacy automation are available elsewhere in the literature.[11–14]

Decentralized Automated Dispensing Devices

Decentralized automated dispensing systems, sometimes referred to as unit-based dispensing cabinets, are secure storage cabinets capable of handling most unit-dose and some bulk (multiple-dose) medications. These devices are typically connected via a real-time interface to the hospital's pharmacy computer system in an attempt to maintain control over drug dispensing. Automated dispensing devices were originally installed in hospitals in the early 1990s to provide increased control over controlled substances and floor stock medications in patient care areas. It is estimated that in 2002 close to 60% of hospitals in the United States incorporated automated dispensing devices for dispensing of medications to inpatients.[9] It is likely that the rate of use has increased since that time. In addition to their traditional uses, many hospitals are now using these devices for storing and dispensing nearly all scheduled doses, thereby eliminating the manual medication cart fill and delivery process.

The primary focus of these automated dispensing systems is to provide prompt, real-time availability of medications for the nurse and patient. They can also help to improve controlled substance accountability, increase productivity, improve charge capture and documentation accuracy, and reduce pharmacy and nursing labor costs. However, the impact of these decentralized automated dispensing systems on medication errors is less clear.[15,16] Decentralized dispensing devices are increasingly incorporating bar code labeling and scanning into the replenishment process, thus improving restocking accuracy and potentially improving medication safety. Also, the use of automated dispensing systems can result in pharmacists not having to check manually filled medication carts and first doses; resulting in the redeployment of pharmacists to direct patient care activities including medication therapy management services.

Automated dispensing systems introduce much potential for medication errors. Some systems allow nurses to choose any patient and dispense any drug they choose. Purchasing an insufficient number of cabinets may preclude an institution's ability to maintain a well-controlled, single-dose access medication dispensing system resulting in a higher potential for product selection and administration errors. Despite increasing pressure from regulatory agencies, some organizations have yet to link their pharmacy computer systems to cabinets in such a way that restricts nurses from obtaining medications that are not ordered for patients. Other medication administration safety concerns with automated dispensing devices include (1) nurses retrieving an incorrect medication because of open access to all drugs in a drawer; (2) carelessness or lack of verification of drug labels due to a belief that the system is computerized and, therefore, not as susceptible to errors (or the belief that pharmacy placed

the drug there and pharmacy does not make mistakes); (3) drugs stocked in the wrong pocket either because one or more doses inadvertently fell into the wrong slot or due to a pharmacy restocking error; and (4) changing the location of the drug in the cabinet can cause errors because the health care professional chooses drugs from particular locations by habit rather than verifying each drug's identity.[17]

Conflicting reports exist in the literature on the impact of automated dispensing devices on medication error rates and provider efficiency.[17-20] Unfortunately, significant capital investments have been made in these systems without full evaluation of the operational changes needed to ensure that efficiency goals were met without compromising patient safety. Automated dispensing devices may improve nurse efficiency for tasks associated with narcotic record keeping, yet increase nursing time requirements for dispensing non-narcotic doses. In the late 1980s and early 1990s, one could set a return on investment (ROI) for this technology based on improved charge capture rates; however, in today's environment of prospective reimbursement, an ROI based on patient charges is rarely sustainable. Regardless of whether or not state regulations exist to assure safe use of automated dispensing systems, it is extremely important that every organization develop, enforce, and continuously improve multidisciplinary policies and procedures to ensure patient safety, accuracy, security, and confidentiality. Table 24-2 provides an extensive list of guidelines and considerations for the safe use of decentralized automated dispensing systems. Table 24-3 provides an extensive list of potential advantages and disadvantages of decentralized automated dispensing systems.

Centralized Robotics for Dispensing Medications

Centrally located automated dispensing devices are designed to automate the entire process of medication dispensing including medication storage, dispensing, restocking, and crediting of unit dose medications. Such systems must be interfaced with the pharmacy information system to provide the system access to each patient's medication profile. Bar coding of medication doses allows dispensing accuracy to approach 100% with centralized robotics technology. Thus, as long as a patient-specific computerized medication profile is maintained in an accurate and timely manner, pharmacist time may be reallocated from medication checking duties to more direct patient care activities.

Centralized robotic dispensing systems were traditionally used exclusively to dispense unit dose, bar

Table 24-2

Guidelines for Safe Use of Decentralized Automated Dispensing Systems

- Assign medications to devices based on the needs of the patient care unit, patient age, diagnosis, and staff expertise

- Create an alert system to flag high-risk medications stocked in devices (such as a maximum dose prompt)

- Develop an ongoing competency assessment program for all personnel with access to the device; include direct observations and random restocking accuracy audits; observe dispensing accuracy as part of the assessment

- Develop a system to locate and remove recalled medications

- Develop clear, multidisciplinary downtime procedures; include procedures in training and ongoing competency programs

- Develop systems to account for narcotic waste; routinely audit controlled substance dispense quantities against patient orders, medication administration record documentation, and waste documentation

- Display allergy reminders for specific drugs such as antibiotics, opiates, and NSAIDs on appropriate medication storage pockets or have them automatically appear on the dispensing screen

- Do not allow nurses to return medications to the original storage pockets/locations; assign a return bin to collect returned medications

- Establish a preventive maintenance schedule with the vendor that does not disrupt workflow

- Establish strict security criteria to limit unauthorized access to devices

- Establish stringent safety criteria for selecting medications that are (and are not) appropriate to store in devices and oversee the process for assigning new drugs to new locations in all care settings

- Incorporate bar code scanning for restocking and medication retrieval

- Limit the numbers of medications not available in profile dispense that may be overridden (dispensed without pharmacist review and verification)

- Maximize the use of unit dose medications in ready-to-administer form, with only a few exceptions

- Only assign medications with minimal harm potential to open access drawers

- Perform routine expiration date checks, as well as concomitantly verifying inventory quantities

- Require all personnel to attend formal training and demonstrate competency prior to accessing the devices

- Require pharmacist medication order review and verification before a medication is accessed for first dose administration (profile dispensing)

- Restrict access to provide single dose (or single drug) availability whenever possible; focus control on high-risk medications and controlled substances (locked lidded pockets)

- Separate sound-alike and look-alike medications; do not stock these medications in the same open-access drawer

coded medications for scheduled medication cart filling; it is now possible to extend the use of this technology to include automation of first dose dispensing. Another recent expanded use of robotic systems is their ability to pick medication doses to be restocked in decentralized automated dispensing cabinets. This has the potential to reduce medication administration errors by improving dispensing cabinet restocking accuracy.

Potential advantages of robotics include reducing pharmacy labor costs, eliminating technical tasks of pharmacists facilitating their redeployment to perform clinical activities, and improving medication dispensing accuracy. No published data are available on these advantages, but in one unpublished study a robot decreased the dispensing error rate from 2.9% to 0.6%.[21] However, this improved dispensing accuracy of robotic technology has never been proven to result in improved patient safety since nurses still have open access to all robot-dispensed medications after they are distributed to patient care areas.

Perhaps the greatest advantage of implementing robotic technology is that all doses dispensed by the robot are bar coded, thus facilitating the implementa-

Table 24-3
Potential Advantages and Disadvantages of Decentralized Automated Dispensing Systems

Advantages	Disadvantages
Ability to add expansion (auxiliary) cabinets to increase capacity	Accurate inventory quantities are difficult to maintain with matrix configurations; results in medication stock outs
Ability to only allow access to a single dose of a medication	Downtimes may impact patient care
Accommodate multiple dosage forms with flexible drawer configurations	Duplicate inventory may increase inventory costs and the amount of expired medications
Automated controlled substance retrieval, inventory reconciliation and the process to resolve discrepancies	If devices are used to replace cart fill, several devices are needed per nursing unit to supply the necessary products and quantities to maintain a safe and efficient system
Automated medication charging increases the amount of charges captured	Inspection and removal of expired medications must be performed manually (devices do not have the software to track expiration dates)
Bar code scanning to improve accuracy of restocking	Multiple dose access still allows for controlled substance diversion and discrepancy follow-up may still be required
Improved medication distribution response time, thus patients may receive the first dose of a medication faster	Poor integration with bedside medication storage systems
Improved nursing satisfaction due to fewer missing doses, fewer delays for first doses, and more nursing control over day-to-day medication distribution activities	Potential cost savings are frequently not realized (labor-neutral for pharmacy technicians)
More pharmacy control versus traditional floor stock system	■ Nursing time saved is difficult to actualize into nursing staff reductions
■ Stocking the device is time consuming (often because medication dispensing can be centrally controlled by an interfaced pharmacy computerized patient profile	Potential for medication errors and suboptimal therapy
Patient-specific medication profiles to direct and control medication administration (profile dispense)	■ Drawers with open access pockets may allow product selection errors
Provide detailed electronic dispensing and usage reports	■ Nurses may access a medications before a pharmacist reviews the order
Redeploy pharmacist to perform patient care activities	Unable to accommodate all medications (limited by medication size, cabinet size, and risk level for a particular medication to be stocked in a device)
Reduce pharmacist time spent towards medication distribution	
Save nursing labor	
■ Eliminate missing or misplaced narcotic drawer keys	
■ Eliminate narcotic counts at shift change	
■ Fewer narcotic discrepancies to resolve	
■ Less narcotic paperwork to handle	

tion of BCMA systems. However, this necessity for bar codes on all medications dispensed by the robot has the potential to introduce new error into the medication-use system. Although some manufacturers provide bar coded medications, most unit dose medications must be accurately repackaged and bar code labeled by the pharmacy department. Many manufacturers offer automation and even full service agreements to assist with this labor-intensive packaging requirement.

Table 24-4 provides an extensive list of potential advantages and disadvantages of centralized robotic dispensing systems.

Table 24-4
Potential Advantages and Disadvantages of Centralized Robotic Dispensing Systems

Advantages	Disadvantages
Accommodates a very large online inventory	Dispensing accuracy is dependent on accurate computer order entry
Automates medication restocking and removal of expired medications	Dispensing accuracy is dependent on accurate repackaging
Automates the credit process for any unused medication doses	Does not accommodate refrigerated items
Easily integrated with bedside medication storage systems	Increased labor requirements for packaging medications because all doses require a bar coded package label
Initial platform for point-of-care bar code medication administration and documentation system	Lack of standard bar codes in health care
Labor saving and improved restocking accuracy by automating the restocking of the decentralized dispensing systems	Nursing acceptance may be mixed
Reduces pharmacist time required to verify technician filled medications, allowing a reallocation of time to focus on patient care activities	■ May not reduce missing doses ■ May still experience delays in receiving first doses ■ Two layers of packaging around most doses
Reduces technician labor required to fill unit dose medication carts and first doses (reductions are easily obtained)	Possible disruption in medication therapy when patients are transferred from one location to another
Theoretical patient safety improvements	Potential to provide more doses than are needed for a single administration time, leading to potential errors
■ Facilitates a pharmacist review of orders before a nurse can administer the first dose of a medication ■ Improved dispensing accuracy	Requires a large amount of space and often physical renovation

Carousel Technology

Carousel automation is a medication storage cabinet with rotating shelves used to automate medication dispensing. Like other centralized robotic systems, the carousel must be interfaced with the pharmacy information system. The carousel utilizes bar code and pick-to-light technology to improve the efficiency and accuracy of pharmacy technicians who pick and restock medications. Rotating shelves within the carousel bring medications to the technician at one working level, where a light identifies the exact location from which the medication is to be picked. Assigning medications into carousel does not need to be in alphabetical order to facilitate locating medications; therefore, carousels can help meet regulatory requirements and reduce errors from sound-alike, look-alike medications. Carousel technology also works to reduce technician travel time, bending, and reaching for medications during the filling process. The rotating shelves allow pharmacies to take advantage of rarely used vertical space to store medications, freeing up space for other uses.

The bar code technology used by a carousel can be a foundation for a patient bedside bar code medication administration, as well as performing perpetual inventory tracking and tracking expiration dates. Accurate inventory levels along with par levels, allow a pharmacy to automate the medication reordering process. By keeping expirations dates accurate, carousels can improve the efficiency with which expired medications are removed from inventory. Carousels can be integrated with automated dispensing cabinets to increase the efficiency of cabinet restocking, eliminating the need for the current paper refill reports and the manual picking process. Comprehensive software within the carousel allows pharmacies to work more efficiently minimizing the number of carousel turns, prioritizing workflow, and processing the most important orders first. Carousel software may also allow pharmacies to set up inventory locations outside of a carousel (e.g., on a shelf or in a refrigerator). Using this feature, pharmacies can process orders through the carousel to take advantage of the carousel's inventory management for items not physically contained within it. Pharmacies also have the option to set up checking stations with bar code scanners to facilitate pharmacist checking of medications dispensed outside of the carousel.

It is clear that an automated medication dispensing system incorporating either centralized robotics or carousel technology will result in improved dispensing accuracy and labor efficiency. However, it is still unclear as to the right configuration of these technologies and how well they complement or unnecessarily duplicate one another. Research is needed to confirm the theoretical benefits of these two systems in stand-alone environments in which these technologies are implemented apart from one another, and in hybrid-approach environments in which these technologies are implemented in synergy to automate the dispensing of most doses from the inpatient pharmacy.

Centralized Narcotic Dispensing and Record Keeping Systems

Accounting for every dose of controlled substance dispensed and administered is one of the most labor-intensive processes in a central pharmacy. There are products that can automate this process, bringing improved efficiency and control into the system. Such systems can record all doses dispensed from a central pharmacy narcotic room or decentralized automated dispensing devices by scanning manufacturer's bar codes, and provide a record of the individual performing every transaction. Additionally, they can interface with decentralized automated dispensing devices to verify that every dose dispensed from the pharmacy is stocked into the intended decentralized automated dispensing device. They can also generate bar coded nursing proof-of-use forms for patient care areas without automated dispensing devices. Lastly, they can suggest reorder quantities based on past usage, provide useful compliance reports for the Drug Enforcement Agency, and facilitate documentation of controlled substance waste. Such systems provide undeniable benefits with regards to tightening up controlled substance inventory maintenance and identifying potential drug product diversion. Hospitals with one or more dedicated narcotic room technicians will likely be able to cost justify the implementation of centralized narcotic dispensing and record keeping systems by reducing personnel time requirements associated with inventory control and record keeping activities. Thus, it is very common to find hospitals that have moved all traditional, narcotic vault drug inventory into automated

dispensing cabinets linked to narcotic inventory control software as a means to improve narcotic inventory control and dispensing accuracy within the hospital.

Drug Administration Systems

Bar Code Medication Administration Technology

The medication administration phase of the medication-use process is perhaps the most error-prone phase of any process in all of health care. Literature demonstrates that error rates are as high as 19% at this phase, meaning that one in five medications are administered in error in today's hospitals.[2] BCMA technology can help to dramatically reduce these errors!

BCMA technology combines a number of hardware and software components to display, receive, and chart real-time patient and medication information, providing caregivers (usually nurses) with the information needed to accurately administer and document medication administration. This technology performs a three-way check at the bedside, linking and checking bar codes on the nurse's identification badge, the dose of medication at the patient's bedside, and the patient's identification wristband. BCMA enables a nurse to administer medications and helps to ensure the five rights of medication administration: right patient, right medication, right dose, right time, and right route. Before administering a medication to a patient, the nurse scans a bar code on their identification badge, a second bar code on the unit dose of medication, and a third on the patient's wristband. When the nurse scans the medication he or she is planning to administer, that medication is electronically compared to the patient's medication profile. The system then either immediately verifies the drug as a match with the ordered drug and instantly documents the medication as administered in an electronic medication administration record (MAR), or warns the nurse that the drug scanned does not match the drug that was ordered for that patient. Specifics of any mismatch are displayed and tracked. The system also verifies the correct patient or immediately warns the nurse of the wrong patient, helping to prevent a serious error. If there is a discrepancy anywhere in the process (drug, dose, time, method or patient), most BCMA systems alert the nurse to the potential problem via a visual and audible alert than an error is about to occur. Each alert must be addressed before the drug may be administered. All avoided errors are documented in the BCMA software. The BCMA system records the time of administration or reason for not giving a medication onto a computerized MAR. Most BCMA technology can also identify and alert the nurse, real time, to any omitted medications

BCMA can provide real-time updates to electronic MARs, enabling all caregivers to view pertinent information about the patient's current and past medication regimens and make judgments about future medication administrations. Most systems use a wireless, radio frequency network and real-time software interface to continuously update hand-held scanners with patient information as well as new, modified, and discontinued medication orders from the pharmacy computer system. Thus, nurses can learn of new and discontinued medication orders almost instantaneously. BCMA systems use various devices applied at the point of care, such as laser bar code scanners and wireless, portable hand-held computers that are linked to pharmacy information system computers via a radio frequency network to maximize portability. BCMA software must receive real-time patient information and medication profiles from the pharmacy computer system in order to be effective. When a medication order is initiated, modified, or discontinued in the pharmacy computer system, the order information is updated into the BCMA point-of-care device. For all scheduled doses the device alerts the nurse when it is time to administer the medication.

This technology offers the potential to dramatically reduce the risk of drug administration errors.[22–24] Organizations that have implemented this technology report up to 87% reductions in medication administration errors, with up to 10% of doses scanned resulting in one of the following discrepancies: wrong patient, wrong drug, wrong dose, or wrong time.[23–25]

Although improvements are being made in BCMA and other electronic medication administration record (MAR) technology, effectively implementing these systems can be costly and complicated. Major limitations to implementing BCMA include (1) cost of the BCMA software; (2) cost of BCMA-related hardware such as portable scanning devices, bedside computers, centralized computer servers, bar code printing systems for patient and caregiver identification tags and bar code medication repackaging systems; (3) all medications must be bar coded in unit-of-use packaging to achieve the optimal safety benefit, usually requiring labor-intensive and potentially error-prone repackaging in the pharmacy; (4) commercially available BCMA products are still at a very early stage of development; (5) nursing workflow redesign issues; (6) elaborate

real-time interfaces between pharmacy and BCMA information systems are necessary to assure accurate patient records within the BCMA system; and (7) installation of a dedicated radio frequency network may be incompatible with certain patient monitoring devices in the hospital. These above stated limitations and incompatibilities have limited the use of BCMA technology in many health care settings. Despite widespread recommendations to use BCMA technology to verify and document medication administration, it is estimated that fewer than 10% of pharmacies incorporate bar codes into their dispensing process and fewer than 2% of hospitals currently use BCMA technology.[26] Although this medical error prevention technology is not yet widespread, it is expected that implementation will rapidly climb secondary to efforts by the Food and Drug Administration, the Joint Commission on Accreditation of Healthcare Organizations, professional societies, and patient safety groups.

Because one of the major limitations of BCMA technology is bar coding all medications, a cursory understanding of the information contained in a bar code is necessary. A bar code is simply a graphic representation of data (alpha, numeric, or both) that is machine-readable. Bar codes are a way of encoding numbers and letters by using a combination of bars and spaces with varying widths stacked side by side in such a way that the scanner interprets the rows as data. Both the lines and spaces are read. Bar codes typically do not contain description data in and of themselves. Each bar code has specific identification encoded in it, and that data is used by a computer/scanner to look up all specific information associated with the data. Bar codes come in many varieties and symbologies. *Symbology* is considered a language in bar code technology. When a bar code is scanned, the symbology enables information to be read accurately. When a bar code is printed, the symbology enables the printer to understand the information that needs to be turned into a label. A critical component of a bar code system exists between the printed bar code symbols on the product and the scanner's ability to interpret the bar code data. The scanner's ability to quickly and accurately interpret the bar code data depends on (1) the quality of the bar code print on the product, and (2) the symbology and configuration of the bar code. Space available on most unit-dose packages is limited, yet many manufacturers have been able to successfully bar code these products. Bar codes on medications contain specific information about that drug, including, but not limited to, the product name, dose, dosage form, route, expiration date, and lot number.

Bar coding of drugs is a useful strategy for reducing errors since it provides a very accurate mechanism to ensure that the drug in hand is indeed the intended one. One historical barrier to implementing bar codes on all medications has been the lack of a consensus among the pharmaceutical manufacturers on the appropriate approach for adding bar coding to unit-dose product labels. No universal standard bar code symbology has been adopted for medications. However, commercially available scanners are able to read most commonly applied unit dose medication linear bar code symbology, and recent federal legislation requires that manufacturers encode the national data code (NDC) number on most prescription and certain OTC products via the use of a linear bar code by April of 2006. Inclusion of the lot number and expiration data remains voluntary at this time. While this regulation is a major stop forward for patient safety, it is increasingly apparent that health-system pharmacies will need the capability to repackage and bar code medications to the unit of use. The bar coding regulation will likely influence some manufacturers to cease production of unit dose product lines, and many manufacturer supplied doses are not provided in the exact dose needed for specific patient populations, requiring local pharmacy compounding and bar code application in order to maximize the theoretical benefits of the BCMA system.

Selecting high-volume unit dose packaging machines can provide pharmacies with significant benefits, including increased efficiency and control over bar coded drug availability. Such technology is increasingly reliable, with greater speed and capacity. Professional packaging systems allow pharmacies to bar code virtually all medication forms, including solids, liquid cups, vials, ampules and syringes. Much literature exists on the successful development and implementation of pharmacy-based bar code packaging operations and distribution systems.[27]

BCMA, by itself, is not an all-encompassing solution for medication safety. With any new process, there exists the potential for new sources of error. New sources of error following BCMA implementation can be numerous, including pharmacy medication repackaging errors, software interface failures, inefficient and inaccurate display of medication order information on the BCMA screen, and nursing workarounds. It is important that organization focus on identifying and managing these new sources of error indefinitely following BCMA implementation to minimize their occurrence. Thus, it is extremely important that adequate resources be allotted to this task, likely requiring dedicated BCMA project management personnel (e.g., nurse and pharmacist labor) throughout the life of the technology. However, the overall benefits of improved patient safety, documentation accuracy, and nurse satisfaction, as well as public and patient relations that can result from a well-designed and implemented BCMA system dramatically outweigh BCMA implementation challenges. Table 24-5 provides an extensive list of advantages and possible limitations with bar code medication administration systems.

Clinical Decision Support-Based Infusion Pumps

Errors associated with the administration of medications through intravenous infusion pumps to critically ill patients can result in adverse drug events. Furthermore, variation in intravenous medication practices is likely associated with increased risk of patient harm.[28] As many as 60% of serious and life threatening errors may be associated with intravenous therapy.[29]

Intravenous (IV) infusion technology has changed tremendously from the first devices offering one infusion channel and simple rate programming, to devices with multiple channels allowing infusion of several medications simultaneously and complex programming for dose calculations and dose delivery (i.e., loading, bolus and maintenance doses). Devices today can signal alerts when air is detected within the infusion line and have moved from general purpose devices to therapy specific devices (i.e., patient controlled analgesia, epidural pumps). Clinical decision support-based infusion pumps (often referred to as *smart pumps*) are taking intravenous medication infusion safety a step further. Such devices are available from several companies, performing clinical decision support at the point of care. The safety software in these devices contains multiple drug libraries that include intravenous medications, concentrations, dosing units, and dose minimum/maximum limits. A nurse programs the pump by selecting the appropriate care area or patient type followed by the drug and concentration of the pump. Programmed doses are automatically checked to determine if they are within the ranges established for each drug. Doses outside the hospital-established limits trigger an alert that must be addressed before the infusion can begin. The software contained in the infusion devices allows institutions the ability to create hospital profiles and drug libraries. Hospital profiles are created to provide

Table 24-5
Potential Advantages and Disadvantages of BCMA Technology

Advantages	Disadvantages
Automated documentation ■ Comprehensive data and reports available "on demand" ■ Facilitates precise pharmacokinetic monitoring ■ On demand view of a patient's history of administered medications ■ Records and verifies in real time the exact time of medication administration information (eliminates missed/incomplete documentation Improved patient safety and accuracy ■ Allergy checks are performed at the bedside ■ Bar code scanning to verify the appropriateness of a medication at the patient's bedside ■ Maintains appropriate packaging and labeling of unit dose medications up to the point of administration, at the patient's bedside ■ Nurse is immediately alerted to discrepancies (wrong drug, dose) ■ Nurse is immediately alerted to missed doses ■ Real-time order and patient information is available to the nurse at the bedside Increased charge accuracy through automation Automates tracking for controlled substances removed from decentralized dispensing devices but never scanned Marketing tool for the organization Nursing convenience ■ Customizable, medication administration planning reports ■ Easy documentation of medication administration criteria and vital signs at the beside ■ Medication administration record is mobile and paperless ■ Small, light weight, wireless hand-held devices	A number of devices are needed for busy or large nursing units, this may be cost-prohibitive for some organizations All medications must be bar coded to ensure a realization of the safety benefits shown Lack of standard bar codes in health care Manual printing of patient medication administration records at discharge for an organization without a fully integrated or interfaced electronic medical record Possible competition among nurses for access to devices (dependent on number of devices an organization can afford) Products are at early stages of development Radio frequency demands may be problematic for some organizations Radio frequency devices are required for real-time updates from pharmacy computer system; may interfere with clinical patient monitoring devices Short battery life requires extra batteries or frequent battery exchanges Success is dependent on nursing's acceptance of the change ■ Implementation causes dramatic changes in how nurses perform their job

specific infusion device operating parameters, programming options, and drug libraries for specific patient populations (i.e., pediatric, pediatric intensive care, neonatal intensive care, adult critical care, adult general care, etc.). Drug libraries are often institutional specific medication lists that contain standard concentrations and preset dosing limits. Institutions often have the option to make dosing limits either hard limits (not an overridable alert) or soft limits (an overridable alert with action). Once the pump is programmed, the smart pump software performs a test of reasonableness against the hospital profile and the drug library to verify the pump has been programmed correctly for the specific patient population and medication.

Along with the test of reasonableness the software has event recording capabilities. Data logs exist to track events such as the number of infusions programmed, the number of times an alert is given, the number of times an alert is overridden and detailed records for programming errors that were averted and could have caused patient harm. Depending on the vendor selected, data logs can often be accessed through downloads from each pump to a computer or pumps can be equipped with radio frequency devices to transmit data in real time. Until recently IV infusion error data was scarcely available, thus new smart pump data logs can help organizations track and trend infusion data in order to identify areas for system improvements.

The literature provides several examples of dramatic reductions in medication infusion error rates as a result of *smart* pump implementation.[28–31] This same literature outlines processes for selecting, implementing, and analyzing data gathered from smart infusion devices. However, smart pump technology is by no means foolproof, and at least one study found no measurable impact on the serious medication error rate following smart pump implementation, likely in part due to poor compliance.[32] Clinicians still have to use their own judgment. Workarounds circumventing the desired safety features of these pumps are common as the design of these pumps make it easy for nurses to bypass the drug library, which contains the drug dosing and rate limits. Alert fatigue is also a consideration if nurses are routinely prompted with alerts that are not considered clinically significant. Convincing nurses to use the safety features of this technology during time-pressed situations can be a challenge. Given that intravenous medication errors and adverse drug events are common and often very harmful, the use of this technology is likely to expand rapidly, perhaps more rapidly than BCMA and CPOE software. Although it has great promise, technological and nursing behavioral factors must be effectively addressed if smart pumps are to achieve their potential for improving medication safety. Unlike traditional infusion pumps, a pharmacist must be very involved in the smart pump selection and implementation process, particularly in the drug library consensus development and programming processes. Pharmacists must also be involved with alert analysis, quality assurance, and drug library upkeep. This technology offers a tremendous opportunity for pharmacist leadership in health systems.

Safety Issues Surrounding the Use of Automation

Ensuring System Accuracy and Reducing Errors

Although information technologies and automated medication systems are widely used in health systems and are integral components of many regulatory and external quality reporting agencies, very little data is available regarding their appropriate use nor on their impact on patient safety.[33] The only exception to this is very limited data on CPOE with computerized clinical physician decision support. Other technologies such as using robotic technology to fill medication doses, bar coding of medications, automated dispensing devices, and BCMA are more widely implemented than CPOE systems, yet their reported impact on reducing medication errors and preventable ADEs is variable. Critical reviews of the safety benefits of various technologies touted to reduce medication errors do exist but are limited.[33] Implementing new technology can create major infrastructure changes, which introduce new sources of error, and vendors routinely market their products without sufficient testing or without being able to fully implement the technology as advertised. Nevertheless, all of these systems intuitively show promise in their medication error reduction potential. If properly integrated, all of these systems should ultimately improve patient safety and would likely be incorporated into most medication-use systems of the future.

Automation has the potential to reduce medication errors by reducing complexity; simplifying and standardizing processes; avoiding overreliance on human memory; and improving efficiency. However, technology by itself will rarely prevent medication errors. Rather, it must be effectively integrated into the existing medication-use system and appropriately managed for it to positively impact patient safety. In fact, if technology is not used properly, it can prolong a system of errors and introduce dangerous new ones. Implementing technology within a previously suboptimal manual system will most often yield a suboptimal automated system. Implementation of automation can be a very complicated process that significant modifies pharmacy, nursing, and medical staff practices, particularly with BCMA and CPOE technologies. Full implementation of these technologies can take years to accomplish and is rarely accomplished without dedicated personnel resources to manage and oversee implementation, training, quality assurance, and ongoing support and maintenance. Without such dedicated oversight, new sources of error will prevail and the automated system may be less safe than the manual system it replaced.

Without a comprehensive system to assure that patients are getting their drugs and dosages correctly and on time, errors will continue to occur. In anticipation of the implementation of new automation, policies and procedures must be modified to assure the continued safe and proper infrastructure exists for medication purchasing, ordering, preparation, dispensing, administering, and monitoring. After all, technology does not preclude the need for safety checks and verification for appropriateness.

Health systems are often unrealistic in what they expect from automation. It can instill a false sense of security leading to carelessness by health care professionals. For instance, health care professionals often neglect to exercise sound double- and triple-checking procedures with medications obtained from automated dispensing devices because of an overreliance on the technology. To avoid such problems, it is critical that all personnel be adequately educated so that they understand that technology cannot completely substitute for human safety checks. Additionally, managers must make certain that staff levels are not overly reduced in response to system automation and that staff are not forced to work at a pace that precludes the ability to deliver safe and effective health care. With all automation, it absolutely critical that appropriate quality control systems exist to assure the accurate and safe use of automation. It is also of the utmost importance to maximize the use of bar codes throughout all automated systems.

Desired Features for Reducing Errors

There is little doubt that the innovative and appropriate use of technology within the medication-use process can significantly improve patient safety. Furthermore, it is reasonable to draw some conclusions about information technology and automation as they apply to preventing medication errors. First, the use of bar coded medications should be maximized throughout the medication-use process including the administration and documentation phase of the medication-use process. Second, information technologies can be used to analyze and prevent medication errors. For instance, sophisticated pharmacy or CPOE systems may be integrated with patient-specific laboratory and clinical documentation systems to identify ADEs and medication errors when they occur. Potential errors prevented and identified by electronic prescribing, BCMA software and smart infusion pumps can be analyzed for common problems to facilitate minimization and elimination of recurring root-causes of potential errors within organizations. Third, automated dispensing systems, especially those incorporating the use of bar code technology, have the potential to improve medication

dispensing and administration accuracy and patient safety, provided the system is managed well. Fourth, aggressive implementation of computer-generated clinical alert and decision support software will improve patient safety, provided the system is properly designed, implemented, and maintained.[34,35] Table 24-6 lists ideal features to assure patient safety throughout the medication-use process, regardless of which automated technologies are employed.

Regulatory Issues

In response to a lack of national standards and regulations for the safe use of automated dispensing systems, The National Association of Boards of Pharmacy (NABP) approved a document entitled *Model State Pharmacy Act and Model Rules* in May of 1997. Thanks to the work of some very forward-thinking pharmacists, the language in this act is very enabling in that it allows the definition of *dispensing* to include the use of automated technology. It provides pharmacists with flexibility in the use of automated devices but appropriately requires that such devices be used only in settings where there is an established program of pharmaceutical care ensuring medication orders are reviewed by a pharmacist in accordance with good pharmacy practice. The act requires pharmacists to have policies and systems in place to assure safe and secure use of such devices but is not very descriptive or restrictive as to how such quality assurance must be completed. This act is intended to serve as a template for individual states to write (or rewrite) their State Pharmacy Practice Acts.

Despite the model act, some State Boards of Pharmacy continue to provide a potential barrier to the appropriate and efficient use of automated devices and technologies. Some states may require pharmacists to check every dose prior to that dose being stocked in an automated dispensing device rather than allowing the pharmacy to develop and document internal quality assurance programs (such as bar coded restocking systems) to assure patient safety. Still other states may require extensive paperwork to be completed, which may be interpreted as a barrier to implementing automated devices. It is important that pharmacists play an active role in assuring that their state's Pharmacy Practice Act contain enabling (rather than restrictive) language related to the use of automated dispensing systems and the transfer of electronic medication (prescription) orders. Developing restrictive language will most certainly be viewed as *self serving* to other health

Table 24-6
Desired Safety Features for Incorporating Automation into the Medication-Use Process

A system must accommodate bar coded unit dose medications and utilize the bar code capability for drug restocking, retrieval, and administering medications

A system should force the user to specify a reason whenever medications are accessed or administered outside of the scheduled administration time or dosage range; all such events are signaled visibly or audibly to the user and are electronically documented and reported daily for follow-up

A unique bar code or user identification code and password are assigned to each user; audit trials of user actions must be reported in an easily viewed format and should include identification of the user, the medication, the patient for whom the drug was dispensed, and the time of the transaction

Bar code medication administration systems must be able to identify and document the patient, the medication, and the person administering using the scanning technology function

Devices are interfaced with the pharmacy computer system only allowing the nurse to view and access those medications that are ordered for a specific patient

Devices need electronic reminders to nurses when a medication dose is due (and by a different mechanism when it is past due)

Hospital admit/discharge/transfer and medication order entry computer systems are interfaced with automation devices to provide caregivers with warnings about allergies, interactions, duplications, and inappropriate doses at the point of dispensing and/or administration

Patient specific information used in the daily care of patients must be timely, accurate, and easily accessible

Pertinent patient- and medication-specific information and instructions entered into pharmacy and/or hospital information systems are available electronically at the point of care (administration), and the system prompts the nurse to record pertinent information before administration may be documented

Real-time integration or interfaces exist for all steps in the medication-use process, starting at the point of prescribing, to order entry and dispensing, and through documentation of medication administration

---

care professionals and health systems and will have negative long-term consequences for the profession. It is also important to note that recent automation-related standards developed the Joint Commission on Accreditation of Healthcare Organizations, particularly those related to the use of automated dispensing devices, are very proactive in assuring the safe use of automation and in requiring pharmacist oversight of automated systems as they relate to the medication-use process.

Quality Assurance

Regardless of whether or not state regulations exist to assure safe use of automated dispensing systems, it is extremely important that every organization develop, enforce, and continuously improve policies and procedures to ensure patient safety, accuracy, security, and confidentiality. Specific areas that should be addressed

in an organization's policies for safe use of automated dispensing systems and technology include accurate inventory and stocking controls, dispensing procedures, security and breach of security, patient confidentiality, reporting, documentation, training of personnel, initial and ongoing competency assessment, routine quality assurance and safety checks, scheduled (and unscheduled) hardware and software maintenance and support, and contingency plans for maintaining safe systems and service in the event of unscheduled downtime.

ASHP Policy and Position Statements

The need for guidance in pharmacy practice has increased greatly with the changes in health care and with the influences from regulatory, accrediting, risk-management, financing, and other bodies. ASHP develops policies, position statements, and guidelines for pharmacy practice in integrated health systems. The policies of ASHP represent a consensus of professional judgment, expert opinion, and documented evidence to provide guidance and direction to pharmacy practitioners and other audiences who affect pharmacy practice. Their content should be assessed and adapted to meet the needs of the specific organization and is very useful in crafting departmental policies and in gaining pharmacist resources for coordination of automation projects within the organization. Policies contain varying levels of detail where positions are short pronouncements on one aspect of pharmacy practice, statements express a basic philosophy, and guidelines offer programmatic advice.

Current ASHP policies for automation and technology include machine-readable coding and related technology (0308), the pharmacist's role in electronic patient information and prescribing systems (0203), regulation of automated drug distribution systems (9813), automated systems (9205), and computerized prescriber order entry (0105). ASHP also provides detailed guidelines on the safe use of automated medication storage and distribution devices.

The machine-readable coding and related technology policy, for example, advocates an industry standard for the placement of bar codes and information contained in a machine-readable bar code for unit dose, unit of use, and injectable drug products. This particular policy statement was very influential in the Food and Drug Administration's final rule requiring the use of a linear bar code to encode the national data code (NDC) number on most prescription drug products by April of 2006. It is also ASHP's position that all medications are identified through machine-readable bar coding, as the use of bar code technology at the point of medication administration will help to ensure safe, accurate, and documented medication administration.

ASHP also advocates pharmacist involvement when key decisions are made in the planning, selection, implementation, and maintenance of electronic patient information systems. Pharmacists are a necessity to facilitate clinical decision support, data analysis, and education of users of electronic patient information systems for the purpose of ensuring the safe and effective medication use. Specific to CPOE, pharmacists are essential during the planning, implementation, and management stages to ensure a safe, effective, and accurate system. To facilitate patient safety all CPOE orders should be part of a single database that is fully integrated with the pharmacy information system and

pharmacists must be able to review and verify order appropriateness before medication are administered to patients. Specific ASHP policy statements that are germane to this chapter are provided below:

Machine-Readable Coding and Related Technology (0308)

To declare that the identity of all medications should be verifiable through machine-readable coding technology and to support the goal that all medications be electronically verified before they are administered to patients in health systems; further, to urge the Food and Drug Administration, other regulatory agencies, contracting entities, and others to mandate that pharmaceutical manufacturers place standardized machine-readable coding that includes National Drug Code, lot number, and expiration date on all manufacturers' unit dose, unit of use, and injectable drug packaging; further, To strongly encourage health systems to adopt machine-readable coding and point-of-care technology to (1) improve the accuracy of medication administration and documentation, (2) improve efficiencies within the medication-use process, and (3) improve patient safety; these systems should be planned, implemented, and managed with pharmacist involvement and should be in all areas of the health system where drugs are used.

Pharmacist's Role in Electronic Patient Information and Prescribing Systems (0203)

To strongly advocate key decision roles of pharmacists in the planning, selection, implementation, and maintenance of electronic patient information systems (including computerized prescriber order-entry systems) to facilitate clinical decision support, data analysis, and education of users for the purpose of ensuring the safe and effective use of medications.

Regulation of Automated Drug Distribution Systems (9813)

To work with the Drug Enforcement Administration and other agencies to seek regulatory and policy changes to accommodate automated drug distribution in health systems.

Automated Systems (9205)

To support the use of current and emerging technology in the advancement of pharmaceutical care; further, to encourage a review and evaluation of the state and federal legal and regulatory status of new technologies as they apply to pharmacy practice.

Computerized Prescriber Order Entry (0105)

To advocate the use of computerized entry of medication orders or prescriptions by the prescriber when (1) it is planned, implemented, and managed with pharmacists' involvement, (2) such orders are part of a single, shared database that is fully integrated with the pharmacy information system and other key information system components, especially the patient's medication administration record, (3) such computerized order entry improves the safety, efficiency, and accuracy of the medication-use process, and (4) it includes provisions for the pharmacist to review and verify the order's appropriateness before medication administration, except in those instances when review would cause a medically unacceptable delay.

Strategic Plan for Selecting Automation within a Health System

Historically, automation had to result in proven cost reduction, quality improvement, improved service, and/or increased efficiency in order to be funded. While expense continues to be one of the major barriers to implementing new technologies, various regulatory and external quality reporting groups and various news media continue to persuade many organizations to prematurely invest heavily in new technologies, which theoretically improve patient safety. Integrated health systems should not view automation and technology as a means to an end, but rather as a series of sophisticated tools to help them optimize the medication-use process. The value achieved by implementing new technology within organizations depends primarily upon three factors: the efficiency of the system being replaced, the level of detail applied to managing and making the most of the system following implementation, and cooperation between departments to assure success of the system.

Within most hospitals, there is consensus that the inpatient medication-use process should be automated, but there are many questions and much debate as to the best way to automate the process. There is no right or wrong answer, and any of the previously discussed approaches can succeed or fail, depending on how well it is managed.[36] Automated systems may either stand alone or be an integrated component of a hospital information system. Suggested characteristics of an ideal system will likely include patient care and safety benefits, responsiveness to customer needs, cost-effectiveness, and ability to leverage the purchase of other existing and pending technologies. It is very important that decision makers evaluate the clinical, cost, and safety advantages and disadvantages of competing technologies, as well as safety claims made by the manufacturer before reaching a final purchase decision. Furthermore, to assure successful selection and hospital-wide implementation of automation and technologies within the medication-use process, it is imperative that pharmacists continuously sell the importance of their role in overseeing and coordinating the use of these systems. Automation selection should include a complete analysis of desired automation system functionality, hardware and software technical requirements, installation and training support, and vendor/system background reference checks. Table 24-7 provides guidelines for pharmacists to use to help guide the automation selection process.

Cost Justification of Automated Systems

Economic Realities in Health Systems

Historically, one could cost-justify the use of new automation if the automation resulted in improved medication charge capture (or reallocated labor to perform new billable services) and charge increases were projected to offset the cost of the technology. Due to declining hospital reimbursement from government and private payers, this scenario is rarely the case any longer. Directors of pharmacy often feel as though they need to "jump through hoops" to gain administrative and financial support for new services and new technologies. Despite even the best cost- and quality-justifications as well as organizationwide support for a new technology, sometimes health systems do not have the available financial resources to purchase new technologies. Many vendors now offer lease options to address this problem. Regardless of an organization's financial situation, a great way to gain administrative approval for financing a new automated technology is to prepare a solid cost-benefit model, which demonstrates that the technology makes good financial sense for the organization. System costs vary dramatically depending on institution size, infrastructure needs, and the number and types of devices, computers, and servers purchased. Initial capital costs dramatically vary; training and other hidden expenses often double these costs, and

Table 24-7
Automation Selection Criteria

Can the vendor provide you with established policies and procedures for integrating the system into the pharmacy's daily workflow, clearly defining pharmacist and technician responsibilities, and clearly defining system downtime procedures?

Cost-Benefit Analysis—Will reduced supply and labor expenses offset the cost of the automation? What is the potential increased revenue as a result of the automation?

Does the system produce useful statistical and managerial reports, and do they provide a report writing and analysis tool?

How does the system utilize bar code technology to improve accuracy of transactions?

How long has the company been in business and how many units do they have in operation?

How much space will the automation require, and is remodeling required?

How much time is required for routine maintenance and equipment servicing? Does the company provide full service, routine and emergency software and hardware maintenance? What is the cost of this maintenance and how is it provided? Will routine maintenance disrupt workflow?

How secure is the system?

Is training interactive and computer-based? How will new users be trained on the system?

Is the automation compatible with the organization's strategic goals?

Is the company willing to guarantee a maximum percent downtime?

Is the system compatible with existing information systems? Has the company interfaced their system with your pharmacy computer system in another organization? If not, what is the cost for building this interface? Who maintains the interface?

What do existing customers say about the accuracy and reliability of the system, ease of use, and unscheduled downtime?

What impact will the automation have on other departments? How are those departments involved in the selection process?

What impact will the automation have on patient safety?

What impact will the system have on controlled substance accountability and overall inventory control?

What sets this company's product apart from their major competitors?

Will the automation enable the provision of new clinical services?

Will the vendor adapt the technology to meet your needs, goals, and objectives rather than expect your system to be redesigned to fit their product?

Will the vendor provide you with a list of all current users?

Will the vendor's training and implementation support meet your expectations and needs?

---

pharmacy involvement in the cost-justification of automated technologies is essential.

Return on Investment Analysis

With the rising costs of health care, the importance or providing an institution with evidence of a technology's ability to positively impact the organization is becoming increasingly more important. There are many drivers for automation including improvements in patient safety, customer service, operational efficiency, revenues, regulatory compliance, and overall quality of care, as well as reduced costs. Whether or not automation saves money is a function of how well the system is managed, the efficiency (or inefficiency) of the manual system being replaced and the extent to which different disciplines cooperate to maximize the system's capabilities. The goal of a return on investment (ROI) analysis is to compare an organization's total costs

Figure 24-1
Model ROI Analysis

	Quantity	Actual Unit Cost	Year 0	Year 1	Year 2	Year 3	Year 4	Year 5	Year 6	Year 7
Capital Purchase										
Hand-held devices	220	$0	$0							
Software and upgrades		$0	$0							
RF Network Installation		$145,000	$145,000							
Total Capital Expenses			**$145,000**							
Ongoing Operating Expenses										
Annual lease expense for software and handhelds, including maintenance				$600,000	$600,000	$600,000	$600,000	$600,000	$600,000	$600,000
Printer and paper suppliesa				$2,500	$2,600	$2,730	$2,867	$3,010	$3,160	$3,318
Additional pharmacy technician labor (FTE) for barcoding and inventory/catalog maintenance	(2 FTE)			$82,701	$86,836	$91,178	$95,737	$100,523	$105,550	$110,827
Nursing project manager	(1FTE)			$102,960	$108,108	$113,513	$119,189	$125,149	$131,406	$137,976
Additional nurse go-live support resources				$75,000	$0	$0	$0	$0	$0	$0
Maintenance (included above)				$0	$0	$0	$0	$0	$0	$0
Batteries for hand-held (included above)				$0	$0	$0	$0	$0	$0	$0
Total Operating Expenses				**$863,161**	**$797,544**	**$807,421**	**$817,792**	**$828,682**	**$840,116**	**$852,122**
Ongoing Savings—Hard										
Printer and paper supply cost avoidance				($22,000)	($22,880)	($23,795)	($24,747)	($25,737)	($26,766)	($27,837)
Bulk drug purchases less than unit dose medications				($92,000)	($95,680)	($99,507)	($103,487)	($107,627)	($111,932)	($116,409)
Net hard savings				**($114,000)**	**($118,560)**	**($123,302)**	**($128,234)**	**($133,364)**	**($138,698)**	**($144,246)**
Ongoing Savings—Soft										
ADE avoidance (see calculation below, conservative estimate applied)				($1,358,450)	($1,358,450)	($1,358,450)	($1,358,450)	($1,358,450)	($1,358,450)	($1,358,450)
Other benefits: nursing satisfaction, improved documentation accuracy, reduced litigation expenses, improved charge capture, patient confidence in care, public relations benefits				$0	$0	$0	$0	$0	$0	$0
Total Savings Potential including soft savings				**($1,472,450)**	**($1,477,010)**	**($1,481,752)**	**($1,486,684)**	**($1,491,814)**	**($1,497,148)**	**($1,502,696)**
Total Net Savings (Loss)—Hard Savings Only			($145,000)	($749,161)	($678,984)	($684,119)	($689,558)	($695,318)	($701,417)	($707,875)
Total Net Savings (Loss)—Hard and Soft Savings			($145,000)	$609,289	$679,466	$674,331	$668,892	$663,132	$657,033	$650,575
Cumulative Net Savings (Loss)—Hard Savings Only			($145,000)	($894,161)	($1,573,145)	($2,257,263)	($2,946,821)	($3,642,139)	($4,343,556)	($5,051,431)
Cumulative Net Savings (Loss)—Hard and Soft Savings			**($145,000)**	**$464,289**	**$1,143,755**	**$1,818,087**	**$2,486,979**	**$3,150,111**	**$3,807,144**	**$4,457,719**

Figure 24-1, continued

ADE Cost Avoidance Calculations at Model Hospital

Assumptions:	Literature method	Conservative method[a]
Annual doses administered per year	3,650,000	3,650,001
Administration error rate before BCMA in manual system	9.10%	9.10%
Total administration errors per year before BCMA in manual system	332,150	332,150
Administration error avoidance as determined via direct observation study	87%	87%
Administration errors avoided per year following BCMA implementation	288,971	288,971
% of medication errors that result in harm or a PADE (per 1995 Bates study)	1%	0.10%
Total harmful errors avoided per year at Model Hospital	2,890	289
Cost of a harmful medication error (per 1995 Bates study)	$4,700	4,700
Total harmful error cost avoidance per year as a result of BCMA	**$13,581,614**	**1,358,161**

[a] Assumes only 1 in 1,000 errors result in harm that add cost to the organization; lowers estimates from 1995 Bates et al. research by tenfold.

---

before and after the implementation of automation and to demonstrate a positive ROI if the decision is made to support the automation.

An ROI analysis is often separated into three distinct sections: capital purchase, ongoing operating expenses, and ongoing savings. For ongoing savings, two components include *hard* and *soft* dollar savings. Hard dollar savings are directly attributable to a reduction in FTEs or the elimination of a direct expense and hard benefits are directly related to an increase in revenue and an increase in reimbursement. Soft benefits include customer service improvements, reduced wait times, reallocating staff to another activity, regulatory compliance enhancement and cost-avoidance. Depending on the institution, soft savings may or may not be included in the ROI analysis. The decision on whether to lease or purchase a technology impacts the placement of those dollars into the ROI analysis. For automation that is purchased, the expense will often be capitalized and appear in year-zero of the ROI analysis. For leased automation the annual lease expense will usually appear as an ongoing operating expense in the ROI analysis. See Figure 24-1 for a model ROI analysis template for cost-justifying a BCMA system.

Every organization will have a slightly different format in which they want ROI information presented, but there are several pieces of information you will need to evaluate regardless of this format. First, clearly state all hardware and software capital, lease, maintenance, and supply (hardware and software) expenses as a result of implementing the new technology. Second, obtain a quote from your Information Systems depart-ment for projected computer system interface expenses. Third, incorporate fixed labor costs (salary, benefits, vacation, sick leave) of any new support activities the automation will require. If the automation you wish to implement is a means of providing a new service (which is often the case in ambulatory settings), then you should be sure to calculate added personnel expense, which will be incurred if the automation is not approved. Fourth, evaluate undeniable minimum expenses that you intend to eliminate from the budget as a result of the new technology. Examples include fixed technician and pharmacist labor costs associated with activities the automation will replace, supply costs, and labor costs savings, which can be achieved in other departments such as nursing. Unfortunately, in most organizations nursing has been protected and most labor savings have been the responsibility of the pharmacy department. Fifth, factor in additional savings the department can commit to as a direct result of implementing the automation. For example, you may wish to propose that pharmacist time saved as a result of the new technology be redeployed to a more direct patient care role where they can assure the appropriate use of medications. Department medication expense reports and clinical literature can help to determine a projected dollar savings for expenses you can reduce as a result of new clinical pharmacy services and target drug programs. At this stage of the analysis, many organizations will allow only those cost savings that will be eliminated from the organization's budget to be factored into the ROI equation. However, over the past few years, journals and literature targeted toward health-system administrators have been filled with reports of the value of clinical pharmacy services on patient care, safety, and reducing total health care costs. Depending on the organization, it may be possible to factor less tangible but real organizationwide cost savings for medication error avoidance into the ROI analysis. Most administrators have probably heard about cost increases in the range of several thousand dollars for every preventable adverse drug event. Since the release of the IOM Report in 1999, patient safety (which was once at the bottom of many organization's objectives versus cost savings) has risen to the top of many organization's priority list, allowing directors of pharmacy to more effectively sell the benefits of error reduction to a higher level. Many insurance companies and employer payers are beginning to select health care facilities based on safety records. If acceptable to an organization's administration, this will make the cost-justification of most dispensing technologies a simpler process. Some less tangible cost savings as a result of redeployed pharmacist time, which may be factored into an ROI analysis, include ordering of fewer laboratory tests, reduced lengths of stay, reduced emergency room visits, and fewer rehospitalizations. Literature supporting such cost savings is plentiful, and an organization's likelihood of successfully incorporating such findings into an ROI analysis depends in a large part to the extent that pharmacy cognitive services have been marketed to and valued by local physicians and administrators. Sixth, projected increased revenues as a result of improved charge capture should be incorporated into the analysis. Most organizations will have a fair understanding of what percent of improved charge capture will actually result in increased income for the organization. Oftentimes organizations have a higher capture rate for ambulatory services, thus increased charge capture should be broken down by inpatient and outpatient areas. Lastly, a good ROI analysis will include a payback period (how long it will take to pay the organization back for their initial investment) and internal rate of return (how much will the money spent on the automation earn the hospital back) in the analysis. The fiscal department in most organizations will be a very valuable resource in helping to perform ROI calculations for new technologies.

Achieving a positive ROI with technologies such as CPOE and BCMA technology is incredibly challenging. These technologies often will not demonstrate hard dollar savings such as reduced personnel expenses, which are tangible to administrators. It is much easier

to show that these technologies are simply the right thing to do and that they will improve patient outcomes. Thus, the ability to translate improved outcomes, fewer errors, and risk reduction into dollars in the eyes of an administrator is an increasingly important skill required of pharmacists. Many health-system pharmacy departments have been successful in cost-justifying advanced automation and technology through the elimination of technical positions and the redeployment of pharmacist time to clinical activities. Technology vendors should be able to provide you with contacts in other organizations that have already completed a similar ROI analysis.

Automation Impact on Pharmacy Manpower

A frequent concern of pharmacists it that the availability of automated dispensing systems will decrease the number of pharmacist positions and consequently the demand for pharmacists. Theoretically, automation (as well as expanded use of pharmacy technicians) increases the amount of work that can be accomplished by the existing work force. In the early and mid 1990s, some pharmacists thought leaders predicted that increased use of automation coupled with a dramatic increase in the use of prescription mail order service would result in a reduced demand for pharmacists. Fortunately, increased organizational recognition of the financial and quality impact of the clinical pharmacist role, the growing population of older Americans who take more and more medications, the soaring number and complexity of medications, and unrecognized theoretical time savings within departments following implementation of automated systems have resulted in quite the opposite trend. However, as automated dispensing and patient monitoring technologies advance, it is very reasonable to predict a reduction in the number of pharmacist and technician positions in which preparing and dispensing pharmaceuticals is the principle activity.

Within health systems, cost-justification of new technologies will likely require a reduction in the number of full-time pharmacy technician positions (and possibly pharmacist and nurse positions also). Technicians will increasingly be expected to oversee automated dispensing systems and even possibly smart IV pump and BCMA systems, which may offset the reduction in technician dispensing positions and help create new patient care technician roles in which pharmacy technician roles are expanded to providing support activities across all phases of the medication-use process. The traditional distributive pharmacist role in the preparation and distribution of medications will most certainly be challenged as technicians and technology become increasingly responsible for dispensing activities. Many pharmacy departments have been very successful in redeploying pharmacist time from distributive to clinical roles. As technology continues to provide pharmacists with opportunities to be more involved with directly taking care of patients, the impact on pharmacist manpower needs will mostly be determined by pharmacists themselves. If pharmacist and pharmacy directors are successful at demonstrating and marketing the quality and economic value of pharmacist patient care services to physicians and administrators, it is reasonable to predict an increase in the number of available health-system pharmacist positions. However, if the patient care role of the pharmacist does not continue to grow and demonstrate overall value, pharmacists may increasingly be displaced by technology. Automation is currently forcing the issue of pharmacists' professional role in the redevelopment of health-systems.

Given that continued automation of the dispensing process is inevitable, future work activities of pharmacists depend primarily on four things: (1) the breadth of tasks a pharmacy technician is legally allowed to perform (and/or allowed to perform by an employer); (2) the extent to which pharmacists are reimbursed for medication therapy management services; (3) the level of productivity that can be achieved through automated systems; and (4) the extent to which pharmacists are able to demonstrate improved quality and overall lower cost of patient care as a result of their role on the patient care team. Existing dispensing automation clearly creates the potential for pharmacists to focus more of their time on direct patient care activities instead of product preparation.

Future Roles of Pharmacy Personnel as a Result of Automation

The transformation of the pharmacist role from distributor of drugs to cognitive provider of care has largely resulted from pharmacists' access to patient-specific information about diagnosis, laboratory results, treatment progress, and the patient's entire drug therapy regimen. Integrated delivery systems and automation will continue to provide pharmacists with opportunities to work more closely with physicians and patients to assure appropriate drug therapy decisions and outcomes. Toward this end, pharmacists must continue to assume increased accountability for understanding patient drug-related needs, identifying, solving and preventing drug-related problems, designing and initiating drug therapy plans, and continuing drug therapy plans once they are initiated. We also have an important responsibility in creating systems to improve the quality and safety of drug distribution and administration. Pharmacists must possess good time management and problem solving skills and be able to focus the majority of their time on issues related to high-risk drugs and high-cost diseases, while paying particular attention to the dosing of high-cost drugs for all patients. Clinical pharmacists in the virtual world may have three primary responsibilities: to assess patient compliance and medication-related outcomes, drug and disease education, and intervention. The optimization of such roles is essential in both inpatient and ambulatory environments to avoid the displacement of pharmacists by automation. Additionally, pharmacists in all practice settings must continue to capitalize on the advances of dispensing technologies in order to maximize pharmacists' potential in providing patient care services that improve patient care and safety.

Summary

Automation is not a panacea. There is no perfect technology, and all systems must be well-managed in order to achieve desired results. No existing automated system fully supports the profession's transition to pharmacist patient care services. To be successful in the future, pharmacists must view automation-induced productivity and efficiency as desired goals, not as threats to their work. Optimized use of automation to perform distributive functions currently performed by pharmacists and technicians is essential in providing pharmacists with additional time to take care of patients in the future. Every change must be implemented with an understanding of human factors engineering and safety science, as even good changes will create unexpected new hazards. It is safe to predict that the capabilities of pharmacy automation will continue to increase at a rapid rate. Efficient electronic physician prescribing systems, fully automated dispensing systems, and virtual patient monitoring systems will be commonplace in the medication-use process of the future, and pharmacists have a choice to make such systems successful or to resist change. Embracing automation, providing leadership within organizations to help assure that automation is implemented safely and efficiently, and continuing to find innovative ways to incorporate automation into pharmacy practice is advisable.

References

1. Kohn LT, Corrigan JM, Donaldson MS, eds. *To Err Is Human: Building a Safer Health System.* Washington DC: National Academy Press; 1999.

2. Barker KN, Flynn EA, Pepper GA, et al. Medication errors observed in 36 health care facilities. *Arch Intern Med.* 2002;162(16):1897–903.

3. Cullen DJ, Bates DW, Small SD, et al. The incident reporting system does not detect adverse drug events: a problem for quality improvement. *Jt Comm J Qual Improv* 1995;10:541–8.

4. Classen DC, Pestotnik SL, Evans RS, et al. Computerized surveillance of adverse drug events in hospitalized patients. *JAMA.* 1991;366:2847–51.

5. Bates DW, Cullen DJ, Laird N, et al. Incidence of adverse drug events and potential adverse drug events. *JAMA.* 1995;274:29–34.

6. Jha AK, Kuperman GJ, Teich JM, et al. Identifying adverse drug events: development of a computer-based monitor and comparison with chart review and stimulated voluntary report. *JAMA.* 1998;5:305–14.

7. Classen DC, Pestotnik SL, Evans RS, et al. Adverse drug events in hospitalized patients: excess length of stay, extra costs, and attributable mortality. *JAMA.* 1997; 277: 301–6.

8. Bates DW, Spell N, Cullen DJ, et al. The costs of adverse drug events in hospitalized patients. *JAMA.* 1997;277:307–11.

9. Louie C, Brethauer B, Cong D, et al. Use of a drug wholesaler to process refills for automated medication dispensing machines. *Hosp Pharm.* 1997;32:367–75.

10. Carroll NV. Changes in channels of distribution: wholesalers and pharmacies in organized health-care settings. *Hosp Phar Report.* 1997;Feb:48–57.

11. Barker KN, Felkey BG, Flynn EA, et al. White paper on automation in pharmacy. *Consultant Pharm.* 1998;13: 256–93.

12. Vermeulen LC, Stiltner RS, Swearingen LL. Technology report revision: automated medication management in departments of pharmacy. Oakbrook, IL: University Hospital Consortium; 1996.

13. Thielke TS. Automation support of patient-focused care. *Top Hosp Pharm Manag.* 1994;14:54–9.

14. Perini VJ, Vermeulen LC. Comparison of automated medication-management systems. *Am J Hosp Pharm.* 1994;51:1883–91.

15. Ray MD, Aldrich LT, Lew PJ. Experience with an automated point-of-use unit-dose drug distribution system. *Hosp Pharm.* 1995;30:18–30.

16. Lee LW, Wellman GS, Birdwell SW, et al. Use of an automated medication storage and distribution system. *Am J Hosp Pharm.* 1992;49:851–5.

17. Barker KN. Ensuring safety in the use of automated medication dispensing systems. *Am J Health-Syst Pharm.* 1995;52:2445–7.

18. Sutter TL, Wellman GS, Mott DA, et al. Discrepancies with automated drug storage and distribution cabinets. *Am J Health-Syst Pharm.* 1998;55:1924–6.

19. Borel JM, Rascati KL. Effect of an automated, nursing unit-based drug-dispensing device on medication errors. *Am J Health-Syst Pharm.* 1995;52:1875–9.

20. Guerrero RW, Nickman NA, Jorgenson JA. Work activities before and after implementation of an automated dispensing system. *Am J Health-Syst Pharm.* 1996;53: 548–54.

21. Weaver PE, Perini VJ, Pierce D. Random sampling process for quality assurance of the Rxobot dispensing system. Presented at: ASHP Midyear Clinical Meeting; 1998;33:289E.

22. Anderson S, Wittwer W. Using bar-code point-of-care technology for patient safety. *J Healthc Qual.* 2004 Nov–Dec;26(6):5–1.

23. Cummings JP. *UHC Technology Report: Bar-Coded Medication Administration.* Oakbrook, IL: University HealthSystem Consortium; 2005.

24. ASHP. Pharmacist's toolkit—implementing a bar coded medication safety program. Available at: http://www.ashp foundation.org/BarCoded.pdf. Accessed July, 2005.

25. Presentation from University of Wisconsin Hospital and Clinics. Bar coding and point of care systems: experiences at UWHC. Available at: http://www.uhc.edu/Web/ COU/RX/RXDec02_mtg/AcuScan.pdf. Accessed July, 2005.

26. Pedersen CA, Schneider PJ, Scheckelhoff DJ. ASHP national survey of pharmacy practice in hospital settings: dispensing and administration—2002. *Am J Health-Syst Pharm.* 2003;60(1):52–68.

27. Ragan R, Bond J, Major K, et al. Improved control of medication use with an integrated bar-code—packaging and distribution system. *Am J Health-Syst Pharm.* 2005;62:1075–9.

28. Bates DW, Vanderveen T, Seger D, et al. Variability in intravenous medication practices: implications for medication safety. *Jt Comm J Qual Patient Saf.* 2005;31(4);203–10.

29. Eskew JA, Jacobi J, Buss WF, et al. Using innovative technologies to set new safety standards for the infusion of intravenous medications. *Hosp Pharm.* 2002;37: 1179–89.

30. Wilson K, Sullivan M. Preventing medication errors with smart infusion technology. *Am J Health-Syst Pharm.* 2004;61:177–83.

31. Williams CK, Maddox RR. Implementation of an i.v. medication safety system. *Am J Health-Syst Pharm.* 2005;62:530–6.

32. Rothschild J, Keohane CA, Cook F, et al. A controlled trial of smart infusion pumps to improve medication safety in critically ill patients. *Crit Care Med.* 2005; 33(3):533–40.

33. Oren E, Shaffer ER, Guglielmo BJ. Impact of emerging technologies on medication errors and adverse drug events. *Am J Health-Syst Pharm.* 2003;60:1447–58.

34. Garg AX, Adhikari NK, McDonald H, et al. Effects of computerized clinical decision support systems on practitioner performance and patient outcomes— a systematic review. *JAMA.* 2005;293(10):1223–38.

35. Degnan D, Merryfeld D, Hultgren S. Reaching out to clinicians: implementation of a computerized alert system. *J Healthcare Qual.* 2004 Nov–Dec;26(6):26–30.

36. Darby AL. Considering a hybrid system for automated drug distribution. *Am J Health-Syst Pharm.* 1996;53: 1128,1134,1137.

Chapter 25

Informatics

James G. Stevenson, Scott R. McCreadie, Bruce W. Chaffee

Definition and Overview of Informatics

Informatics is a broad term that can be defined as the application of computer and information sciences to the management and processing of data, information, and knowledge.[1] To broaden the definition, one can define informatics as the science concerned with the gathering, manipulation, classification, storage, and retrieval of recorded knowledge; the techniques and practices used to manage and operate information systems and technology.

In health care, informatics can be divided into subsets such as medical informatics, pharmacy informatics, nursing informatics, biomedical informatics, and other specialty areas.[2] Medical informatics limits the definition to informatics involving the support of medical research, education, and patient care while pharmacy informatics limits the definition to those areas involving the medication management system within the health care environment.[3] The other areas focus on aspects of informatics specific to those specialties.

This chapter will be focusing primarily on pharmacy informatics by exploring several topics that are pertinent to pharmacies within health care institutions. Topics include information security and confidentiality, educational applications, operations and clinical applications, systems integration, and finally opportunities and training for those interested in pharmacy informatics.

Pharmacies have often been in the forefront of using technology to improve medication dispensing, ordering, record keeping, safety, and billing. Pharmacies have been using computers for profile management for many years. Computerized profiles improve the efficiency and safety of the medication-use system by reducing legibility and transcription errors. More recently, dispensing technologies have advanced to include point of use devices such as automated dispensing cabinets and robots. Further advances in technologies have been seen in IV compounding machines and inventory management of pharmaceuticals.

Many different computing devices are used in health care environments. On the back end, large ser-

vers running advanced operating systems with multiple processors power many of the software applications used in the care of patients. Clinicians use a variety of devices including personal desktop computers, laptops, tablet PCs, personal digital assistants (PDAs), and cell phones. The devices chosen often support the practice area through mobility, screen size and computing ability. One can also think of many health care machines as computing devices. The medication system may incorporate robotics, compounding machines, syringe pumps, and others devices in the provision of patient care.

Today, information technology is increasingly focused on the complete medication management cycle from prescribing through administration. The cycle includes prescriber order entry, integration with pharmacy systems and dispensing devices, and electronic documentation of administration. Health systems are rapidly adopting these technologies to improve patient safety, reduce errors and improve the efficiency of the process.

Pharmacy informatics is a broad and rapidly growing field. Looking ahead, pharmacists will continue to use informatics to provide care for patients in inpatient and ambulatory environments. Electronic prescribing, currently a high priority for implementation in many health care organizations, eliminates the manual handwriting of prescriptions and significantly enhances the pharmacist's ability to partner with physicians in providing care. Pharmacists can provide more focus on the appropriateness of therapy for the patient rather than the mechanics of drug distribution.

Data, Information and Knowledge Management

To understand informatics, one must understand the differences between data, information and knowledge.[4] Data are simply discrete and objective facts about a subject or an event. Good examples in health care are patient laboratory values, drug orders for a patient or the patient's weight. Data are easy to capture and store in media such as databases and files.

Information is often defined as data that has relevance and purpose. Information has meaning whereas pure data does not because information is contextualized, categorized, calculated, corrected, or condensed. In health care, examples of information are the patient's weight defined in kilograms or pounds or knowing that a particular laboratory result was high or low from reference values (Figure 25-1).

Figure 25-1
Relationship of Data, Information, and Knowledge

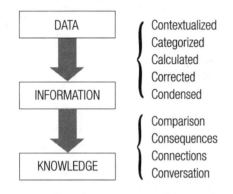

Knowledge is broader, deeper, and richer than data and information. Knowledge is combining information with framed experiences, norms, and contextual understanding. Information is transformed into knowledge through comparison between the current situation and another similar one, understanding the consequences of the information, knowing how the information connects to other information, or understanding what people think about the information. Knowledge is very difficult to capture as it often resides in people's heads. In health care, having knowledge means that a clinician knows the consequences of a particular laboratory test or knows whether the drug therapy prescribed for a patient is adequate to treat the condition being treated. Knowledge is often transferred tacitly though teaching, one-on-one interactions, experience, and practice norms.

Why is this important in the field of informatics? Informatics focuses on the use of technology to improve the use of data, information, and knowledge. Tools and technologies used to improve these areas vary considerably whether the focus is on data storage, retrieval and transfer, information gathering and sharing, or knowledge sharing. Understanding the differ-

ences helps the informatics pharmacist best utilize tools and technologies to solve the business problem at hand.

Information Security/Confidentiality

Information security may be defined as reasonable protection from risk of loss, risk of inappropriate access, or doubt regarding authenticity of information. These data security concerns can be referred to as confidentiality, authentication, and nonrepudiation.[5] Confidentiality ensures that the data is readable only by the intended recipients. Authentication provides protection against unauthorized access or forgeries. Nonrepudiation ensures that someone cannot deny having conducted a transaction. Vulnerabilities and threats to information security may consist of internal failures of hardware or software, human errors, deliberate attacks on information security, and natural catastrophes. Pharmacists responsible for informatics must ensure that security design in all pharmacy information systems support the prevention, detection, and correction of these vulnerabilities and threats.

Approaches to securing information and systems vary depending on the degree of sensitivity of the information. One of the first steps is to ensure that the physical location where servers are stored has been secured. Access to a network should be limited to those who need it and control must be exercised by a combination of security methods (e.g., passwords, smartcards, and/or biometric identification). These methods provide for authentication of individuals accessing information to help assure that only authorized individuals access the data. Furthermore, they provide for a history of access that can be examined if there are ever questions about who accessed certain data or was involved in specific transactions. Passwords are ubiquitous in current systems. However, a disadvantage is that they do not provide positive identification of individuals (passwords may be shared by multiple individuals). Biometrics, such as fingerprint recognition or retinal scanning, are becoming more prevalent due to their ability to provide a more positive authentication of an individual.

One key component of security in pharmacy systems is the ability to back up data so that it can be restored in event of internal hardware or software failures. Backing up data sets may be accomplished by replicating the data in an alternate medium and site. Media that may be used include hard drives, tapes, CDs or DVDs, to name a few. The availability of adequate back-up systems is essential to protect against natural disasters as well as hardware or software failures. Critical applications are often created with redundancies built to protect against such failure.

Another key security issue that has arisen with the advent of electronic transmission of prescriptions between physicians and pharmacies (and, in particular, Internet pharmacies) has been the authenticity of the involved parties and the electronic signature. In response to public concern for the safety of pharmacy practices on the Internet, the National Association of Boards of Pharmacy (NABP) developed the Verified Internet Pharmacy Practice Sites (VIPPS) program in the spring of 1999.[6] A coalition of state and federal regulatory associations, professional associations, and consumer advocacy groups provided their expertise in developing the criteria which VIPPS-certified pharmacies follow.

Pharmacies displaying the VIPPS seal have demonstrated to NABP compliance with VIPPS criteria. To achieve accreditation, a pharmacy practice site must comply with the licensing and inspection requirements of the states in which it does business and must demonstrate to NABP compliance with VIPPS criteria including patient rights to privacy, authentication and security of prescription orders, maintenance of a quality assurance and improvement program, and provision of meaningful consultation between patients and pharmacists.

Systems such as VeriSign™ are available to encrypt prescription or other protected health information during the electronic transmission of these data. This prevents the interception and unintended disclosure of confidential patient information during these transactions. Any pharmacy systems that involve transmission of patient data need to have a reliable and effective encryption process to assure confidentiality and authenticity.

While maintaining patient confidentiality and the security of patient information has long been a tenet of practice among pharmacists, the requirements of health care providers were increased with the passage and implementation of the Health Insurance Portability & Accountability Act (HIPAA).[7] Two goals of this legislation were to improve efficiency in health care delivery by standardizing electronic data and interchange and to protect the confidentiality and security of health data through setting and enforcing standards. The impact of HIPAA on institutions has been an increased awareness of the security and confidentiality

of protected health information. Health systems must conduct detailed assessments of their computer systems to assure that appropriate privacy protections are in place and that the security of systems is adequate. In many cases this has resulted in updating information systems to safeguard protected health information (PHI) and to enable the use of standard claims and other electronic health transactions. From a security perspective, HIPAA requires institutions to ensure the confidentiality, integrity, and availability of all electronic PHI that the institution creates, receives, maintains or transmits. It requires the hospital to protect against any reasonably anticipated threats or hazards to the security or integrity of this information and to ensure that rules and safeguards are in place to prevent inappropriate disclosure of this information. Within HIPAA, disclosure of PHI is limited to the minimum needed for health care treatment, business operations, and quality improvement.

One technique that may be useful when handling protected health information is to use encryption of patient identifiers. Encryption involves replacing identifiers that are traceable to an individual with another set of letters or numbers which cannot be linked back to individual patients. This technique of deidentification is very useful when doing analyses of aggregate data sets, examining overall prescribing trends, and evaluating drug utilization when there is no need to identify patients specifically.

Information Retrieval/Knowledge Sources

Automated retrieval and information systems have been a great advance in enhancing the availability of information and knowledge. They offer benefits with regard to information access as well as education for health care providers and patients alike. Historically, pharmacists have used hard-copy references to access drug information and other knowledge resources. However, today pharmacists are increasingly utilizing electronic information sources. The advantages of electronic information include availability of information from almost anywhere within the health care system and at the point of service (especially with the availability of intranets and wireless networks), reduced space requirements for storing information, and significant advances in the efficiency of information retrieval. Increased availability of information should lead to better decision making and improvements in the quality of care provided.

A wide variety of information retrieval and knowledge sources are currently available. According to a recent estimate, more than 100,000 websites provide health information today.[8] While it is not feasible to list all of them, some of the most frequently used sites and types of sources are indicated in the following table (Table 25-1). The easy and convenient access to the literature, drug information databases, and online continuing education help enable pharmacists (even in remote areas) to maintain their professional knowledgebase and to assist them in their practice.

The next several generations of knowledge systems will likely include information availability with increased customization and decision support. That is, when a question is asked about a drug there will be the capability of providing information within the context of the patient or clinical scenario as well. This will allow the knowledge source to return information that is specific to that particular patient or clinical situation. For example, instead of reporting the usual dosage range of a particular drug, the information provided might be a dosage recommendation specific to a patient of a given age and creatinine clearance.

One clear impact of the Internet is the enabling of more educated patients than ever before. Patients frequently will present to a health professional with a stack of printed material about their condition from the Internet. This can raise concerns about the validity of information available online. Because of the common knowledge of the deficiencies in much of the information available through the Internet, some health systems are providing patients with a list of endorsed, reliable health information links.[9] Furthermore, the Commission of the European Communities has published criteria to assure quality in health-related websites (Table 25-2).[8]

Table 25-1
Information Retrieval/ Knowledge Sources

Electronic databases and search engines
Medline, *International Pharmaceutical Abstracts*
Electronic journals
Electronic drug information resources (Micromedex, Multum, ePocrates, Lexicomp, Facts and Comparisons eFacts, etc.)
Electronic textbooks
The Natural Medicines Comprehensive Database

Table 25-2
Important Quality Criteria for Health-Related Websites

Transparency and honesty
Transparency of provider of site, purpose, and objective of site
Target audience is clearly defined
Transparency of all sources of funding
Authority
Clear statement of sources for all information and date of publication
Privacy and data protection policies
Clear and regular updating of information with date clearly displayed
Accountability for information
Process for user feedback and appropriate oversight responsibility
Editorial policy has clear statement on process used for selection of content
Guidelines on accessibility, searchability, readability

Source: Adapted from Reference 8.

Practice Applications of Informatics

Operational

Informatics plays many roles in the daily operation in health care pharmacies. Computer systems manage drug profiles and histories for patients allowing pharmacists to better manage care. Label generation and patient billing are tied to these systems to automate many of the tasks required for providing pharmaceutical care. Batch processing capabilities of a pharmacy system allows production runs for manufactured products or filling of patient orders in advance.

The complexity of health care systems requires that a number of interfaces be present to leverage the information stored in multiple systems. Interfaces allow patient information to flow directly into the pharmacy system from a patient management system which allows the pharmacy not to hand enter patient data. Interfaces to laboratory systems allow easy retrieval of patient laboratory results and addition of rules to promote safe and effective use of drugs. Interfaces to external devices such as IV compounders, automatic dispensing cabinets and robots increase the efficiency of the overall operations of the pharmacy.

Clinical

More and more, informatics is now playing a role in clinical pharmacy activities. A key area is the improved access to information. Without informatics, it is difficult to collect information about the patient and their care. The tools to collect data, filter results, provide decision support and record pharmacist activities are becoming more available to all pharmacies. These applications are now available using clinical mobility devices such as PDAs and tablet PCs.

One clinical area that is important for pharmacies is the documentation of clinical pharmacy activities. The methods to document pharmacists' interventions and patient care activities have changed significantly as technology has improved. Initial efforts to document pharmacists' interventions involved the use of paper forms and handwritten notes.[10–12] Paper documentation was cumbersome, time consuming, and the handwritten forms had the potential to be lost or unreadable and was difficult to compile.[11–12]

As technology improved and became more available, reports were published highlighting the development of computerized methods to document interventions.[11,13,14] Some of these systems required pharmacists to record their interventions on paper and later enter them into the computer. This process did not completely eliminate the drawbacks of manual documentation; however, it did make data interpretation more efficient.[13] Advantages include reduced time needed for documentation and improved ease of use, accessibility, time efficiency, and general acceptance.[14]

The ease of use, portability, and wealth of available programs has made hand-held computers, including personal digital assistants (PDAs), increasingly popular among health care professionals. Interventions are entered into the PDA and later downloaded into a database for evaluation. The small form factor was the greatest benefit for practitioners. Downsides include the small screen size, difficulty in capturing much detail and lack of real-time synchronization with other health care systems.

Tablet PCs or other wireless laptops are also being used for clinical pharmacist documentation. While the size is larger and heavier than a PDA, the clinician benefits from real-time access to patient data and other resources.

Administrative

The management of pharmacy services has improved greatly through technology and informatics. Managers have information tools that allow them to better assign resources to meet workload requirements, identify opportunities for cost savings, and justify new services. Medication system automation tools have allowed managers to move pharmacists into clinical roles and increase the overall safety of the medication-use system. A number of administrative applications of informatics are in Table 25-3.

Workflow and Process Improvement

Technology improvements have had significant impacts on workflow and process improvement within pharma-

Table 25-3
Administrative Uses of Informatics

Item	Benefit
Drug usage reporting	■ Compliance with policies and standard practices
Inventory management systems	■ Control inventory costs and turns
	■ Monitor purchasing activities
	■ Manage recalls and drug shortages
	■ Monitor compliance with regulatory requirements for controlled substances
Scheduling systems	■ Manage employee schedules
	■ Manage personnel costs
Portals	■ Dissemination of information
	■ Creation of knowledge sources regarding drug therapy
Workload reporting	■ Measure efficiency and productivity of processes

cies. Automation has permitted change in historically important pharmacist functions such as dispensing and has allowed these functions to be accomplished by robots, automated dispensing cabinets, and compounding devices, thus allowing the pharmacist to apply their knowledge to patient-specific health issues. Pharmacists, in part due to technology improvements, are much more able to participate in patient care teams and exercise clinical skills to improve patient care.

Process improvement is also often seen through improved knowledge sharing. Technology, including email and the web, has made sharing knowledge much easier and lower in cost. Clinical guidelines, disease management approaches, formularies, and more rich content are easily accessible to the pharmacist. Portable clinical computing advances in the forms of PDAs, wireless laptops, and tablet PCs have brought this knowledge closer to the patient and the care plan.

Perhaps the most important improvement seen with technology and automation is increased safety. Technologies such as bar codes and linking of disparate clinical systems have helped ensure that the right medication is for the right patient at the right time. As technology and information systems continue to improve, health systems will continue to see improvements in safety.

Systems Integration and Interfacing

Pharmacist-Computer Interactions

There are many different types of software that are used in health care informatics and pharmacists have varying ways in which they work with software. Software can be a simple, unchangeable system program solely designed to operate a piece of equipment or medical device or it can be a complex application designed for data entry, storage, exchange, and retrieval. Most pharmacists generally do not get involved in software programming, especially for the complex applications required in today's health care environment. The primary interaction hospital pharmacists have with software is directing the software to perform various tasks via the user interface on the display screen of the computer or device. This interaction can consist of activities such as programming infusion rates, entering orders, entering compounding volumes, or extracting reports for various equipment, devices and systems, such as pharmacy information systems (PIS) or computerized prescriber order entry systems (CPOE).

Beyond this day-to-day interaction pharmacists have with the user interface, pharmacists and other health care professionals can get more involved in the intricacies of an information system by working with system analysts or by directly working with the system, to define the business logic required for configuring a system to meet workflow needs and/or policies using the system's software configuration options. These activities require computer skills generally acquired through specialized training and experience obtained by working with the various automation and information systems that are discussed in the chapters dealing with information systems, automation, and the electronic medical record and prescriber order entry systems found in this text.

Access to and Use of Information

One of the most important aspects of any information system is the benefit it provides an organization in terms of accurate and efficient information storage and retrieval. Modern software applications contain a database tier where information is stored as a result of user input into the application's user interface. Depending on the complexity of the application, there may be thousands of discrete data elements stored in the application's database management system. The majority of data stored in the database includes input patient level data such as dispensing, billing, facility, and audit information.

While most information retrieval is conducted from within the application, these data may also be useful for activities external to the originally intended use of the system. For example, data in a PIS contains useful historical utilization information about commonly used drugs, dose forms, doses, and frequencies of administration that can be useful for making informed decisions about drug use policies within an organization. These data may be retrieved using a vendor-supplied report writer within the PIS database or, depending on the accessibility of the database, using report writing software. Such information can be invaluable to pharmacy managers and clinical pharmacists in addressing the administrative, clinical and patient safety needs of the department.

A second manner in which data contained in an information system may be useful beyond its original intent is when data may need to be imported from, exported to, or exchanged with another information system. A few of the many situations where this may occur include: input of patient-specific status and location data acquired from a patient management system (e.g., patient admission, discharge, and transfer information), integration of laboratory information into the pharmacy information system for the purposes of providing pharmacy staff with important clinical data for use in context with medication orders, provision of pharmacy utilization information to the hospital financial system for the purposes of billing, and clinical integration between a PIS and CPOE system to ensure accurate and complete medication profile information.

Integrating Information Systems with Work Activities

There are several methods for integrating information systems into existing pharmacy processes. One of the most widely used systems in pharmacy practice is a pharmacy information system (PIS). In addition to the many clinical features contained in a PIS, the PIS often serves as the backbone for pharmacy work activities by automating and organizing the daily workflow. Printed cart fill lists and intravenous medication labels allow the pharmacy department to sort and perform work activities in batches based upon patient location, type of medication, anticipated administration time, and/or via other sorting features. Similarly, PIS-generated medication administration records (MARs) can help nurses organize activities related to the medication administration process. MARs are designed to provide the nurse with sufficient information so that the nurse can safely and accurately provide the medication to the patient according to the time schedule desired by the prescriber.

CPOE systems are also used to organize work activities. Most contemporary CPOE systems contain patient lists, profiles, demographic information, electronic medication administration documentation, order forms, and other features. Orders made using the system can generate electronic or printed work lists or tasks for a wide variety of departments or individual health care providers.

The pharmacy department is the recipient of a large proportion of physician orders. The format for receipt of these orders can be quite different from one hospital to another depending on a number of factors, including work flow patterns, extent of technology deployment, physical size and layout of the hospital, type of facility, and practice-base of the physician (e.g., independent practice, group practice, hospitalist, or resident). Pharmacy orders can be: (1) handwritten or electronic; (2) individual or grouped (e.g., single sheet of paper or order set); (3) entered by physicians or a physician agent (e.g., nurse or clerk); or (4) delivered manually, via facsimile machine, via document imaging technology, or electronically from the CPOE system to the PIS. Once orders are delivered to the pharmacy, it becomes the pharmacists' responsibility to ensure that the orders are accurately placed on the patient's electronic profile in the PIS. In general, computerized prescriber-entered orders that are delivered to the pharmacy via a dedicated orders printer or an electronic interface to a PIS are more likely to be legible, complete, and delivered in a timely manner when compared to handwritten orders.

Types of Electronic Interfaces

There are several options for handling orders that are electronically delivered to the pharmacy department. The first option is for the pharmacist to take printed copies of the order and reenter the orders into the PIS. A second option is to transmit orders electronically from a CPOE system to the PIS via a one-way interface. A third option is to transmit orders from the CPOE system to the PIS or from the PIS to the CPOE system via independent one-way interfaces. The fourth option is for orders to be transmitted back and forth between systems using a bi-directional orders interface (Figure 25-2).

There are many advantages and disadvantages to each of these solutions.[15] The biggest advantage to an electronic transmittal of the order is that most orders, if correctly mapped, will not have to be entered into the pharmacy system, eliminating the potential for a transcription error, entry on the wrong patient, or omission due to the order being lost. A one-way or unidirectional interface consists of a transmission of orders from the CPOE system to the PIS. There are several advantages to this model, including direct mapping of the ordered medication on the CPOE side to the dispensed product on the PIS side of the interface, similar appearance of the ordered medication information and its appearance in the PIS and in downstream automated dispensing machines, and reduced overall design complexity. Disadvantages to a unidirectional interface include the need for prescribers or the pharmacist to reenter problem orders in the CPOE system when changes are required, the appearance of medication ordering information inconsistent with the manner in which physicians typically order medications, and the need for elaborate procedures in the event of CPOE system downtime.

Figure 25-2

Possible Computerized Prescriber Order Entry System (CPOE) Interfaces with a Pharmacy Information System (PIS)

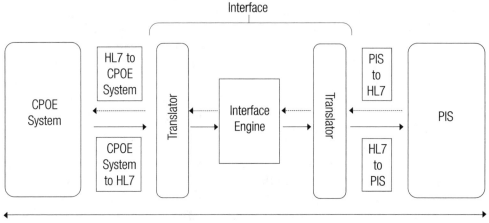

Solid arrows = CPOE to PIS; dashed arrows = PIS to CPOE; both = bidirectional interface

Source: Adapted from Chaffee BW, Bonasso J. Strategies for pharmacy integration and pharmacy information system interfaces, part 2: scope of work and technical aspects of interfaces. *Am J Health-Syst Pharm.* 2004;61(5):506–14.

Integration of a CPOE system with a PIS using two unidirectional interfaces allows the pharmacist to discontinue a CPOE order and then reenter the order properly in the PIS. The prescriber then will receive notice that there is a new order and can verify the accuracy of it. In some cases, this may create confusion and require discussion between the prescriber and the pharmacist to resolve any concerns that may arise. In addition, if the CPOE system is down, handwritten orders can be used and entered into the PIS for label generation and use by downstream technologies (e.g., automated dispensing machines). Once the CPOE system comes back up, the orders queue can be used to repopulate the patient's profile and MAR in the CPOE system.

Implementation of a bidirectional orders interface is a very complex undertaking, but it can offer some advantages over two unidirectional interfaces. If the two systems are sufficiently robust to handle the transaction details, changes made in the PIS can be sent back across the interface and will update the order information stored in the CPOE system. This eliminates the need for deletion of an incorrect order and reentry of the order in the CPOE system. Further, if either the CPOE system or the PIS system is down for

significant periods of time, the interface engine can be used to queue the orders on the live system until such time as the system that is down is able to be placed back into production. The major problem with a bidirectional orders interface is the complexity—there are three possible components that can be down: the CPOE system, the PIS, and the interface itself. Further, like the unidirectional interface, it may be difficult to create medication orderable items that are physician friendly, yet containing sufficient details to be efficiently mapped to products on the PIS.

Clinical Decision Support

The term *clinical decision support* (CDS) represents the features and functions of an information system that passively or actively convey clinical knowledge content to health care professionals so that choices can be made that are in the best interest of patient care. There are many methods for providing system users with clinical knowledge. Passive conveyance of clinical knowledge content occurs as a result of system design features and choices made during system configuration.[16,17] This can include providing users with links to knowledge sources as mentioned earlier in the section on information retrieval and knowledge sources.

Another passive method for providing basic CDS is the use of structured data elements for medication ordering in a PIS or CPOE system (Table 25-4). During system configuration, tables are built for each drug entity that define the allowable drug order choices that users of system users can select during order entry. Many systems will allow the institution to select the appearance and order of selections and even provide default selections. By limiting the choices a prescriber can make, the institution can help prevent the errors that occur from ordering medication doses, routes of administration, or frequencies that are unsafe, subtherapeutic, excessively costly, nonstandard, or inconsistent with institutional policy. By passively directing choices in this manner, it is more likely that patients will receive safe, effective, and cost-efficient therapy.

Table 25-4
Examples of Basic Structured Data Elements

- Generic drug name
- Dose amount
- Unit of measure (e.g., mg, units, mg/kg, mEq/L, etc.)
- Route of administration
- Frequency or rate of administration
- Prn
- Prn reason
- Dispensing dosage form (tablet, capsule, suppository, etc.)
- Dispensing strength
- Dispensing dispensed

The use of structured order entry also ensures that key clinical information contained in the PIS or CPOE system can be coded.[18] Coding of structured information is important for expansion of the CDS capabilities to include clinical checking for allergy problems, drug interactions, abnormal doses, therapeutic duplication, intravenous drug admixture incompatibilities, therapeutic indication problems, and other rules. For some of these basic types of decision support, there needs to be clinical knowledge content available that uses the coded drug entity or entities to identify situations that may cause a clinical problem. This clinical content is most often provided by commercially available products that are designed to be easily incorporated into the CDS

offerings of CPOE systems or PIS. The CPOE or PIS vendor will then imbed proprietary code or rules into their software to use this content for these basic alerts.

Clinical Data Repositories

In addition to the availability of commercial clinical knowledge content, there are other key prerequisites for expanding CDS to include rule-based alerts. The most important piece is the presence of a repository of patient-specific clinical data often referred to as a clinical data repository (CDR). CDS rules often require data from other ancillary systems, such as the laboratory or dietary systems. Rather than make many system-to-system database interfaces and creating multiple, redundant repositories of these data in ancillary system databases, many institutions choose to create an organizational CDR. Data can then be imported into the CDR from ancillary systems and extracted from the CDR when necessary for use by ancillary departments. Often, organizations choose to use the CPOE system database as the organizational CDR because it already contains the largest amount of clinical data and typically contains additional storage capacity for ancillary data. Larger organizations may choose to create and maintain their own CDR using a large database management software program. In either case, having a central source of valid clinical data is key to successful implementation of rules. Data contained within the CDR is often useful beyond the CDS activities. Data within the CDR is often useful for clinical or administrative reporting purposes or for use in other applications.

A CDS rule is a coded program incorporated into the CPOE system, the PIS, or a standalone CDS system in order to identify specific clinical care or business-related situations for the purposes of alerting specified users of the need to address a particular situation. CDS rules can be imbedded rules created by the vendor or rules conceived by a hospital's employees. The end product of rules is most frequently seen by clinicians in the context of patient care alerts. Rules can take information from disparate systems, perform calculations, and/or incorporate logic to determine whether or not an alert should occur and then invoke that alert via a user-defined alert process.

Alerts and Knowledge Source Links

There are massive amounts of data available in the medical literature—old and new, substantive and meaningless, evidence-based and anecdotal. It is very difficult, if not impossible, for clinicians to stay adequately informed about best practices on their own. Hospitals can utilize the collective knowledge of all of their physicians and departments to create best practice guidelines for the majority of high volume diseases. CDS alerts and links to both internal and external knowledge sources can be used to provide clinicians with warnings, supportive prompts, or access to clinical content to ensure that clinicians have the best tools at their disposal to care for their patients.

Active conveyance of clinical knowledge content is generally provided through alert and warning screens provided to the user but can also include notification of alerts via printed documents, electronic mail, and pagers. CDS alerts can be imbedded as a part of most any clinical information system, but it is most frequently seen in pharmacy information systems (PIS), inpatient or ambulatory care computerized prescriber order entry systems (CPOE), or as standalone expert systems that use data from existing clinical databases for supporting the diagnosis, surveillance, and/or treatment of disease. The proper use of CDS requires not only the wisdom and experience of health care professionals but also an understanding by these clinicians of the capabilities, limitations and deficiencies of CDS within their environment.

There are two main types of alerts that can be presented to users.[19] Synchronous alerts represent warning screens that are invoked based upon specific actions taken by a user of the system. An example of a synchronous alert might be the appearance of a drug dosing warning alert notification screen when a user attempts to enter an excessive dose of a medication. The action taken by the user could be selecting a *submit* button, which invokes a check of the dose against defined criteria within the system. Asynchronous alerts generally occur as a result of an imbedded rule. Data introduced to the CDS system, for example reported laboratory results, are examined to see if they are included as part of a rule. If so and if the rule criteria stipulate that an alert should occur, then the system will present the alert to a given user or category of users. An example of an asynchronous alert could be having a flag placed on a users electronic work list, patient list, or system inbox when an abnormal laboratory value is manually entered or electronically transmitted to the CPOE system for a blood chemistry test.

Clinical Informatics Pharmacist

Pharmacist positions in clinical informatics are positions that have evolved in response to contemporary pharmacy practice needs rather than positions which have a clear academic and training path. Informatics education does not appear often in the curricula at colleges of pharmacy in the United States. In general, pharmacists who accept these roles either have a strong interest in informatics or have developed a specific informatics aptitude on the job.

Roles and Responsibilities

Pharmacists who specialize in informatics generally are responsible for one or more of the following activities:

- Inpatient pharmacy information systems
- Outpatient pharmacy information systems
- Robotic unit-dose dispensing machines
- Automated medication dispensing machines
- Point-of-care bar code medication administration
- Automated intravenous admixture devices
- Inpatient computerized prescriber order entry systems
- Outpatient computerized prescriber order entry systems
- Clinical decision support
- Packaging machines
- Programming
- Report writing
- Inventory control systems
- Pharmacy intranets
- Customized pharmacy applications
- Desktop and application support
- Staff training and education

Education and Training

Pharmacists who wish to pursue a position in pharmacy informatics can accomplish this in several ways. One option is to take specific courses or obtain a degree in computer science, information systems, and/or business information technology. Useful coursework would include areas such as network administration, basic programming, database management, and heuristics. Another option available to pharmacists would be to complete an advanced residency in pharmacy informatics. Several sites for informatics residencies have emerged in recent years and they offer the resident a wide array of learning opportunities not generally available to most pharmacists or pharmacy practice residents. A third way is to volunteer to assume an informatics role at one's current place of employment. This can be done by indicating an interest in informatics, to volunteering to take responsibility for one or more aspects of informatics and/or obtaining as much on-the-job experience as possible, including taking coursework through local community colleges, attending certified training courses, attending vendor training courses, attending informatics-related conferences, and learning from colleagues. The field of pharmacy informatics is constantly evolving. Many pharmacists have found applying their clinical knowledge with information technology skills for the purposes of bettering patient care to be very a very satisfying and rewarding career.

Summary

Pharmacy informatics is a broad and growing area. While the formal organization of pharmacy informatics is not as developed as is seen in other disciplines, pharmacists have played a leading role to date in the adoption of technologies to improve the medication-use system. Much work is yet to be done. Technology tools in the hands of properly trained pharmacists have the potential to greatly improve the safety and efficiency of the medication-use system in health care organizations.

References

1. Healthnet BC Glossary. Available at: http://healthnet.hnet.bc.ca/tools/glossary/. Accessed November 12, 2004.

2. Nursing Informatics Frequently Asked Questions. Available at: http://nursing.umaryland.edu/~snewbold/sknfaqni.htm. Accessed November 12, 2004.

3. Definitions of Medical Informatics. Available at: http://www.veranda.com.ph/hermant/definitions.htm. Accessed November 12, 2004.

4. Davenport TH, Prusak L. *Working Knowledge*. Boston: Harvard Business School Press; 2000.

5. A Structure for Discussing Application Security Requirements. Available at: http://enterprise.state.wi.us/home/strategic/sec.htm. Accessed November 12, 2004.

6. Verified Internet Pharmacy Practice Sites (VIPPS) Program. Available at: http://www.nabp.net/vipps/intro.asp. Accessed November 12, 2004.

7. Tribble DA. The health insurance portability and accountability act: security and privacy requirements. *Am J Health-Syst Pharm.* 2001;58:763–70.

8. Commission of the European Communities: eEurope 2002. Quality criteria for health related websites. *J Med Internet Res.* 2002;4:e15.

9. UMHS-Endorsed External Sites. Available at: http://www.med.umich.edu/pteducation/links.htm. Accessed November 12, 2004.

10. Bearce WC, Willey GA, Fox RL, et al. Documentation of clinical interactions: quality of care issues and economic considerations in critical care pharmacy. *Hosp Pharm.* 1988;23:883–90.

11. Zimmerman CR, Smolarek RT, Stevenson JG. A computerized system to improve documentation and reporting of pharmacists' clinical interventions, cost savings, and workload activities. *Pharmacotherapy.* 1995;15:220–7.

12. Haslett TM, Kay BG, Weissfellner H. Documenting concurrent clinical pharmacy interventions. *Hosp Pharm.* 1990;25:351–5,359.

13. Narducci WA, Norvell MJ. Development and use of an automated pharmacy services documentation system. *Hosp Pharm.* 1989;24:184–9,204.

14. Schumock GT, Hutchinson RA, Bilek BA. Comparison of two systems for documenting pharmacist interventions in patient care. *Am J Hosp Pharm.* 1992;49:2211–4.

15. Chaffee BW, Bonasso J. Strategies for pharmacy integration and pharmacy information system interfaces, part 1: history and pharmacy integration options. *Am J Health-Syst Pharm.* 2004;61:502–6.

16. Teich JM, Merchia PR, Schmiz JL, et al. Effects of computerized physician order entry on prescribing practices. *Arch Intern Med.* 2000;160:2741–7.

17. Senholzi C, Gottlieb J. Pharmacist interventions after implementation of computerized prescriber order entry. *Am J Health-Syst Pharm.* 2003;60:1880–2.

18. Broverman C, Kapusnik-Uner J, Shalaby J, et al. A concept-based medication vocabulary: an essential requirement for pharmacy decision support. *Pharm Pract Manage Q.* 1998;18:1–20.

19. Galanter WL, Polikatis A, DiDomenico RJ. A trial of automated safety alerts for inpatient digoxin use with computerized physician order entry. *J Am Med Inform Assoc.* 2004;11:270–7.

Chapter 26

Electronic Data Management: Electronic Health-Record Systems and Computerized Provider Order-Entry Systems

James R. Knight, Stephen K. Huffines, S. Trent Rosenbloom

Introduction

Electronic health record (EHR) systems are computer-based applications designed to store, manage, and display health care related records, including all clinical and administrative information entered by all practitioners involved in health care delivery.[1] Today, despite a clear understanding by health care providers and system developers of the composition and role of EHR systems, adoption remains limited.[2,3] Many reasons for limited adoption have been postulated in the scientific and lay literature. These reasons likely include problems related to how the systems collect, organize, store, interpret, analyze, and report patient data, the technical limitations inherent in the software and hardware supporting EHR systems, and the high cost of developing and implementing such systems.

Computerized provider order entry (CPOE) is the process by which health care providers place clinical orders (such as prescriptions and laboratory testing requests) using a computerized system. The *p* in CPOE is traditionally attributed as *physician;* in our experience, health care *provider* is the more accurate description since multiple health care providers serve in a prescribing role—physicians, nurse practitioners, physician assistants, and pharmacists. While only about 10% of hospitals currently use CPOE systems, the number is expected to grow due to national mandate, industry incentives, and stakeholder pressure.[3–6] Although CPOE systems support multiple order types (i.e., radiology, dietary, and laboratory), the focus of this chapter will be on the medication component.

To cover these main issues, this chapter is divided into two sections. The first section focuses EHR systems including the evolving definition of EHR systems, the information contained in an EHR system and, the role of an EHR system in health care. The second section introduces CPOE concepts to the pharmacist so that these systems might be properly deployed and positioned.

Definitions

CPOE—Computerized provider order entry is the process by which health care providers electronically place clinical orders (such as prescriptions, laboratory, and radiology requests).

EHR—An electronic health record is an electronic version of the patient's paper-based medical record but often takes on additional functionality.

HIPAA—Health Insurance Portability and Accountability Act enacted in 1996. To improve portability and continuity of health insurance coverage in the group and individual markets, to combat waste, fraud, and abuse in health insurance and health care delivery, to promote the use of medical savings accounts, to improve access to long-term care services and coverage, to simplify the administration of health insurance, and for other purposes.

History and Definition of EHR Systems

The history of EHR systems began in the early 1960s with early pioneers developing programs to assist in documenting patient history, physical examinations, and radiology reports.[7–9] Some of the earliest EHR systems include The Medical Record (TMR), developed in 1970 at Duke University, the Regenstrief Medical Record System (RMRS), first developed in 1972, and the HELP system in Utah.[1,9–12] Since then, many EHR systems have been developed in academic settings across the country. Examples include the COSTAR project at Massachusetts General Hospital and systems at Stanford, Johns Hopkins, Columbia, and Vanderbilt.[13] In addition, the U.S. government has developed EHR systems for the Veterans Administration, the Department of Defense, and the Indian Health Service, and many commercial vendors have been creating or licensing additional systems in the private sector.[14]

In general, EHR systems are designed to replicate the information found in paper-based medical records but often take on greater functionality.[15] EHR systems are tools that provide secure, real-time, point-of-care and patient-centered information for all health care providers, according to early developers.[16] This means that they make patient care information available wherever it is needed, 24 hours a day, seven days a week. In the best cases, EHR systems can help to manage multiple aspects of patient care (e.g., clinical documentation, medication and allergy management, laboratory results tracking) and promote better decision making by providing accurate and timely clinical information. Modern EHR systems can enable patient care to be coordinated across different sites of health care delivery, can support administrative functions related to scheduling patients' admissions or appointments, and can organize information according to what is needed and when it is needed. Information extracted from EHR systems can also provide data for quality assurance monitoring and for medical research. In the United States, EHR systems must now also be designed to meet HIPAA patient privacy requirements.

Comprehensive EHR systems generally contain several core components: a patient *data repository*, user interfaces (which may be task- and user role-specific), a care provider order-entry system, clinical decision support tools, clinical note capture tools, and rules engines. A data repository is generally a type of database that contains patient information, including lists of medications, allergies, laboratory and radiology testing results, clinical documents, demographic information such as age, gender, and address, and orders. The information available in a patient data repository can be displayed in or inform the functioning of other tools within an EHR system. *User interfaces* allow health care providers who are not necessarily computer experts to interact with the data in a patient data repository. User interfaces can permit entry of new orders or prescriptions, viewing of recent laboratory reports, scheduling clinical visits or admissions, and managing lists of diagnoses, among others. *Clinical decision support tools* provide guideline- or knowledge-based information to health care providers as they are generating clinical orders to improve their decision making. The knowledge and content that inform decision-support tools can come from local medical libraries, national professional societies, and national governmental services. Decision support can be as simple as providing lists of the available dosage forms as the health care provider

is entering the dose, and as complicated as therapy advisors for total parenteral nutrition or chemotherapy, which must balance recent laboratory results, current diagnoses, and concurrent medications. *Clinical note capture tools* assist health care providers in documenting their clinical decision making and patient interactions. *Rules engines* apply specific algorithms to data available from any of these systems to ensure that it conforms to system standards and to drive additional functionality (such as decision support). Often, an EHR system is made up of component tools developed in isolation from the others, and each serving one or more of the functionalities described above. When this occurs, a comprehensive EHR system may also include software to manage the data flow among the different tools.

Benefits of ER Systems

EHR systems provide a number of direct benefits to all categories of health care providers, including physicians, nurses, pharmacists and therapists. Key benefits result from the distributed nature of EHR systems (i.e., patient information is not tied to a single location as it is with a paper chart), the powerful processing capabilities of computers, and the imposition of legibility and clarity on clinical data, while simultaneously generating data to support administrative functions and quality improvement monitoring. By improving data availability, clarity and correctness, EHR systems can minimize the number of times health care providers are uninformed about a patient's history and current or recent treatment plans. As a result of computer power and more structured data compliance with any institutional rules or pathways EHR systems can support both clinical decision making and actions by providing relevant medical knowledge within the workflow. EHR-based tools that support decision-making can assure that health care providers select the best therapy, while tools that support clinical actions can verify that the therapy is administered to the right patient at the right time, at the right dose and interval.

From an institutional standpoint, one of the major benefits of the use of EHR systems is the wealth of automated solutions and data that they can provide for quality assurance and continuous improvement efforts.[13] Clinical documentation tools, for example, can improve legibility and reduce medication and documentation errors. EHR systems can aggregate performance information by disease, by health care providers, and patient-care area. Such performance information can identify where clinical practice benchmarks are not being met. In some cases, EHR systems connected to medical devices such as infusion pumps or heart monitors can trigger alerts when patients have a significant change in status.[17] EHR systems may also help to improve compliance with regulatory society standards, such as those published by the Joint Commission on Accreditation of Healthcare Organizations (JCAHO) by increasing the ability to manage and store data.[18]

EHR systems may also benefit research efforts. Without an EHR system, gathering information necessary for individual research protocols from clinical documents is a manual process prone to inefficiency and error. Generally, research personnel isolated from the clinical encounter abstract data related to research from these notes onto semistructured forms. Chart abstracters working with handwritten or typed documents, clinical forms, and a dispersed medical record may encounter additional problems with poor handwriting, vaguely documented concepts, and variability in their ability to interpret what is written. Because data abstraction usually occurs after the patient encounter is finished, it expends additional resources and generates data that cannot be used in real time to modify the care the patient receives. EHR systems can improve the process by prompting health care providers to be complete, automatically abstracting data relevant to research, and providing real-time research-related feedback. In addition, using relevant patient data, EHR systems can automatically identify patients meeting inclusion criteria for research trials, thereby improving targeted recruitment.[17]

Information Content and Data Issues with an EHR system

Wagemann recently outlined some key information that should be incorporated in an EHR system.[19] According to his model, EHR systems should include the following:

- Problem list, history and physical exam information, any allergies to drugs or food, current and past medications, laboratory orders, past and planned procedures, radiology results and current nutrition orders
- Health care provider orders (including drug-therapy orders)
  - Order-entry tools that enable providers to input orders directly
  - Order sets and/or collaborative pathways for the diseases most frequently seen in each practice site
  - Tools for outlining evidence-based or guideline-based clinical practice
  - Decision-support systems that drive order-generation based on institutional practice, patient-specific data, and corollary information from other orders
- Nurse documentation of patient observations and order completion
- Other ancillary professional documentation, including respiratory therapy, nutrition, physical/occupational/speech pathology, and pharmacy consult services
- Patient daily charges information
- Practice variance, quality assurance, continuous quality improvement, and risk management data in the format desired when it is needed
- Access to electronic knowledge sources, such as the National Library of Medicine (NLM)

Although there is general agreement on what information/data is contained within an EHR system, two commonly identified problems relate to entering information into an EHR system and sharing information between systems. As EHR systems have developed, input methodology has greatly improved but not resolved. Once in the computer systems, information cannot always be shared with other systems; multiple solutions, including data standards, exist but are incompletely adopted.

The difficulties with data entry have been known since the first EHR components were being developed, were again articulated by McDonald in 1972, and remain to this day.[1,2,8,9,16] Most EHR systems provide a number of different ways to input patient data.[19] The earliest EHR systems permitted input using manual punch cards, which many system users believed were preferable to typed entry.[9,16] Other developers experimented with patient-entered data using simple electronic questionnaires.[20] Ultimately, the keyboard has evolved as the primary means of data input. Other common methods of data entry include direct interfaces with other computers that generate data (e.g., digital laboratory test analyzers, some blood glucose monitors), point and click entry into a computer-form using a computer mouse or a touch-screen monitor, dictation and transcription, drawing, using a specialized digital tablet, and scanning of handwritten documents.

Each method for data input has relative strengths and weaknesses. Typing, for example, may be efficient and acceptable for skilled users and relatively simple for data entry needs, but it is time consuming for others and limits the type of data that can be entered to what fits on a standard keyboard. Dictation/transcription is useful for those who cannot type efficiently, but it is expensive, error-prone, and inefficient. Point and click entry into structured forms can be very fast for simple data entry tasks, but it can become difficult if the user cannot find what they need to document. Handwriting and scanning offers providers tremendous flexibility and ease but may lead to reduced legibility and data availability.

Closely related to data input problems, the difficulty sharing data contained in one EHR system with others has played a major role in limiting system-interconnectivity (called "interoperability"). This problem arises when different systems (or tools within a single system) encode the same information using different words, codes, or narrative structure. For example, system users may expect to type a patient's weight only once and have it subsequently available to all connected EHR component systems. A component pharmacy system may store the patient weight and call it by the name "Weight," while the order-entry system calls it "Wt.," and the physician's clinical note contains the unstructured narrative, "the patient weighs..." Sharing the patient's weight between these different systems is very difficult—if not impossible—without extensive programming. The problem recurs for every potential piece of patient data, including medications, allergies, clinical findings, diagnoses, lab results, and orders.

One solution to the problem of sharing information between systems is data standardization. Standardization defines a regular format for the data, the terms used to represent it, and the configuration it should take. For example, one standard would state that physical measurements, such as weight, must include the measurement name (e.g., weight), the value (e.g., 175) and the units (e.g., pounds), a corollary standard would state that weight must always be represented in EHR systems by the term "weight," and a formatting standard would state that the three must follow a certain configuration (e.g., '<measurement=weight, value=175, unit=pound>'). A major standards organization, Health Level 7 (HL-7), has been widely adopted as an industry data interchange standard. HL-7 primarily defines standards for data formatting and configuration. Data

from two HL-7 compliant systems can communicate with relative ease and minimal additional programming. HL-7, however, generally stops short of defining standard terms for data exchange. The United States National Committee on Health and Vital Statistics (NCVHS) recently identified several core clinical vocabularies as terminology standards; however, these terminologies are inconsistently available or adopted by system developers.[21]

An additional component solution for data exchange among EHR systems involves enterprise information architecture. Originally, information resources were managed separately; each clinical and administrative department would use different computerized systems that met different information and workflow needs. In an information architecture focused on the enterprise as a whole, individual programs are managed as components of a single application and are supported by common information resources. This architecture can minimize the amount of data standardization required by reducing interfaces between different systems within a single enterprise. To handle the specific needs for the different clinical and administrative departments, user interfaces can be developed to provide context-sensitive information views and data entry forms, while transaction engines can manage the information generically for the entire enterprise information system. The problem is that integration within an enterprise may not be the final answer to the integration issue.[10] Few commercial systems have adopted the enterprise-information architecture that distinguishes the user application from the underlying data.

Promoting Expansion Of EHR Systems: Issues and Solutions

At present, only 5–39% of U.S. health care systems, office-based physician practices, hospitals, and clinics (excluding the Veterans Administration) have implemented EHR systems.[2,3] As previously discussed, there are many reasons for poor adoption, including difficulties related to data entry and interoperability. In addition, there is tremendous variability among systems in terms of functionality, ease of use, integration with other health care applications, data security, and ability to conform to clinical workflow needs. Health care providers and organizations must also expend resources to manage local knowledge-based rules and guidelines for their decision support and order entry systems. Furthermore, most EHR systems are expensive to purchase, implement, and maintain, and the physician may not realize any direct benefit from their investment in such systems. To remove the negative forces created by these problems, there must be some realignment of incentives for office-based physician practice. Incentives that can help offset the EHR system purchasing costs include improved reimbursement from third-party payers and/or governmental support.

Currently, industry and the U.S. Department of Health and Human Services (HHS), Congress, Food and Drug Administration (FDA), and Centers for Medicare and Medicaid Services (CMS) have high expectations for EHR systems. A recent announcement from the former Health and Human Services Secretary, Tommy Thompson, detailed a proposed 10-year plan that addresses the need for standards for EHR functionality, privacy, and interoperability, with the overarching goal of stimulating EHR system adoption.[22] Secretary Thompson stated, "Health information technology can improve quality of care and reduce medical errors, even as it lowers administrative cost. It has the potential to produce savings of 10% of our total spending on health care, even as it improves care for the patients and provides support for the health care team. Ten percent of the total health care spending represents savings of $150 billion." This plan was prepared by the new National Coordinator for Health Information Technology, David J. Brailer, MD, Ph.D., who clearly defines the broad steps that need to be taken to ensure that every patient's medical information is managed in an up-to-date EHR. This plan specifies regional grants and low interest loans to offset the expense of purchasing EHR systems and improved regulations to produce common standards for drug e-prescribing. Under this plan Medicare would provide additional reimbursement for health care systems that implement EHR systems and share patient information with other health care providers. Other third-party payers would also be encouraged to provide incentives for demonstration projects showing how EHR systems can reduce resource utilization.

The Future of EHR in the United States

Since the early adoption of EHR systems in the 1970s, experts have often believed that EHR systems would be used throughout all health care settings. However, problems with implementation have limited widespread adoption. In 2005, experts again are optimistic that use of EHR systems will greatly expand. One of

the very positive signs of possible expansion is that former Secretary Thompson announced the government's plan to expand the implementation of EHR systems because it focuses on all of the current problems that must be addressed to enable widespread use of EHR systems. Other positive drivers are younger physicians, pharmacists, and nurses who are more accepting of using computers and the Internet to enable them to provide the best patient care and patients who are becoming more familiar with the risk of errors in health care that can be minimized with EHR systems. Government and other private payers and EHR systems must make the positive changes to enable greater adoption of EHR systems.

Finally, patients' knowledge of the high risk of errors in the health care system may be the most forceful driver of increasing the safety in providing health care though implementation of EHR systems. On the negative side this initiative involves changes in all of the players in health care today. Changes will be required in the government, the providers of health care, and the payers. For this expansion to come true, all of these programs must achieve the outcome that the changes are designed to produce. The results over the next 10 years will indicate whether these changes produce the outcomes that will enable widespread expansion of EHR systems.

CPOE History and Background

In 2000, the Institute of Medicine published its first report on medical error, *To Err is Human*.[6] This report garnered a great deal of attention and galvanized many health care organizations to make patient safety the top priority. A second report, *Crossing the Quality Chasm: A New Health System for the 21st Century*, highlighted the importance of electronic health record (EHR) systems and the use of CPOE to eliminate many of the preventable adverse events in the provision of care.[25] Since medication errors are the most prevalent medical error, many CPOE systems focus on the reduction of adverse drug events. Various studies are now validating this approach. The Leapfrog Group made CPOE one of the three recommended goals to improve quality in hospitals providing care to more than 34 million consumers.[4] The business roundtable seeks to improve quality and enhance efficiency, thereby increasing its purchasing power and limiting the dramatic increase in health care costs. The presidential administration of George W. Bush has demonstrated support by establishing the Office of the National Coordinator for Health Information Technology (ONCHIT) and by awarding more than $139 million dollars in grants and contracts to regional projects that support the adoption of health information technology.[26,27]

In their earliest forms, CPOE systems date back to the mid-1970s. Early systems allowed health care providers to enter orders directly into the system but provided little decision support to alert drug-drug interactions, allergy warnings, etc. System functionality, hardware limitations, and readiness of institutions limited early adoption. Over subsequent years, technical advancement and the necessity for tools to assist professionals in delivering ever-increasing complex care to patients have led to further adoption of CPOE.

In spite of these efforts, CPOE has not moved far beyond the first adopters; however, according to recent surveys and reports, interest in deployment of CPOE systems is high on the agenda of many facilities. In a 2003 survey of 786 hospitals, Leapfrog reports that 22% of respondents are committed to implementing CPOE by 2004; however, Leapfrog reports that only 4.3% of respondents had CPOE fully available in 2003.[28] Ash et al. report that 9.6% of the 626 hospitals responding to a survey have CPOE completely available in 2002.[3] According to a report prepared by First Consulting Group for the American Hospital Association and the Federation of American Hospitals, an estimated 5% of hospitals use CPOE.[3] Regardless of the exact number of facilities who have CPOE, the statistics validate the difficulty and the time required to implement CPOE in complex health care facilities. Even in the hospitals who report CPOE is installed, full integration of systems including clinical decision support is even more unlikely.[29] This again speaks to the complexity and the onsite development that is required to fully deploy these systems in the hospital environment. Figure 26-1 (adopted from Abernathy and Utterback) illustrates the technology curve that one would expect for this application and the authors' proposed timeline Figure 26-2.[30] These graphs demonstrate the use of CPOE in the early life cycle of this technology. In addition, Figure 26-2 illustrates the product innovations that precede the process innovations. CPOE will not be maximized until these process innovations are fully integrated into the process workflow.

The primary reasons generally cited for lack of diffusion of this tool are (1) belief that physicians would not use computerized ordering, (2) products available from vendors have not been perfected, and (3) technical and process complexities of implementing CPOE translate into a significant investment with no guarantee of success.[31,32] Lack of standardization in practice across health care facilities is also cited as an additional barrier.[29]

As one begins the journey, one should note that it would be hard to overestimate the positive impact of a properly employed CPOE system on care provided to patients and enhancing the practice of pharmacy. Likewise, the opposite is true for a poorly implemented system.

Goals of a CPOE System

Advocates of CPOE systems promote them based on their potential to reduce adverse events related to prescribing by alerting health care providers to potential errors (including drug interactions and patient allergies). Enthusiasm for CPOE has extended throughout the health care industry and into pharmacy circles in recent years. This interest comes from many different directions including health care facility leadership, standard and regulatory organizations, informatics professionals, software vendors, and within the pharmacy profession.

While the implementation of a CPOE system impacts every hospital department, the pharmacy often becomes disproportionately involved in the process. This is due to the complexity of the medication module, volume of transactions, and perceived value of CPOE on the medication order process.[23] CPOE implementation is generally too massive for the pharmacy to initiate; however, the pharmacy must be prepared and positioned to provide leadership in the medication component of these systems. The pharmacist is well-prepared and has historically demonstrated clinical and process skills in utilizing pharmacy computer systems.[24] These skills must be combined with innovation and an insatiable desire to provide solutions.

The goals of CPOE should be clearly defined before initiating the project and must be realistically aligned with the functionality of the product, the resources available to develop the product and commitment to make needed clinical process redesign. Development of realistic goals with a reasonable timeline is critical and will significantly enhance the potential for success. The goals of CPOE system implementation usually include the following:

Figure 26-1
Technology Life Cycle—CPOE

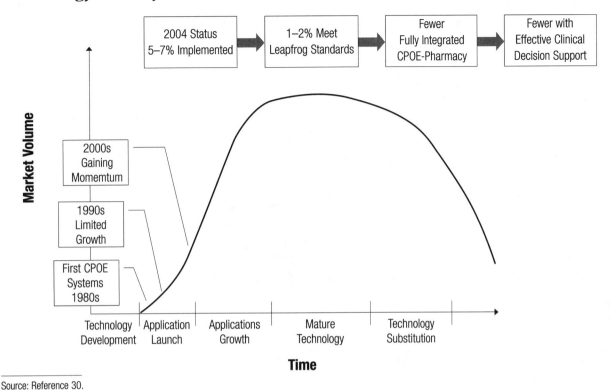

Source: Reference 30.

- Improve patient safety
- Increase timeliness of care
- Facilitate use of current medical knowledge via clinical decision support
- Improve the process and coordination of care
- Limit the missed opportunities for preventive care
- Research capability for epidemiological studies
- Control or reduction of cost

Overcoming Barriers to CPOE

It becomes obvious when surveying successful models for CPOE implementation that one must aggressively address barriers that are most commonly faced with implementation of CPOE. A survey of senior management at U.S. hospitals by Poon et al. found similar results as the California Healthcare Institute.[31] Three general areas were identified that must be overcome before implementing CPOE.[33] The three areas identified were (1) physician and organizational resistance

most often associated with perceived negative impact on workload, (2) the high CPOE cost and lack of capital, and (3) the product/vendor immaturity.

Managing Change

Implementing CPOE systems can lead to profound workflow changes within an institution. Nancy Lorenzi et al. have effectively defined the importance of managing change with the introduction of extensive informatics systems into complex health care environments.[33] She states, "As our new systems affect larger, more heterogeneous groups of people and more organization areas, the major challenges to systems success often become more behavioral than technical." Certainly, the system must be technically and functionally sound; however, proper attention must be invested in managing the change in behavior and process.[33]

During the planning phase, careful review of the complete medication process should be performed. The tendency is to focus on the technology and the complex steps to get this into place; however, significant investment must be made into the integration of this

Figure 26-2
Product Life Cycle—Process Innovations

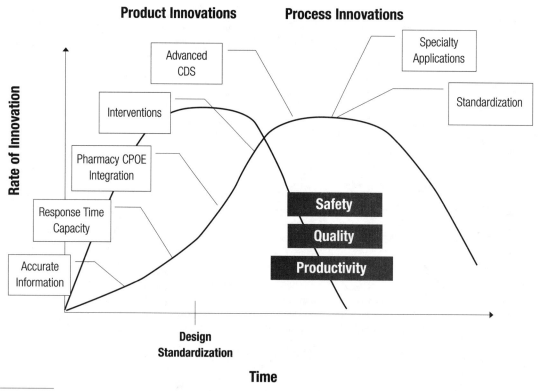

Product Innovations   **Process Innovations**

Rate of Innovation

- Advanced CDS
- Specialty Applications
- Standardization
- Interventions
- Pharmacy CPOE Integration
- Response Time Capacity
- Accurate Information

Safety

Quality

Productivity

Design
Standardization

Time

technology with the systems and people. Flowcharts should be updated to remove processes that will be eliminated while adding those new process steps. This process will reveal the extensive changes to the medication-use process that CPOE introduces and provide a clear indication of the processes that must be closely monitored in the new environment. The pharmacy must also model a sampling of all medication order types in the CPOE system, making certain that each order type can be ordered effectively and passed to the pharmacy system.

One should also review the literature and other facilities' experiences to understand successes and difficulties with deploying CPOE. An effective discussion of Reasons for Contemporary System Failures is presented in Figure 26-3.[33] Although few implementation failures are documented in the literature, many are discussed and well-known in professional circles. Most recently, Cedars Sinai's difficulty in sustaining the implementation of a CPOE system was widely communicated with commentary in a number of circles.[34,35]

The alarm sounded in this highly visible project was the time and resources invested and the lack of success on the initial try. The lay press has also shown interest in describing the opportunities and challenges in the area.[36–38] To be used effectively, the technology must meet the needs of the users rather than accommodating technical needs of the system.

Likewise, successes must be evaluated and elements of this success incorporated into the implementation plan.[39] Pharmacists will find colleagues eager to share their experience with these systems and the success and failure of their introduction. The science and the art required for implementing CPOE make sharing among colleagues essential to maximize use of limited resources and to learn from past successes and failures.[35]

Prior to Implementing CPOE

Review of the literature and the authors' personal experience reveal the critical importance of executive vision and support in the ultimate success of a CPOE

372   HANDBOOK OF INSTITUTIONAL PHARMACY PRACTICE

Figure 26-3
Lessons Learned—Why Do Systems Fail?

Communications	Ineffective outgoing communication Ineffective listening Failure to effectively prepare the staff for the new system
Culture	Hostile culture within the information systems organization Hostile culture toward the information systems area No strategies to nurture or grow a new culture
Underestimation of Complexity	Missed deadlines and cost overruns Lost credibility
Scope Creep	Failure to define and maintain original success criteria Failure to renegotiate deadlines and resources if criteria do change
Organizational	No clear vision for the change—unintended consequences Ineffective reporting structure—staff turnover and/or competency Provision of a technical "fix" to a management problem Lack of full support Roles & responsibilities not clearly defined—several people vying to be "in charge" Adequate resources not available from the beginning Failure to benchmark existing practices—inability to measure success
Technology	System not dependable—system too technology oriented Lure of the leading (bleeding) edge—Inadequate testing
Training	Inadequate or poor quality training Poor timing of training—too early or too late
Leadership Issues	Leader too emotionally committed—leader's time over committed Too much delegation without control—failure to get ownership in the effort Leader's political skills weak—"lying" to get initial approval

Source: Reprinted with permission from Reference 33.

project. The magnitude and complexity of the project will demand strong executive and project leadership. In a publication prepared by the California HealthCare Foundation and First Consulting Group, project leaders were asked to consider critical elements for success.[40] Some of these elements include executive vision and involvement; strong medical executive committee and physicians leading the effort and; spirit of collaboration among medical staff, administration, pharmacy, nursing and information management. The importance of strong physician leadership cannot be overemphasized. Physician champions must be involved in the development and planning for each phase of implementation, each providing expertise from their specialty area. Without this involvement, successful deployment will be at considerable risk.

Planning for CPOE and Pharmacy Role

As previously mentioned, the scope of this project demands careful, meticulous planning and, critical decisions about timing and strategy. The pharmacist is well-prepared to play a critical role in this project given the longstanding background in clinical skills relating to medication therapy, managing pharmacy information systems, managing automated dispensing systems, managing drug databases, knowledge from reviewing all mediation orders, maintaining medication administration records, and the integration of these systems that is required.[24] The pharmacist also possesses corporate knowledge relating to mediation safety and the interplay between systems and potential medication errors. No one else possesses this skill set in the organization.

The initial effort of the pharmacy administration must be to (1) educate oneself and leaders of the pharmacy on CPOE and impact on the pharmacy, (2) fully understand the scope of the project, (3) make certain the pharmacy is adequately represented at all levels of the project and on all relevant working groups, (4) obtain funding approval for appropriate resources to successfully implement the project, and (5) establish a multidisciplinary team to address pharmacy centric issues and impacts.

CPOE Education

Educating one's self and the pharmacy team must be led by a pharmacy informatics specialist who is experienced in the terminology and management of existing pharmacy systems and integration of these systems into the larger HIS landscape. A number of good references are now available to provide education and general introduction. These include *FCG Computerized Physician Order Entry in Community Hospitals: Lessons from the Field* and *A Primer on Physician Order Entry*.[40,41] Additional references are found at the end of this chapter. *Hospital Pharmacy* (www.hospitalpharmacyjournal.com) contains a series of articles on CPOE planning and implementation by Alicia White et al. and a series of articles on implementation of CPOE in a *Children's Hospital* by Alison Grisso et al. These articles are very helpful and should be reviewed by pharmacists prior to beginning CPOE. Professional networking and meetings are good sources of information from the field that will yield a slightly different perspective. We found visiting sites who had previously implemented CPOE successfully to be invaluable; these visits helped to mold our concept for CPOE at our facility. More recently, various list serves and online information can also be helpful.

Scope of Project

The scope of the CPOE project can be overwhelming; therefore, it must be clearly defined at the outset. The pharmacy must understand how the scope of the project will impact the process and service provided by the department. It has been our experience as well as the experience of other pharmacists that the planning for these systems may underestimate the impact on the pharmacy.[35] This may result from lack of understanding, direction of focus in other areas or our past success in managing projects, and our business in the organization. Scope creep, has been defined as a challenge with projects the magnitude of CPOE, can derail momentum and enthusiasm. It is well-documented in the literature that many times objectives are unrealistic and are not achievable in the timeframe allotted, with the system chosen and/or with the staff resources available.[33] Realistic goals aligned with system capability and resources available are essential to the ultimate success of CPOE. The pharmacist must advocate for the proper scope and goals relating to the medication component of the system. This brings us to the importance of being a player in these decisions.

Pharmacy Representation

The responsibility for selection of a CPOE system will rest with a multidisciplinary team outside the pharmacy, although the pharmacy must be involved early on in the selection process.[29] The pharmacy must be represented in groups dealing with the following:

- Planning and implementation
- Training and support during go live
- Process and safety evaluation
- Clinical decision support
- Integration and interfaces
- Assessing effectiveness

Representation at the many work groups requires a sizeable investment but is rewarded in the end.

Pharmacy Resources

One of the common questions from pharmacy directors relates to the pharmacy personnel resources that will be required for planning, developing and maintaining CPOE. Unfortunately, one must begin the response with, "it depends." This question cannot be answered categorically due to many variables that each institution will present; however, two concepts regarding allocating pharmacy resources are worthy of mention before listing specifics. First, the complex system development and file-building tasks requiring pharmacy personnel will be virtually the same whether for a 50- or a 500-bed hospital. Second, if resources are properly deployed and focused in the development and integration and clinical decision support, there is probably no more effective use of the pharmacist. The return on this investment can benefit patient care 24 hours a day, 365 days a year, and in all areas of the institution. This expanded *coverage* of the pharmacist, heretofore not provided, can be achieved only with the use of automated systems and clinical decision support. As mentioned elsewhere in this chapter, this basic coverage liberates the pharmacist from the more routine interventions and permits the pharmacist to practice at a higher level to impact patient care.

While intense resource support will be required during planning, development, and implementation, it is obvious that the increasing reliance on informatics and automation necessitate commitment of permanent resources to this endeavor. Mistakenly, the authors believed 10 years ago that much of the committed resource would be temporary in nature. A recent survey of eight hospitals with CPOE reveal 0.5 to 4 FTE pharmacists were required in the building process for CPOE.[42] Similar numbers are required in an ongoing basis to support CPOE. Even in light of this, some have even voiced concern that CPOE will reduce the number of pharmacists required. This is certainly not the case at our site or others described in the literature.[43]

Once implemented, CPOE, as any other major system, demands constant development. But much more, the innovative professionals utilizing CPOE will discover important new applications and demand that functionality be added in the name of patient care and safety. This innovation from the users is essential and builds support for the longer term success of CPOE at any institution. Nowhere is the importance of continuous improvement more evident than with CPOE.

One must assess each of the areas to determine the estimated resources. Having multiple persons involved in each step is important, although many times considered a luxury, to enhance decision making and to avoid single points (or persons) of failure. Limited numbers of individuals are involved and could in turn pose significant risk to the system and care of patients. Once again, the resources are driven based on goals and expectations of the system.

Planning and Learning

Identifying appropriate time for planning and understanding the products and goals of the project should not be overlooked. The project team should be involved in this process and should use all resources at their disposal. Of special note is the learning from other sites and colleagues. Both successes and failures should be evaluated.

Building the System/Maintaining the Databases

The building of the CPOE drug database and related tables is a major project. In the worse case-scenario, the database would be duplicative of the pharmacy database and require cooperative efforts to link these files to the pharmacy database if the systems are to be interfaced. This is labor intensive and, more importantly, conducive to errors. Ideally, both the CPOE and

pharmacy systems will utilize the same core drug content database. In this model, maintenance is required in only one file to drive both the CPOE and pharmacy systems. This permits the use of the drug database already developed for the pharmacy system.

Training and Implementation Support

Training is required for all pharmacy staff relating to operational, clinical, and technical changes introduced. As noted above, significant training must occur relating to process and procedure change. Comprehensive training is required due to the complexity of the medication pathway and the reliance that others will have on the pharmacy's expertise. Implementation support must be considered for internal pharmacy operations and external support of medication order entry. A team approach for implementation is required to support physicians and nurses during the initial phases of implementation. A pharmacist was found to be an invaluable member of this team at our institution. Support with medication order entry on the patient care unit greatly facilitates learning and acceptance of the system.

Clinical Decision Support Systems (CDSS)

The installation and development of CDSS is ultimately critical to the success of CPOE and can demand significant pharmacy resources. See section below.

Pharmacy Project Team

The team must provide oversight for the medication component both internally and externally. The team should be composed of the individuals who can provide expertise in the following areas operational, technical, clinical, regulatory, and financial. The team should report to the director of pharmacy, the larger CPOE structure, and the P&T Committee.

Integration of the Pharmacy Module

A seamless (at least from the perspective of the end user) integration of the pharmacy application or medication order process with the CPOE system must be the ultimate goal of a mature ordering system. While this integration is critical, maintaining the functionality of a prescribing system (CPOE) and a dispensing system (pharmacy system) is also essential. Having stated integration as the ultimate goal, one must fully understand the options of integration and possible stages of integration as the scope and goals of the project are planned. This includes a clear enunciation of the advantages and disadvantages of various levels of integration.

Proper integration of the medication ordering process is a required component to create the necessary functionality for a safe and efficient system. An effective CPOE system and an effective pharmacy system are only the beginning pieces of the puzzle, but the true value is created with the effective integration of these two systems. Failure to achieve full integration will invariably limit the overall effectiveness of the system. It must be noted this integration is currently posing challenges for many pharmacy departments. Figure 26-4 depicts varying levels of integration of a dispensing and prescribing system.

Pharmacy integration options can be broadly classified as follows: (1) no integration of the CPOE and pharmacy systems, (2) an integrated all in one system, (3) a unidirectional interface with most frequently the CPOE system passing an electronic order to the pharmacy system, and (4) a bidirectional interface, which adds the ability to pass an order electronically from the pharmacy system to the CPOE system or, at a minimum, confirms that the order has been processed in the pharmacy system.[44] It must be noted that each of these levels of integration provide advantage over manual systems, have varying levels of risks to successfully complete, and have the capacity to deliver a wide range of benefit.

When the CPOE and pharmacy system are not integrated most commonly a printed order will be immediately transmitted to the pharmacy. This certain-ly provides advantage over manual written systems in that the receipt of the order is immediate and the order is legible. In past years this would be thought of as a breakthrough given the long history of problems and delays with medication order receipt. Currently, this option can be viewed only as a transitional way station (and should be brief) in the journey to integration.

An integrated all-in-one system provided by a single vendor would seem to be the logical solution to this complex integration; however, given the early development phase of these systems this does not seem to borne out in the market place.[45] This arrangement has the potential to limit the complex linking of databases and construction of interfaces; however, all too often this comes at the expense of a compromise in functionality of one or both systems. While it appears this would be the ultimate goal of vendor solutions, at this point in time one must carefully evaluate the functionality of the all-in-one system, especially if this requires a change in pharmacy information systems. An in-depth gap analysis closely comparing functional requirements is essential.

A unidirectional interface typically infers the electronic transmission of medication orders from a CPOE to pharmacy system. The CPOE and pharmacy system may be provided by the same vendor or may be considered "best of breed" and provided by multiple vendors. The flexibility to retain or purchase a dedicated pharmacy information system appears to offer the highest level of functionality. The electronic transmission offers many advantages including immediate access of the order, prior selection of the patient, and the selection of a predefined default drug product in the pharmacy system. It is highly advisable in this environment for each system to utilize the same drug database and the same drug knowledge content database. This limits the maintenance required and facilitates consistency between the two systems. This environment also requires the maintenance of two separate patient medication profiles, one each in the CPOE and pharmacy systems. This can be time-consuming and provides the potential for error; therefore, it requires an electronic comparison of the two databases with production of an exception report. A key factor in this and the bidirectional interface (described below) is an intelligent interface between the two systems to aid in mapping/converting orders. If well done, this provides assurance of synchrony of the patient medication profiles. The authors have 10 years experience with this method of integration. The experience validates the effectiveness

Figure 26-4
Levels of Integration (CPOE—Pharmacy Order Communication)

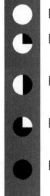

No integration—receive printouts

Dispensing order communicated to pharmacy electronically

Prescribing order communicated to pharmacy electronically with manual conversion

Prescribing order translated to dispensing order via intelligent interface

Prescribing order translated to dispensing order via intelligent interface with order confirm sent back to CPOE system of this model as long as the intelligent interface exists.

A bidirectional interface includes all functionality of the unidirectional model and adds a return loop, commonly referred to as *closed loop*, from the pharmacy system to the CPOE system. This has two major advantages: (1) providing reverse link to ensure that the patient medication profile is the same in both systems, and (2) theoretically provides an excellent backup system for order entry in the event the CPOE (or interface) is down because reentry of these orders would not be necessary. It should be noted that the reverse interface will require additional development and maintenance in similar ways as the inbound interface between the CPOE and pharmacy system. While maintenance of these intelligent intermediaries can be extensive, the dividend makes this a worthwhile investment. Figure 26-5 illustrates a basic schematic of a bidirectional interface. For more extensive information on technical aspects of pharmacy integration, the reader is referred to the article by Chaffee and Bonasso.[46]

Implementation Strategies and Pharmacy Support

A number of options are available for implementing CPOE, which the pharmacy must be prepared to support. Most sites find it essential to implement a pilot unit to evaluate the readiness of the system and the needed refinements prior to moving throughout the facility.[47] Ideally, the pilot unit will be self-contained such that patients do not frequently transfer into and out of the unit. As mentioned above, a physician champion practicing in the pilot areas is critical.

The pace of the implementation is often debated and must be individualized for the institution. The extensive changes introduced by CPOE seem to beg for a multiple-phase implementation where one is dealing with specific services or physicians with each phase. A *big bang* approach is not advisable due to the extraordinary complexity and the learning curve that is required at all levels and departments in the organization. While a phased-in implementation offers advantages, the pharmacy is required to support dual systems, likely, for an extended period of time. For example,

Figure 26-5
Medication Order Flow (Basic)

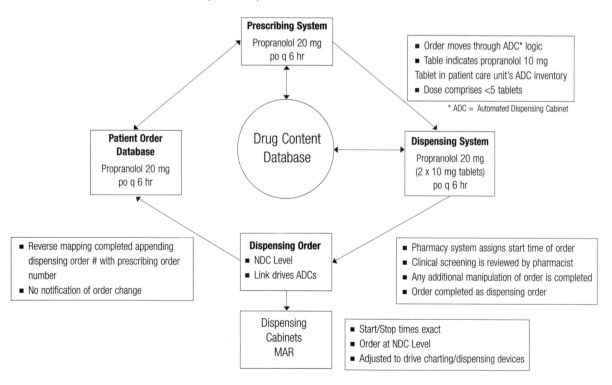

receipt of orders would occur electronically on the implemented patient care units and via the fax or pneumatic tube on non-CPOE units, therefore, requiring the management of order flow from two disparate processes. All areas of dual processes must be carefully evaluated and planned to minimize opportunity for mistakes and inefficiencies.

The pharmacy must also be prepared to support CPOE implementation with support staff both externally and internally. The clinical or decentralized pharmacist is invaluable in supporting the provider's entry of medication orders. They must be well-versed on the CPOE system as should all pharmacists who might be consulted relating to order entry. Likewise, support internally for order-entry and process questions will be required throughout the learning process. Maximum efficiency will not be gained for 3–6 months after implementation and is dependent on the ability of the site to address identified problems or needed changes in the functionality.

One of the most important decisions during the deployment of CPOE is the level of support for the entry of medication orders when not entered by the physician. If order entry is not required by the physician or the system is unavailable, procedures must be in place for entry of these orders. From the authors'

experience, the pharmacy must provide this support. This can be labor intensive in the event of poor participation by physicians or frequent downtimes and can place a burden on the pharmacy staff.

Clinical Decision Support

A clinical decision support system (CDSS) is a set of tools that facilitates the decision-making capabilities of the prescriber at the decision point. Clinical decision support (CDS) brings together the information shown in Figure 26-6 to promote the correct clinical decision for the individual patient in a timely manner. CDS ranges from simple (a field edit) to complex (algorithms) to recommend or change therapy. While early CPOE systems focused on process, much of the recent work has been in the area of CDS. This is a rapidly developing area with tremendous potential for improving the quality of care delivered.

Pharmacy systems have long employed clinical decision support as a core module. Functionality has traditionally included allergy checking, duplicate-therapy checking, drug-interaction checking, and dose-range checking. This has proven an important safety tool for the pharmacists in managing ever more complex drug therapy; however, most would admit that

Figure 26-6
Decision Support Integrated Into Workflow

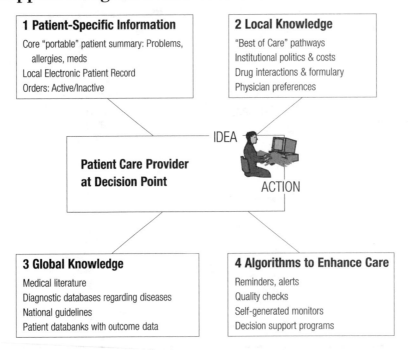

these tools must be improved to be effectively utilized in a CPOE system. No longer can we accept CDS that overloads the practitioner with alerts that are of little clinical significance or important alerts that are not properly evaluated in the care of the patient.

A missing ingredient with decision support in pharmacy systems has been extensive patient demographic information, disease information, and laboratory values. Certainly EMRs and CPOE make this information available and effective if properly integrated with the CPOE system.

All CPOE systems will provide a basic level of CDS, although this functionality varies greatly with the product. Increasingly, CDS is recognized as the cornerstone of improving quality and safety with CPOE systems. Typically, this module must be carefully evaluated before implementation since these systems should not be considered mature and tested. They require manipulation and integration at the individual institution for true effectiveness. CDS can be provided in a passive means or in a more active method. Passive interventions generally present relevant patient-specific information to the prescriber without recommending a change in therapy. Examples would include nonformulary alerts, drug shortages, and order sets. Active alerts utilize specific patient information combined with other content knowledge to recommend or change therapy. Examples include recommendation of dosing, allergy warnings, and safer therapy, or less expensive treatment options.

A critical decision in deploying CDS is the speed with which this tool is implemented. An incremental approach is highly recommended to build confidence in the system and to avoid alert fatigue which can occur unless interventions are strategically utilized.

CPOE vendors provide drug-content modules (i.e., First Data Bank, Multum, Micromedex) with their products which serve as the core of medication CDS. These systems do not effectively function as a turnkey system and must be modified to function properly with the CPOE system and provide the level of decision support deemed appropriate.[29] This is a critical function of the pharmacist.

Assessing the Impact

Measures of success should also be clearly defined for the CPOE system with methods to track and evaluate these measures of success. The extraordinary commitment required for deployment of a CPOE system sometimes leaves little time available for assessing its effectiveness. Still, one must devote time to strategically evaluate the use of the system to make certain that desired goals are attained.

In addition, particular focus should be given to the process change introduced by CPOE. Multiple sources cite the importance of aggressively integrating the systems into the process. CPOE must not overlay the process but be an integral part, supporting the intended result and the professionals.

Potential areas of evaluations are the following:

- Medication safety and adverse drug events
- Response time for medication processing
- Pharmacy resource needs
- Drug cost reductions and achieving financial targets
- Downtime and availability of system
- Response time of system
- Clinical alerts and action taken by provider

As with any new complex system, it is imperative to monitor the performance, make needed adjustments, and provide feedback to the user. This encourages support of the system and continuous improvement of the system. A change of this magnitude will introduce new opportunities for errors. Systems must be in place to quickly identify these issues so they can be managed aggressively.

Summary

Figure 26-7 demonstrates a schematic on the positioning of CPOE in pharmacy practice. CPOE and other systems are critical tools for the effective delivery of pharmaceutical care as health care grows more complex. CPOE implementation is a long and difficult process with the medication component being one of the more difficult modules. The pharmacy must be prepared to take a leadership role and provide its expertise in systems and medication therapy to ensure the success of the medication component of CPOE. It is essential that pharmacists share their experience with colleagues and advocate for standardization to enhance the successful diffusion of this powerful tool. CPOE provides new opportunities for pharmacists in the area of system integration and clinical decision support systems and demands that more formalized training for pharmacists be available. A good CPOE system properly deployed provides strategic advantages to the institution and, most importantly, improved care to patients.

Figure 26-7
Pharmaceutical Care Pyramid

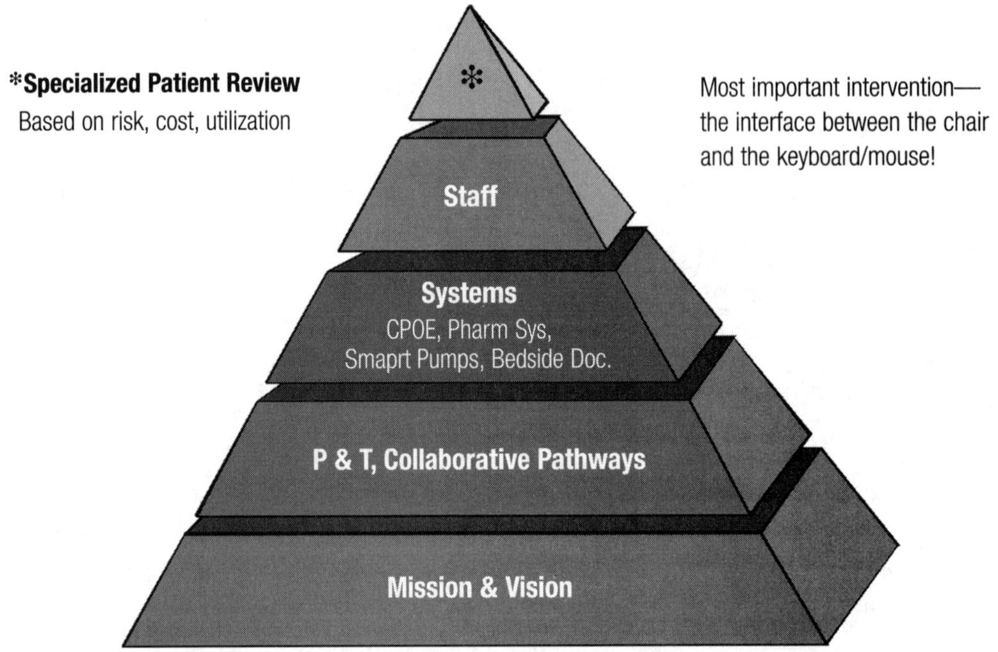

*Specialized Patient Review
Based on risk, cost, utilization
*
Most important intervention—
the interface between the chair
and the keyboard/mouse!
Staff
Systems
CPOE, Pharm Sys,
Smaprt Pumps, Bedside Doc.
P & T, Collaborative Pathways
Mission & Vision

Source: References 3, 4–6, 24–47.

References

1. McDonald CJ, Tierney WM, Overhage JM, et al. The Regenstrief medical record system: 20 years of experience in hospitals, clinics, and neighborhood health centers. *MD Comput.* 1992;9(4):206–17.
2. Ash JS, Bates DW. Factors and forces impacting EHR systems adoption: report of a 2004 ACMI discussion. *JAIMIA.* October 18, 2004.
3. Ash JS, Gorman PN, Seshadri V, et al. Computerized physician order entry in U.S. hospitals: results of a 2002 survey. *J Am Med Inform Assoc.* 2004;11(2):95–9.
4. The Leapfrog Group. Available at: http://www.leapfrog group.org/media/file/CPOE_FactSheet011305.pdf. February 2005.
5. Bates DW, Leape LL, Cullen DJ, et al. Effect of computerized physician order entry and a team intervention on prevention of serious medication errors. *JAMA.* 1998;280(15):1311–6.
6. Kohn LT, Corrigan J, Donaldson MS. Institute of Medicine (U.S.). Committee on Quality of Health Care in America. *To Err is Human: Building a Safer Health System.* Washington, DC: National Academy Press; 2000.
7. Slack WV, Peckham BM, Van Cura LJ, et al. A computer-based physical examination system. *JAMA.*1967;200(3):224–8.
8. Slack WV, Hicks GP, Reed CE, et al. A computer-based medical-history system. *N Engl J Med.* 1966;274(4):194–8.
9. Hammond WE. How the past teaches the future: ACMI distinguished lecture. *J Am Med Inform Assoc.* 2001;8(3):222–34.
10. Stead WW, Miller RA, Musen MA, et al. Integration and beyond: linking information from disparate sources and into workflow (see comments). *J Am Med Inform Assoc.* 2000;7(2):135–45.
11. McDonald CJ. The barriers to electronic medical record systems and how to overcome them. *J Am Med Inform Assoc.* 1997;4(3):213–21.
12. Gardner RM, Pryor TA, Warner HR. The HELP hospital information system: update 1998. *Int J Med Inform.* 1999;54(3):169–82.
13. Barnett GO. COSTAR, a computer-based medical information system for ambulatory care. *Proc IEEE.* 1979;67:1226–37.
14. Brown SH, Lincoln MJ, Groen PJ, et al. VistA—U.S. Department of Veterans Affairs national-scale HIS. *Int J Med Inf.* 2003;69(2–3):135–56.
15. Handler T, et al. *Electronic Health Record Definition Model Version 1.0. Health Information and Management Systems Society.* Chicago IL: HIMSS; 2003.

16. Collen MF. *A History of Medical Informatics in the United States, 1950 to 1990.* Indianapolis, IN: American Medical Informatics Association; 1995.

17. McDonald CJ, Tierney WM. Computer-stored medical records. Their future role in medical practice. *JAMA.* 1988;259(23):3433–40.

18. Sado AS. Electronic medical record in the intensive care unit. *Crit Care Clin.* 1999;15(3):499–522.

19. Waegemann CP. The year of the EHR? *Health Manag Technol.* 2004;25(5):66, 65.

20. Stead WW, Heyman A, Thompson HK, et al. Computer-assisted interview of patients with functional headache. *Arch Intern Med.* 1972;129(6):950–5.

21. Lumpkin JR. Uniform data standards for patient medical record information. Washington DC: National Committee on Vital and Health Statistics; 2003.

22. Brailer DJ. Decade of Health Information Technology. Washington DC: U.S. Department of Health and Human Services; 7/21/2004 2004.

23. Carpenter JD, Gorman PN. What's so special about medications: a pharmacist's observations from the POE study. *Proc AMIA Symp.* 2001:95–9.

24. Gouveia WA, Shane R, Clark T. Computerized prescriber order entry: power, not panacea. *Am J Health-Syst Pharm.* 2003;60(18):1838.

25. IOM. *Crossing the Quality Chasm: A New Health System for the 21st Century.* Washington, DC: National Acacemy Press; 2001.

26. Bush GW. Executive Order Establishing Office of the National Coordinator for Health Information Technology (ONCHIT). Available at: http://www.white house.gov/news/releases/2004/04/20040427-4.html.

27. Brailer D. Dr. Brailer's Address to HIMSS Conference. 2005.

28. Young D. CPOE takes time, patience, money, and team-work. *Am J Health-Syst Pharm.* 2003;60(7):635, 639–40, 642.

29. Schiff GD. Computerized prescriber order entry: models and hurdles. *Am J Health-Syst Pharm.* 2002;59(15):1456–60.

30. Abernathy W, Utterback J. Patterns of industrial innovation. *Technology Review.* 1978;80(7):40–7.

31. Poon EG, Blumenthal D, Jaggi T, et al. Overcoming barriers to adopting and implementing computerized physician order entry systems in U.S. hospitals. *Health Aff (Millwood).* 2004;23(4):184–90.

32. Doolan DF, Bates DW. Computerized physician order entry systems in hospitals: mandates and incentives. *Health Aff (Millwood).* 2002;21(4):180–8.

33. Lorenzi NM, Riley RT. Managing change: an overview. *J Am Med Inform Assoc.* 2000;7(2):116–24.

34. Morrissey J. An info-tech disconnect. Even as groups such as Leapfrog push IT as an answer to quality issues, doctors and executives say, 'not so fast'. *Mod Healthc.* 2003;33(6):6–7, 36–38, 40.

35. Shane R. CPOE: the science and the art. *Am J Health-Syst Pharm.* 2003;60(12):1273–6.

36. Connolly C. Cedars-Sinai doctors cling to pen and paper. *Washington Post.* March 21, 2005:A01.

37. Freudenheim M. Many hospitals resist computerized patient care. *New York Times.* April 6, 2004:C1, C6.

38. Perez-Pena R. Bronx hospital embraces online technology that others avoid. *New York Times.* April 6, 2004:C6.

39. Ash JS, Stavri PZ, Kuperman GJ. A consensus statement on considerations for a successful CPOE implementation. *J Am Med Inform Assoc.* 2003;10(3):229–34.

40. Metzger J FJ. Computerized physician order entry in community hospitals: lessons from the field. Available at: http://www.chcf.org/documents/hospitals/CPOE CommHospCorrected.pdf. Accessed February 16, 2005.

41. Metzger J. A primer on physician order entry. Available at: http://www.chcf.org/documents/hospitals/ CPOEreport.pdf. February 2005.

42. ASHP. CPOE Listserve Resources Survey; 2004.

43. Seger AC, Hanson CM, Fanikos JR. Benefits of CPOE. *Am J Health-Syst Pharm.* 2004;61(6):626–7.

44. Chaffee BW, Bonasso J. Strategies for pharmacy integration and pharmacy information system interfaces, part 1: history and pharmacy integration options. *Am J Health-Syst Pharm.* 2004;61(5):502–6.

45. Gray MD, Felkey BG. Computerized prescriber order-entry systems: evaluation, selection, and implementation. *Am J Health-Syst Pharm.* 2004;61(2):190–7.

46. Chaffee BW, Bonasso J. Strategies for pharmacy integration and pharmacy information system interfaces, part 2: scope of work and technical aspects of interfaces. *Am J Health-Syst Pharm.* 2004;61(5):506–14.

47. Computerized physician order entry: costs, benefits and challenges. Available at: http://www.fcg.com/research/ serve-research.asp?rid=36. Accessed February 16, 2005.

Chapter 27

Medication Distribution Systems

Stephen F. Eckel, Fred M. Eckel

Introduction

Providing the patient with an appropriate medication in an acceptable dosage form to facilitate easy administration has always been the role of the pharmacist. At different times in pharmacy's evolving responsibilities, some of these activities seemed to receive more attention. The hospital pharmacist working with other professionals accepted responsibility to purchase or prepare drug products approved for use in the hospital by the Pharmacy and Therapeutics Committee. These products were then distributed by the pharmacist so they were available to the nurse to administer to the patient as prescribed by the physician. Finally, the drug's therapeutic effects were monitored to assure the desired effects were achieved and undesirable effects were minimized. The evolving drug distribution system used by hospital pharmacists reflects the expanding pharmacist's role, the advancement in technology, and the increasing complexity of drug products.

What transformed the hospital pharmacist into an integral member of the health care team is the unit dose system.[1] The system required the pharmacist to receive individual patient medication orders. The pharmacist would prepare patient-specific doses in a ready-to-administer form by reviewing the medication order. This allowed the hospital pharmacist to accept responsibility for a patient's drug therapy. Over the past 40 years, there have been many improvements to the unit dose system, mostly through advancement in technology.

This chapter will provide a brief overview of the history of the medication distribution system leading to unit dose, a discussion of the unit dose system, an analysis of different technologies that assist drug distribution today, and thoughts on the future of medication distribution.

History of Medication Distribution Systems Leading to the Unit Dose Concept

The role of the hospital pharmacist 50 years ago was primarily confined to the basement.[2] This location reflects the role the pharmacist had in the medication use cycle. The space was small and the personnel were few. The pharmacist's primary role was to purchase or prepare the desired drugs. The pharmacist prepared medications to be used on the nursing unit. The physician would prescribe the medication and the nurse would administer it to the patient. The pharmacist rarely decided whether the therapy was appropriate for the patient or not, they would simply make sure that the nurse had a supply of medication for the patient. If this required repackaging or compounding of the medication, the pharmacist accepted responsibility for this function with the exception being IV admixtures, which were usually prepared by the nurse on the nursing unit.

There were at least two distinct distribution methods the pharmacist would utilize for the nurse to obtain the medications for patient use.[2] One was referred to as the floor stock system and the other was the patient prescription system.

Floor Stock System

The floor stock system was the more common method. In essence, it was a duplication of a small pharmacy on the nursing unit where drugs were stored prior to the nurse preparing drugs to administer to patients. The pharmacist was responsible for stocking the nursing unit. The pharmacist would place bulk containers of medications on the unit, often called the drug room. There were multiple doses in each bottle to supply all patients receiving that drug on the nursing unit. The nurse was the professional responsible for preparing the patient-specific medications for both oral and intravenous use. The nurse would read the physician order, go into the drug room to select the drug and prepare it, and then administer it to the patient. In this selection process, the nurse could choose from many different medications. If a medication needed to be refilled or a patient was started on a different drug, the nurse would request the new medication to be stocked on the nursing unit. The pharmacist would likely never see the physician order but would stock the medication on the floor solely from the nursing request. This system was utilized because it required few pharmacy personnel. It was assumed that this distribution system was safe. Patients were only charged for the drugs administered to them or were billed a daily fee, also termed per diem, for the drugs.

Patient Prescription System

The patient prescription system involved the pharmacist to a greater extent by requiring a review of the patient order. After the physician wrote the order, the nurse would transcribe the medication order and send it to pharmacy for preparation. The pharmacist would prepare a 2- to 5-day supply of medication for the patient and charge the patient for the medications dispensed. The nurse would store the medication on the nursing unit. This system still required the nurse to prepare the individual dose for the patient. When the drug needed to be refilled, the nurse would contact the pharmacist who would prepare it and send it to the floor for continued use. When the drug was discontinued or the patient was discharged, the prescription bottles were returned to the pharmacy and the unused drugs were credited to the patient's account. Even though the pharmacist had the opportunity to review the patient order, the pharmacist would place only limited judgment on whether it was correct or appropriate for the patient. This was because the pharmacist did not have access to pertinent patient information and because it was not expected of them.

Unit Dose System

Several researchers studied the medication use process and found that the floor stock system and individual prescription system were error-prone.[3–5] Because it was believed that the hospital pharmacist could play a larger role in the medication use cycle, a few hospitals began experimenting with the unit dose system because it seemed a safer system.[4,6] This placed the pharmacist in a position to begin affecting a patient's medication therapy.

The unit dose system is defined as a pharmacy-coordinated method of dispensing and controlling medications in health care institutions.[7] This system is characterized by medications contained in unit dose packages, dispensed in ready-to-administer form, and not more than 24-hour supply being delivered or available on the patient care unit at any time. This is very different than the previous methods discussed. The pharmacist dispenses patient-specific medications to be administered, not prepared, by the nurse.

The U.S. General Accounting Office concluded in 1971 that the unit dose system was the most cost-effective of any distribution system—more cost-effective in fact than any other pharmacy system when the entire medication use cycle is considered.[2] Other articles have evaluated the reduction of medication errors when transitioning from the floor stock system to the unit dose system.[3–5] Table 27-1 lists a comparison of some of these studies and their specific outcomes.

Advantages

When utilizing the unit dose method, it has been noted that the advantages are the following[7]:

- Reduction in medication errors
- Decrease in total cost of medication-related activities
- More efficient use of pharmacy and nursing personnel
- Improved drug control and drug use monitoring
- More accurate patient billing for medications
- Minimization of credits for drugs
- Greater control by pharmacist over work patterns and scheduling
- Reduction of inventories maintained on nursing units

A survey was conducted to determine the extent of unit dose services in 1975.[8] This study demonstrated that only 17.5% of the hospitals in the sample had a unit dose system for 90% or more beds and 10.2% had a unit dose system for less than 90% of beds. At this point in time, only about one in four hospitals had transitioned to a unit dose system. This survey was repeated every few years. It tracked the growth of the unit dose system, with 38.2% of hospitals completely adopting it by 1978, 61.1% using it in 1982, 62.4% in 1985, and 73.8% by 1987.[9] In 1987, only 2.9% of hospitals reported no use of a unit dose system at all. In the 12-year span of these surveys, there was virtually a complete adoption by hospitals of the unit dose system. This demonstrates the impact that the original studies of unit dose had on the practice of pharmacy and how quick places were to adopt the system.

Increased Pharmacist Involvement

Not only is unit dose less expensive and safer for the patient when considering its entire impact on medication distribution and patient safety, but it placed the

Table 27-1
Incidence of Medication Errors[3]

| | Type of Distribution System | | | |
| | Traditional | | Unit-Dose | |
	Number of Doses Observed[a]	Error Rate[b]	Number of Doses Observed[a]	Error Rate[b]
University of Florida (Gainesville)	607	13.9%	-	-
General hospital in Arkansas	9,704	6.7%	-	-
University of Arkansas (Fayetteville)	11,015	13.3%	3,043	1.9%
University of Iowa (Iowa City)	32,985	7.74%	42,578	5.88%
University of Kentucky (Lexington)	-	-	6,061	3.52%
Ohio State University Hospitals (Columbus)	3,678	5.33%	3,447	0.64%

[a] Number of doses = number of doses administered plus number omitted.
[b] Time not considered as source of errors.

pharmacist in a better position to be involved in patient care. Now the pharmacist was reviewing medication orders and could intervene prior to the first dose being available to the nurse. Even though this was a new role for the pharmacist, it was a much better use of their knowledge and training.

This increased role of the pharmacist to be able to evaluate the patient order helped propel clinical pharmacy services, whereby the pharmacist began impacting patient drug therapy. Instead of being focused solely on making sure the drug was correct on the nursing unit (for nurse selection and administration), the pharmacist began evaluating whether this drug was appropriate for the patient. The unit dose system requires the pharmacy to have and maintain a patient medication profile.[10] This activity was new to hospital pharmacy, but it allowed the pharmacist to gain access to patient-specific information. The legible medication order that pharmacy received should contain the following[10]:

- Patient's name and location
- Generic name of medication
- Dosage in metric system, where feasible
- Frequency of administration
- Route of administration
- Signature of the physician
- Date and hour the order was written

These orders could be received by the pharmacy in various ways. Some hospitals have couriers that routinely go to the nursing unit to collect orders and deliver medications. Others in the centralized model of distribution rely on pneumatic tube systems for order delivery or facsimile devices for order transmission. Institutions that utilize decentralized models have pharmacy satellites close to the nursing unit or have pharmacy personnel (technicians and pharmacists) that work directly on the nursing unit for immediate access to orders and patients. In the near future, these orders will all be electronic. As hospitals begin to implement computerized physician order entry, orders will immediately print at the location of choice. Once computer systems evolve further and are able to communicate with one another, there will be no need for paper transmission. Every action will be electronic, with the transfer of patient-specific information.

Also by receiving the medication order, it requires the pharmacist to directly follow-up with the physician for clarification. If an order was written incorrectly or was inappropriate for the patient, the pharmacist needed to notify the physician regarding the inaccuracy. This created an opportunity for the pharmacist to recommend an alternative for the patient. The implementation of clinical pharmacy began as the pharmacist took responsibility for the patient's medication regimen.

After the order is reviewed and deemed appropriate for the patient, the medication is entered into the pharmacy computer system. A label is usually generated for enough doses until the next cart fill. Most institutions utilize a 24-hour cart-fill, whereby they process a medication batch for a specified time period each day. Doses for a patient are filled for the time period and delivered to the floor for administration. New medications that are begun on a patient between cart exchanges to last until the next scheduled cart exchange, and then the next cart will contain the subsequent doses. However, cart exchange times are hospital-specific and the type of drug ordered determines the method of distribution and dispensing. A pharmacy technician fills the medication from the label, but they are not delivered to the medication cart on the floor until the pharmacist has checked it for accuracy and appropriateness. Table 27-2 lists a sample of delivery methods and doses needed for a typical tertiary care hospital.

A copy of the physician order is transcribed at the nursing unit to a medication administration record (MAR) or is computer generated from the pharmacy profile. The MAR is a record of all the medications that are prescribed for the patient, including administration times. Prior to giving the new medication to the patient, the nurse will double-check the MAR against the patient order to ensure that it is appropriate. After patient administration, the nurse will initial the MAR to denote that the drug was given and at what time. In order to ensure consistency between the pharmacy record and the MAR, most pharmacy departments generate the MAR and deliver them to the nursing unit every 24 hours or at cart exchange.

Besides actively placing the pharmacist in the middle of the medication use process, the unit dose system also changed the process and form of medication distribution. Each medication is placed in a *unit of use* package.[2] This is designated as the correct dose for the patient in a ready-to-administer form, not requiring any preparation or selection by the nurse. The medication will have a label that bears the patient name, the name of the medication, the corresponding strength, and expiration date. The thought process that did occur at the nursing level prior to administering the dose was shouldered by the pharmacy in preparing doses in this manner. Also, only enough medication that covered a certain period of time was sent to the patient (usually 24 hours). Presently, manufacturers will produce medications already in unit dose packaging. This was not true at the time of the development of this concept. Pharmacy technicians, in a highly supervised role by the pharmacist, prepared these for distribution.

On the nursing unit, these medications were stored in locked medication carts. It was inappropriate for them to be stored on the unit without any control. Each patient bed had a separate compartment where the medications were stored. The pharmacy would place them in the correct bin in the cart. These medications were secured and could only be accessed by a nurse or other appropriate representative. The cart had wheels, but was usually kept stationary. It also had a flat surface for the nurse to use for preparation prior

Table 27-2[2]
Medication Delivery from Pharmacy to Patient Care Unit (PCU)

Medication Category	Delivery Method
1. Stable scheduled medications	24-hr supply in patient-specific bin on medication cart
2. Unstable scheduled medications	Automatic delivery to PCU 1 hr before administration time
3. Scheduled IV/TPN solutions	Automatic delivery to PCU 1 hr before administration time
4. PRN medications	Limited supply in patient-specific bin on medication cart; limited floorstock supply; delivered by pharmacy in response to request by PCU
5. Controlled medications	Limited patient-specific supply secured on medication cart; limited floorstock supply
6. STAT medications	Delivered by pharmacy in response to request from PCU
7. Emergency medications	Emergency drug kits located on PCU; delivered by pharmacy in response to request from PCU
8. Investigational medications	Per dispensing protocol

to administering the dose and for documentation needs. The medication cart could also store supplies required when preparing doses.

Each day, this cart was exchanged with a new one that contained medications for the day. Yesterday's cart was returned to pharmacy and the medications that were not given were evaluated as to why they were not given and were credited to the patient. Following this, the cart replenishment process started again, where medications were placed in the cart for the next day. The carts were filled by the pharmacy technician but were checked by a pharmacist before being exchanged. If done properly, this cart replenishment would be done accurately and efficiently in a short period of time.[11] In some states, technicians filled the unit dose cart and another technician could check the filled cart.

If the pharmacy received a new medication order for a patient or a dose request from the nurse, the pharmacist provided the medication to the floor before the next cart exchange. This could be delivered to the floor either through a courier or pneumatic tube system.

This process was different for narcotics and PRN (as needed) medications. Schedule II narcotics, because of Drug Enforcement Agency requirements, cannot be stored in the individual patient bins in a medication cart. This does not provide the necessary security for control. These were usually stored in a locked cabinet with limited access. Pharmacy would place bulk medications into this locked area and the nurse could obtain needed doses. Prior to giving the dose, the nurse had to take an accurate inventory of the medication and document doses removed. Pharmacy would reconcile the number of orders against the number of medications given, to minimize the chance of diversion. Even though this system was effective in reducing diversion, it was time intensive to keep up with the paperwork and provide the necessary oversight.[12,13] This also mandates a requirement that nurses assume proper accountability from shift to shift for controlled substances in Schedule II.

As needed (PRN) medications were handled differently. One method was to keep them in the pharmacy and dispense them upon request. This system had the most control over medication distribution. However, it was time intensive for the nurse and pharmacist and led to delays in administration. Another method was to send up a small amount of medication for each patient in their medication drawer. If the patient requested a dose, the nurse would retrieve the medication from the medication cart. The downside to this process is that many doses went up per day and then were returned because they were not used. This produced inefficiency.[14,15] Most hospitals began using a limited floorstock system. Medications that had a low potential for misuse and patient harm (laxatives, antacids) were stored in small quantities in the medication cart. If the patient requested the dose, the nurse would remove the medication from the drawer and administer it to the patient. These medications would remain in the cart upon cart exchange and be readily available for the patient if needed. These medications would be in unit dose form and pharmacy would regulate the appropriate use. This system minimized the work needed for patient use in using commonly prescribed medications.

A final area that required pharmacy oversight was the distribution of emergency medications for emergencies. Medications need to be available instantly, in order to assist with reviving the patient. Any delay could be harmful. A selective number of medications were provided in a tray or kit in ready to administer form. These were available on all nursing units for immediate access. Presently, pharmacists are more involved in patient emergencies beyond just making sure medications are available. They are assisting in the drug selection, preparation, and administration.[16,17]

Methods of Unit Dose

There are two main ways that a pharmacy can be structured in order to provide unit dose services: centralized and decentralized model. A *centralized* model emanates from the main pharmacy (a centralized location). The medication order is received in the central pharmacy, and all of the processing for patients occurs there: order processing, drug packaging, cart fill, and medication dispensing. The advantages of this model are that all resources can be localized into one area and drug inventory can be minimized. The biggest disadvantage is that the pharmacist is not able to directly interact with the physician and nurse. Clinical services are limited since the pharmacy is not closely located to patient care areas.

The *decentralized* model is characterized by pharmacy satellites distributed evenly throughout the institution.[18] A physician order is routed to this satellite. The pharmacist there processes the order and dispenses the first dose of the medication directly to the nursing station. Since they are closely located to patient care areas, it is very easy for a health care professional to stop by to ask a question. The pharmacist can also go into the patient care areas to speak with a patient or provide clinical services. In addition to the pharmacy satellite, a centralized pharmacy still exists to provide cart fill and serve the decentralized satellites. Also, the centralized pharmacy remains open all the time, providing services for the satellites when they close. These satellites can be focused on pediatrics, oncology, critical care, the emergency room, and the operating room.[19–23] The advantages with a decentralized model compared to a centralized model include reduced turnaround time, increased physician and nursing satisfaction, expansion of clinical services, fewer dispensing errors, and decreased floor stock.[24]

Rise of Technology to Assist Drug Distribution

As medication options continued to expand, the personnel demands of maintaining the unit dose method increased. Also, the use of technology and computers had a drastic impact on the manual system that was in use. New ways emerged to make drug distribution safer and less manual.

The original attempt to automate the drug distribution system was the Brewer system.[25,26] This system, described in 1961, was located on the nursing unit and it provided individual doses with labels, charge slips, and an accounting report. It was credited in reducing medication errors by 30–51%.

Another automatic dispensing unit was the Baxter ATC-212. This machine, located in a central place, packaged individual doses upon demand. Early studies with this technology demonstrated that it was 99.98% accurate compared to technicians manually completing a cart fill, who were only 92.62% accurate.[27] This system interfaces with the computer containing the fill list. This information is transferred to the machine, which instructs it to package and dispense medications in the order it is generated. It is usually operated by technicians. This system has been demonstrated to significantly reduce technician time with cart fill, by saving 0.36 technician FTE and significantly reducing error rate (from 0.84% to 0.65%). It had no effect on reducing pharmacist time in cart checking.[28]

Another device that has widespread utilization is the use of robots. These are a centralized automated dispensing devices used to fill medication carts. It contains a medication selection station, a bar-code reader, and packaging and bar-coding equipment. Through the use of bar-code scanning, the robot will select the appropriate medication and number of doses for a medication drawer.[29] This type of technology supports a centralized model of drug distribution, whereby cart fill is conducted in one location. The computerized information from the pharmacy system was transferred to the robotic dispensing system before filling. Once started, a bar-code label for each patient was generated from the system. These were placed on a medication bin for each patient. These bins were placed on a conveyor belt and the patient label was read by a scanner. The robotic filling device would immediately recognize what that specific patient's medication needs were for the next period. It would then proceed to pick those medications for that patient and place them in the bin. Once completed, the conveyor belt would start and advance the next bin and the process would start all over again. This process would go until all medication carts were filled.

The benefit of the system is that it replaced the manual activity of the cart fill. The assumption is that this would also be a more accurate system, since it is completely bar-code driven. It removes confusion over sound-alike drug names, skipping a medication, or choosing the wrong strength. It also freed up technician and pharmacist time to become more involved in other activities within the institution. Finally, because the inventory of the medications is located in one place, the overall cost of carrying these medications is less.[26]

All of the medications have to be prepared to be loaded into the robotic filling system. As mentioned, they are unit dosed in a sleeve containing the medication name and a bar code. Many medications did not come from the manufacturer prepared this way, so pharmacy departments had to do it themselves or they outsourced this activity. Just keeping the robotic filling device stocked was a time consuming process. The other large issue is how to handle down time. When a system of this magnitude is not functional, it requires the pharmacy to hand fill medication carts.

One study attempted to analyze the staff attitudes and employee perceptions with the implementation of a robotic system.[29] Overall, the staff expressed favorable opinions on job security and professional impact. Technicians were the most concerned with these categories and the impact on them. Another study demonstrated that a complete return on investment was realized through the reduction of medication errors and increasing efficiency.[26]

The other technological device that had a large

impact on medication distribution is automated dispensing cabinets (ADCs). These are a type of medication cart located on the nursing unit, except that all drugs that are stored there are not patient-specific. A single strength of a medication is stored in one pocket. Instead of the nurse going into a patient drawer to retrieve the dose, the nurse goes into the pocket, which keeps the specific medication needed. In its crudest form, ADCs are a modified floor stock system. Instead of bulk bottles of medications for the nurse to prepare the dose, the drug is packaged in a unit of use container. Also, the nurse has to enter the system to get the medication from it (and being barred from others), as opposed to entering a room that has all of them on the shelf.

The advantage to the system is that pharmacy could minimize its filling and delivery of medication carts. The vast majority of the medications needed for the patient were in the ADC, depending on the storage capacity and location. The ADCs could be configured to meet many of the needs of the specific floor. Pharmacy technicians started to refill the ADC instead of filling a patient-specific medication cart. The other major advantage of an ADC is that the nurse will only remove a dose if it is needed. This provides more accurate patient charges and minimizes the number of credits processed, since doses are administered upon removal. The major disadvantage of the system is that it is similar to the floor stock system, a system many hospitals migrated away from because of medication errors. The other major disadvantage is that it places more medications on the floor for the nurse to choose between when giving a dose and increases inventory.

The first ADC systems that were developed had a static inventory and did not communicate with the pharmacy computer system. As technology and networks advanced, these ADCs were able to communicate with the pharmacy computer system. This is referred to as *profiled*, containing an accurate, up-to-date patient specific profile. When a nurse wants to remove a dose to administer, the nurse logs into the system with a unique password or by using bio-ID scanning of fingerprint, it recognizes the user. The nurse selects the patient of interest and all of the medications that this patient is currently receiving appear. There is also a designation on whether this specific medication and strength is contained in this ADC. If the drug is located there and the nurse wants to use it, the nurse would select the drug by touching the screen and the correct drawer where the medication is located

opens. The screen also gives the nurse a description on the exact pocket to choose. Once the nurse removes the drug, they would close the drawer. At this time, the patient is charged for the dose and the inventory is decremented by what was removed. This allows for accurate patient bills and a perpetual inventory. This feature is extremely important with narcotics. The ADC can provide the tracking required by the DEA and can store the narcotics in a place where distribution is limited. In configuring these machines, there are different drawer types that can be used. These range from very restrictive (only housing the medication of interest) to less restrictive (gaining access to all of the medications in this drawer, trusting the nurse to choose the correct medication).

The effectiveness of the ADC in improving the distribution of medications has been evaluated. One study determined that by placing the ADC on a nursing unit, medications were 2.3 times more likely to be administered on schedule.[30] This is intuitive because the medication is already located on the floor, eliminating the time it takes pharmacy to send the dose. Another study demonstrated the effectiveness of an ADC in collecting charges.[31] The mean monthly charge for noncontrolled floorstock medications increased from 63% to 97% through the addition of an ADC. However, pharmacy personnel time increased per nursing unit from 7.17 minutes to 48.96 minutes per day due to the addition of the ADC. Another study demonstrated that the introduction of this technology increased the clinical time of the pharmacist from 36.5% to 49.1% in one unit and from 27.9% to 35.1% in another unit.[32] Finally, other studies have evaluated the ADC for its role in reducing medication errors. One study found that the implementation of an ADC decreased the medication error rate from 16.9% to 10.4%.[33] This study counted wrong administration time as an error, detecting this for over 80% of the occurrences in the ADC group.

ASHP has provided important guidelines as it relates to the safe use of automated medication storage and distribution devices.[34] Goals for the use of the devices are balanced between having medications readily available and accessible to meet patient needs within safety and security needs and minimizing the vulnerabilities to medication errors. To do this, ASHP recommends that performance standards for safety, accuracy, timeliness, and costs be determined. Also, a written plan for safe and effective use of the system should be developed. Finally, a pharmacist should review all medication orders prior to removal in order to check against appropriateness for the patient and dose.

Future of the Medication Use System

Technology will continue to develop that will take over the many manual tasks that are involved with the medication distribution system. It still takes time to fill the medication cart (if it is done manually), replenish the robotic dispensing device, or refill the ADC. Automation will be developed that will further decrease the number of people involved with the dispensing of medications. Another area that will further develop is the role of the wholesaler. Many institutions are outsourcing more of the distributive functions. Presently, wholesalers are taking a role in delivering totes specific for an ADC. Depending on various state laws, this could expand for them to take on an even larger role by going to the nursing unit and replenishing the ADC, reducing the amount of time that a pharmacy department needs to be involved. Perhaps the wholesaler may even own the inventory and charge for it when the patient uses it. Bar-code technology will also further change medication distribution. Hopefully, more doses will come from the manufacturer with a bar code on the package before the use of this technology becomes more widespread. This product, when scanned, will assist in making sure the correct product is sent to the patient or loaded in an ADC. The bar code will also help the nurse in making sure the proper dose is given to the patient. Studies will need to be conducted to demonstrate the success of the bar code in reducing medication errors, but the potential for having a large impact on the patient seems evident.

The role of the technician will continue to play a larger role in the medication distribution system. Studies have been conducted that demonstrate that a tech-check-tech system for checking unit dose carts is as good as, if not better than, pharmacist checking a technician.[35,36] The professional judgment of the medication distribution system lies in the profiling of medication orders and the administration of the drug. Making sure that the drug and dose is appropriate for the patient and that no drug interactions are occurring is important in a patient's regimen. It is also extremely important that the patient gets the drug administered appropriately, and that someone is monitoring that it is effective. The technician can manage the distributive aspects of it, while the pharmacist cares for the patient. Pharmacists could also get more involved in taking medication histories and discharge counseling, a role that is usually filled by physicians and nurses. This is called reconciliation, whereby medications are reconciled across the continuum of care. If the pharmacist can be freed up from the routine of the distribution system (assuming that tech-check-tech is as good, if not better than having a pharmacist involved) then the pharmacist can further evolve into these other roles. It is still unsure if pharmacists will expand into these roles, but the potential exists.

Summary

In summary, the unit dose system and the development of automation for drug distribution has had a profound impact on elevating the practice of hospital pharmacy. The unit dose system reduced medication errors and aided in the introduction of the concept of clinical pharmacy. Technology has further enhanced the distribution of medications, allowing pharmacists to become more involved with patient care. The future of technology should further reduce medication errors while maintaining the pharmacist oversight of the process and allow the pharmacist to better care of patients.

Suggested Reading

American Society of Hospital Pharmacists (ASHP). ASHP technical assistance bulletin on single unit and unit dose packages of drugs. *Am J Hosp Pharm*. 1985;42: 378–9.

ASHP statement on the pharmacist's responsibility for distribution and control of drug products. In: Deffenbaugh JH, ed. *Practice Standards of ASHP 1996–97*. Bethesda, MD. American Society of Health-System Pharmacists; 1996.

Barker KN. Ensuring safety in the use of automated medication dispensing machines. *Am J Hosp Pharm*. 1995;52:2445–7.

Barker KN. The effects of an experimental medication system on medication errors and costs—part one: introduction and errors study. *Am J Hosp Pharm*. 1969;26;324–33.

Barker KN, McConnell WE. The problems of detecting medication errors in hospitals. *Am J Hosp Pharm*. 1962;19;360–9.

Barker KN, Pearson RE, Hepler CD, et al. Effect of an automated bedside dispensing machine on medication errors. *Am J Hosp Pharm*. 1984;41:1352–8.

Botwin KJ, Chan J, Jacobs R, et al. Restricted access to automated dispensing machines for surgical antimicrobial prophylaxis. *Am J Hosp Pharm*. 2001;58:797–9.

Klibanov OM, Eckel SF. Effects of automated dispensing on inventory control, billing, workload, and potential for medication errors. *Am J Hosp Pharm*. 2003;60:569–72.

Latiolais CJ. A pharmacy coordinated unit dose dispensing and drug administration system—philosophy, objectives, and pharmaceutical implications. *Am J Hosp Pharm.* 1970:27;886–9.

Max BE, Itokazu G, Danzinger LH, et al. Assessing unit dose system discrepancies. *Am J Hosp Pharm.* 2002;59:856–8.

Oren E, Griffiths LP, Guglielmo BJ. Characteristics of antimicrobial overrides associated with automated dispensing machines. *Am J Hosp Pharm.* 2002;59:1445–8.

Schwarz HO, Brodowy BA. Implementation and evaluation of an automated dispensing system. *Am J Hosp Pharm.* 1995;52:823–8.

Sutter TL, Wellman GS, Mott DA, et al. Discrepancies with automated drug storage and distribution cabinets. *Am J Hosp Pharm.* 1998;55:1924–6.

References

1. Black HJ. Unit dose drug distribution: A 20-year perspective. *Am J Hosp Pharm.* 1984;41:2086–8.

2. Black HJ, Nelson SP. Medication Distribution Systems. In: Brown TR. *Handbook of Institutional Pharmacy Practice.* 3rd ed. Bethesda, MD: American Society of Hospital Pharmacists; 1992:165–74.

3. Shultz SM, White SJ, Latiolais CJ. Medications Errors Reduced by Unit-Dose. Hospitals. *JAHA.* 47, March 16, 1973:106–12.

4. Barker KN, Heller WM. The development of a centralized unit-dose dispensing system for UAMC—part VI: the pilot study—medication errors and drug losses. *Am J Hosp Pharm.* 1964;21:609–25.

5. Hynniman CE, Conrad WF, Urch WA, et al. A comparison of medication errors under the University of Kentucky unit dose system. *Am J Hosp Pharm.* 1970;27:802–14.

6. Black HJ, Tester WW. Decentralized pharmacy operations utilizing the unit dose concept. *Am J Hosp Pharm.* 1964;21:344–50.

7. American Society of Hospital Pharmacists (ASHP). ASHP Statement on Unit Dose Drug Distribution. *Am J Hosp Pharm.* 1975;32:835.

8. Stolar MH. National Survey of Selected Hospital Pharmacy Practices. *Am J Hosp Pharm.* 1976;33:225–30.

9. Stolar MH. ASHP National Survey of Hospital Pharmaceutcal Services—1987. *Am J Hosp Pharm.* 1988;45:801–18.

10. American Society of Hospital Pharmacists(ASHP) ASHP technical assistance bulletin on hospital drug distribution and control. *Am J Hosp Pharm.* 1980;37:1097–103.

11. McGovern D. Print, prepare, check, and deliver a 24-hour supply of unit dose medication for 600 patients in one hour. *Hosp Pharm.* 1981;16:193–206.

12. Woller TW, Roberts MJ, Ploetz PA. Recording schedule II drug use in a decentralized drug distribution system. *Am J Hosp Pharm.* 1987;44:349–53.

13. Norvell MJ, McAllister JC, Bailey E. Cost analysis of drug distribution for controlled substances. *Am J Hosp Pharm.* 1983;40:801–7.

14. Baker GE. Reducing the handling of prn doses in a unit dose drug distribution system. *Am J Hosp Pharm.* 1987;44:2255–6.

15. Woller TW, Kreling DH, Ploetz PA. Quantifying unused orders for as-needed medications. *Am J Hosp Pharm.* 1987;44:1347–52.

16. Shimp LA, Mason NA, Toedter NM, et al. Pharmacist participation in cardiopulmonary resuscitation. *Am J Health-Syst Pharm.* 1995;52:980–4.

17. Gonzalez ER, Ornato JP. Cardiopulmonary resuscitation documentation: a survey of 135 medical centers. *Drug Intell Clin Pharm.* 1988;22:559–62.

18. Kelly WN, Meyer JD, Flatley CJ. Cost analysis of a satellite pharmacy. *Am J Hosp Pharm.* 1986;43:1927–30.

19. Tisdale JE. Justifying a pediatric critical-care satellite pharmacy by medication-error reporting. *Am J Hosp Pharm.* 1986;43:368–71.

20. Sauer KA, Nowak MM, Coons SJ, et al. Justification and implementation of a cancer center satellite pharmacy. *Am J Hosp Pharm.* 1989;46:1389–92.

21. Caldwell RD, Tuck BA. Justification and operation of a critical-care satellite pharmacy. *Am J Hosp Pharm.* 1983;40:2141–5.

22. Powell MF, Solomon DK, McEachen RA. Twenty-four hour emergency pharmaceutical services. *Am J Hosp Pharm.* 1985;42:831–5.

23. Vogel DP, Barone J, Penn F. Ideas for action: the operating room pharmacy satellite. *Top Hosp Pharm Mgt.* 1986;6(2);63–81.

24. Rascati KL. Brief review of the literature on decentralized drug distribution in hospitals. *Am J Hosp Pharm.* 1988;45;639–41.

25. Manzelli TA. Utilization of the Brewer System in the controlled distribution of medication within the hospital. *Am J Hosp Pharm.* 1961;18:560–6.

26. Perini VJ, Vermeulen LC. Comparison of automated medication-management systems. *Am J Hosp Pharm.* 1994;51:1883–91.

27. Kratz K, Thygesen C. A comparison of the accuracy of unit-dose cart fill with the Baxter ATC-212 computerized system and manual filling. *Hosp Pharm.* 1992;27:19–22.

28. Klein EG, Santora JA, Pascale PM, et al. Medication cart-filling time, accuracy, and cost with an automated dispensing system. *Am J Hosp Pharm.* 1994;51:1193–6.

29. Crawford SY, Grussing PG, Clark TG, et al. Staff attitudes about the use of robots in pharmacy before implementation of a robotic dispensing system. *Am J Hosp Pharm.* 1998;55:1907–14.

30. Shirley KL. Effect of an automated dispensing system on medication administration time. *Am J Hosp Pharm.* 1999;56:1542–5.

31. Lee LW, Wellman GS, Birdwell SW, et al. Use of an automated medication storage and distribution system. *Am J Hosp Pharm.* 1992;49:851–5.

32. Guerrero RM, Nickman NA, Jorgenson JA. Work activities before and after implementation of an automated dispensing system. *Am J Hosp Pharm.* 1996;53:548–54.

33. Borel JM, Rascati KL. Effect of an automated, nursing unit-based drug-dispensing device on medication errors. *Am J Hosp Pharm.* 1995;52:1875–9.

34. American Society of Health-System Pharmacists (ASHP). ASHP guidelines on the safe use of automated medication storage and distribution devices. *Am J Hosp Pharm.* 1998;55:1403–7.

35. Ness JE, Sullivan SD, Stergachis A. Accuracy of technicians and pharmacists in identifying dispensing errors. *Am J Hosp Pharm.* 1994;51:354–7.

36. Andersen SR, St. Peter JV, Macres MG, et al. Accuracy of technicians versus pharmacists in checking syringes prepared for a dialysis program. *Am J Health-Syst Pharm.* 1997;54:1611–3.

Chapter 28

Sterile Preparations and Admixture Programs

Philip J. Schneider, E. Clyde Buchanan

Introduction

Patient safety is a crucial component to patients receiving the most benefit from their medications. Pharmacists have historically played a critical role in protecting patients from harm that may result from drug therapy. Increased attention has been devoted to the use of high-risk medications—those that have the greatest potential to cause adverse drug events when used. High-risk medications are most commonly defined according to the drug toxicity but may also be defined by the route by which they are administered. Focusing on both high-risk medications and high-risk methods of administering these medications can narrow the scope of work. Cohen has an excellent chapter titled "High-Alert Medications: Safeguarding against Errors" in his text *Medication Errors*.[1] Sixteen medications or drug categories are listed, 14 of which can or are administered by the intravenous route. Kaushaul et al. found that the intravenous route of administration was the most common in medication errors detected in pediatric inpatients.[2] In their annual report, USP reports that "the intravenous route of administration often results in the most serious medication error outcomes" based on the reports submitted to MEDMARX[SM] in the year 2002.[3] We do not need a formal failure mode analysis to know that intravenous drug administration is a high-risk area of medication use, and needs more attention.

The intravenous route of administration bypasses three physiologic safeguards—the gut, liver, and skin. The gut may break down medications before they are ever absorbed, or the drug may not even be absorbed by through the gastrointestinal tract. The liver protects patients from many toxic doses of medications and can safeguard patients through the first pass effect when medications are administered orally. The skin protects patients from infections that might be caused by pathogenic microorganisms that are in the environment, especially the hospital.

Reports about problems with the safety of intravenous drug therapy were reported in the late 1960s.

Patterson et al. expressed concerns about drug incompatibilities and the length of time between preparation and administration of medications prepared at the bedside after finding that 60% of intravenous fluids used at their hospital contained more than one drug, and many were administered more than an hour after preparation.[4] These authors recommended that pharmacy assume responsibility for compounding intravenous admixture doses to resolve these problems. Flack et al. reported being asked for "technical help from the pharmacy service" by the surgeons investigating the effectiveness and safety of parenteral nutrition to resolve problems of contamination and incompatibilities with the formulas that were being "hand mixed in open laboratory surroundings."[5] Thur et al. observed nurses preparing parenteral admixtures in patient care areas and reported an error rate of 21%. The rate of wrong dose prepared was 9%, incompatible drugs mixed was 6%, wrong drug or solution used was 3%, and preparation of drugs not ordered was 3%. Deviations from accepted sterile technique was observed, with counters not being cleaned (99%), hands not washed (97%), touching sterile areas of the IV container (47%), and vial or bottle tops not being cleaned (31%).[6] O'Hare et al. used a disguised observer method to evaluate error in preparation and administration of intravenous medications by physicians and nurses. They found that physicians made at least one error in 98% of the doses prepared and 83% of these doses were administered by nurses.[7]

Even if properly ordered, errors can occur in preparation that can cause harm to patients. Thompson et al. evaluated the concentrations of admixed medications delivered to patients and found evidence of incomplete mixing of medications in IV solutions prepared at the bedside. The also found that there were fewer differences in the uniformity of concentrations of potassium chloride when these doses were prepared in the pharmacy.[8] Calculation errors are also a root cause of error in preparing medications. Perlstein et al. found that one of 12 doses calculated by nurses had an error that resulted in a tenfold dose compared to that ordered. Pediatricians made errors in one of 26 computations. Pharmacists made fewer errors that nurses and physicians.[9]

As a result of these reports, pharmacy-based centralized intravenous admixture programs have emerged as a fundamentally safer medication-use system. According to ASHP National Surveys of Pharmacy Practice in hospital settings, this system is present in the vast majority of U.S. hospitals.[10] Indeed, ASHP has developed and promoted guidelines for quality assurance for pharmacy-prepared sterile products.[11] There is some evidence that complacency can arise in pharmacies blunting the purported benefits of a pharmacy-based intravenous admixture program. Sanders et al. reported that pharmacists had an error rate of 7.24% and a contamination rate of 7%.[12] These errors and contamination rates were higher than that observed for pharmacy technicians. Pharmacists made fewer errors and contaminated fewer IV preparations when they knew they were being observed, suggesting the emergence of complacency and the need for continuing vigilance.[13] High error rates in pharmacy-based intravenous admixture programs were also reported by Flynn et al. They found an error rate of 9% in five hospital pharmacies studied using an observation-based method.[14]

Recent reports of patients being harmed by pharmacy-compounded sterile medications, including intravenous admixtures have resulted in public concern about patient safety. The recent publication of an enforceable standard, USP Chapter <797> and attention to this by the Joint Commission on Accreditation of Healthcare Organizations (JACHO) points out the importance of taking responsibility for compounding sterile preparations seriously.[15,16] The intent of this chapter is to summarize the requirement for doing this.

Definitions

Ante Area or Anteroom—Any area adjacent to buffer or clean room where unsterilized products, in-process components, materials, and containers are handled (see also controlled area).

Aseptic Technique—The methods used to manipulate sterile products so that they remain sterile.

Biological Safety Cabinet (BSC)—A primary environmental control used for the preparation of hazardous drugs when the product, personnel, and environment must be protected according to National Sanitation Foundation Standard 49.

Buffer Room—The space that is designated for compounding sterile preparations (see also cleanroom).

Clean Room—A room in which the concentration of airborne particles is controlled and which is constructed and used in a manner to minimize the introduction, generation, and retention of particles inside the room and in which other relevant parameters (e.g., temperature, humidity, and air pressure differentials) are controlled as necessary.

Closed System Transfer—A method of transferring one sterile component to another without contaminating the final preparation.

Cold Storage Conditions (Refrigerator)—2–8°C (36–46°F).

Components—The individual ingredients that are used to compound a sterile preparation.

Compounded Sterile Preparation (CSP)—A dose of medication that is prescribed for a specific patient that must be prepared for administration and is sterile.

Controlled Area—The space designated for compounding sterile preparations. This is referred to as the buffer zone (i.e., the cleanroom in which the laminar-airflow workbench is located) by USP Chapter <797>.

Critical Area—Any area in the controlled area where sterile preparations, surfaces, or containers are exposed to the environment.

Garb—Clothing worn by those compounding sterile preparation to minimize particulates and possible contamination of final preparations during compounding.

Isolator—An isolator is a controlled environment that is defined by fixed walls, floor, and ceiling. Transfers of materials into and out of the environment as well as the interaction technologies are separated by barriers such as gloves, sleeves, and airlocks.

Laminar Air Flow Workbench (LAFW)—A controlled environment created by a high-efficiency particulate air (HEPA) filter to retain airborne particles and microorganisms, and its use decreases the chance of contamination during compounding sterile preparations.

Standard Operating Procedures (SOPs)—A set of instructions or steps someone follows to complete a job safely, with no adverse impact on the environment (and which meets compliance standards), and in a way that optimizes operational and production requirements.

Quality Assurance in Compounding Sterile Preparations

Preparations to be used for parenteral, ophthalmic, and irrigation purposes must be free from chemical and physical contaminants, accurately and correctly compounded, sterile and pyrogen-free, stable until their beyond-use date, and properly packaged and labeled.

Components

The majority of compounded sterile preparations are comprised of components that are clean, sterile, and pyrogen-free as purchased from pharmaceutical manufacturers. Nevertheless, USP Chapter <797> states that the pharmacist is ultimately responsible for the quality of sterile preparations compounded from commercially available ingredients. High-risk compounding involves the use of components that are neither sterile nor pyrogen-free. The extemporaneous compounding of concentrated morphine HCl solutions is an example. In high-risk compounding, it is essential to use a USP grade chemical or to obtain a certificate of quality analysis from the supplier of the chemical, since the pharmacy is usually not equipped or qualified to perform chemical analyses. Assuming that the certificate is judged to be reliable and the substance meets acceptable standards, like those of the USP, the pharmacist can take the responsibility for using the chemical. Subsequent compounding procedures must be developed so that the final preparation meets the standards required for a sterile preparation, including sterility, freedom from pyrogens, and an acceptable particulate level. For high-risk preparations, the pharmaceutical characteristics must be produced as a consequence of the compounding and processing steps. Sterility must be achieved, usually by appropriate filtration through sterile, disposable, nonreactive, 0.2 micron porosity membrane filter devices. During filtration, particulate matter will be removed to very low levels and to below visible sizes, rendering the solution clear. Removing pyrogens will be more difficult; the best approach is to obtain raw materials that are free from pyrogens as supplied. When pyrogens are present, appropriately charged filters may remove them, but determinations must be made to be sure that required molecules in the formulation are not also removed. A more complex technique is the use of ultrafiltration, which removes molecules selectively by size.

For low- and medium-risk preparations, assuring that the preparation has the required characteristics is primarily a matter of maintaining the quality level built into the product by the commercial supplier.

Compatibility and Stability

Responsibility for the compatibility and stability of formulated preparations also rests on the pharmacist. Detailed compatibility and stability information may not be readily available for high-risk compounding. Lacking the facilities to perform research and testing, pharmacists are challenged to draw upon their basic chemical and physical knowledge, experience in compounding, and awareness of available literature resources. Probably the most widely used reference is Trissel's *Handbook of Injectable Drugs*.[16] Other information may be available from the commercial supplier of a component and from other literature resources.

Unexpected compatibility problems may be visible immediately or within a few hours of compounding, but not all incompatibilities are visible. All incompatibilities affect the stability of a preparation. However, stability considerations are broader and include overall assurance that the activity and chemical/physical integrity of the formulation is maintained until the preparation is administered to a patient.

Facilities

The facilities in which the compounding of sterile preparations is performed must be designed and operated in a manner conducive to achieving/maintaining the quality characteristics of the finished preparation. USP Chapter <797> requires that all sterile compounding, regardless of risk level, be done in a an ISO Class 5 environment (i.e., fewer than 100 air borne particles larger than 0.5 microns per cubic foot) that is maintained in a horizontal laminar airflow workbench (LAFW), a suitable biological safety cabinet (BSC) or a suitable isolator. Because LAFWs and BSCs draw air from the surrounding room, USP Chapter <797> requires a clean room environment that meets ISO Class 7 (i.e., fewer than 10,000 air borne particles larger than 0.5 microns per cubic foot). Low- and medium-risk preparations may be compounded in facilities where there is no physical separation between the ante area and the buffer room. High-risk preparations require an anteroom separate from the buffer room. See schematic Figures 28-1 and 28-2.

The surfaces of all clean room ceilings, walls, floors, shelving, cabinets, and work surfaces should be smooth, impervious, free from cracks and crevices, and nonshedding, making them easy to clean and sanitize. Junctures of ceilings to walls, walls to walls, and floors to walls should be coved or caulked to make them easier to clean. There should be no dust-collecting ledges, pipes, or similar surfaces. Work surfaces should be constructed of durable, smooth, and impervious materials, such as stainless steel or molded plastic. Carts should be of stainless steel wire or sheet construction with good quality, cleanable casters, and should be restricted to the buffer room. The key equipment unit is the LAFW, designed to continuously sweep the work area with HEPA-filtered air at a velocity of 90 feet per minute. The 99.97% efficiency of an HEPA filter should render the air stream clean and approaching sterility, if LAFW or BSC remains properly validated. Still, this 90 foot/second air flow velocity can easily be overcome with adverse air currents, even by the expelled breath from compounding personnel talking; thus, the critical

work area must be protected from inappropriate activities of personnel (to be discussed later). The HEPA filter should be protected from damage during use and its efficiency validated at least every 6 months. BSCs should be used to maintain sterility of the preparation and to protect compounding personnel when hazardous drugs are being compounded.

Clean airflow should be outward from the critical area through the buffer room, then through the anteroom by means of cascading differential air pressures, starting with the highest pressure from HEPA-filtered air in the buffer room. These or similar structural design considerations, along with planned cleaning programs, sanitizing of all surfaces, and traffic control of personnel and supplies, make it possible to protect the critical area.

A newer approach to environmental control is an isolator (see Figure 28-3). Basically, the unit isolates the ISO Class 5 critical area from surrounding air. Compounding personnel maintain the interior of the isolator's cleanliness by sanitizing its inside surfaces.

Figure 28-1
Schematic Example of Clean Room Floor Plan Suitable for Low- and Medium-Risk Level Compounded Sterile Preparations

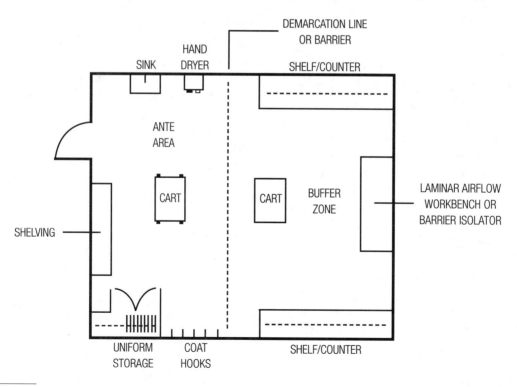

Source: Reference 14.

Figure 28-2

Schematic Example of a Clean Room Floor Plan Suitable for High-Risk Level Compounded Sterile Preparations

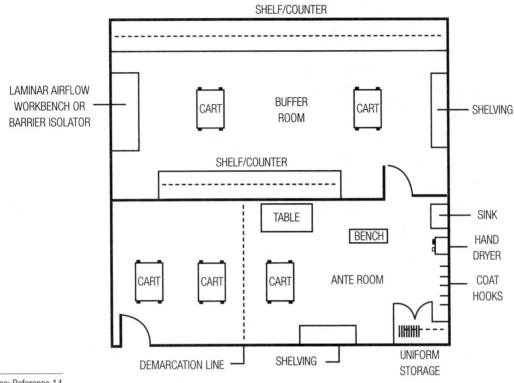

Source: Reference 14.

Access is provided for personnel through glove ports or half-suits sealed in the walls. Components are introduced through pass-through chambers. The advantages of such a system are that the critical area can maintain a high level of cleanliness and personnel preparation and gowning requirements are greatly reduced. While the USP prefers a clean room environment for isolators, it is not required unless the requirement for a clean room is stated by the isolator manufacturer. The most apparent problem is the contamination risk associated with the introduction of supplies into the isolator and the removal of finished preparations.

Environmental Control

Proper utilization of the facilities described is fundamental to adequate control of the working environment, with the ultimate focus on the critical area. However, without proper use of the controlled area, the LAFW or BSC alone would be inadequate to provide a critical work area that could assure the sterility of

preparations in any of the three risk levels. Since, by definition, a HEPA filter will deliver an air stream that has had particles of 0.5 microns and larger removed with an efficiency of 99.97%, there is a 0.03% probability of particles passing through, a small portion of which could be microorganisms. Therefore, the risk of any microbial contaminant in that air stream gaining ingress to a preparation is very low, particularly for low-risk preparations. The operational challenge is to prevent contaminants from entering the critical area; such an effort constitutes environmental control—keeping the critical area at least an ISO Class 5 environment. Environmental control encompasses several areas:

- *Cleaning and Sanitizing*—Surface contamination can be expected, even in the LAFW, BSC or isolator. Therefore, written standard operating procedures (SOPs) should be developed and followed for cleaning and sanitizing all surfaces within the ante area/room and buffer room. Cleaning outside of the LAFW, BSC, or isolator

Figure 28-3
Compounding Pharmacy Technician Working in an Isolator

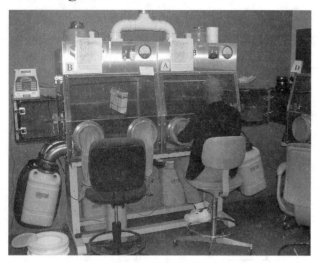

Source: Winship Cancer Institute of Emory Healthcare, Atlanta GA.

should be performed with a mild detergent in purified water using a nonshedding, absorbent wipe or sponge. This should be followed by wiping surfaces with an effective sanitizing agent (disinfectant). A commercial agent can be used, sometimes combined with a detergent, provided adequate evidence of effectiveness is available. All shelving, supply carts, and countertops in the remainder of the controlled area should be cleared of supplies and then cleaned in a similar manner at least monthly. Cleaning should be followed by wiping with a sanitizing agent more aggressive than IPA. Floors in these areas should be cleaned and sanitized daily, working from the cleanest area outward. The detergent and/or sanitizing agent solution should be replaced with fresh solution at frequent intervals during floor cleaning. All reusable cleaning tools should be restricted to the controlled area and thoroughly cleaned and sanitized after each use.

Cleaning in the LAFW, BSC or isolator may be done with a nonshedding wipe or sponge dampened with Water for Injection (WFI), with or without a mild detergent. This step should be followed by sanitizing, most often with sterile-filtered 70% isopropyl alcohol (IPA), allowed to

remain inside surfaces for at least 30 seconds before wipe-off. Alternatively, cleaning and sanitizing may be accomplished with IPA alone, at least at the beginning and ending of each shift and whenever spillage occurs.

■ *Traffic Control*—The flow of supplies and personnel through the ante area/room and buffer room for operations in the critical area must be rigidly controlled to prevent carrying contamination inward. No personnel should be allowed to approach the LAFW unless properly garbed and adequately trained. All supplies should be externally cleaned and sanitized during the movement through the ante area/room to the buffer room.

An arrangement in which supplies are brought into the ante area/room external to the demarcation is preferred. At this point, they are unboxed, cleaned, sanitized and transferred to a clean cart restricted to the buffer room. This step serves as a barrier to many of the natural contaminants on the outside of large volume parenteral (LVP) bags, vials, syringe pouches, transfer set packages and other required supplies.

A further transfer barrier step should occur as supply items are introduced into the LAFW, BSC or isolator. Whenever possible, an external wrap would be removed (such as syringe pouches) at the edge of the LAFW or BSC. Vials and other items not packaged in an outer wrap should be carefully sanitized by wiping with a wipe dampened with a sanitizing agent, most commonly IPA. The supply items introduced into the LAFW should be limited to those required for the planned procedure and should be arranged so as not to obstruct the HEPA airflow pattern and to provide for efficient processing—that is, to the right and left of the work site in a horizontal LAFW and around the perimeter in a BSC.

These barrier steps during the introduction of supplies should be recognized as only sanitizing, not sterilizing, steps, and their effectiveness depends on the techniques of the operator and on the sanitizing agent used. Any residual contaminants on the surfaces of supply items may be transferred to the sterile gloves of an operator and then be present for possible touch contamination transfer to the preparation. This risk of contaminating a preparation will increase progressively from low-risk to high-risk preparations.

- *Environmental Testing*—While all the elements so far mentioned, pursued with dedication, should provide a controlled environment, a testing program should be developed to verify that the control is achieved and maintained. The focus of testing should be on detecting the presence of microbial contaminants in the environment. Both surface testing, for the deposit of microorganisms on exposed surfaces over time, and air-volume sampling, for microorganisms suspended in the air, should be performed. In principal, baseline (minimal) microbial counts should be determined when the environment is under control. A monitoring program should then be designed to detect loss of control evidenced by increases in the microbial counts. Such increases signal the need to determine the cause and correct it. The USP has a microbiologic evaluation process for clean rooms that should be considered.[17]

Compounding Personnel

Compounding personnel in the ante area/room and buffer room should be limited to those adequately trained and validated for aseptic technique (to be discussed later) and to the minimal number required for the planned procedures. Since the human body is constantly shedding particles, many of which are viable microorganisms, an effort must be made to reduce the ingress of these particles into the buffer room but, particularly, into the critical area. This is accomplished by good personal hygiene, thorough washing/sanitizing of hands, following good aseptic technique, and by donning garb to confine the particles as much as possible.

Training and Evaluating Compounding Personnel

To achieve good sterile compounding practice, personnel must be adequately trained and the effectiveness of the training validated. This is the most significant factor contributing the assurance of quality in sterile preparations, for personnel are recognized as the primary source of contaminants, both viable and nonviable, shed in the clean room environment. Therefore, compounding personnel must be taught to understand this natural phenomenon and how they can control particulate shedding while compounding. Considerable information regarding proper training will be found in ASHP's text and video programs on compounding sterile preparations.[18–20]

Pharmacists and technicians who compound sterile preparations in a pharmacy must practice excellent aseptic technique, and they should understand good compounding practice. Training should make clear that sterile preparations must have the highest level of quality and purity of all dosage forms because they are given by injection, irrigation, or ophthalmically, therefore bypassing the first line of defense of the human body against the invasion of toxic substances—the intact skin. The secondary body defenses have much less capacity to neutralize the effects of hazardous substances or microbial toxins. Trainees should be instructed in the nature of contaminants and the means for achieving the required level of purity, maintaining stability during the required beyond-use dating of the preparation, and evaluating the required characteristics. Pharmacists should be sufficiently familiar with the principles of sterilization to work with technicians who perform autoclaving or hot-air sterilization of supplies or preparations. The validation of these processes for their bactericidal effect is highly critical and requires considerable expertise.

While pharmacists and technicians are not expected to be engineers, they should know the specifications for facilities in which they must perform. This includes the selection of equipment (for example, an LAFW) from external suppliers or working with in-house engineers to assure proper clean air flow into the ante area/room and buffer room. An understanding of some engineering principles is needed to achieve required environmental standards. For example, the dynamics of air flow through a HEPA filter to achieve laminar air flow and the clean sweep of the critical area. It is also necessary to know how to achieve the air pressure differentials to produce the cascading effect from the buffer room out through the less-clean ante area/room.

The use of barriers to interrupt the ingress of contaminants into the critical area must be understood, whether these are physical barriers such as walls or curtains or interruption barriers (e.g., removing supply items from a cart, cleaning and sanitizing, and transferring to another restricted-area cart). Another interruption barrier is the washing of hands and the donning of clean garb before entering the buffer room. The selection of the sanitizing agent must be based on knowledge of the antimicrobial action of the agent.

Trainees must have a basic understanding of microbiology. They need to know that microorganisms are ubiquitous and, therefore, are present in the work environment, even in the critical area. They must know these organisms will multiply rapidly (about every 20 minutes) by when moisture, the proper temperature, and nutrients are present.

Compounding personnel should understand the principles of environmental evaluation (i.e., how to determine the effectiveness of the environmental controls used). This means knowing and selecting methods for detection of viable microorganisms in the environment, what the methods selected will detect, how samples should be gathered and incubated, proving that any viable microorganisms present will grow, and what the results signify, including when and if action is required.

Aseptic Technique

Typically, manipulations by compounding personnel are used in small-scale compounding of sterile preparations in the buffer room for low and medium-risk preparations. Medium-risk preparations may require automated compounding devices for the addition of small-volume additives to total parenteral nutrition (TPN) solutions. Compounding personnel must set up such devices, connect fresh stock containers, fill the final preparation containers, and generally monitor the operation. High-risk preparations are particularly exposed to the environment and to compounding personnel.

Because of the inherent shedding of viable and nonviable particles from the body of compounding personnel (as many as 1 million particles of 0.3µm and larger per min with average arm and upper-body movement from a sitting position dressed in a long-sleeved, nonshedding coat), serious efforts must be made to control this shedding. Means used include garbing, designed to confine most of the discharge within the garb; planning movements while using aseptic technique to minimize losing particles from the body; and removing human beings as far as possible from the critical area. One of the advantages of isolators is the fact that the bodies of compounding personnel are isolated from the critical area by the use of sealed rubberglove ports or half-suits.

The generally accepted garb for compounding personnel working at an LAFW or BSC in either a sitting or standing position would be clean hair cover, face mask, long-sleeved (with elastic or snaps at the wrists) nonshedding knee-length coat or gown, shoe covers, and sterile gloves. Working at an isolator, the operator normally would wear clean street clothing, unless the isolator is located in a buffer room.

The following lists some elements of good aseptic technique:

1. Practice good personal hygiene; be organized and level-headed.

2. Be healthy, without eczema or other skin rashes, and free from allergies or other conditions causing sneezing or coughing.

3. Wash hands and arms thoroughly or disinfect with foamed alcohol.

4. Put on garb properly, avoiding contaminating the outside of the clean/sterile gowns.

5. Replace garb or parts of garb that become contaminated while gowning or working.

6. Put on sterile gloves as the final garbing step.

7. Sanitize all internal surfaces of the LAFW (except the HEPA filter face) with an appropriate sanitizing agent, usually IPA.

8. Sanitize gloves (usually with IPA) as frequently as necessary while performing aseptic technique to maintain the aseptic condition of the outer surfaces.

9. Replace gloves with new sterile ones if they become punctured or torn.

10. Move with slow, smooth, gentle motions.

11. Do not talk unnecessarily.

12. Do not disrupt HEPA-filtered laminar air flow within the critical area.

13. Do not interpose arms or any other nonsterile object above a critical site in vertical laminar air flow (VLAF) or behind a critical site in horizontal laminar air flow (HLAF).

14. Do no spray or splash disinfectants where the liquid might enter a preparation container or reach other preparation contact sites.

15. Do not introduce any packages into the buffer room unless they have been adequately sanitized or sterilized externally.

16. Minimize in and out movement at the LAFW, BSC or isolator.

17. Arrange sterile supply items in the critical area so as not to interrupt the laminar air flow and to provide for efficient processing of the preparation(s).

18. Resanitize gloves with IPA after handling any package if the outside had uncertain sterility or surfaces such as switches of mixing pumps.

19. Cooperate with other compounding personnel and mutually assist in maintaining proper aseptic technique.

20. Pass through doorways, plastic curtains, or other passageways slowly and carefully to minimize the generation of potentially contaminating air currents.

21. Do not leave open vials, tanks, or other critical sites exposed to the environment during breaks or other delays in operation.

22. Inspect all supply items before using and the finished preparation after preparation for evidence of defects.

23. Remove used supply items and clean/sanitize work area as needed.

24. Prepare and apply appropriate labels and complete documents away from the critical area or, preferably, pass preparation outside so that a second person can perform the paperwork.

25. Remove used garb carefully to avoid distributing accumulated body contamination before exiting the gowning room.

26. Leave the HEPA filter blower operating at all times.

Packaging and Labeling

The final container for a compounded sterile preparation needs to be sterile and maintain the sterility of the preparation during to the beyond-use date. It should also protect the final preparation from chemical degradation, especially if the preparation is light sensitive. The choice of package for sterile preparation should take into account the use of the preparation. For example, ophthalmic medications need to be packaged in a way where drops can be instilled in the eye. Irrigation solutions need to accommodate administration sets, if necessary, and ideally not be confused with intravenous drug administration containers. Plastic containers are now preferred for most sterile medications because of cost and to prevent breakage, but this material should not be used if the preparation is not compatible with plastic (e.g., hydrochloric acid) or if heat sterilization of the final preparation is needed.

Proper labeling is an important component of safe medication systems because it enables identifies the medication, quantity of medication, and beyond use date. If the preparation is patient-specific, it also associates the medication with the patient for whom it is intended and the dose that is prescribed. Labels may also include supplementary information to help assure the dose is administered properly, such as how to store the preparation, when to administer the dose, and how to prepare the dose for administration. Special techniques can be used to highlight important characteristics of drug names or doses to avoid confusion that might result from look-alike or sound alike drug names or doses. Examples are bold letters, larger font, color, or capital letters (so called *tall man* lettering) for drug names or concentrations or doses. As a caveat, it is important not to include too much information on a label so that the user cannot or does not read the information.

There are specific requirements for labeling compounded sterile preparations included in USP Chapter <797>.[14] They include the following:

- Name and amounts or concentrations of ingredients
- Total volume of the compounded sterile preparation
- Beyond-use date
- Appropriate route of administration
- Storage conditions (e.g., refrigerate, protect from light)
- Other information for safe use (e.g., cautionary statements, initials of responsible pharmacist, disposal instructions)

Patient specific labeling may include additional information to assure proper drug administration. This includes the following:

- Patient name and identification number
- Patient location
- Name and amount of drug(s) added and the name of the admixture solution
- Time and date of scheduled administration
- Time and date of preparation
- Administration instructions
- Initials of the persons who prepare and check the IV admixture

Verification of compounding accuracy and sterility

There are two components of compounded sterile preparations that are important—the accuracy of the content, and sterility. Manufactured products cannot be used before these two factors are assured. It is not possible to wait for the results of tests to measure content or sterility for compounded preparations because of the urgency of clinical need. Therefore, more indirect methods of quality assurance are needed.

Measures of compounding accuracy are directed toward assuring the content of the admixture matches what is ordered and printed on the label. This can be done for parenteral nutrition formulations by weighing an admixture. The weight of the final preparation can be calculated using specific gravity of the components. Deviations from the calculated weight would suggest that a wrong base solution or the wrong volume of one or more of the base solutions was used to compound the preparation. Another method for evaluating parenteral nutrition and electrolyte preparations is refractometry. A small drop of the final compounded preparation is placed in a hand-held refractometer. The index measured can be compared to a theoretical value for a preparation with the intended content. More commonly, the staff preparing an admixture is asked to place the syringes and vial/ampules used to compound the preparation on a tray with the final admixture for checking by a pharmacist. These supplies are checked to verify the use of the proper component(s) and volume (based on syringes drawn to the amount used) for each admixture.

Sterility is best evaluated through process validation. This is a method where the staff that compound sterile preparations are asked to simulate the procedures used with media that support microbial growth (usually trypticase soy broth). The final preparation containing the growth media is incubated for 14 days. Positive growth indicates a problem with aseptic technique that should be evaluated. It is suggested that process validation be used after initial training to validate technique, and periodically (every 6 months to yearly) to evaluate technique on an ongoing basis.

Storage and Beyond Use Dating

Two important considerations in assuring the quality of pharmacy compounded sterile preparations are the condition under which the preparation is stored and the time that elapsed between compounding and administration. These are important considerations because of both chemical stability and sterility considerations. Chemical stability issues can be determined from the package insert, a reliable reference such as *Extended Stability for Parenteral Drugs,* the *Handbook of Injectable Drugs,* or other published literature.[16,21]

Sterility considerations are defined in USP Chapter <797>.[14] In the absence of passing a sterility test, USP requires beyond use dating of 48 hours at controlled temperature, 14 days at cold temperature, and 45 days in solid frozen state at -20°C or colder for low-risk level CSPs. For medium-risk CSPs, this dating is shorter— 30 hours at controlled temperature, 7 days at cold temperature but still 45 days frozen For high-risk preparations, beyond-use dating should not exceed 24 hours at controlled temperature or 3 days at cold temperature and 45 days frozen unless sterility testing provides evidence to the contrary.

To protect the patient, the beyond use date should be provide on the label of the compounded sterile preparation.

Maintaining Quality after the Preparation Leaves the Pharmacy

Assurance of proper storage conditions can pose a challenge after the CSP leaves the pharmacy. Temperature requirements can be compromised during delivery to the patient or patient care area. Proper storage after the dose is received in patient care areas must be assured. Usually this means CSPs are stored in a refrigerator. To accomplish this, it may be desirable for the pharmacy to assume responsibility for delivery and storage of CSPs after they leave the pharmacy. If this is not possible, shorter beyond use dating should be used.

Another challenge to maintaining quality after CSPs leave the pharmacy is the reuse of the preparation for patient other than the one for whom the original preparations was compounded. Redispensing of CSPs is often a way to avoid waste but requires oversight by pharmacy to avoid administering doses that might be contaminated or after the beyond-use date. USP requires that pharmacy must have the sole authority for determining whether a CSP not administered as originally intended can be used for another patient.[14] Some examples of considerations that need to be considered in making this decision include the following:

- CSP was maintained under continuous refrigeration

- CSP was protected from light
- No evidence of tampering
- Time remaining before originally assigned beyond-use date and time

Standard Operating Procedures

USP requires that the pharmacy should have written and approved standard operating procedures (SOPs) to assure the quality of the environment and operator technique use to compound sterile preparations.[14] There are specific components to these SOPs that are recommended:

- Access to the buffer or clean area
- Decontamination of supplies in the anteroom area
- Storage of supplies not needed for scheduled operations
- Use of carts to transfer supplies and preparations
- Use of particle generating objects, such as pencils, cardboard, and paper
- Traffic flow
- Policy for jewelry
- Procedures for hand washing
- Policy for food items
- Procedures for cleaning surfaces in the compounding environment
- Policy for maintaining ISO class 5 critical area conditions
- Handling of supplies within the critical area
- Inspection and final preparation checking procedures
- Removal of preparations and supplies from the critical area
- Environmental monitoring

Readers are referred to USP Chapter <797> for a more detailed summary of the appropriate content of SOPs.[14]

Summary

Centralized, pharmacy IV admixture programs are a best practice for minimizing the risks of patient harm with intravenous drug therapy. This system should be in place for compounding all IV medications for routine use in the health system. There are cases where the urgency of clinical need is too critical for the time required for a dose to be compounded in a centralized, pharmacy IV admixture area. In these cases, doses may need to be prepared extemporaneously in patient care areas, often by nonpharmacy personnel. In these cases, greater vigilance is needed to assure the accuracy of calculations and technique used to prepare the dose. Alternatively, premixed, frozen, or point of care activated devices may be used to assure accuracy and maintenance of sterility when a dose is needed quickly. In these cases, the double check the physicians order by a pharmacist is often bypassed. Health care professionals need to work collaboratively to choose the right system to optimize the benefits of IV therapy.

The authors recognize the significant contributions that Kenneth E. Avis, D.Sc. made to this chapter.

References

1. Cohen MR, Kilo CM. High-alert medications: safeguarding against errors. In: Cohen, MR, ed. Medication Errors. Washington DC: American Pharmaceutical Association; 1999.
2. Kaushal R, Bates DW, Landrigan C, et al. Medication errors and adverse drug events in pediatric inpatients. *JAMA*. 2001;285:2114–20.
3. Hicks RW, Cousins DD, Williams R. *Summary of information submitted to MEDMARX℠ in the year 2002. The Quest for Quality.* Rockville, MD: UPS Center for the Advancement of Patient Safety; 2003.
4. Patterson TR, Nordstrom KA. An analysis of IV additive procedures on nursing units. *Am J Hosp Pharm.* 1968;25:134–7.
5. Flack HL, Gans JA, Serlick SE, et al. The current status of parenteral hyperalimentation. *Am J Hosp Pharm.* 1971;28:326–35.
6. Thur MP, Miller WA, Latiolais CJ. Medication errors in a nurse-controlled parenteral admixture program. *Am J Hosp Pharm.* 1972;29:298–304.
7. O'Hare MCB, Bradley AM, Gallagher T, et al. Errors in the administration of intravenous drugs. *Br Med J.* 1995;310:1536–7
8. Thompson WL, Feer TD. Incomplete mixing of drugs in intravenous solutions. *Crit Care Med.* 1980;8:603–7.
9. Perlstein PH, Callison C, White M, et al. Errors in drug computations during newborn intensive care. *Am J Dis Child.* 1979;133:376–9.
10. Pedersen CA, Schneider PJ, Scheckelhoff DJ. ASHP national survey of pharmacy practice in hospital settings: dispensing and administration—2002. *Am J Health-Syst Pharm.* 2003;60:52–68.

11. American Society of Health-System Pharmacists (ASHP). ASHP Guidelines on Quality Assurance for Pharmacy-Prepared Sterile Products. *Am J Health-Syst Pharm.* 2000;57:1150–69.

12. Sanders LH, Mabadeje SA, Avis KE, et al. Evaluation of compounding accuracy and aseptic technique for intravenous admixtures. *Am J Hosp Pharm.* 1978;35:531–6.

13. Flynn EA, Pearson RE, Barker KN. Observational study of accuracy in compounding i.v. admixtures in five hospitals. *Am J Hosp Pharm.* 1997;54:904–12.

14. Chapter <797> Pharmaceutical Compounding—Sterile Preparations. In: *United States Pharmacopeia, 27th rev./National Formulary, 22nd ed.* Rockville, MD: United States Pharmacopeial Convention; 2004.

15. Thompson CA. JCAHO gears up to survey sterile compounding practices. *Am J Health-Syst Pharm.* 2004;61:980–1.

16. Trissel LA. *Handbook on Injectable Drugs.* 13th ed. Bethesda, MD: American Society of Health-System Pharmacists; 2004.

17. Chapter <1116> Microbiological evaluation of clean rooms and other controlled environments. In: *United States Pharmacopeia, 27th rev./national formulary, 22nd ed.* Rockville, MD: United States Pharmacopeial Convention; 2004.

18. Buchanan EC, Schneider PJ, eds. *Compounding Sterile Preparations.* 2nd ed. Bethesda, MD: American Society of Health-System Pharmacists; 2005.

19. Compounding Sterile Preparations: Video Training Program (with companion workbook VHS/DVD). Bethesda MD: American Society of Health-System Pharmacists; 2005.

20. Kastango E. Compounding Sterile Preparations Software. Version 2: Multimedia Learning Tool. Bethesda MD: American Society of Health-System Pharmacists; 2005.

21. Bing C, ed. *Extended Stability for Parenteral Drugs.* 2nd ed . Bethesda, MD: American Society of Health-System Pharmacists; 2003.

Chapter 29

Contemporary Compounding

Christina Martin Barnett, Gus Bassani, William Letendre, Renee Remmert Prescott

Introduction

Compounding is a professional prerogative performed by pharmacists since the beginning of the profession. In references to pharmacy the King James version of the Bible includes compounding: "And thou shalt make an oil of the holy ointment, an ointment compounded after the art of the apothecary; it shall be an anointing oil."[1] Even today, definitions of pharmacy include the "preparing, preserving, compounding, and dispensing of medical drugs."[2,3]

The heritage of pharmacy, spanning some 5,000 years, has centered on the provision of pharmaceutical products for patients. Pharmacists are the only health professionals possessing the knowledge and skills required to compound and prepare medications to meet unique needs of patients. The responsibility to extemporaneously compound safe, effective prescription products for patients who require special care is fundamental to the pharmacy profession.[4]

For a period of 150 years (1800–1950), the role of the pharmacist in America was to "mix-and-make" formulas according to prescriber orders. Compounded formulas were the primary source for medications. In the mid-20th century, the manufacturers' role of providing medication therapies became more predominant and the services of a compounding pharmacist diminished proportionately. The transitional decade was in the 1960s. By 1970, nearly 100% of all prescriptions dispensed were commercially manufactured.

In the last decade, as the role of the pharmacist shifted from primarily drug product distributor to that of medication therapy manager, the responsibility to offer compounded alternatives grew in need. This new paradigm, known as *pharmaceutical care*, practiced in the community pharmacy identified a significant noncompliance problem with traditional medications.[5] As a medication therapy manager, the pharmacist was called upon to provide alternatives to assist the patient to become compliant with the prescribed therapy. It was evident that as the commercially available pharmaceutical therapies increased in pharmacokinetic efficiency, they oftentimes precipitated patient compliance problems. Since most commercially available medications are limited in available strength, dosage form, and flavor, the only means available to patients and prescribers to overcome noncompliance problems is to rely upon customized options. Although the role of compounding as an integral alternative to successful medication therapy had lain dormant for more than three decades, it became increasingly obvious that prescribers required these services to overcome the gap in therapy options for noncompliant patients. Therefore, the role of the compounding pharmacist evolved from mix-and-make to that of a problem-solving specialist. Using fundamental pharmaceutics knowledge, compounding pharmacists invested time and effort to create dosage form alternatives to enhance therapy compliance for difficult patients. No other health professional is capable of bringing to the pharmacotherapeutic decision-making table such concepts as pH, particle size, partition coefficient, protein binding, structure activity relationships, economics, and epidemiology to assist a prescriber in overcoming a medication therapy noncompliance problem. Realizing that such services were available, patients and prescribers alike sought out these specialists in order to assist them to overcome compliance problems with traditional commercially available therapies.

Another significant reason why the need for compounding services has grown is the increase in shortages of commercially manufactured products. These drug shortages can cause significant turmoil in the marketplace. Therefore, prescribers have turned to the compounder for temporary relief in overcoming manufacturer supply problems. Although the U.S. Food and Drug Administration (FDA) bans the compounding of commercially available products in its Compliance Policy Guideline (CPG), it does allow compounders to offer such products temporarily when a manufacturer shortage occurs.

The focus areas that have benefited the most with the availability of customized compounded formulations include: pain management, pediatric and geriatric medicine, wound care, andropause, menopause, sports medicine, dermatology, ophthalmology, sterile products, and veterinary medicine.

Definitions

Compounding—the preparation, mixing, assembling, packaging, or labeling of a drug or device (1) as the result of a practitioner's prescription drug order or initiative based on the practitioner/patient/pharmacist relationship in the course of professional practice, or (2) for the purpose of, or as an incident to research, teaching, or chemical analysis and not for sale or dispensing. Compounding also includes the preparation of drugs or devices in anticipation of prescription drug orders based on routine, regularly observed prescribing patterns.[6]

Manufacturing—The production, preparation, propagation, conversion, or processing of a drug or device, either directly or indirectly, by extraction from substances of natural origin or independently by means of chemical or biological synthesis and includes any packaging or repackaging of the substance(s) or labeling or relabeling of its container and the promotion and marketing of such drugs or devices. Manufacturing also includes the preparation and promotion of commercially available products from bulk compounds for resale by pharmacies, practitioners, or other persons.[6]

Impact on Therapeutic Outcomes

Compounding pharmacy has adjusted to the evolving needs of patients through the decades. Some barriers to optimal health care, however, stand the test of time. As those hurdles become more resolute, the opportunities and solutions afforded by compounding pharmacy become even more significant and essential.

Regardless of the constant advancements in medical technology and pharmacotherapy, patients struggle to complete their regimens. A report published by the World Health Organization (WHO) in 2003 states that only 50% of patients with chronic disease states adhere to treatment recommendations.[7] Complete adherence to short-term therapy may be even more difficult since the temporary disruption of a patient's daily pattern is invasive and inconvenient. Fortunately, the pharmacist has the opportunity to improve patient adherence to medication regimens, a notion that has long been upheld and examined. A review of 30 studies published between 1969 and 1994 concluded that, while the

styles of communication, means of analysis, and reporting techniques varied, the vast majority of studies showed a distinct and positive relationship between patient-pharmacist communication and patient adherence.[8] After extensive discussion with a patient, a compounded product can be tailored to the patient's individual needs to account for daily schedules and habits, preferences, and personal concerns about privacy and confidentiality.

It is far more reasonable to tailor a dosage form to fit into a patient's lifestyle than to ask a patient to adjust his or her lifestyle for the duration of therapy. For instance, it may be much easier for a patient to remember to apply a topical or transdermal cream at bedtime when they may already have a similar habit, rather than asking the patient to remember to take an oral dosage form. More discreet and portable dosage forms, such as troches (lozenges) and topical products packaged in small glide-on or roll-on devices, enable patients to carry medications with them, making multiple daily doses more accessible and realistic. Patients with specific preferences or aversions to tastes can easily be accommodated: palatability of products can be increased by masking the taste of the drug itself, changing the viscosity of the product, altering the response of the taste receptors, and creating complementary flavors. Most practitioners believe that a more involved patient is a more adherent patient: "Since it is the patient who decides how to use the therapy, his or her involvement in the process of explaining and understanding it is the key to improved compliance."[9] Patients who are actively involved in the decision-making process of their regimens—whether that involvement be as complicated as discerning an appropriate dose based on symptomatology, or as simple as selecting a preferred flavor—are more invested, more educated, and generally more adherent.

Satisfactory therapy completion and results are also compromised by a patient's anticipation and experience of potential adverse effects. Compounded products can offer—to both prescribers and patients—the avoidance of such effects. Patients may be sensitive to common preservatives such as parabens, food dyes such as tartrazine (FD&C Yellow No. 5), or sweeteners like aspartame, yet those chemicals can be found in many commercially available over-the-counter and prescription products. A compounded product can be designed to eliminate such ingredients. Lactose intolerance, for instance, can make it difficult for patients to take the majority of manufactured tablets and capsules, while compounded capsules can be formulated using numerous alternative inert fillers.

Adverse effects can be instigated by a host of causes other than patient-specific sensitivities. They are frequently caused by chemical derivatives produced during first-pass metabolism. Utilizing nonoral routes of administration eliminates such metabolism, which can result in possible decreases of adverse effects and, in some cases, decreased doses of medication. Gastrointestinal upset, a common side effect of oral medications, can range from transient and mild to persistent and hazardous but can be eliminated by employing alternative dosage forms. Targeting the drug's site of action, rather than relying on systemic absorption and effects, can improve patient outcomes, whether that is measured in hospital days, time for wound healing, pain rating, quality of life, etc. Transdermal gels and creams formulated with penetration enhancers allow for local delivery of drug for effects at the *site of need*. An example of transdermal application is the use of nifedipine to increase circulation in the feet of diabetic patients. In some instances, numerous medications with synergistic mechanisms of action can be incorporated to not only alleviate discomfort, but also treat the cause of the problem. For example, arthritic and injury-related joint pain has been treated using transdermal dosage forms that incorporate several analgesics to help alleviate numerous types of pain (skeletal, muscular, neuropathic, etc.) as well as agents to decrease inflammation. A study published in 1996 examined drug levels of ketoprofen after application to the back, the arm, or the knee. It was determined that systemic ketoprofen concentrations after transdermal application were about 20 times lower than typical systemic concentrations seen after standard oral dosing. In addition, systemic concentrations after transdermal dosing were 100 times lower than the local concentration at the site of application. These data, along with the adverse effects seen with transdermal dosing (which included only mild, topical effects), lend credence to the concept that the transdermal route is effective in delivering medication directly to the site of action without incurring systemic effects and consequent adverse effects.[10]

Local therapy can also provide more rapid results with fewer adverse effects. Urethral suppositories, or inserts, can be used to deliver local treatment as well as anesthesia and pain control for such ailments as urinary tract infections; urinary muscle spasms and incontinence; and urethral and bladder cancers. Especially for chemotherapeutic agents, the prevention of

systemic activity, combined with a more concentrated, local effect, makes such alternative dosage forms ideal for accelerated, improved treatment.

The distinction between doses that provide therapeutic efficacy and doses that cause adverse effects can be faint; manufactured drugs may not offer the ideal dose to match that distinction. Manufactured combination medications can increase patient compliance, but the fixed doses of each ingredient may be limiting. For instance, the total daily dose of a combination hydrocodone and acetaminophen tablet is limited by the acetaminophen component, which may lead to inadequate hydrocodone dosing. By decreasing the quantity of acetaminophen in a compounded product, a regimen that optimizes the hydrocodone therapy can be followed. In addition, some medications must follow tapered dosing to begin or end therapy or to determine the therapeutic dose. The accuracy and consistency of dosing when tablets are split or broken have long been debated. A 1998 study showed that weight variations between 1,752 split tablets varied by more than 10% in 41.3% of the tablets, and a variance greater than 20% was seen in 12.4% of tablets.[11] Compounded dosage forms can overcome all these concerns since they are formulated for a specific need and can also be adjusted as required by the patient, symptoms, or disease state.

Compounding allows the pharmacist to exercise knowledge and creativity to augment a patient's health care. Understanding of drugs' pharmaceutical and pharmacokinetic characteristics can generate unique therapies with rational pharmacological foundations. For instance, tamoxifen is a nonsteroidal antiestrogenic drug used primarily to treat breast cancer. Its known effects include the ability to decrease cell proliferation; alter transcriptional synthesis; arrest cells in the G1 phase of development; and modulate the production of multiple polypeptide growth factors including transforming growth factor (TGF) and TGF-β, epidermal growth factor, etc. The TGF and TGF-β are known components in the formation of keloid scars.[12] Tamoxifen's down-regulation of TGF-β expression has led to its successful use in the topical treatment and prevention of keloid scars.[13]

Often, patients, physicians, and pharmacists work together to achieve a desired outcome with a pharmacologic regimen, only to learn that the central medication has been discontinued by the manufacturer. In some cases, these discontinuations are due to safety concerns; far more often, however, they are prompted by concerns about economic feasibility, patient demand, or issues relating to the large-scale manufacturing process. Drugs that are used to treat small patient populations and transient disease states requiring only short-term therapy are particularly prone to such decisions. In other cases, the chemical itself is not suited to the lengthy procedure of manufacturing, distribution, and delivery of the drug to the patient. Chemical properties such as stability, light-sensitivity, hygroscopic nature, etc., may make such extensive processes unfeasible. Medications that are not pursued by manufacturers remain essential to patients' health care, and the unavailability of those products can greatly alter the quality and even length of life for those patients. Drugs in pharmaceutical grade chemical form that are still considered safe and effective by the FDA can be obtained by a compounding pharmacist to provide not only that medication, but also a dose, dosage form, and regimen best suited to the patient's needs.

The *traditional* responsibilities of pharmacists are being shifted to other health care professionals: physicians are able to dispense, and nursing staff frequently counsel their patients on medication use. Compounding remains as one skill—indeed, one art form—that will not be delegated. As the *team approach* to medical care becomes mainstream, pharmacists are more recognized as an essential member of those teams, and the focus broadens from disease state-specific to whole-patient awareness. Compounded products lend themselves to this perspective because the individualized care of the patient must be all-encompassing. The success of any therapy, especially those that are compounded, relies on the patient/pharmacist/prescriber triad, and specifically, the involvement and participation of the patient. Compounders must act as consultants for both the patient and the health care providers in order to elucidate and confirm the unique role compounded medications play in medical care.

Patient Consultations

Throughout the profession of pharmacy, the role of pharmaceutical care is being emphasized. Many pharmacists have expanded their traditional dispensing pharmacy practice to include patient consultations. Consulting by pharmacists is not a new idea. The Omnibus Budget Reconciliation Act of 1990 (OBRA 90) requires pharmacists to counsel all their patients on prescribed medications. However, those laws address the minimum expectation of all pharmacists.

Compounding pharmacists spend extra time with their patients to discuss the proper use of the patients' dosage form as well as to counsel the patients on their medication. Many times a private consultation is warranted in order to further discuss disease states and wellness management with patients. Private consultations are most common in the areas of bioidentical hormone replacement therapy, pain management, diabetes care, and men's health. A professional, one-on-one environment similar to a doctor's office setting is typically used. This provides the patient and pharmacist privacy thereby allowing patients to be more comfortable with sharing information regarding health than they typically would feel in a check-out counter setting.

There are multiple goals of the consultation. A primary goal is to educate the patient about his/her disease state and discuss the therapy in detail including the importance of being compliant with the therapy. Additional goals include providing information to the patient on lifestyle modifications and health maintenance. In order to provide such a service, pharmacists must thoroughly educate themselves on the disease state(s) they wish to provide consultations on. Many pharmacists also provide supplemental information for the patient to read to help them better understand the disease state and treatment. Above all, the pharmacist is an invaluable resource in helping the patient achieve his/her treatment goals.[14]

Clinical Applications

The compounding pharmacist is well-equipped, trained, and positioned to solve unique patient problems. It is impossible, however, to fully comprehend the impact of compounding without examining *real-life* practice settings and case examples. It is critical to note that, due to the specialized nature of this form of care, much of the clinical information is anecdotal or drawn from the professional experiences of the authors. When available, information published in peer-reviewed or scientific journals is utilized. The compounding pharmacist is continually challenged with clinical scenarios that fall outside the realm of commercially available solutions. Therefore, one must rely on his or her knowledge of pharmaceutics, pharmacology, pharmacokinetics, and chemistry to formulate answers to clinical issues. Compounders must never deviate from the quality assurance standards set forth by their respective State Boards of Pharmacy, as well as the pertinent chapters of the United States Pharmacopeia (USP).

Creativity that is harmoniously meshed with wise, scientific judgment can broaden the therapeutic window. However, effective communication between the prescriber, patient and pharmacist is the most vital component of a compounding practice.

Hospice—Case Study

LT is a 52-year-old female admitted to hospice with uncontrolled nausea/vomiting and inadequate pain control. She has a five-year history of battling breast cancer, which has recently turned metastatic. The Hospice nurse reports that the patient has tried prochlorperazine, promethazine, ondansetron, and a "few others" for her nausea without success. The nurse would like to try a compounded suppository commonly referred to as *RBD,* which is an acronym for Reglan®, Benadryl®, Dexamemthasone. However, the patient and her family are reluctant to insert medication rectally on a regular basis. LT also reports significant pain (6 out of 10) on her lower spine and hip. The physician suspects that this is due to bone metastasis. Recently her pain regimen was switched from oral sustained–release morphine to a fentanyl patch due to nausea/ vomiting. She reports that the patch "takes the edge off" but does not control her pain. She requires 5 to 6 prn doses of morphine liquid every day, which she has difficulty keeping down due to the volume and taste. At the multidisciplinary meeting, the attending physician and nurses turn to the compounding pharmacist for medication suggestions. The pharmacist recommends a transdermal gel containing metoclopramide, diphenhydramine, dexamethasone, and haloperidol for LT's nausea. This gel is applied, after a warm moist compress, to LT's inner wrist every 4 to 6 hours as needed. The gel is designed to deliver the medication through the skin and into the systemic circulation. Because LT is having difficulty with her prn morphine doses, the pharmacist also recommends compounding a more concentrated solution of morphine and flavoring as per LT's request. This should reduce the volume required for each dose and improve the taste. The pharmacist remembers that NSAIDs are often beneficial for metastatic bone pain and suggests another transdermal gel containing ibuprofen, which is applied locally to the area of pain every 4 hours. With the aid of the compounding pharmacist, LT's nausea improved and her pain was dramatically reduced (2 out of 10).

Patients in the hospice setting consistently present with formidable drug therapy challenges. Swallowing difficulties, limited or nonexistent intravenous access, complicated pain syndromes, and unresponsive nausea are just a few examples of issues seen every day. In many instances practitioners have "tried everything" with little success.

When medication cannot be administered orally, the rectal route is often employed. This creates a problem because the vast majority of drugs are not commercially available in a rectal dosage form. The oral medication is either extemporaneously prepared in a suppository by a compounding pharmacist or administered rectally in its original form (i.e., inserting a tablet or capsule rectally). Compounders can combine multiple drugs into an individual suppository as well, making drug therapy more acceptable and efficient for both the patient and caregiver. While the rectal route is a viable alternative to oral delivery, it can be stressful and uncomfortable for the patient and family. Many pharmacists have utilized transdermal gels to deliver medications through the skin and into the systemic circulation. Early studies on the use of lecithin organogels and poloxamer gels as vehicles for the transdermal delivery of medications have made it possible for patients to receive medications in a noninvasive and nonstressful manner.[15,16] Many hospice patients have benefited from the transdermal delivery of opiate analgesics, antinausea medications, anticholinergics, corticosteroids, and antiepileptics to name a few.[17] Transdermal gels prepared by the pharmacist are easily customizable dosage forms that are well-received by patients, families, and physicians.

Preparing oral solutions of medications in higher concentrations than commercially available can be extremely valuable. For example, preparing a morphine sulfate solution in a concentration of 50 mg/mL instead of 20 mg/mL will reduce the required volume of administration. Simple issues, such as the flavor of an oral solution, can be significant deterrents to successful pharmacotherapy. Compounding pharmacists have the ability to prepare an oral solution or suspension that is more palatable.

The difference between adequate pain control and excessive somnolence can be a fine line. With the aid of a compounding pharmacist, a dosage form can be prepared that delivers the exact amount of medication required for pain control and nothing more. For example, imagine a patient that is on oral morphine for pain control. The patient has had success using a commercially available oral sustained-release formulation but is caught *in between* strengths. Pain control is not achieved at 100 mg, but increasing the dose to 200 mg eliminates the ability to communicate or stay awake. The compounding pharmacist is able to prepare a sustained-release capsule of morphine sulfate that is 135 mg, which controls the pain and enables the patient to be cognizant.

Customization is an invaluable tool in the hospice environment. As part of the hospice multidisciplinary team, the compounding pharmacist has the opportunity to interact with a variety of professionals, all focused on the individualized care of the patient. With the help of compounding, hospice patients and their families have more options.

Wound Care—Case Study

RC is a 78-year-old bedridden man in a local nursing home. A nurse phones the pharmacy and reports that RC has a decubitis ulcer that has not responded to therapy. She states that the gels she has applied do not stay in place long enough to "do the job" and that the ulcer is causing him pain. It has also developed a significant odor. The patient's physician requested that the nurse call the compounding pharmacist for suggestions. The pharmacist suggests a powder dosage form that is designed to adhere to wet surfaces. She tells the nurse that she can incorporate specific active ingredients, such as metronidazole (for the bacteria causing the odor), phenytoin (for wound healing) and lidocaine (for pain). The powder is lightly "puffed" onto the wound after dressing changes and is then lightly sprayed with water for irrigation to finalize gel formation. Later the nurse reports that the odor is gone and the patient is out of pain. The wound appears to be improving.

Physicians and nurses are continually challenged in the area of wound care. One issue that can be troublesome is adherence of products to the site. Often gels and creams do not adhere to the wound, especially if it is purulent or *oozing*. Some pharmacists have incorporated active ingredients into powder dosage forms that are designed to stay at the site of application. This powder, which is sometimes referred to as the *polyox mucosal bandage* can be prepared with active ingredients such as phenytoin (healing properties, collagen stimulator), misoprostol (healing), aloe vera (healing), local anesthetics (pain), and antibiotics (if necessary).[8,19] The powder is simply puffed onto the wetted wound and then lightly sprayed with water for irrigation to complete gel formation. Astringents such as tannic acid can be added if there is a problem with bleeding.

With tissue damage often comes pain, and there have been studies investigating the role of peripheral opioid receptors in pain perception. In some instances, pharmacists have prepared low concentration morphine sulfate solutions that can be applied to the wound for pain control.[20] This compounded preparation targets the peripheral opioid receptors that are exposed in the wound, and there is no systemic action.

Pain Management—Case Study

BM is a 65-year-old female complaining of a "burning and itching" pain that radiates from her waist to her toes. Two years ago she fell from a second story while cleaning a window. Her hip was broken and she sustained injury to her lower spine. Over the past 2 years the pain in her legs has progressively worsened. Her physician prescribed oral nortriptyline and eventually added oral gabapentin for her neuropathic pain. She states that the medications help the pain but make her somnolent and give her extreme dry mouth. She is seeking alternatives, so the physician calls the compounding pharmacist for suggestions. After consultation with the patient and the physician, the pharmacist suggests a combination of gabapentin, ketamine, ketoprofen, and baclofen in a topical gel. This gel is applied to either side of the spine in the lumbar-sacral region four times a day and every 2 hours as needed. This is designed to achieve high concentrations of these drugs locally, with minimal systemic levels.

Along with the customized oral and transdermal dosage forms previously discussed, there is considerable need for efficacious neuropathic pain therapies. Neuropathic pain is a complex multineurotransmitter mediated problem that often requires multiple drugs to achieve results. By utilizing topical gels, the pharmacist and physician can target these nerve endings locally with multiple medications, thus reducing the chances of systemic side effects.[21] For example, gabapentin, ketamine, and amitriptyline can be applied topically to achieve high tissue concentrations around specific nerve endings, while potentially achieving negligible systemic concentrations. Each of these drugs, when taken orally, can be very sedating and can have many undesirable side effects, such as dry mouth or nightmares.

Pediatrics—Case Study

SG is a 6-year-old boy who presents to the pediatrician

with otitis media. SG has suffered with otitis media over six times in the past 9 months. The pediatrician decides to place him on a chronic antibiotic. Sulfamethoxazole-trimethoprim is the choice, but SG refuses the medication due to taste. Other antibiotics are tried, but SG refuses. In a state of frustration, the pediatrician calls the compounding pharmacist to discuss the problem. The pharmacist asks if the parents know of a flavor or type of treat that the child enjoys. The parents state that SG "really likes chocolates." Using creative pharmaceutics, the pharmacist decides to calibrate a bear mold in order to make sulfamethoxazole-trimethoprim chocolate bears. A small number of SMZ-TMP bears are made as a trial. SG has no problems taking the bears and states that they are "yummy!" Thanks to the creativity of the compounding pharmacist, SG's ear infections are controlled.

Children can be some of the most challenging patients. Palatability is one the most critical aspects of pediatric dosage forms. In some cases the formulation may only require the addition of a sweetening agent such as acesulfame potassium, stevioside, saccharin, or aspartame. Increased sweetness can, in some cases, eliminate bitterness.[22] The right flavor or flavor blend is also critical. Since taste is subjective, the ability of the compounding pharmacist to individualize flavor is tremendously desirable. Many artificial and natural flavors are available for compounding pharmacists to utilize in their practices. Novel dosage forms can be of value in pediatrics as well. Examples of this would be lollipops, flavored troches or lozenges, and gummy bears.

Children with disabilities or other special needs may require specialized dosage forms as well. Pediatric dentists, for example, may have a need for sedative *cocktails* with difficult patients prior to procedures. Transdermal delivery of medication, as stated previously, may also be valuable in this patient population. For example, the use of antinausea medication in transdermal gels may provide a desirable alternative to suppositories. This may lead to greater compliance and efficacy.

Geriatrics—Case Study

AB is an 89-year-old male currently living in a nursing home. AB has a feeding tube and is unable to take medication orally. The nurse on staff calls the compounding pharmacist to see if there is way to "make all of AB's medication into liquids." Currently the nursing staff is required to crush his medication and flush them down the feeding tube. The nurse states that sometimes the tube becomes "clogged" due to powder agglomeration. After consulting stability data on AB's medication, the pharmacist ascertains that he can compound suspensions of all the medications in question. Since the drugs are going down a tube, flavor is not a potential issue. Therefore, aqueous suspensions with methylcellulose are prepared for AB's medication. This saves time for the nursing staff and helps prevent clogging of the tube.

The extemporaneous preparation of oral suspensions is one the most common requests that a compounding pharmacist will receive. This is especially common in the nursing home environment. It is important to consult available reference texts regarding the stability of medication in the desired vehicle before preparing the suspension. An example of this type of text is *Trissel's Stability of Compounded Formulations*.

The use of NSAIDs in the elderly population is often desired, but concerns about GI side effects and renal toxicity limit their overall usefulness. Topical NSAIDs offer the potential advantage of achieving high tissue concentrations and low systemic absorption.[9G,10G] This would allow a patient to apply a ketoprofen gel, for example, to his arthritic knee with a decreased concern for GI ulcers. Topical preparations containing NSAIDs such as ketoprofen and diclofenac have been available commercially in other countries for many years. For example, Voltaren Emulgel® (Novartis Consumer Health Australasia Pty Ltd) is a topical formulation of diclofenac that is manufactured in Germany. Compounding pharmacists have recognized the need for topical anti-inflammatories and have been helping geriatric patients with these types of compounds since the early 1990s.

Ophthalmology—Case Study

TR is a 42-year-old male who presents to the ophthalmologist with a severe fungal infection of the right eye. Based upon TR's physical exam, the ophthalmologist decides to empirically start amphotericin B as an eye drop while awaiting culture and sensitivity results. Since amphotericin B is not commercially available as an ophthalmic drop, the physician calls the compounding pharmacist for assistance. The pharmacist utilizes an injectable form of amphotericin B to prepare an eye drop for TR.

Ophthalmologists encounter a number of issues that may require customized dosage forms. Enough ophthalmic preparations have been compounded over the years that, at one time, there was a textbook in publication entitled *Extemporaneous Ophthalmic Preparations* by Lois Reynolds and Richard Closson. This text contained over 50 compounded ophthalmic formulations. In many cases the injectable form of a drug is utilized in the preparation of an eye drop. One example may be the preparation of an eye drop with a unique combination of antibiotics from the injectables. Stability of these combinations may not be long enough for a manufacturer to justify bringing the product to market. Therefore, the only source of this treatment would be the pharmacist. Compounding pharmacists regularly prepare eye drops with a variety of ingredients, including antibiotics, antifungals, corticosteroids, anesthetics, and NSAIDs. Preparing eye drops and intraocular injections requires the use of aseptic technique and compliance with State Board regulations regarding aseptic compounding.

Dermatology—Case Study

JB is a 33-year-old female who presents to the dermatologist with dermatitis on her face and arms. After many sensitivity tests, it is determined that JB has an allergy to several common preservatives used in cosmetics and the food industry. JB is in need of a topical corticosteroid cream, as well as a moisturizing cream that does not contain preservatives. Since manufacturers do not produce creams without preservatives, the dermatologist calls upon the compounding pharmacist to prepare the emulsions from scratch without preservatives.

Dermatologists regularly encounter patients with environmental sensitivities that may require a customized topical preparation. For example, making a cream that is preservative-free, or free of a particular ingredient, could mean the difference between therapeutic success and failure. The compounding of a cream is probably the most recognized aspect of compounding. Most pharmacists recall levigating creams as part of a pharmaceutics laboratory course. However, compounding for dermatologists can be much more technical than this simple levigation. Compounding pharmacists may use equipment such as ointment mills or electronic mortar and pestles to mix topical preparations. Examples of common dermatologic compounds include topical anesthetics for laser hair removal, acne preparations with multiple ingredients, antiaging or antiwrinkle creams, and topical formulations for warts.

Sports Medicine/Physical Therapy—Case Study

SW is a compounding pharmacist who developed a professional relationship with a physician who is on staff with a local professional sports team. Muscle injuries are commonplace with this patient population, and having a medication that is easy to administer is highly desirable. The team physician commonly calls upon SW to prepare transdermal gels containing anti-inflammatory agents such as ketoprofen and muscle relaxants such as cyclobenzaprine or guaifenesin. These gels are conveniently applied by the athlete or trainer, and the players have been happy with the results.

A recent study regarding the effect of topical ketoprofen on delayed onset muscle soreness, as well as current information regarding the behavior of NSAIDs when applied topically, point to the therapeutic potential of transdermal NSAID gels.[23–25] Sports medicine specialists and physical therapists continually seek out creative and convenient methods for delivering medication to athletes. The ability to administer potent anti-inflammatory medication directly to the site of injury without the need for systemic administration can be very valuable for the patient from a cost as well as satisfaction standpoint. The compounding pharmacist may widen the therapeutic window for this practice niche. For instance, physical therapists often require the preparation of customized phonophoresis gels and iontophoresis solutions. Examples include hydrocortisone phonophoresis gel and dexamethasone iontophoresis solutions.

Dentistry—Case Study

MJ is a 14-year-old female who presents to the dentist with severe recurrent aphthous stomatitis. She has multiple ulcers in her mouth that are making it difficult to eat, drink, and speak. The dentist has tried commercially available mouth pastes with triamcinolone, but adherence is a problem. The pastes only provide a few minutes of relief. Anesthetic rinses numb the entire mouth, which MJ does not like. The dentist calls the compounding pharmacist for suggestions. The pharmacist recommends a powdered mucosal bandage that is puffed onto the surface of the ulcer, using a puffer device. The powder contains an anesthetic, corticosteroid and an antibiotic. When the powder comes in contact with the wet mucosal surface, it forms a sticky adherent gel that does not move. It also provides a protective barrier over the ulcer, which reduces MJ's pain as well.

The needs of dentists are very unique. Whether it is the compounding of a dry socket paste or an adherent powder for recurrent aphthous stomatitis, compounding pharmacists can have a positive influence in the care of dental patients. A common problem in the treatment of mouth ulcers is the wet environment of the oral cavity. Many products have a difficult time adhering to the oral mucosa, thus diminishing the contact time of the drug at the site of action. The use of a *denture powder* type dosage form that is impregnated with active ingredients such as anesthetics, antivirals, antifungals, corticosteroids, or antibiotics may be desirable to the dentist.[26,27] This improves adherence properties and increases the contact time of the drug to the site of action. Dentists commonly request paste formulations for dry sockets with a variety of active ingredients. Commercial availability of products specific to the needs of dental patients is limited. Other commonly prescribed dental compounds include anesthetic gels designed for application prior to an injection, anesthetic solutions for the gums, lip balms or ointments with a variety of active ingredients, bleaching gels, etching gels, and mouthwashes.

Veterinary—Case Study

WS is a local veterinarian who works with exotic animals at the city zoo. The zoo's families of orangutans are fighting a case of lethal tularemia, and the vet calls the compounding pharmacist inquiring about the best method to administer doxycycline. The animals are very finicky and are refusing medication. The pharmacist asks the vet about their favorite foods. The vet states that the orangutans really enjoy peanut butter and jelly sandwiches, specifically with grape jelly. The pharmacist recognizes that doxycycline has limited shelf life in an aqueous environment (refrigerated), but it is much more stable if frozen. So, the pharmacist recommends a doxycycline grape jelly paste that is prepared with grape jelly and a hydroxypropyl methylcellulose gel. Additional sweeteners are added for bitterness suppression. The paste is unit-dosed in oral syringes, and the syringes are stored in the freezer until administration time. The vet squirts the paste onto a slice of bread with peanut butter, and the animals take the drug without conflict. Thanks to the pharmacist, these precious animals are saved.

Many pharmacists do not realize that there is a desperate need for customized dosage forms in veterinary medicine. Commercial products are lacking in the veterinary world. Combine this fact with the large variety of species, and the therapeutic void becomes obvious. Producing drug products that are palatable to a large number of animals is impossible for drug manufacturers. Compounding pharmacists have the ability to make suspensions, for example, in a variety of flavors ranging from chicken to liver to cheese. Every animal is different, including those within the same species. It is logistically impossible for the manufacturing arena to solve all of the drug therapy problems encountered in the veterinary world. Compounding pharmacists are well-positioned and trained to assist veterinarians in the treatment of animal patients.

Women's Health—Case Study

DB is a 56-year-old healthy woman who reports to her physician complaining of hot flashes, night sweats, "foggy thinking," vaginal dryness, fatigue, and diminished libido. She also reports that she has not menstruated in almost a year. Her physician decides to check DB's hormone levels. The results indicate low estradiol, estrone, progesterone, and testosterone levels. The physician states the results are consistent with menopause. DB is an avid reader and vocalizes to her doctor that she is apprehensive about taking synthetic or animal derived estrogens and progestins such as those used in the Women's Health Initiative (WHI) study. The physician mentions to the patient that a compounding pharmacist can prepare a formulation that consists of hormones identical to what the body normally produces, which is sometimes referred to as *bioidentical*. Satisfied with this option, the patient agrees to therapy. The physician calls the compounding pharmacist to discuss DB's clinical situation and hormone levels. After consulting the pharmacist, the physician prescribes a Bi-Estrogen (estradiol and estriol), progesterone, and testosterone cream to replace DB's low levels. The physician prefers topical administration in order to bypass first pass hepatic metabolism of the hormones. Four weeks after initiating therapy DB reports a "dramatic" reduction in symptoms and improved energy. The physician instructs DB to continue therapy and return in 2 months for a follow-up evaluation and hormone levels.

Physicians and patients commonly seek out alternatives to synthetic estrogens, progestins, and androgens for hormone replacement therapy. Compounding pharmacists have been called upon to prepare formulations containing *bioidentical* hormones, which are structurally identical to those produced in the human body. Some practitioners liken this therapeutic philosophy to the use of human insulin in diabetes instead of animal derived insulin. Compounding pharmacists also have the ability to customize the hormone dose in order to meet the individual needs of the woman. Topical creams, oral capsules, troches, sublingual drops, vaginal creams, and suppositories can be prepared by the pharmacist. Each woman's clinical situation may be different and, therefore, may require a completely unique pharmacotherapeutic approach. Compounding broadens the available treatment options for these patients and physicians.[28]

Quality Assessment/Quality Control

Regulatory agencies such as the FDA, the Occupational Safety and Health Administration (OSHA), and the State Boards of Pharmacy are paying more attention to the practice of compounding pharmacy. In recent years, many new regulations and standards of practice have been implemented mandating that compounding pharmacies practice at a higher level of quality. These regulations were put in place to ensure patients receive more safe and effective medications. Pharmacies therefore have had to change the way they operate to account for these new regulations. In order to comply, various quality assurance and quality control mechanisms are being put in place by compounding pharmacies across the country. It is the responsibility of the pharmacist to compound prescriptions that are not only packaged and labeled correctly but also of acceptable strength, quality, and purity.

Continuous quality improvement in all steps of the compounding process is necessary to assure regulations are being followed. For instance, in the preparatory phase, the pharmacy staff must take great care in the donning of proper safety attire as well as the selection of proper equipment to be used for the prescription at hand. The compounding laboratory and equipment also must be properly cleaned and calibrated before the compounding phase can begin. During the compounding phase, in order to assure quality, the compounder should prepare the prescription according to the formula record and utilize appropriate compounding techniques. In the final check phase, continuous quality improvement procedures are essential for ensuring the prescription is of good quality. It is the responsibility

of the pharmacist to perform a comprehensive review of the preparation including appropriateness of the physical characteristics, weight variance, percent strength, physical tests, and beyond-use dating. Continuous quality improvement is important as well in the last steps of the compounding process. Documentation and records must be kept on each compound, and the patient or caregiver must be counseled on the proper use of the medication as well as signs to look for regarding evidence of instability.[29]

One way to ensure more safe and effective compounded preparations is to have a policy and procedure manual in place in each pharmacy. Policy and procedure manuals provide step-by-step written guidelines that must be followed by pharmacy personnel on a daily basis. The manual should include policies ranging from reference books in the pharmacy library to daily monitoring of the temperature in the compounding laboratory, as well as quality control checks for each compound that is prepared and accurate handling of medications in order to protect the safety and welfare of not only the patient but also the pharmacy staff. It is important to ensure that each pharmacy employee is familiar with all the policies and understands what tasks must be done to comply with the policies that have been put into place. Each employee thereby knows what is expected of them and the quality of products and services they should provide. A policy and procedure manual will also assist the pharmacy in maintaining appropriate records and reports. One example of this is a maintenance form check list that includes duties that must be performed daily, weekly, and monthly. At the end of the specified period, the maintenance form can be filed for documentation of duties performed in case of inspection by regulatory agencies. Having a policy and procedure manual and ensuring that those policies are carried out is a very important tool in helping the pharmacy prepare compounds that are of the highest quality and are safe and effective for the patient.

The implementation of safety precautions in the compounding laboratory is a crucial factor in the quality control process. Safety precautions are designed to protect both the compounder and the patient. Personnel engaged in compounding should wear safety apparel such as gloves, masks, and hair covers in addition to a laboratory jacket. Safety equipment for the compounding laboratory is recommended as well. For example, HEPA (High Efficiency Particulate Air) filtered powder flow hoods are designed to decrease the risk of exposure to potentially harmful chemicals. OSHA regulations require pharmacies to have a Hazard Communication Program in place if there is any potential for personnel to be exposed to hazardous chemicals. This program is based on the belief that every employee has a right to know the hazards of the chemicals they are exposed to while at work. Part of this program includes a requirement for material safety data sheets (MSDS) to be readily accessible to each employee. Another aspect of the program includes the orientation and training of employees on safety and the use of hazardous chemicals, as well as measures the pharmacy has taken to reduce or prevent exposure by using appropriate work practices and personal protective equipment.[30]

Another important quality assurance and quality control technique utilized by pharmacies is the testing of compounded medications for stability. Stability is the extent to which a dosage form retains, within specified limits and throughout its period of storage and use, the same properties and characteristics that it posed at the time of its preparation. There are five different types of stability: chemical, physical, microbiological, therapeutic, and toxicological. There are many factors that can affect the stability of a preparation including temperature, light, air, the packaging of the preparation, and qualities of the chemicals themselves such as pH and particle size.[31] The stability information determined by the pharmacy in conjunction with guidelines set forth in USP <795> *Pharmaceutical Compounding—Nonsterile Preparations* will assist the pharmacist in determining an appropriate beyond-use date.

Besides stability testing, pharmacists also have the responsibility to ensure the prescriptions dispensed are of an acceptable strength, purity, identity, and quality. Outsourcing the testing of finished preparations to an independent analytical laboratory to perform these tests is ideal because the pharmacy likely does not have the appropriate equipment to complete such tests. Routine testing of random samples is performed using instrumentation such as a High-Performance Liquid Chromatograph (HPLC).

It is important however to maintain testing that can occur both in the pharmacy as well as in an outsourced laboratory. Product testing outside of the pharmacy is considered a quality assurance technique whereas product testing within the pharmacy is considered a quality control technique. Quality control techniques include tests such as observance of physical characteristics, individual and average dosage form weights, pH, and use of organoleptic technique. Organoleptic testing involves the use of one's senses including taste, smell, and sight to check the quality of the product.

Quality control procedures can easily be performed on a daily basis within the pharmacy. The quality assurance and control techniques employed at each site may vary; however, testing is considered an integral part of the compounding process.[32]

Determination of an appropriate beyond-use date must be done before the prescription is dispensed to the patient. The beyond-use date is the date after which a compounded preparation is not to be used and is determined from the date the preparation is compounded. Even in the absence of stability testing, pharmacists can determine a compound's beyond-use date. One way to do this is to apply information gathered from drug-specific and general stability documentation. Other considerations that the pharmacist should take into account are the packaging, storage conditions and intended duration of therapy. The USP lists recommendations for maximum beyond-use dates when no other information is available.

A final step in the quality control process involves the completion of documentation and record keeping. By maintaining thorough documents, another compounder will be able to reproduce the preparation exactly as was originally prepared. The formulation record and the compounding record are two important forms of documentation that will help accomplish this goal. The formulation record details step-by-step how the compound is prepared, dispensed, and checked for quality. The compounding record documents items such as ingredients, quantities, number of dosage units compounded, name of the compounder, and name of the pharmacist who approved it.[31] Additional records that are important to maintain include laboratory and equipment maintenance records. These records may include daily monitoring of the drug product refrigerator temperature as well as the daily calibration of the electronic balance. All compounding pharmacies must comply with the record-keeping requirements of their individual State Board of Pharmacy.

Compounded Sterile Preparations

The majority of the information on sterile compounding techniques will be discussed in another chapter in this book. The focus of this section is high-risk level sterile compounding based on the regulations set forth in USP <797> *Pharmaceutical Compounding—Sterile Preparations*. The emphasis in USP <797> is the quality assurance program that must be formally put in place by the pharmacy. The program should include information on maintenance of the compounding environment, monitoring of outcomes, and requirements for documentation and record-keeping. Many of the quality assurance and quality control measures put in place for nonsterile compounding hold true for sterile compounding as well.

High-risk level compounding is a type of sterile compounding commonly performed in a community practice setting. The most common example of a high-risk level compound is dissolving nonsterile bulk drug powders to make solutions that must eventually be sterile. Other examples include measuring and mixing sterile ingredients in nonsterile devices before sterilization is performed, as well as the exposure of sterile ingredients, devices, and mixtures to an environment with air quality inferior to ISO Class 5.

Some of the requirements for high-risk level sterile compounding remain the same as the requirements established for low-risk and medium-risk levels. For example, pharmacists who compound high-risk level preparations may do so in a clean room inside a Laminar Airflow Workbench (LAFW) that has met the standards for low-risk and medium-risk levels. Many pharmacists performing high-risk level compounding alternately choose to use a barrier isolator glove box located in a Class 7 area rather than a LAFW inside a clean room to help conserve space in the pharmacy. The barrier isolator boxes must meet the same USP requirements as LAFW.

High-risk level compounding has an increased level of quality assurance associated with it as compared to low- and medium-risk levels. In addition to following all quality assurance steps associated with low-risk level compounding, high-risk level compounding requires a semi-annual media fill evaluation of compounding personnel technique that simulates the most challenging condition experienced and requires simulation of each high-risk level compounding sterilization process.

All high-risk level compounded sterile preparations that are prepared in groups of 25 identical individual, single-dose packages or in multiple-dose vials for administration to multiple patients or exposed longer than 12 hours at 2–8°C and longer than 6 hours at warmer than 8°C before they are sterilized must be tested to ensure that they do not contain excessive bacterial endotoxins, according to USP <85> *Bacterial Endotoxin Test*, and also must be tested to ensure they are sterile, according to USP <71> *Sterility Test*, before being dispensed or administered. USP also requires that any pharmacy compounding sterile preparations regularly establish its own contamination rates using

media-fill simulations for the various types of dosage forms it prepares.

Along with testing of preparations, pharmacies also must evaluate the quality of the compounding environment. This is accomplished by measuring the total number of particles and the number of viable microorganisms in the controlled air environments of the compounding area. Evaluation of airborne microorganisms must be performed at least weekly if high-risk level sterile compounding is performed. The importance of performing these quality control checks is to establish an acceptable baseline and then watch for trends. A sufficient increase in numbers over time should lead to a reevaluation of cleaning and operational procedures as well as air filtration efficiency in the compounding area.

Compliance with USP <797> is essential and pharmacies may be subject to inspection against these standards by their State Boards of Pharmacy. Pharmacists must understand their role in the importance of preparing a sterile product that is safe and effective. The individual criteria set forth by USP <797> are not meant to stand alone; rather they are part of an entire quality control system. Dependable quality control systems must be in place to ensure the sterility and accuracy of the prescriptions dispensed or administered to patients.[31]

Regulatory Criteria

As a resource to assist each State of Board of Pharmacy in promulgating practice regulations for compounding pharmacy, the National Association of Boards of Pharmacy (NABP) published the *Model Pharmacy Rules—Good Compounding Practices*. This guideline provided recommendations as to what are considered minimum current good compounding practices for the preparation of drug products by State-licensed pharmacies for dispensing and/or administration to humans or animals. Of significant note, the definitions of compounding and manufacturing were published. These NABP definitions remain the cornerstone for delineation of the two functions (see Definitions).

The key factor to differentiate compounding and manufacturing is the existence of the *Triad Relationship*—practitioner/patient/pharmacist, which results in an individual patient's medication order to be compounded for the patient.[6]

Although the State Boards of Pharmacy have exclusive jurisdiction over the practice of pharmacy in the United States, in 1992 the FDA determined that compounding pharmacists may use this new problem-solving role to circumvent the new drug application process. To avoid any misunderstanding of the differentiation between manufacturers and compounders, the FDA published a Compliance Policy Guideline (CPG 7132.16 and later renumbered 460.200) to be used by its enforcement staff as reference when inspecting pharmacies. Since several segments of the CPG were regarded as being too restrictive by the compounding pharmacy community, a lawsuit was filed to rescind the guideline. After 3 years of litigation, the lawsuit was dismissed upon appeal in the circuit court. Thus, the CPG was allowed to stand. Since the restrictions in the CPG were not struck down by the courts, the pharmacy profession rallied and sought legislation that would expressly exempt pharmacy compounding activity from the provisions of the Federal Food Drug and Cosmetic Act (FFDCA) of 1938. This effort resulted in the passage of Section 127 of the Food and Drug Administration Modernization Act (FDAMA) of 1997, codified as 21 U.S.C. Section 353a.[33] This legislation set forth requirements that, if complied with by a compounding pharmacy, would prohibit the FDA from determining that the pharmacy was engaged in the manufacturing of an unapproved drug.

One of the requirements in FDAMA was to prohibit the pharmacy from advertising or promoting the compounding of a particular drug, drug class, or drug type, although the pharmacy could advertise and promote its general compounding skills and services. A lawsuit was filed by a group of compounding pharmacists alleging those restrictions created an unconstitutional restraint of free speech guaranteed by the First Amendment of the United States Constitution. The result of this lawsuit that eventually went to the United States Supreme Court was to rescind all sections of FDAMA. The Court's opinion was that one section was inherently connected to all sections and could not be severed from the Act. Therefore, since one section was unconstitutional, it was decided that the whole Act was invalid.[34] In response to the Supreme Court decision, on June 7, 2002, the FDA reissued CPG 460.200 to provide guidance regarding the FDA enforcement policy on pharmacy compounding. This CPG states that the FDA believes that an increasing number of pharmacies are engaged in manufacturing and distributing unapproved new drugs in a manner clearly outside the bounds of traditional pharmacy practice and in violation of the FFDCA. If upon inspection such activities were discovered, the FDA would hold those pharmacies to the same regulatory requirements as drug manufacturers. The specific activities listed in the CPG that may initiate enforcement action include the following:

- Compounding drugs in anticipation of receiving prescriptions, except in very limited quantities in relation to the amounts of drugs compounded after receiving valid prescriptions

- Compounding drugs that were withdrawn or removed from the market for safety reasons

- Compounding finished drugs from bulk active ingredients that are not components of FDA approved drugs without an FDA sanctioned investigational new drug application (IND)

- Receiving, storing, or using drug substances without first obtaining written assurance from the supplier that each lot of the drug substance has been made in an FDA-registered facility

- Receiving, storing, or using drug components not guaranteed or otherwise determined to meet official compendia requirements

- Using commercial scale manufacturing or testing equipment for compounding drug products

- Compounding drugs for third parties who resell to individual patients or offering compounded drug products at wholesale prices to other state-licensed persons or commercial entities for resale

- Compounding drug products that are commercially available in the marketplace or that are essentially copies of commercially available FDA-approved drug products. (In certain circumstances, it may be appropriate for a pharmacist to compound a small quantity of a drug that is only slightly different from an FDA-approved drug that is commercially available. In those circumstances, the FDA will consider whether there is documentation of the medical need for the variation of the compound for an individual patient.)

- Failing to operate in conformance with applicable state law regulating the practice of pharmacy

The FDA further states that this list is not exhaustive and that other factors may be appropriate for consideration in a particular case.[35] In press releases from the FDA in 2004, it was reported that a revised CPG will be forthcoming based on public comments in opposition to the 2002 version. As of this writing, the use of the 2002 CPG for enforcement action has not been recorded in published reports.

Compounding Accreditation

With the increased role of compounding services, United States regulatory agencies have demanded accountability as a means to protect the welfare of the patient. To satisfy some of these concerns, a coalition of pharmacy organizations has founded the Pharmacy Compounding Accreditation Board (PCAB) for the express purpose of raising standards and offering a specialist accreditation status to compounding pharmacies. PCAB is expected to use the USP <795> and <797> standards to measure the competencies of the pharmacies that promote the availability of compounding services. This initiative will most likely be the foundation of the future for compounding pharmacy in the United States. Once the pharmacy accreditation program has been implemented, a pharmacist credentialing program is expected to follow.

The role of compounding pharmacy will grow in the next decade based on the assumption that new therapies will fail to meet the needs of all patients. As the number of patients requiring pharmacy services continues to grow, so will the requests for customized alternatives. It is a bright future for those who understand the marketplace dynamics of this extremely rewarding segment of pharmacy practice. With the launching of the PCAB credentialing initiative, it is expected that the FDA and State Boards of Pharmacy concerns with safety issues will be ameliorated. The credentialing process may foster the recognition of compounding pharmacy as a specialty area of practice in the profession.

References

1. Exodus 30:25. *The Holy Bible,* King James Version. Chicago: Moody Press; 1978.

2. Merriam-Webster Online Dictionary. Available at: http://www.merriam-Webster.com/cgibin/Dictionary?book=Dictionary&va=pharmacy&x=19&y=13. Accessed September 15, 2004.

3. *The Compact Oxford English Dictionary.* Ed 2. New York: Oxford University Press Inc.; 1991.

4. Allen L. The decision to compound. *IJPC.* 1997;1(2).

5. Hepler CD, Strand LM. Opportunities and responsibilities in pharmaceutical care. *Am J Hosp Pharm.* 1990; 47(3):533–43.

6. NABP Model State Pharmacy Act—Good Compounding Practices. Available at: http://www.nabp.net. Accessed September 15, 2004.

7. *Adherence to Long-Term Therapies: Evidence for Action.* World Health Organization; 2003.

8. de Young, M. Research on the effects of pharmacist-patient communication in institutions and ambulatory care sites, 1969–1994. *Am J Health Syst Pharm.* 1996 Jun 1;53(11):1277–91.

9. Claesson S, Morrison A, Wertheimer AI, et al. Compliance with prescribed drugs: challenges for the elderly population. *Pharm World Sci.* 1999 Dec; 21(6):256–9.

10. Shah AK, Wei G, Lanman RC, et al. Percutaneous absorption of ketoprofen from different anatomical sites in man. *Pharm Research.* 1996;3(1):168–72.

11. McDevitt JT, Gurst AH, Chen Y. Accuracy of tablet splitting. *Pharmacotherapy.* 1998;18(1):193–7.

12. Younai S, et al. Modulation of collagen synthesis by transforming growth factor β in keloid and hypertrophic scar fibroblasts. *Ann Plast Surg.* 1994 Aug;33(2):148–54.

13. Chau D, et al. Tamoxifen downregulates TGF-β production in keloid fibroblasts. *Ann Plast Surg.* 1998 May;40(5):490–3.

14. Kuntz RL, Remmert RM. A new trend in pharmacy practice: private consultations. *IJPC.* 2001;5(3):170–2.

15. Chi SC, et al. Release rates of ketoprofen from poloxamer gels in a membraneless diffusion cell. *J Pharm Sci.* 1991;80(3):280–3.

16. Willimann H, et al. Lecithin organogel as matrix for transdermal transport of drugs. *J Pharm Sci.* 1992;81(9):871–4.

17. Allen LV Jr. Dexamethasone/lorazepam/haloperidol/diphenhydramine and metoclopramide in PLO, fentanyl/promethazine in PLO. *IJPC.* 2000;4(4):297–9.

18. Kincaid MR. Options in wound care. *IJPC.* 2002;6(4):92–5.

19. Torsiello MJ, Matthew HK. Transdermal nifedipine for wound healing: case reports. *IJPC.* 2000;4(5):356–8.

20. Twillman RK, et al. Treatment of painful skin ulcers with topical opioids. *J Pain Symptom Manage.* 1999;17(4):288–92.

21. Jones M. Chronic neuropathic pain: pharmacological interventions in the new millennium a theory of efficacy. *IJPC.* 2000;4(1):6–14.

22. Kloesel LG. Flavoring: compounding a treat. *IJPC.* 2001;5(1):13–6.

23. Cannavino CR, et al. Efficacy of transdermal ketoprofen for delayed onset muscle soreness. *Clin J Sport Med.* 2003;13(4):200–8.

24. Franckum J, et al. Pluronic lecithin organogel for local delivery of anti-inflammatory drugs. *IJPC.* 2004;8(2):101–5.

25. Heyneman CA, Lawless-Liday C, Wall GC. Oral versus topical NSAIDs in rheumatic diseases: a comparison. *Drugs.* 2000;60(3):555–74.

26. Vail J. Compounding for diseases of the oral cavity: a discussion with Stu Sommerville, R.Ph. *IJPC.* 2002;6(1):16–8.

27. Bassani G, et al. Compounding for the dental patient: a focus on ulcers of the mouth. *IJPC*. 2004;8(6):436–40.

28. Gillson GR, et al. A perspective on HRT for women: picking up the pieces after the women's health initiative trial—part 1. *IJPC*. 2003;7(4):250–6.

29. Allen LV. *The Art, Science, and Technology of Pharmaceutical Compounding*. Washington, DC: American Pharmaceutical Association; 2002.

30. United States Department of Labor Occupational Safety and Health Administration. Guidelines for employer compliance—1910.1200 App E. October 29, 2004.

31. The United States Pharmacopeia, 27th rev., and The National Formulary, 22nd ed. Rockville, MD: The United States Pharmacopeial Convention; 2004.

32. Kupiec TC. Ensuring compounding excellence: quality control or quality assurance? *IJPC*. 2002;6(2):160.

33. Food and Drug Administration Modernization Act of 1997 (FDAMA). Available at: http://www.fda.gov/cvm/fdama/fadma.html. Accessed September 15, 2004.

34. Smith LK. Regulatory and operational issues of founding a compounding pharmacy. *IJPC*. 2002;6(6):434–7.

35. Guidance for FDA staff and industry: compliance policy guides manual. Sec. 460.200 Pharmacy compounding. Available at: http://www.fda.gov/ora/compliance_ref/default.htm. Accessed September 15, 2004.

Chapter 30

Investigational Drugs in the Hospital

Scott M. Mark, Karl F. Gumpper

Introduction

Since hospitals are the primary centers for clinical investigations on new or investigational drugs, it is likely that hospital pharmacists will at some time be involved in the handling of these special drugs. The extent of the involvement will depend on the type of hospital facility, the willingness of the pharmacist to accept responsibility for investigational drugs, and the amount of service required. In order to carry out this role effectively, it is important for the pharmacist to know the laws governing the use of investigational drugs and the general methodology for handling and evaluating new drugs.

This chapter deals with a review of the current Food and Drug Administration (FDA) regulations regarding the clinical investigation of new drugs and attempts to describe the role of a hospital pharmacist in handling these special drugs. The discussion of the role of the pharmacist is presented in two parts: the basic functions involving the usual hospital pharmacy facilities, and a further, expanded role that involves specialized services and equipment in a hospital pharmacy.

Definitions

Adverse Drug Reaction (ADR)—In preapproval clinical experience with a new medicinal product or its new usages, particularly since the therapeutic dose(s) may not be established, all noxious and unintended responses to a medicinal product related to any dose should be considered adverse drug reactions. Responses to a medicinal product means that a causal relationship between a medicinal product and an adverse event is at least a reasonable possibility (i.e., that the relationship cannot be ruled out).

An ADR to a marketed medicinal product is a response to a drug that is noxious and unintended and that occurs at doses normally used in humans for prophylaxis, diagnosis, or therapy of diseases or for modification of physiological function.

Adverse Event (AE)—An AE is any untoward medical event that occurs in a patient or clinical investigation subject administered a pharmaceutical product and that does not necessarily have a causal relationship to this treatment. An AE can, therefore, be any unfavorable and unintended sign (including an abnormal laboratory finding), symptom, or disease temporally associated with the use of a medicinal (investigational) product, whether or not related to the medicinal (investigational) product.

Audit—A systematic and independent examination of trial related activities and documents to determine whether the evaluated trial-related activities were conducted and the data were recorded, analyzed, and accurately reported according to the protocol, sponsor's standard operating procedures, good clinical practice, and the applicable regulatory requirements.

Case Report Form—A printed, optical, or electronic document designed to record all of the protocol-required information to be reported to the sponsor on each trial subject.

Clinical Trial or Study—Any investigation in human subjects that is intended to discover or verify the clinical, pharmacologic, or other pharmacodynamic effects of an investigational product, to identify any adverse reactions to an investigational product, or to study absorption, distribution, metabolism, and excretion of an investigational product with the object of ascertaining its safety, efficacy, or both. (The terms clinical trial and clinical study are synonymous.)

Direct Access—Permission to examine, analyze, verify, in the evaluation of a clinical trial. Any party (e.g., domestic and foreign regulatory authorities, sponsors, monitors, and auditors) with direct access should take all reasonable precautions within the constraints of the applicable regulatory requirements to maintain the confidentiality of subjects. identities and sponsors. proprietary information.

Independent Ethics Committee—An independent body (institutional, regional, national, or supranational review board or committee), constituted of medical or scientific professionals and nonmedical or nonscientific members, whose responsibility it is to ensure the protection of the rights, safety, and well-being of human subjects involved in a trial and to provide public assurance of that protection by, among other things, reviewing and approving or providing favorable opinion on the trial protocol and the suitability of the investigators, the facilities, and the methods and material to be used in obtaining and documenting informed consent of the trial subjects.

Informed Consent—A process by which a subject voluntarily confirms his or her willingness to participate in a particular trial, after having been informed of all aspects of the trial that are relevant to the decision to participate. Informed consent is documented by means of a written, signed, and dated form.

Investigator's Brochure—A compilation of clinical and nonclinical data on an investigational product that are relevant to the study of the product in human subjects.

Protocol—A document that describes the objectives, design, methods, statistical considerations, and organization of a trial. The protocol also usually gives the background and rationale for the trial, but these could be provided in other protocol-referenced documents. (Throughout the ICH GCP Guideline, the term protocol refers to protocol and protocol amendments.)

Serious Adverse Event or Serious Adverse Drug Reaction—Any untoward medical event that occurs in a patient or subject receiving a drug at any dose and results in death, is life-threatening, requires inpatient hospitalization or prolongation of existing hospitalization, results in persistent or significant disability or incapacity, or is a congenital anomaly or birth defect.

Source Data—All information in original records and certified copies of original records of clinical findings, observations, or other activities in a clinical trial that is necessary for the reconstruction and evaluation of the trial. Source data are contained in source documents (original records or certified copies).

Source Documents—Original documents, data, and records (e.g., hospital records, clinical and office charts, laboratory notes, memoranda, subjects. diaries or evaluation checklists, pharmacy dispensing records, recorded data from automated instruments, copies or transcriptions certified after verification as being accurate and complete, microfiches, photographic negatives, microfilm or magnetic media, roentgenograms, and

subject files and records kept at the pharmacy, the laboratories, and the medico-technical departments involved in the clinical trial).

Sponsor—An individual, a company, an institution, or an organization that takes responsibility for the initiation, management, or financing of a clinical trial.

Sponsor-Investigator—An individual who both initiates and conducts, alone or with others, a clinical trial, and under whose immediate direction the investigational product is administered to, dispensed to, or used by a subject. The term does not include any person other than an individual (e.g., it does not include a corporation or an agency). The obligations of a sponsor-investigator include both those of a sponsor and those of an investigator.

FDA Regulations

At the present time the clinical investigation and marketing of new drugs is governed by the 1938 Federal Food, Drug and Cosmetic Act and the Kefauver-Harris Amendments of 1962.[1,64] These statutes have been implemented by a series of FDA regulations that were published in the Federal Register and the Code of Federal Regulations. In essence, these laws and regulations define the conditions under which clinical investigational drugs may be shipped in interstate commerce and delineates the evidence for the claimed safety and efficacy of the drug which needs to be provided prior to its marketing.[2,50]

Before a new drug is first shipped interstate for clinical use, the sponsor (a pharmaceutical firm, a nonprofit institution, or an individual investigator) must submit a Notice of Claimed Investigational Exemption for a New Drug (FDA Form 1571), commonly called an IND, to the FDA. Form 1571 contains 15 points of information including the following[3,4,6,8]:

1. Complete composition of the drug, its source, and manufacturing data
2. Results of all preclinical investigations including animal studies
3. Background information regarding the training, experience, and facilities of each clinical investigator and of the individual charged with monitoring the progress of the investigation
4. Copies of informational materials supplied to each investigator
5. An outline (or protocol) of the phase or phases of the planned investigation (see The Clinical Investigations below)

6. A statement that the sponsor will notify the FDA if the investigation is discontinued and the reasons why

7. A statement that the sponsor will notify each investigator if a new drug application (NDA) is approved, or if the investigation is discontinued

8. Assurance that the clinical studies will not begin until 30 days after the FDA acknowledges receipt of the IND

Sponsors, Research Bases, and the Investigators

When investigators perform clinical trials, there are two key groups, the sponsor of the trial and the research base. The activity of private pharmaceutical companies has increased dramatically in recent years. We also discuss the vital role of the research base in support of the investigator. As is the case with all types of research, clinical trials cannot take place without a substantial institutional commitment.

Sponsor

The development of new pharmaceutical agents is a long and complex process, but successes have been significant. The process of new agent development is often divided into preclinical and clinical components. In the United States, clinical research with experimental agents is carefully regulated. The ultimate authority for assuring the safety of the public in matters relating to investigational agents and medical devices rests with the Food and Drug Administration (FDA). Additionally, the Public Health Service Act mandates a number of safeguards for the rights and welfare of individuals who are involved as subjects of the research. Regulations of the Department of Health and Human Services (DHHS) administered by the Office for Human Research Protections (OHRP), DHHS, specify the requirements to ensure adequate protections for human subjects. Clinical investigators and institutions taking part in the clinical trials network are responsible for meeting the requirements of the HHS regulations.

Sponsors of an investigational agent are responsible for seeing that clinical trials proceed safely and rationally from the initial dose-finding studies through to a definitive evaluation of the role of the new agent in the treatment of one or more specific illnesses. Collaboration between sponsors and the pharmaceutical industry may occur at any step along the new agent development process. Private companies often submit compounds for testing and joint development.

Research Bases and Investigators

A research base is an entity that assumes a broad range of responsibilities and functions for the support of clinical trials conducted under its name. Examples of research bases include Cancer Centers and Cooperative Groups. The research base supports the investigator in developing, organizing, implementing, and analyzing clinical trials. It assumes responsibility for the quality of the research, both in concept and execution, and has an important role in assuring patient safety. An effective research base enhances the investigator' research in several specific ways. It provides assistance in developing protocols and obtaining approval by sponsoring agencies. It often offers centralized data management and statistical consultation. An effective research base should also provide the opportunity for internal peer review and quality assurance. Obviously, the research base enhances its own scientific credibility by assuming responsibility for the quality of the scientific ideas and the care with which they are tested. These activities may also be an economical way of supporting multiple clinical investigations simultaneously. In short, a research base provides an institutional source of support and assistance for the activities of protocol chairs and investigators.

Investigational New Drug Applications (INDs)

Any organization seeking to sponsor clinical trials with experimental agents must first submit an IND to the FDA.[15] The IND is the legal mechanism under which experimental agent research is performed in the United States. No experimental agents may be administered to patients for research in the U.S. without an IND. All IND sponsors have obligations which are specified in the regulations of the FDA.

The use of the term *sponsor* is generally reserved for organizations assuming broad responsibilities for the development of a new agent. It is also possible for an individual investigator to hold an IND. In addition, an IND must be submitted to perform clinical studies under the following conditions:

- When an investigational agent is manufactured in one state or country and transported to another state or country for clinical use

- When the bulk material (or components of the agent) is manufactured in one state or country and transported to another state or country for further processing, formulation, or for final fill

Although situations arise in which an agent is manufactured and tested within a state, technically, if any component of that clinical product (from the diluent to the vials and labels) is obtained from another state or country, the FDA could require an IND to be submitted and all the requirements to be adhered to.

Preclinical Development

Preclinical development refers to the extensive research that is done on compounds before therapeutic indications are found. Millions of compounds are tested in an attempt to find one that may have a pharmaceutical or medicinal use.

The Clinical Investigation

The clinical investigation of a new drug is divided into three phases and is directed toward producing substantial proof for the safety and efficacy of the drug.[3]

Phase 1

Clinical pharmacology studies represent the initial introduction of the new drug into man. Phase 1 trials determine a safe dose for Phase 2 trials and define acute effects on normal tissues. In addition, these trials examine the agent's pharmacology and may reveal evidence of biologic activity. The purposes of these studies include the determination of human toxicity, absorption, metabolism, elimination, pharmacodynamics, preferred route of administration, and safe dosage range. Phase 1 studies involve a small number of persons (20–80) and should be conducted under carefully controlled circumstances by qualified clinical pharmacologists.[5]

Therapeutic intent is always present in Phase 1 trials; indeed, agents are not tested in patients unless preclinical activity studies have already demonstrated evidence of significant activity in laboratory models.

Animal toxicology studies carried out prior to Phase 1 trials provide the investigator with

- estimates of a starting dose for clinical trials
- prediction of the likely effects of the agent on normal tissues

These data provide the investigator with clues that help focus clinical observation of the patient. The dose is increased gradually by some defined procedure until a level is found that produces limiting but tolerable adverse events and/or clear signs of therapeutic activity. Phase 1 trials define acute effects that occur with a relatively high frequency on normal tissues. Continued careful observation during Phase 2 and 3 trials is essential to identify less frequent acute adverse effects, as well as cumulative and chronic adverse events.

Phase 2

Clinical pharmacology studies are conducted on a limited number of patients (100–200) for the treatment or prophylaxis of a specific disease.[5] Phase 2 studies are conducted by clinicians familiar with the methods of drug evaluation, as well as the disease being treated, and drugs currently in use for this condition. These carefully supervised studies are designed to demonstrate the new drug's efficacy and relative safety.

Each sponsor must devise and implement a plan for Phase 2 trials of new agents. An adequate Phase 2 plan, while conceptually straight-forward, is often difficult to execute. A reasonable plan presupposes answers to the following questions:

- What doses and schedules that have emerged from Phase 1 ought to be carried forward into Phase 2?
- What diseases should be targeted for testing?
- How to integrate full scientific investigation with NDA- or BLA-directed trials?
- How to perform Phase 2 studies if there are limited supplies of the new agent?
- What important laboratory correlates can be made within the context of a clinical trial?

A Phase 2 study

1. determines whether an agent has pharmacologic activity
2. estimates the response rate in a defined patient population

In addition, well-designed Phase 2 trials do not permit the entry of more patients than are necessary to ensure detection of a medically significant level of activity.

Phase 2 studies are disease-oriented. The various diseases are tested in Phase 2 as distinct clinical entities, as each has differing prognostic factors, eligibility requirements, and patterns of responsiveness to a particular agent. The goal of these initial Phase 2 trials is to determine whether the new agent has activity against a particular disease. These trials, therefore, serve as a screen for further study. For this reason, every effort should be made to avoid false results. Although false-positive results are certainly undesirable, false-negative Phase 2 results are especially misleading, as the discovery of a potentially useful agent may be significantly delayed or overlooked altogether.

Guidelines should be adopted concerning eligibility requirements based on patient characteristics that appear to have a particular impact on likelihood of response. Specifically, for initial Phase 2 studies, investigators should seek trials that restrict patient eligibility to the minimum extent of prior therapy consistent with ethical medical practice.

Phase 3

Studies for this phase, involving extensive clinical trials, may be initiated if the information obtained in the first two phases demonstrates reasonable assurance of safety and effectiveness, or suggests that the drug may have a potential value outweighing possible hazards. The Phase 3 studies are intended to assess the drug's safety, effectiveness, and most desirable dosage in treating a specific disease in a large group of subjects. The studies should also be carefully monitored, even though they are extensive.

The FDA should receive constant reports on the progress of each Phase. If the continuation of the studies appear to present an unwarranted hazard to the patients, the sponsor may be requested to modify or discontinue clinical testing until further preclinical work has been done.

If significant activity is observed in any disease during Phase 2, further clinical trials usually compare the efficacy of the experimental therapy with that of a standard or control therapy. If reasonable standard treatment can be defined for the disease in question, we generally wish to know whether the new agent or therapy constitutes a significant contribution in terms of patient benefit. A variety of trial designs may be suitable, according to the state of the art treatment in the particular disease. The most satisfactory ones are the controlled trial that compares the new agent to a standard single agent or a standard regimen plus the experimental agent to the standard regimen alone. Whatever design is selected, however, an appropriate control group must exist and relevant endpoints must be used to measure relative effects. Of greatest medical importance, of course, are relative survival and quality of life. Other measures, such as complete remission rate or disease-free survival, may also be of interest.

These studies, which attempt to isolate the role of a new agent in the treatment of a specific disease, are of obvious importance to industrial sponsors, because the results are pivotal in applications to register the agent for commercial distribution. The results of such trials may be of great medical importance as well. If the control group is properly selected and the experimental treatment is constructed as imaginatively as possible, such trials may yield valuable information for the care of patients.

Every protocol must contain a section that discusses the study design and the plan for evaluation of the data. The major objectives of the study should be stated as hypotheses to be tested, and a target sample size should be clearly specified. Justification for the sample size goal, in terms of precision of estimation or of levels of type I and type II error, should be provided. In a Phase 3 study, it is insufficient simply to give the number of patients to be accrued on each arm. The protocol should specify the test to be used to compare the treatment groups, and the probabilities of drawing incorrect conclusions when performing this test with the proposed sample size should be given. The magnitude of improvement in outcome that can be reliably detected using the planned sample size should also be specified. The accrual rate of eligible patients per year that can be realistically anticipated should be stated and documented. The protocol should describe specific statistical plans for interim analysis of accumulating data. The committee for monitoring interim results should also be indicated.

If evaluation of treatment effect will require use of nonrandomized controls, a thorough description of the control group to be employed should be part of the protocol. This description should include a detailed discussion of comparability issues and analytic techniques.

Phase 3 trials may be submitted from any source eligible to submit a Phase 2 trial Because the sample sizes required for such studies are usually quite large, however, a multicenter approach is frequently the only feasible one. It is expected, therefore, that the clinical Cooperative Groups will be the major research bases for such trials. Proposals for Phase 3 studies from single institutions should be very specific in documenting adequate accrual potential. Furthermore, if the proposal includes collaboration with institutions not formally affiliated with the research base, the protocol should include a description of the procedures by which the collaborating institutions will manage the conduct of the protocol.

Qualifications of Investigators

The sponsor (usually a pharmaceutical manufacturer) of an investigational new drug will ask the clinical investigator to supply the following information before shipping the investigational drug to the investigator: a statement of his education, training, and experience and information regarding the hospital or other medical institution where the investigation will be conducted; special equipment and other facilities. This information will be supplied on form FDA 1572 (Figure 30-1) for clinical pharmacologists engaged in Phase 1 or 2 trials, or form FDA 1573 for physicians engaged in Phase 3 clinical trials.[7]

The training and experience required will vary, depending upon the kind of drug and the nature of the investigation. In Phase 1, the investigator must be able to evaluate human toxicology and pharmacology. In Phase 2, the investigator should be familiar with the conditions and the methods of human toxicology and pharmacology evaluation. In Phase 3, in addition to the experienced clinical investigators, other physicians not regarded as specialists in any particular field of medicine may serve as investigators. At this stage, a large number of patients may be treated by different physicians to obtain a broad background of experience with the drug.

Obligations of Investigators

The investigator, when he or she signs the FD 1572 and FD 1573, agrees to do the following[6,7,16]:

1. To maintain adequate records of the disposition of all investigational drugs including dates and quantities received and their use, and to return any unused supply of drug when the investigation is completed, terminated, or suspended

2. To prepare and maintain adequate and accurate individual case histories designated to record all observations and other pertinent data

3. To furnish progress reports to the sponsor; the sponsor collects and evaluates the results from various investigators and submits progress reports to the FDA at intervals not exceeding 1 year

4. To report adverse reactions to the sponsor promptly so that the FDA and other investigators can be notified

5. To submit annual progress reports and comments regarding disposal of the drug when studies are discontinued

6. To maintain records of disposition of drugs and case histories for a period of 2 years following the date a New Drug Application (NDA) is approved, or if the NDA is not filed or approved, 2 years after the investigation is discontinued

7. To certify that the drug will be administered only to subjects under his or her personal supervision or under the supervision of physicians responsible to him or her

8. To certify that informed consent will be obtained from all patients on whom the drug is to be tested before the test is made, including any person used as a control, or from their representatives, except where this is not feasible or, in the investigator's professional judgment, is contrary to the best interests of the subject. For subjects in Phase 1 or Phase 2 studies, this consent must be in writing. In Phase 3 it is the responsibility of the investigator, taking into consideration the physical and mental state of the patient, to decide when it is necessary or preferable to obtain consent in other than written form.

9. To give assurance that for investigations involving institutionalized subjects the studies will not be initiated until the institutional review committee has approved the study

It should be noted that the FDA does not give formal approval to the submissions in the IND, but it does monitor and review them. The sponsor is notified of any deficiencies, and if a safety problem exists, the IND will be terminated.[5]

So much for our review of the regulations; now to their practical application. With knowledge of the regulations, the hospital pharmacist can inform and advise a physician or clinical investigator who is planning to use investigational drugs how to file a Notice of Claimed Investigational Exemption of a New Drug (IND) with the FDA. The responsibility to inform the FDA on all aspects of the investigation depends on who becomes the sponsor, the pharmaceutical company or the physician (principal investigator) must provide the manufacturer with the following information: a clinical protocol approved by the physician's institutional review committee, a *curriculum vitae* and bibliography of each physician participating in the study, and depending on whether the study is Phase 1, 2, or 3, a signed form FD 1572 or 1573. As the sponsor, the pharmaceutical manufacturer then has the responsibility to communicate with the FDA and holds the IND.

Figure 30-1
Form FDA 1572

DEPARTMENT OF HEALTH AND HUMAN SERVICES FOOD AND DRUG ADMINISTRATION **STATEMENT OF INVESTIGATOR** *(TITLE 21, CODE OF FEDERAL REGULATIONS (CFR) PART 312)* (See instructions on reverse side.)	Form Approved: OMB No. 0910-0014. Expiration Date: January 31, 2006. *See OMB Statement on Reverse.*
	NOTE: No investigator may participate in an investigation until he/she provides the sponsor with a completed, signed Statement of Investigator, Form FDA 1572 (21 CFR 312.53(c)).

1. NAME AND ADDRESS OF INVESTIGATOR

2. EDUCATION, TRAINING, AND EXPERIENCE THAT QUALIFIES THE INVESTIGATOR AS AN EXPERT IN THE CLINICAL INVESTIGATION OF THE DRUG FOR THE USE UNDER INVESTIGATION. ONE OF THE FOLLOWING IS ATTACHED.

☐ CURRICULUM VITAE ☐ OTHER STATEMENT OF QUALIFICATIONS

3. NAME AND ADDRESS OF ANY MEDICAL SCHOOL, HOSPITAL OR OTHER RESEARCH FACILITY WHERE THE CLINICAL INVESTIGATION(S) WILL BE CONDUCTED.

4. NAME AND ADDRESS OF ANY CLINICAL LABORATORY FACILITIES TO BE USED IN THE STUDY.

5. NAME AND ADDRESS OF THE INSTITUTIONAL REVIEW BOARD (IRB) THAT IS RESPONSIBLE FOR REVIEW AND APPROVAL OF THE STUDY(IES).

6. NAMES OF THE SUBINVESTIGATORS *(e.g., research fellows, residents, associates)* WHO WILL BE ASSISTING THE INVESTIGATOR IN THE CONDUCT OF THE INVESTIGATION(S).

7. NAME AND CODE NUMBER, IF ANY, OF THE PROTOCOL(S) IN THE IND FOR THE STUDY(IES) TO BE CONDUCTED BY THE INVESTIGATOR.

FORM FDA 1572 (3/05)   PREVIOUS EDITION IS OBSOLETE.   PAGE 1 OF 2

Figure 30-1, continued

8. ATTACH THE FOLLOWING CLINICAL PROTOCOL INFORMATION:

☐ FOR PHASE 1 INVESTIGATIONS, A GENERAL OUTLINE OF THE PLANNED INVESTIGATION INCLUDING THE ESTIMATED DURATION OF THE STUDY AND THE MAXIMUM NUMBER OF SUBJECTS THAT WILL BE INVOLVED.

☐ FOR PHASE 2 OR 3 INVESTIGATIONS, AN OUTLINE OF THE STUDY PROTOCOL INCLUDING AN APPROXIMATION OF THE NUMBER OF SUBJECTS TO BE TREATED WITH THE DRUG AND THE NUMBER TO BE EMPLOYED AS CONTROLS, IF ANY; THE CLINICAL USES TO BE INVESTIGATED; CHARACTERISTICS OF SUBJECTS BY AGE, SEX, AND CONDITION; THE KIND OF CLINICAL OBSERVATIONS AND LABORATORY TESTS TO BE CONDUCTED; THE ESTIMATED DURATION OF THE STUDY; AND COPIES OR A DESCRIPTION OF CASE REPORT FORMS TO BE USED.

9. COMMITMENTS:

I agree to conduct the study(ies) in accordance with the relevant, current protocol(s) and will only make changes in a protocol after notifying the sponsor, except when necessary to protect the safety, rights, or welfare of subjects.

I agree to personally conduct or supervise the described investigation(s).

I agree to inform any patients, or any persons used as controls, that the drugs are being used for investigational purposes and I will ensure that the requirements relating to obtaining informed consent in 21 CFR Part 50 and institutional review board (IRB) review and approval in 21 CFR Part 56 are met.

I agree to report to the sponsor adverse experiences that occur in the course of the investigation(s) in accordance with 21 CFR 312.64.

I have read and understand the information in the investigator's brochure, including the potential risks and side effects of the drug.

I agree to ensure that all associates, colleagues, and employees assisting in the conduct of the study(ies) are informed about their obligations in meeting the above commitments.

I agree to maintain adequate and accurate records in accordance with 21 CFR 312.62 and to make those records available for inspection in accordance with 21 CFR 312.68.

I will ensure that an IRB that complies with the requirements of 21 CFR Part 56 will be responsible for the initial and continuing review and approval of the clinical investigation. I also agree to promptly report to the IRB all changes in the research activity and all unanticipated problems involving risks to human subjects or others. Additionally, I will not make any changes in the research without IRB approval, except where necessary to eliminate apparent immediate hazards to human subjects.

I agree to comply with all other requirements regarding the obligations of clinical investigators and all other pertinent requirements in 21 CFR Part 312.

INSTRUCTIONS FOR COMPLETING FORM FDA 1572
STATEMENT OF INVESTIGATOR:

1. Complete all sections. Attach a separate page if additional space is needed.

2. Attach curriculum vitae or other statement of qualifications as described in Section 2.

3. Attach protocol outline as described in Section 8.

4. Sign and date below.

5. FORWARD THE COMPLETED FORM AND ATTACHMENTS TO THE SPONSOR. The sponsor will incorporate this information along with other technical data into an Investigational New Drug Application (IND).

10. SIGNATURE OF INVESTIGATOR

11. DATE

(WARNING: A willfully false statement is a criminal offense. U.S.C. Title 18, Sec. 1001.)

Public reporting burden for this collection of information is estimated to average 100 hours per response, including the time for reviewing instructions, searching existing data sources, gathering and maintaining the data needed, and completing reviewing the collection of information. Send comments regarding this burden estimate or any other aspect of this collection of information, including suggestions for reducing this burden to:

Department of Health and Human Services
Food and Drug Administration
Center for Drug Evaluation and Research
Central Document Room
5901-B Ammendale Road
Beltsville, MD 20705-1266

Department of Health and Human Services
Food and Drug Administration
Center for Biologics Evaluation and Research (HFM-99)
1401 Rockville Pike
Rockville, MD 20852-1448

"An agency may not conduct or sponsor, and a person is not required to respond to, a collection of information unless it displays a currently valid OMB control number."

Please DO NOT RETURN this application to this address.

FORM FDA 1572 (3/05)   PREVIOUS EDITION IS OBSOLETE.   PAGE 2 OF 2

If the sponsor is a physician, his institution must provide the FDA with the following: a clinical protocol approved by the institutional review committee, a *curriculum vitae* and bibliography of each physician participating in the study, a signed form 1572 or 1573, depending upon whether the study is Phase 1, 2, or 3, a signed form FD 1571, and manufacturing information.

FDA Authority in the Investigational Use of Commercially Available Drugs

It should be stressed that the FDA has no authority over the practice of medicine and cannot require a physician to prescribe or not to prescribe a drug for a particular illness. However, physicians are encouraged to submit an IND when they use a drug regularly for purposes other than those approved by the FDA. The FDA can then accumulate data on the safety and efficacy of the drug for such treatment and can share the information with other physicians.[3,52]

IRB APPROVAL

The Institutional Review Board (IRB) is an administrative body established to protect the rights and welfare of human subjects (including patients) recruited to participate in research activities.[79] In accordance with the Federal Policy regulations (45 CFR 46) of the Department of Health and Human Services (DHHS) and the applicable regulations (21 CFR 50,56) of the Food and Drug Administration (FDA), the IRB has the authority to approve, require modifications in (in order to approve), or disapprove all research activities involving humans that fall under one or more of the following jurisdictional criteria:

1. The research is sponsored by the organization.

2. The research is conducted by or under the direction of any employee or agent of the organization in connection with his or her institutional responsibilities.[3]

3. The research interventions or interactions are performed at or on an organization property and/or the research involves the use of this institution's nonpublic information.

Information related to the study proposal is submitted to the IRB Investigators and each investigator must meet the requirements of the Federal regulations for human subject assurances and informed consent and for Investigational Review Board (IRB) review and approval. Submissions are generally done on an IRB Cover Sheet or an IRB Service Request Form and contain key elements of the study (Figure 30-2.) Each investigator must also report to his or her IRB any problems, serious adverse events, or proposed changes in the protocol that may affect the status of the investigation and the willingness of patients to participate in it. The investigator must also give a report to the IRB at intervals appropriate to the degree of risk in the study, but no less frequently than once a year, or at study closure.

The Role of the Hospital Pharmacist

The extent of the role of the hospital pharmacist in the handling of investigational drugs will depend upon the type of hospital, its facilities, equipment, specialized services, and the expertise of the pharmacy department. Before discussing the extent of the different roles of the hospital pharmacist, we should discuss what is the minimal or basic involvement of all hospital pharmacists using investigational drugs in their hospitals. This basic role includes the registration, control, storage, dispensing, maintenance of disposition records, and drug information of every investigational drug. In order for the hospital pharmacists to carry out even this basic role, it is imperative that the hospital adopt certain policies for the use and storage of investigational drugs.

Although the FDA does not require that investigational drugs be stored and dispensed through a hospital pharmacy, many hospitals require that all clinical investigational drugs be registered and stored by the hospital pharmacy for dispensing on orders from specifically authorized investigators.[9] The advantages of this policy, which should be stressed to physicians, include the following: drugs can be stored, dispensed, accounted for; they can be observed for shelf-life and stability and returned to the manufacturer if need be by the pharmacy. In addition, some hospitals have established a policy that no investigational drug be administered to a patient by a nurse or physician unless it bears a pharmacy department control or registration number. Armed with these two policies the hospital pharmacists can now exert some effective control over the use of investigational drugs in the hospital.[29,30,49,61–63,71,72]

Usually when the clinical investigator has written the clinical research protocol (which describes the use of the investigational drug) and has obtained the investigational drug from a manufacturer, they meet with a pharmacist to discuss the handling and dispensing of

Figure 30-2
IRB Cover Sheet/IRB Service Request Form

IRB COVER SHEET/IRB SERVICE REQUEST

Reason for Submission New Project [ ] Responding to Comment [ ] Reconsideration [ ] Disapproval Resubmission [ ] Modification [ ] Renewal [ ] Adverse Event Report [ ] Date of Submission:	IND #: IDE #: If there is an IND or IDE number, please include 4 copies of the investigation drug/device brochure	IRB #: **IRB Use Only:** DATE STAMP:

PART A – PROTOCOL/INVESTIGATOR/COORDINATOR INFORMATION
Title of Study:
Principal Investigator: Title of Principle Investigator:
Address of Principal Investigator: School: Department: Division Phone Number: e-mail address:
FAX NUMBER(S) WHERE THE APPROVAL LETTER SHOULD BE SENT: NOTE: HARD COPIES ARE NOT SENT UNLESS THERE IS NO FAX NUMBER LISTED
Co-Investigators:
Coordinator's Name: Address: Phone Number: e-mail address:

PART B-LEVEL OF RISK/TYPE OF REVIEW REQUESTED			
Level of Risk:	[ ] Minimal	[ ] Moderate	[ ] High
Type of Review Requested:	[ ] Full Board	[ ] Expedite	[ ] Exempt

PART C-RECRUITMENT INFORMATION
Would you like recruitment information related to this study placed on the web site established by the Office of Clinical Research? [ ] Yes [ ] No *If yes, please complete the Clinical Research Website Form and attach it to this submission. **Is this a multi-center study?** [ ] Yes – Indicate number of subjects to be enrolled at multi-center sites: [ ] No **If yes, please include 4 copies of the multi-center protocol** **Number of subjects to be enrolled at this site:** Please note: the IRB considers a subject to be enrolled if s/he signs an informed consent document. If a higher number of subjects must be enrolled for screening in order to hit a targeted number of subjects completing the study, please indicate the higher number. Gender: [ ] Male   [ ] Female   Age Range for all Subjects: **Duration of Study Per Subject:**   **Duration of Study (entire study):** **Sites where research procedures will be performed:**

Figure 30-2, continued

PART D-SOURCE OF SUPPORT
Indicate all applicable sources of support and the sponsor: [ ] Federal* - Sponsor: Awardee Institution: _____ (NOTE: If the University is the awardee institution, submission of one copy of the grant is required.) [ ] Commercial** - Sponsor: [ ] Foundation – Sponsor: [ ] Other (specify) – Sponsor: [ ] No support *If federal funding, please provide a copy of the entire grant application. **If commercial funding, please provide either a check, a payment form from the IRB website or a waiver request.
PART E – CONFLICT OF INTEREST
Does the principal investigator or any co-investigator or research coordinator involved in this study (or in aggregate with his/her spouse, dependents or members of this/her household): a. possess an equity interest in the entity that sponsors this research or the technology being evaluated that exceeds 5% ownership interest or a current value of $10,000? [ ] Yes [ ] No b. receive salary, royalty or other payments from the entity that sponsors this research or the technology being evaluated that is expected to exceed $10,000 per year? [ ] Yes [ ] No c. possess a license agreement with the University or an external entity that would entitle sharing the current or future commercial proceeds of the technology being evaluated? [ ] Yes [ ] No If yes, please attach detailed information to permit the IRB to determine if such involvement should be disclosed to potential research subjects.
PART F - RESEARCH COSTS
1. will testing, services, procedures be performed, samples obtained or hands-on care be provided? [ ] Yes [ ] No 2. Will these be done at a University facility?   [ ] Yes   [ ] No If response to both questions is yes, a University review is required. If the patient does not visit any University facility OR if the study involves only data analysis, interviews, or questionnaires, fiscal review is not required. The IRB and//or University also have the authority to require a University fiscal review based on their review.
PART G – ADDITIONAL APPROVALS REQUIRED

1. Has this protocol been reviewed by a prior scientific review committee?
    [ ] Yes (Please attach an approval letter)   [ ] No (Indicate the reason)
2. Does this research involve the administration, for research purposes, of a drug (investigational or FDA approval)?
    [ ] Yes* [ ] No
    *(Please attach written notification of receipt/review from the Investigational Drug Service)
3. Does this protocol involve the exposure of human subjects to ionizing radiation (excluding the use of standard diagnostic or treatment procedures, performed in a routing clinical manner and frequency)? [ ] Yes (Attach approval letter) [ ] No
4. Does this research study involve the deliberate transfer of recombinant DNA (rDNA) or DNA or RAN derived from rDNA into human subjects?
    [ ] Yes* [ ] No
*If yes, attach written notification of prior approval by the University Biosafety Committee

PART H: CREDENTIALING – DEPARTMENT/DIVISION CHAIR APPROVAL
FOR RESEARCH PROCEDURES CONDUCTED WITHIN A UNIVERSITY FACILITY: I have reviewed this human subject research proposal and have determined that 1) the listed investigators are members or associates of the medical staff of the hospital where the research will be conducted and have been appropriately granted hospital privileges to perform the procedures outlined in the research proposal; and/or 2) the listed investigators are employees of the hospital whose job descriptions and competencies qualify them to perform the procedures outlined in the research proposal.   _____   _____ Department/Division Chairman   Date

the drug.[77,78] It is at this initial encounter that drug delivery, control, labeling, ordering, storage, disposition, and authorized coinvestigators are discussed.[73] Specifically the following information should be obtained: (1) name of drug (chemical and other), (2) dosage form and strength, (3) pharmacology, (4) purpose of the investigation, including a copy of the protocol or outline for the study approved by the Institutional Review Committee, (5) route of administration, (6) dosage, (7) side effects, toxicity, and any known antidote, (8) storage conditions, (9) stability of product, (10) pharmaceutical manufacturer and name of its medical director with knowledge of the drug, (11) names of the principal investigator and coinvestigators authorized to prescribe, (12) nursing units, (13) name of sponsor and IND number for the drug, (14) how the drug will be written for (what it will be called), (15) need to relabel product if necessary. Also, product must contain Caution: New Drug—Limited by Federal (or United States) Law to Investigational Use, and (16) arrangements for obtaining additional drug along with tentative utilization rate should also be discussed at this time.

The information enumerated above should be recorded on an Investigational Drug Service Request form (Figure 30-2), which facilitates the registration process and ensures that complete and consistent information is obtained. The physician should also be told that the pharmacy will be preparing an Investigational Drug Fact Sheet for the nurses and pharmacists and that it will be cleared through them prior to distribution. After the pharmacist meets with the physician, the product is labeled with a control number, a disposition record is prepared, and the drug is stored. The clinical investigator can then initiate the use of the investigational drug by writing a drug order on a duplicate Doctor's Orders form in the patient's chart (if such a form exists in the hospital). The nurse on the unit then sends a copy of the duplicate order to the pharmacy. Prior to filling the order the pharmacy checks the disposition record to see if the physician writing the order is an authorized investigator; if so, the order is filled for a specified number of days, generally either a 7-day supply of the drug for inpatient studies, or a 30-day supply for ambulatory studies. Such a procedure would thus establish another hospital policy: all investigational drug orders must be reviewed and rewritten at least every 7 days (or 30 days in the case of ambulatory studies).[10]

Single- and Double-Blind Studies

Pharmacists can be extremely helpful in establishing single-and double-blind studies.[11] Blinded studies are extremely important as part of a clinical trial and are continually emphasized by the FDA to eliminate as far as possible subjective evaluations of drug efficacy. The hospital pharmacy can play an integral role with the investigator in the initiation of these studies because the pharmacist has been trained to design such studies and can act as a consultant to the investigator.

Blinded studies objectively evaluate an investigational drug by comparing its actions to those of a placebo or another drug. In a single-blind study, the patient's course of drug therapy is unknown to him or her. In some cases it is also unknown to the person (either the nurse or nonprescribing physician) evaluating the patient's response to the drug. In a double-blind study the patient, nurse, and prescribing physician are unaware of which therapy the patient receives.

The pharmacist can develop a simple system for coding drugs for single-blind studies. This system involves assigning, after consulting with the investigator, a series number and letters to the drug or drug and placebo. For example, the drug may be assigned letters A, C, and T and the placebo letters B, E, and Y in compound series 492. If the physician wanted to prescribe the drug for the patient he would have three choices and could write a prescription for compound 492A, 492C, or 492T, Likewise, the physician has three choices to prescribe for the placebo: compound 492B, 492E, or 492Y. More letters and numbers can, of course, be assigned if needed to keep the study blinded.

Occasionally there may be a need to break the blind of a study. This is generally only done in the case of an emergency when it becomes medically necessary to know if the patient is on an active drug and the characteristics of the drug.[67,69] For example, it may be necessary to provide emergent medical attention and the choice of therapy may have a significant drug interaction with one of the study medications. When it becomes medically necessary to break the blind of a study, a pharmacist should determine the reason and who is requesting the action be taken. Every effort should be made to minimize who has access to the information and the appropriate study investigators and sponsors should be notified.

Double-blind studies are generally more objective than single-blind studies, since the patient's courses of drug therapy are randomized. This randomization helps to eliminate bias and to give more validity to data generated from these studies. For simple double-blind studies, a pharmacist can use a table of random numbers or a calculator with a random number generator to set up the study. For example, a double-blind study may involve 10 patients, each of whom is to receive a 2-week course of either drug or placebo. To create the random sequence or treatment regimens, one begins by arbitrarily assigning label numbers 1–5 to treatment regimen A (drug) and label numbers 6–10 to treatment regimen B (placebo).[12] Ten consecutive random numbers are then obtained and the first random number is assigned label number 1; the second random number is assigned label number 2; etc. The random numbers are then rearranged in numerical order and the corresponding label numbers provide the random sequence of the treatment regimens.

If the study is more involved, the use of a statistician is imperative, for example, if a study is divided into phases and the patient receives a placebo in one phase and the drug in the other or if the patient population is divided into special groups. This kind of study design ensures the validity of the study. The consultant statistician may meet with the pharmacist or discuss the study with the physician and then prepare the randomization. In the latter case, the physician presents the pharmacy with the randomization in a sealed envelope. In some cases where a pharmaceutical company is sponsoring the study, the randomization, packaging, and matching placebo are all provided. Here the pharmacist is only involved in the drug distribution, data collection, and record maintenance aspects of the study.

At the meeting between the pharmacist and the physician to prepare a double-blind study, certain basic information must be obtained. At first the study is assigned a name. This is to alert the pharmacy personnel that this is a special study when they receive a copy of the physician's order sheet. The study is usually named after the drug being used or the disease being treated. The pharmacist then ascertains the number of patients to be studied, the number and frequency and courses of therapy, the randomization (as discussed above), and the directions to the patient. If the directions to the patient will not change throughout the study, a preprinted label may be prepared. The pharmacist then explains to the physician the format in which the order should be written. This format should be standard for all physicians participating in the study, and the importance of adhering to this format should

be stressed. The more rigid the format, the less likely an error may occur.

A form for use in the preparation of a *double-blind* study in which simple randomization (sometimes referred to as the *urn method*) is seen in Figure 30-3. This randomization sheet can be designed to provide whatever information is needed. Randomization can also be done using a random number table or through the use of an Interactive Voice Randomization System (IVRS). IVRS systems are often used when the randomization involves physiological parameters such as blood pressure. The pharmacist calls the phone system, inputs an identity code and then enters patient-specific information related to their condition. The computer then randomizes the patients to the appropriate treatment group.

Marketing Application

After clinical trials have shown that the new agent is safe and effective, there is reason to make the agent generally available to patients and physicians. The formal process in the U.S. by which this occurs is the approval by FDA of a marketing application (New Drug Application or a Biologic License Application for biological agents). The applicant seeks approval from FDA for one or more specific indication(s). Review and approval of an NDA or BLA are based on the demonstration of safety and efficacy assessed from detailed reports of the clinical trials; particularly randomized controlled studies. The contribution of a new agent in the treatment of a disease is demonstrated unambiguously if the agent is the only variable between the treatments. The specific endpoints that constitute satisfactory evidence of efficacy (e.g., response rate, quality of life, survival) have been addressed in a published paper prepared by FDA and NCI entitled *Commentary Concerning Demonstration of Safety and Efficacy of Investigational Anticancer Agents in Clinical Trials*. The approval of the NDA or BLA is a critical milestone not only for the pharmaceutical company but also for the clinical investigator, and the general public. An affirmative decision by the FDA permits the pharmaceutical company to market and promote the agent for the approved indication(s). Once an agent is marketed, no Federal regulation prevents any licensed physician from prescribing it for any indication he or she deems appropriate.

For the practicing physician, NDA or BLA approval means that the agent is readily available for routine

Figure 30-3
Randomization Sheet

Patient Number	Patient Name	Course 1	Date Received	Course 2	Date Received
1		Drug		Placebo	
2		Placebo		Drug	
3		Drug		Placebo	
4		Placebo		Placebo	
5		Placebo		Drug	
6		Drug		Drug	
7		Drug		Drug	
8		Drug		Placebo	

treatment of patients. The practitioner no longer has to devise acceptable protocols with research intent, simply for the purpose of obtaining the agent for patient care. No longer must he or she use the cumbersome procedures for obtaining compassionate INDs from the FDA to treat individual patients. For the clinical investigator, NDA or BLA approval means that it may be more difficult to recruit patients for further clinical trials with the agent, since use of the agent is no longer restricted to patients on research protocols. For the general public, NDA or BLA approval means that a new effective agent is now available on the widest possible basis. It is admittedly also true that an agent that was formerly available without cost for research purposes is no longer free to the patient after NDA or BLA approval.

Protocol Development

Many research bases have procedures for review of the science of a clinical trial, either at the concept stage or at the time a protocol is written. This review is distinct from the task of the Institutional Review Board (IRB), which may or may not view as part of its charge a critical scientific review. Ideally, a scientific review assists the investigator in focusing his or her ideas and perhaps in identifying other useful scientific resources within the research base. This process should facilitate research and assist in the testing of new ideas. Careful review may be particularly important for Phase 3 trials, because of the very substantial commitment of time, patients, and resources involved.

Biostatistical Consultation

The design of any clinical trial should be based on sound statistical principles. Issues such as sample size, stopping rules, endpoints, and the feasibility of relating endpoints to objectives are pivotal to a successful trial. Statistical expertise should be provided by a research base.

Protocol Administration

Since most protocols require multiple levels of approval, and since policies of the various sponsoring agencies may differ and change with time, a research base can provide valuable assistance to the investigator in obtaining these approvals. Establishment of a centralized mechanism for submitting and tracking a protocol through the necessary approvals, including the IRB, saves individual investigators a very large expenditure of time and effort that is much better directed elsewhere. A research base with multiple sponsored protocols could efficiently assume the responsibility for communicating status changes, amendments, results reports, publications, and other pertinent protocol administration information.

Letters of Intent

The Letter of Intent (LOI) is an investigator's declaration of interest in conducting a Phase 1 or 2 trial with a specific investigational agent in a particular disease. LOIs are often used when the supply of a particular agent is limited. It helps the vending agency maximize the efficiency and fairness by which experimental agents are allocated to investigators for study. For the investigator, the LOI system also promotes much saving of time and effort, because its use should spare him or her the writing of a protocol that might not be approved. The LOI system also is used for the submission of combination pilot studies. In these cases, reviews typically focus on the rationale for combining the agents, the proposed sample size, and the adverse events of each agent when given alone.

Content of LOIs

In order to review the LOI properly, it must have the following information:

- Principal investigator
- Lead group/institution
- Other participating groups/institutions
- Patient characteristics, including extent of prior therapy, performance status, and abnormal organ function permitted (if any)
- Phase of study
- Treatment plan—agents, doses and schedule of administration
- Rationale/hypothesis
- Laboratory correlate
- Endpoints/statistical considerations
- Proposed samples size
- Estimated annual accrual
- Accrual documented by prior (similar) trials
- List of competitive studies

A letter should also accompany the LOI that explains in greater depth the rationale, where not obvious, or any unique features of the study.

Informed Consent

Each patient should complete a document referred to as informed consent. The purpose of this document is to educate patients on the known risks of each therapy or procedure.[58–60] Each informed consent document must be protocol-specific and contain the elements required by Federal regulation. These regulations do not specify the language of the document but provide a list of elements that must be addressed in the text of the consent form.

Protocol authors should be certain that the description of expected adverse events is complete and balanced and reflective of the treatment plan to be used. Adverse events of other modalities used in the study (e.g., radiotherapy, surgery) must also be described.

In response to concerns that many informed consent documents for clinical trials have become complex, lengthy, and difficult to understand, working groups of medical, ethical, communication, and consumer experts along with officials from the FDA were convened. The result of this initiative is the development of guidelines for writing consent documents that are more understandable to prospective research participants.

Many have asked about the legality of review of a patient's primary medical record by outside individuals. The answer is straightforward. No Federal law prohibits external review of a patient's medical record. The regulations of informed consent do require, however, that the patient be informed of "the extent to which confidentiality of records will be maintained."[80] This means that there is no rule against chart review by outsiders but that the patient must be told what will be done.

Drug Information

Before an investigational drug is administered to a patient, the nurse should have basic information concerning the drug, including dosage forms and strengths available, actions, and uses, adverse effects, toxicity, and antidote. This information can be provided in the form of an Investigational Drug Data/Fact Sheet (Figure 30-4). The data on the sheets is approved by the Principal Investigator prior to its release and is updated by the pharmacy as more information becomes available. In addition to providing the data sheets to the nurses, they may be distributed to other pharmacists and authorized personnel. The Joint Commission on Accreditation of Healthcare Organizations (JCAHO) specifically lists investigational drugs in standard MM 3.20 as an example of an order type which must have specific institutional policies on file to govern their use. Standard MM 1.10 further states that information must be readily accessible to all involved staff. For this reason, information related to an investigational drug should be kept in a patient's chart so that it is available to any health care provider not familiar with the product.[27,32,59]

The pharmacy may also maintain an information file on each investigational drug that is registered and used in the hospital. Such a file is very useful in helping to answer any inquiries about the drug. Included in each file is the registration form, copy or outline of the protocol, drug fact sheet, drug disposition records,

Figure 30-4
Investigational Drug Service/Drug Data Sheet

UNIVERSITY MEDICAL CENTER
DEPARTMENT OF PHARMACY
INVESTIGATIONAL DRUG SERVICE
DRUG DATA SHEET

SMM-16

How does this medication WORK?
- SMM-16 is an immunoconjugate created by conjugation of the cytotoxic maytansinoid to a humanized version of the murine monoclonal antibody.

What is the investigational USE of this medication?
- Evaluation of the efficacy and safety in small cell lung cancer, CD56+ small cell carcinomas

What DOSAGE FORMS are available? What is the usual DOSAGE RANGE?
- SMM-16 is available as a 20 mL buffered solution for injection; concentration 1 mg/mL; pH 6.0 – 7.0.
- Each cycle of therapy for Study #2006 will be 60 mg/m² weekly x 4, then off 2 weeks. May be repeated up to 6 cycles

What are frequent ADVERSE EFFECTS that have been observed?
- Retroperitoneal hemorrhage
- Pancreatitis
- Aseptic meningitis
- Peripheral sensory neuropathy

What CAUTIONS need to be taken with this medication?

What DRUG-DRUG INTERACTIONS are there?
- None Known

How should this medication be PREPARED and ADMINISTERED?
- Withdraw solution from vial using a low-protein binding 5 micron filter and add drug to an empty 150 – 250 mL Viaflex bag
- IV solution should be administered within 8 hours of preparation.
- IV solution should be administered to the patient using a 0.22 micron filter
- SMM-16 should not be diluted or administered with any other IV fluids (the infusion tubing may be primed and flushed with either D5W or NS

What are some of the PHARMACOKINETIC properties of this medication?
- Half-life – 21.6 hours (based on 6 pts @ 60mg/m²)
- Clearance – 61.8 mL/hr/m²

What STORAGE CONDITIONS are necessary for this medication? What is the STABILITY/COMPATIBILITY of this medication?
- Vials of SMM-16 should be stored in the refrigerator at 2 - 8° C (35 - 47° F)
- Do not freeze or shake solution
- Protect from direct sunlight
- Prepared drug dose must be administered to the patient within 8 hours

Who is the MANUFACTURE/SUPPLIER for this medication?
- DrugCo, Inc
  Pittsburgh, PA

For what STUDY is this medication being used?	Who are the PRINCIPAL INVESTIGATORS?	Who are the STUDY CONTACTS?
A Phase I Open-Label Dose Escalation Study of Weekly Dosing with SMM-16 followed by a Phase II Efficacy Study	Aaron Joseph, MD; Medical Oncology Evan Jonathan, MD; Medical Oncology	Olivia Lauren, RN Phone: 4-2689 Pager: 259-8690

Investigational Drug Service:

Laura Kristeen, M.S., Pharm.D,
Ext: 4-2698; Pager: 259-8691

RETAIN THIS INFORMATION IN PATIENT CHART

correspondence regarding the drug, and any pertinent articles published on the drug.

An Expanded Role for the Hospital Pharmacist

The handling of investigational new drugs can result in a possible expanded role for the pharmacy department: (1) the reordering of investigational drugs, (2) design of single- and double-blind studies, (3) the formulation, development, and preparation of the finished dosage form, (4) carrying out of stability studies, and (5) the preparation of drug identity documents for the FDA. Whether or not the hospital pharmacy accedes to this expanded role will depend on the need for these services, the equipment, expertise, and commitment of the department.[21–26]

The participation of pharmacists in investigational drug programs can also result in significant savings to institutions.[56,57,66,68,70,74–76] Often there are hidden costs associated with IDS programs. It is helpful to perform an economic assessment of each program to determine the total financial impact of an IDS to the organization.[51]

Reordering of Investigational Drugs

Although the principal investigator usually reorders the investigational drug, he or she may wish to delegate this responsibility to the pharmacist because the pharmacy is already involved in the acquisition, storage, disposition, and maintenance record of the drug. The pharmacy knows when additional supplies are needed and can notify the pharmaceutical company directly. The pharmaceutical company can then send the drug directly to the investigator or, preferably, to the pharmacy with reference to the appropriate protocol number.[14] In the past, the company would send the drug to the pharmacy with the words "for the use of Dr._____," but given the volume of protocols now, this practice is seldom seen anymore. However, it should be noted that while most pharmaceutical companies readily accept orders from pharmacies, a few prefer to deal directly with the clinical investigator.

Formulation, Development, and Preparation of the Dosage Form

When an investigator wishes to conduct a study with a new drug in which no manufacturer is interested in preparing or sponsoring, he or she can often obtain assistance for the development and formulation of the dosage form from a pharmacist.[13] The service the pharmacist can provide varies from the reformulation of commercial tablets into matching drug and placebo capsules, to the preparation of a suitable effective dosage form from a bulk powder. If this service is needed, the investigator will meet with the pharmacist and discuss the study and provide them with certain information. The information is recorded on the investigational service drug form, which is the same document used for the registration of a drug (in the finished dosage form) obtained from the pharmaceutical manufacturer sponsoring it. The portion of the form marked "service and packaging requested" will include specifics: dosage form, potency per dose, route of administration, quantity, method of packaging and labeling, and certificate of analysis, and any other information, chemical or otherwise that may be available about the drug.

Initially, the analytic and quality control section in the pharmacy conducts studies to ensure the identity, strength, quality, and purity of the compound. With this information, and guided by the investigator's stated desire, the pharmacist is ready to proceed with the formulation. To provide an optimum rate of absorption in the body, the pharmacist concerns him/herself with particle size, solubility, pH, disintegration and dissolution time, and other factors. The pharmacist will reject distasteful or objectionable combinations, because a medication is useless if the patient cannot or will not take it. Therefore, the physical form and dose, possible pain on injection, the odor, and appearance of the drug is considered. The pharmacist must also test for a parenteral drug's sterility, pyrogenicity, and safety.[17,20] All pharmacy instructions are included on the Pharmacy Dispensing Instruction Sheet (Figure 30-5). This sheet contains all information regarding the drug supply, the preparation procedures, drug stability, storage instructions, and a copy of the pharmacy label.

If the clinical investigator is satisfied with the dosage form the pharmacist can now prepare the formulation on pilot plant batch. It should be noted that if no suitable assay method for the active ingredient is available, another pharmacist from the quality control section may monitor the manufacturing to provide a double check, thus ensuring that the proper amount of active drug is used. However, if an assay method does exist, or has been developed, then the pharmacists in the quality control section will determine the active

Figure 30-5

Pharmacy Dispensing Instructions

Pharmacy Dispensing Instructions

**A Phase I Study of Markarubicin in Combination with Gumppamycin
in Patients with Relapsed or Refractory Hematologic Malignancies (Study #2005)**

Investigator(s):	Aaron Joseph, MD; Medical Oncology Evan Jonathan, MD; Medical Oncology
Study Contact(s):	Olivia Lauren, RN; Clinical Trials Office Ext: 4-2689; Pager: 259-8690
Objective(s):	To determine the MTD, specific toxicities & dose-limiting toxicity of the combination of Markarubicin & Gumppamycin in patients with AML or NHL
Patients:	Pts ≥ 18 yr of age with histologically or cytologically confirmed AML (Stratum I) or B-cell NHL (Stratum II) who meet all protocol criteria
Study Design:	Phase I; open-label; dose-escalating
Treatment Duration:	Patients may receive up to twelve 21-day cycles if evidence of objective response is present
Orders:	Orders will be written on the standard chemotherapy order form or entered into COE & then processed by standard departmental procedures
Randomization:	None required; Dose level will be assigned by the Clinical Trials Office

Study Drug(s):	**Gumppamycin (with EPL diluent)**	**Markarubicin**
Supply	<u>STUDY</u> supply	<u>STUDY</u> supply
Availability	Gumppamycin: Single-use concentrate vials containing 50mg in 2ml dimethylsulfoxide EPL diluent: 48ml single-use vial	3.5 mg single-use vials for reconstitution; For IV use
Dose	100-250 mg/m^2/day IV (over 60 minutes) on Days 1, 4, 8 & 11 of a 21-day cycle immediately before Markarubicin Dosage may be reduced or delayed per protocol for toxicity *See dose escalation table on the next page*	0.5-1.3 mg/m^2 IV push (over 3-5 seconds) on Days 1, 4, 8 & 11 of a 21-day cycle immediately after Gumppamycin (except Cycle 1 is on Days 4, 8, & 11 only) Dosage may be reduced or delayed per protocol for toxicity *See dose escalation table on the next page*
Computer Entry	Pharmacy Computer = **/Gumpp2005** Change/enter needed dose and the final total volume	Pharmacy Computer = **/Markar2005** Change/enter ordered dose & volume
Preparation	1) Sign out the needed vials of Gumppamycin on the accountability record 2) Sign out an equal number of EPL diluent vials on the accountability record 3) Thaw the drug concentrate vial(s) at room temperature (takes about an hour) or roll the vials in the hands to expedite thawing. 4) *It is very important that the concentrate is at **ROOM TEMPERATURE** before withdrawing.* 5) Withdraw 2ml of the drug concentrate and add to the 48ml vial of EPL diluent yielding a <u>1 mg/ml</u> final concentration 6) Mix gently until a clear solution is obtained. To avoid foaming, DO NOT SHAKE! 7) Draw up the needed dose and add to an <u>empty **glass** evacuated bottle</u>. No further dilution is needed. 8) Affix IV label 9) No special infusion set is required so a NTG set will be used since it is vented for use with glass bottles	1) Sign out needed vials(s) on drug accountability record 2) Reconstitute each vials with 3.5 ml normal saline to yield a <u>1 mg/ml</u> concentration 3) Draw up needed dose/volume into a syringe 4) Place black luer tip onto the end of the syringe 5) Affix label to syringe
Stability	• Vial stability (Gumppamycin & diluent) as per NCI • Prepared infusions should be used within 8hr of mixing	• Reconstituted solution is stable for 43 hr at room temperature but it is recommended that it be used within 8 hr since the product contains no antibacterial preservatives • Vial stability as per manufacturer recommendation
Storage	• Store Gumppamycin vials in the <u>freezer</u> (-10 to -20° C) • Refrigerate EPL diluent (2-8° C). Do not freeze	• Intact vials should be stored at 2-8° C in the investigational drug refrigerator

Figure 30-5, continued

Record Keeping: Drug accountability records for Gumppamycin <u>and</u> EPL diluent as well as for Markarubicin

Special Notes:
- **Gumppamycin Drug Data Sheet** is on the pharmacy intranet
- Dose escalation will be performed independently in patients with AML (Stratum I) and NHL (Stratum II); Starting dose level is Level 1
- Stage 1 of the study is dose escalation. Stage 2 is using the recommended phase II dose (determined from Stage 1) in an expanded number of patients.
- Treatment may be administered on an outpatient basis at the physician's discretion
- Patients should not take any agent that alters CYP3A4 activity (See Appendix B of protocol for list)
- Since Gumppamycin is formulated using egg phospholipids, patients with a history of serious allergic reactions to eggs should not receive the agent.

Dose Level	**Gumppamycin** $(mg/m^2$ over 60 min) Days 1, 4, 8 & 11 of a 21-day cycle	**Markarubicin** $(mg/m^2$ over 3-5 seconds) Days 1, 4, 8 & 11 of a 21-day cycle
-1	100	0.5
0	100	0.7
1	150	0.7
2	200	0.7
3	200	1
4	200	1.3
5	250	1.3

Sample Pharmacy Label(s):

```
DOE, JOHN              08888 999999999 UNITX
ORD:  1-1    DUE:  1/01/05 10:00   U-XXXX-A

                 CYTOTOXIC
GUMPPAMYCIN (2005)                   200 MG
EVACUATED CONTAINER 250 ML       1
SET, NITRO CLEAR 2C8851           1
IN TOTAL VOLUME                     200 ML


FRQ PRN                    INFUSE OVER 60 MIN
INFUSE OVER 60 MIN; INVESTIGATIONAL USE ONLY
DO NOT START AFTER 1/01/05  14:00
CHECKED BY: _____
           UNIVERSITY MED. CENTER
```

```
DOE, JOHN        XX XXXXXXXXX XX   UNIT
ORD  XXX                          IDTEST
"INVESTIGATIONAL DRUG SUPPLY      1
MARKARUBICIN (2005)               1.4 MG
IN TOTAL VOLUME                   1.4 ML
PRN                     ROUTE: IV PUSH
GIVE IVP OVER 3-5 SECONDS; INVESTIGATIONAL USE ONLY
DUE: XX/XX/XX  10:00   CHECKED BY: _____
MC       DO NOT START AFTER XX/XX/XX 10:00
```

drug content. This group also determines pharmaceutical quality and specifications for the drug. The specifications for the fill weight for hard-filled gelatin capsules and tablets, pH, and specific gravity, when appropriate, should be included. When the formulation is complete, dispensing is recorded on the Drug Accountability Log (Figure 30-6) and all lot numbers and expiration dates are recorded. There is also a section to record returned product to ensure that all drug product in a study has been properly accounted. Signatures for verification are also recorded. This process has been automated now in some studies and accountability is done through the Internet or by a phone messaging system.

Stability

Along with the preparation of the drug dosage form some knowledge of its stability is required in order to use it effectively. The definition of drug stability in the USP is the extent to which a product retains, within specified limits and throughout its period of storage and use, the same properties and characteristics that it possessed at the time of its manufacture. The stability of the formulated product or maintenance of the stated potency should, therefore, be determined. To do this the pharmacist may study the rate and mechanism of the drug's decomposition, develop assay methods, and predict long-range stability under various storage conditions. He may have to experiment further with the formulation and packaging to achieve the desired stability.

If possible, a stability profile should be obtained at every stage in the formulation in order to support the standards of identity, strength, quality, and purity being proposed for the drug. The analytical methods used to obtain this data should be capable of measuring characteristic physical and chemical properties associated with the intact drug. Stability characteristics of the drug under extreme conditions of temperature (e.g., 5, 50, and 75°C), humidity (90% RH at 25°C), and light (UV 3,500 to 4,000 A°) could be carried out to satisfy FDA requirements of stability and shelf-life if the sponsor, in this case the physician, is filing for the IND. The degradation products encountered during stability studies should be quantitatively and qualitatively identified, if possible, and the source (e.g., reactants) and mechanisms considered. The stability studies of the dosage form subsequently developed should include the behavior of the degradation products as well as other impurities associated with the drug. The test methods should be capable of distinguishing the intact molecule from the degradation products.[18]

Drugs that are susceptible to heat, light, and air should be carefully monitored, and any change in manufacturing procedures may introduce trace quantities of metal, which may affect stability of the drug product.

Figure 30-6
Drug Accountability Log

DRUG ACCOUNTABILITY LOG

SPONSOR:	SPONSOR STUDY NO:
INVESTIGATOR NAME:	STUDY CONTACT (S):
INVESTIGATIONAL DRUG:	DILUENT MANUFACTURER:

Patient initials: Randomization Number:

Drug description:								Batch Number:							
PREPARATION FOR SUBJECT								BAG/BOTTLE RETURN				VERIFICATION			
Vial	Used	Date	Time	Diluent Lot Number	Diluent Expiration Date	Label Complete	Prepared By Initials	Date	Time	Received By Initials	Stored 2-8°C	Vial	Bag/Bottle	CRA	Date
1	Y N					Y N					Y N				
2	Y N					Y N					Y N				

Comments:

_____

_____

_____   _____   _____   _____
Investigator Designee Name   Title   Signature   Date

The most carefully produced dosage form can be no better than the quality of the container in which it is held. The safety, effectiveness, and stability of the product depends to a significant extent upon the suitability of the packaging materials and the adequacy of the packaging. Therefore, stability studies that do not include temperatures and conditions beyond room temperature with the drug form in its container are usually not satisfactory.

Drug Accountability and Storage

Although FDA regulation places the responsibility for maintaining accountability for the use of investigational agents with the investigator, an institution may assume these responsibilities for the investigators on its staff and assure itself of compliance with Federal requirements.[19,41–46]

The intent of the agent accountability procedures described in this section is to assist the investigator in making certain that agents received are used only for patients entered onto an approved protocol. The investigator is responsible for the proper and secure physical storage and record keeping of investigational agents. The record keeping described in this section is required under FDA regulation. Investigators are responsible for the use of investigational agents shipped in their name. Even if a pharmacist or chemotherapy nurse has the actual task of handling these agents upon receipt, the investigator is the responsible individual and has agreed to accept this responsibility by signing the FDA.

Specifically, the investigator must do the following:

- Store the agent in a secure location, accessible to only authorized personnel, preferably in the pharmacy

- Maintain a careful record of the receipt, use and final disposition of all investigational agents received

- Maintain appropriate storage of the investigational agent to ensure the stability and integrity of the agent

- Return any unused investigational agents to PMB at the completion of the study or upon notification that an agent is being withdrawn (Should not be a bullet point for this)

- Store each investigational agent separately by protocol. If an agent is used for more than one protocol, there should be separate physical storage for each protocol.

- Account for each agent separately by protocol. If an agent is used for more than one protocol, there should be a separate Drug Accountability Record Form (DARF) for each protocol.

- Maintain a separate DARF for each agent in a multiagent protocol

- Maintain separate accountability forms for each different strength or dosage form of a particular agent (e.g., an agent with a 1-mg vial and a 5-mg vial would require a different DARF for the 1-mg vial than for the 5-mg vial)

- Use the DARF at each location where agents are stored (e.g., main pharmacy, satellite pharmacy, physician's office, or other dispensing areas)

- Use the DARF to accommodate both dispensing records and other agent transaction documentation (e.g., receipt of agent, returns, broken vials, etc.)

The Disposition Records

The physician/clinical investigator is allowed by FDA to delegate authority to the hospital pharmacist to maintain the investigational drug disposition records.[9] Although the records will differ with each hospital, they usually include the name of the drug, quantity and date received, the dosage form and strength, the name of the manufacturer, lot or control number, and expiration date. As each drug order is filled, the date, patient's name, serial number of the prescription, and name of the prescribing investigator and quantity dispensed are recorded on the form. In addition, a list of the authorized coinvestigators, the pharmacology of the drug, the maximum dose and route of administration of the drug, and a description of the dosage form should be included on the form. This form can also be used as an inventory record by maintaining a running balance as each drug order is filled.

Case Report Forms

Information about patients is recorded on case report forms (or in a computerized clinical trials database) that incorporate all patient data stipulated in the protocol. The case report document should not be the same as the patient's primary medical record. The former ultimately serves as the formal and fixed data base on which the study is reported. A well-designed case report form will assist the investigator and assistants in collecting and recording all data called for in the protocol. The patient's chart, although the primary medical record, is generally not organized for purposes of research and does not reliably contain the judgments of the treating physician on the effects of the protocol treatment. For these reasons, a separate research record (i.e., case report form or well-designed clinical trials database) should be maintained on each protocol patient. Case research records are best maintained concurrently with the medical record. A research record should include not only the actual data, but the responsible physician's assessment of the treatment effect (e.g., response category) and judgment as to whether any medical events in the patient's course were treatment-induced (i.e., agent-related adverse events). Unfortunately, adverse events are often underreported, particularly if the effect is well-described.

Study Summary Forms

The study summary is a tabulation and analysis of the collated individual patient data. It includes not only objective tabulations of data, but the assessment of the protocol chair concerning each case, with particular attention to eligibility, evaluability, and interpretation of the observations.

Drug Identity Documents

The analytic and quality control section is also responsible for the preparation of drug identify and purity documents for submission to the FDA to support an IND.[13] These documents or data sheets are prepared both for the bulk investigational drug and the finished product. The data for the bulk drug may include the clinical and other names, the empirical and structural formula, molecular weight, solubility, melting point, pH, identification assay, packaging, and storage. The document for the finished product may include source and batch or control of bulk drug, control or research number of finished dosage form, the manufacturer, and such characteristics as pH, weight variation, and disintegration time (if applicable), sterility, and pyrogenicity, identification, assay, moisture determination (if applicable), stability testing and shelf-life, packaging, and storage.[28]

All assay and stability studies to determine expiration date and shelf-life of the finished dosage form, including its use in intravenous additive mixtures, are carried out by the analytic and quality control section. The effects of variables, such as temperature, air, light, and autoclaving are considered. Accelerated storage conditions are used such as elevated temperatures,

increased humidity, or exposure to ultraviolet light. Although data obtained in this way may not be translated directly into shelf-life data, they serve as guides for immediate working conditions.

Retention of Records

FDA regulations require that all research records (including patient charts, case report forms, x-rays and scans that document response, IRB approvals, signed informed consent documents and all agent accountability records) must be kept by the investigator for at least 2 years after an NDA or BLA has been approved for that indication or the study has been closed.

Data Management and Statistics

Since most clinical trials involve professional staff other than the protocol chair, adequate collection of clinical data is a complex task that must be integrated into the medical practices of the institution. Furthermore, data collection is best done as data are generated; this practice promotes protocol compliance and permits the protocol chair to monitor the study's progress. For these reasons, data management organized and supported at the department or institution level is usually more efficient and reliable than that which is left to the individual investigator.[53]

The accrual goals of a study should be specified in advance, with a maximum number of patients stated explicitly. Justification for the target sample size, in terms of precision of estimation or levels of type I and type II error, should be provided. Multistage designs for distinguishing an unacceptable level of response from a promising level are recommended. The accrual rate of eligible patients that can be *realistically* anticipated should be given. Mechanisms should be in place for early stopping of negative trials. Statistical considerations for Phase 2 trials of combinations should base unacceptable and promising levels of response on activity levels of the components or other combinations. References to those levels should be cited.

Analysis and Quality Control

Some comments about the need for an Analysis and Quality Control section in the pharmacy when dealing with the preparation of dosage forms and the filing of an IND for the physician are needed.[13] The analytic and quality control section of the pharmacy can ensure the identity and quality of an investigational drug. Its primary objectives should be to determine methods for testing the bulk investigational materials and the chemical formulation. The physician or clinical investigator, pharmaceutical manufacturer, or screening group supplying the bulk investigational material is requested to submit information on the chemical and physical properties of the drug. The analytic and quality control section then conducts a literature search on the assay methodology for the major component, anticipated minor components, and degradation products. When possible, the bulk material may be examined by gas-liquid chromatography and thin-layer chromatography to detect unexpected minor components. Other data sought for a given material may include the results of elemental analyses, heavy metals determination, loss on drying, optical rotation, infrared, ultraviolet, and nuclear magnetic resonance spectra, and the results of functional group or minor component determinators. A pharmacist then reviews the data for each lot before it is used. Any bulk supply stored for 6 months or more is reexamined before it is formulated for clinical testing.

If possible, the analytic group defines a standard reference sample of known purity. This can be used in preparing specifications for the drug when it is processed for clinical formulation and for eventual large-scale manufacturing.

A quality assurance program permits the research base to satisfy itself that each participating investigator is fulfilling his or her responsibilities.[36,48] It also provides the research base with data about the quality of execution of its clinical research, and it provides the investigator an opportunity to learn from an external evaluation of his or her performance. In its most constructive form, this process constitutes a peer review of performance and improves the quality of clinical research.

Sponsors and research bases must monitor their clinical trials. In assuring the quality of data, monitoring is a key component of any clinical trials program. Quality assurance and monitoring are concerned with the execution of a trial, rather than its conception, and with the quality of the data that support the scientific conclusions. Many individual activities are part of quality assurance, and investigators have recognized some of them as vital to the integrity of clinical trials for years. More recently, investigators have increasingly recognized the importance of verifying the accuracy of other classes of data.

The importance of verifying the accuracy of the basic data elements used in the analysis of study endpoints is obvious. Data accuracy is assessed during on-site audits by comparison of the research record (e.g., flow sheets) with the primary patient record.

Verification of Compliance

Compliance with procedures to ensure proper agent usage will be reviewed during site visits conducted under the monitoring program. Specifically, site visitors will check that the agent accountability system is being maintained, and will spot-check the agent accountability records by comparing them with the patients' medical records to verify that the agents were administered to a patient entered in the recorded protocol.[34,35,37,38]

Summary

The hospital pharmacist has a definite role in the handling and monitoring of all investigational drugs by virtue of their expertise in the labeling, storage, and dispensing of all drugs in the hospital. Also, the pharmacy is the logical place for the central repository for all investigational drug information, including the IND numbers. The basis services that could be provided by the pharmacist in the handling of investigational drugs are the registration, control, storage, dispensing, maintenance of disposition records, and drug information for every investigational drug evaluated for use in humans. If the drug dosage form is prepared in the hospital, the pharmacist plays an even large role: in the capacity of advisor on filing of drug information, date to the FDA as well as manufacturer of the drug product. The latter role will depend upon the pharmacist's expertise in formulation, development, and preparation of finished drug dosage forms, ability to assay the drug and confirm its identify, and to prepare documents as the manufacturer for submission to the FDA in support of the IND. The pharmacist also has a responsibility to provide information to the physician on how and what to submit to the FDA in compliance with the new drug regulations. This includes information for both roles the physician plays, that is, as a coinvestigator and as the sponsor. As long as investigational drugs are used in the hospital some type of pharmacy involvement will be needed.

References

1. Kelsey, F. The Kefauver-Harris amendments and investigational drugs. *Am J Hosp Pharm.* 1963;20:515–7.
2. Abrams, W.B. Introducing a new drug into clinical practice. *Anesthesiology.* 1974;35:176–92.
3. Food and Drug Administration. Clinical Testing for safe and effective drugs, DHEW Publication No. (FDA) 74-3015. Washington, DC: U.S. Government Printing Office.

4. Food and Drug Administration. Notice of claimed investigational exemption for a new Drug, FD Form 1571 (04/05).

5. Kumkumian, C.S. Manufacturing and controls, guidelines for INDs and NDAs. Presented at: 15th Annual International Industrial Pharmacy Conference; February 24, 1976; University of Texas, Austin, Texas.

6. Food and Drug Administration. Statement of Investigator, Form FD 1572 (4/05).

7. Food and Drug Administration. Statement of Investigator, Form FD 1573 (4/05).

8. Food and Drug Administration. Instructions for Submitting FD Form 1571, A Notice of Claimed Investigational Exemption for a New Drug by Individual Investigator (Investigational New Drug Application).

9. Bureau of Medicine, Food and Drug Administration. Investigational drug circular. *Am J Hosp Pharm.* 1965;22:69–70.

10. Kleinman LM, Tangrea JA, Gallelli JF. Control of investigational drugs in a research hospital. *Am J Hosp Pharm.* 1974;31:368–71.

11. Kleinman LM, Tangrea JA. Involvement of the hospital pharmacist in single- and double-blind studies. *Am J Hosp Pharm.* 1974;31:979–81.

12. Raff MS. [personal communication]. Bethesda, MD: BRB, National Heart and Lung Institute.

13. Gallelli JF, Skolaut MW. Pharmaceutical development: new concept in pharmacy service. *Hospitals.* 1967 Dec 16;41(24):95–101.

14. Armistead JA, Zillich AJ, Williams KL, et al. Hospital and pharmacy departmental policies and procedures for gene therapy at a teaching institution. *Hosp Pharm.* 2001;36:56–66.

15. Davis WM, Walters IW, Vinson MC. New drug approvals of 1999: part 1. *Drug Topics.* 2000;144(3):82–100.

16. National Institutes of Health, Office of Recombinant DNA Activities. Documents-recombinant DNA. Protocol list (PDF format); protocol list table (PDF format). Available at: http://www.od.nih.gov/oba/protocols.pdf.

17. Weber DJ, Rutala WA. Gene therapy: a new challenge for infection control. *Infect Control Hosp Epidemiol.* 1999;20:530–2.

18. DeCederfelt HJ, Grimes GJ, Green L, et al. Handling of gene-transfer products by the National Institutes of Health Clinical Center pharmacy department. *Am J Health-Syst Pharm.* 1997;54:1604–10.

19. National Institutes of Health, Office of Recombinant DNA Activities. Guidelines for research involving recombinant DNA molecules, May 1998. Appendix B: classification of human etiologic agents on the basis of hazard. Available at: http://www.nih.gov/od/orda/ toc.htm.

20. Evans ME, Lensnaw JA. Infection control in gene therapy. *Infect Control Hosp Epidemiol.* 1999;20:568–76.

21. Mutnick AH, Armistead JA, Cooley TW, et al. A Survey of Investigational Drug Services at Academic Health Centers. *P&T.* 2002;27(12);623–5.

22. Phillips M. Clinical research: ASHP guidelines and future directions for pharmacists. *Am J Health-Syst Pharm.* 1999;56:344–6.

23. Rogers SD, Lampasona V, Buchanan EC. The financial impact of investigational drug services. *Top Hosp Pharm Manage.* 1994;14:60–6.

24. Marnocha R. Clinical research: business opportunities for pharmacy-based investigational drug services. *Am J Health-Syst Pharm.* 1999;56:249–52.

25. Anandan J, Isopi M, Warren A. Fee structure for investigational drug services. *Am J Health-Syst Pharm.* 1993;50:2239–43.

26. Gajewski L, Vanscoy G, Dean J, et al. The development of a computerized LAN-based investigational drug information database. *Hosp Pharm.* 1995;30:1113, 1116–8.

27. Wermeling D, Nowak-Rapp M, Sitzlar S. Computer-assisted investigational drug information and testing mechanism for nurses. *Hosp Pharm.* 1994;29:745–6, 748–50.

28. Vlasses P. Clinical research: trends affecting the pharmaceutical industry and the pharmacy profession. *Am J Health-Syst Pharm.* 1999;56:171–4.

29. Rockwell K. Pharmacy-based investigational drug services: a national survey. *Top Hosp Pharm Manage.* 1993;13:1–15.

30. Rockwell K, Bockheim-McGee C, Jones E, et al. Clinical research: a national survey of U.S. pharmacy-based investigational drug services—1997. *Am J Health-Syst Pharm.* 1999;56:337–44.

31. Shehab N, Tamer H. Dispensing investigational drugs: regulatory issues and the role of the investigational drug service. *Am J Health-Syst Pharm.* 2004;61:1882–4.

32. Joint Commission on Accreditation of Healthcare Organizations (JCAHO). Medication management, Sec. 1. In: *Comprehensive Accreditation Manual for Hospitals: The Official Handbook.* Oakbrook Terrace, IL: Joint Commission on Accreditation of Healthcare Organizations; 2004:MM1-20.

33. American Society of Health-System Pharmacists (ASHP). Guidelines on clinical drug research. In: Deffenbaugh JH, ed. *Best Practices for Health-System Pharmacy: Position and Guidance Documents of ASHP, 2001–2002.* Bethesda, MD: American Society of Health-System Pharmacists; 2002:294–300.

34. Rockwell KA, Marnocha RS. Audit tool for investigational drugs dispensed in clinics. Presented at: ASHP Annual Meeting; June 1994; Reno NV.

35. Truelove KE, Ferolie ER, Ossing MM. Pharmacist auditing of investigational new drugs used in studies not dispensed by pharmacy. Presented at: ASHP Annual Meeting; June 1995; Philadelphia, PA.

36. Petrich JM, Suttles CC, Shermock KM. The impact of a quality control program within an investigational drug service. Presented at: ASHP Midyear Clinical Meeting; December 2002; Atlanta, GA.

37. Siden R, Tankanow RM, Tamer HR. Understanding and preparing for clinical drug trial audits. *Am J Health-Syst Pharm.* 2002;59:2301–6.

38. Food and Drug Administration. Institutional review board inspections. IRB operations and clinical investigation information sheet. Available at: www.fda.gov/oc/ohrt/irbs/operations.html. Accessed April 15, 2005.

39. Food and Drug Administration, International Conference on Harmonization. Good clinical practice consolidated guidelines. *Fed Regist*. 1997;62:25692–709.

40. National Cancer Institute. Investigator's handbook. Part 16.5. Available at: http//ctep.cancer.gov/forms/Hndbk.pdf. Accessed April 5, 2005.

41. Anticipating an audit. In: Ginsberg D, ed. *The Investigator' Guide to Clinical Research*. 2nd ed. Boston: CenterWatch, Inc.; 1999:154–6.

42. FDA inspections. In: Iber FL, Riley WA, Murray PJ, eds. *Conducting Clinical Trials*. New York: Plenum Medical; 1987:315–23.

43. Curran CF. Preparing a clinical site for a clinical investigator inspection by the FDA. *Drug Inf J*. 1999;33:253–6.

44. 21 C.F.R. 312.59.

45. 21 C.F.R. 312-61.

46. 21 C.F.R. 312-62.

47. American Society of Health-System Pharmacists (ASHP). Guidelines on clinical drug research. In: Deffenbaugh JH, ed. *Best Practices for Health-System Pharmacy: Position and Guidance Documents of ASHP 2001–2002*. Bethesda, MD: American Society of Health-System Pharmacists; 2002:294–300.

48. Food and Drug Administration. Compliance program guidance. Manual for FDA staff. Part III—inspectional. Available at: www.fda.gov/ora/compliance-ref/bimo/7348-811. Accessed April 1, 2005.

49. Seybert CD. Are investigational drugs getting you down? One hospital's solution to the increasing number of clinical research studies. *Hosp Pharm*; 2003;38:140–3.

50. American Society of Health-System Pharmacists (ASHP). ASHP guidelines for the use of drugs in clinical research. *Am J Health-Syst Pharm*. 1998;55:369–76.

51. Marnocha RM. Clinical research: business opportunities for pharmacy-based investigational drug services. *Am J Health-Syst Pharm*. 1999;56:249–52.

52. Wermeling DP. Clinical research: regulatory issues. *Am J Health-Syst Pharm*. 1999;56:252–6.

53. Chan DS. Computerized worksheet for tracking pharmacy costs for an investigational drug service. *Am J Health-Syst Pharm*. 1995;52:208–9.

54. American Society of Hospital Pharmacists (ASHP). ASHP guidelines for pharmaceutical research in organized health-care settings. *Am J Hosp Pharm*. 1989;46:129–30.

55. American Society of Hospital Pharmacists (ASHP). ASHP guidelines for the use of investigational drugs in organized health-care settings. *Am J Hosp Pharm*. 1991;48:315–9.

56. LaFleur J, Tyler LS, Sharma RR. Economic benefits of investigational drug services at an academic institution. *Am J Health-Syst Pharm*. 2004;61:27–32.

57. McDonagh MS, Miller SA, Naden E. Costs and savings of investigational drug services. *Am J Health-Syst Pharm*. 2000;57:40–3.

58. U.S. Food and Drug Administration. International Conference on Harmonisation; good clinical practice: consolidated guidelines; notice of availability. *Fed Regist*. 1997;62:25691–709.

59. Hoffman RP. The use of investigational drugs—JCAHO. *Hosp Pharm*. 1988:23:905–9.

60. Dipiro JT, Talbert RL, Yee GC, et al., eds. *Pharmacotherapy: A Pathophysiologic Approach*. 4th ed. Stamford CT: Appleton & Lange; 1999.

61. Stolar MH, ed. *Pharmacy-Coordinated Investigational Drug Services*. Revised ed. Bethesda MD: American Society of Hospital Pharmacists; 1986.

62. American Society of Health-System Pharmacists (ASHP). ASHP guidelines: minimum standard for pharmacies in hospitals. *Am J Health-Syst Pharm*. 1995;52:2711–7.

63. American Society of Hospital Pharmacists (ASHP). ASHP statement on the use of medications for unlabeled uses. *Am J Hosp Pharm*. 1992;49:2006–8.

64. Federal Food, Drug, and Cosmetic Act (21 U.S.C. 301 et seq.) 1938, as amended.

65. Food and Drug Administration, Department of Health and Human Services. International conference on harmonization; good clinical practice consolidated guideline. *Fed Regist*. 1997;62:25692–709.

66. Wermeling DP, Piecoro LT, Foster TS. Financial impact of clinical research on a health system. *Am J Health-Syst Pharm*. 1997;54:1742–51.

67. Bailey EM, Habowski SR. How to apply for emergency use of an investigational agent. *Am J Health-Syst Pharm*. 1996;53:208–10.

68. Rogers RD, Lampasona V, Buchanan EC. The financial impact of investigational drug services. *Top Hosp Pharm Manage*. 1994;14(1):60–6.

69. Fink J. Liability threat should be considered when conducting drug investigations. Paper presented at: American Pharmaceutical Association Annual Meeting; March 12, 1990; Washington, DC.

70. Mehl B. Investigational drug protocols—hidden costs. *Hosp Pharm*. 1991;(5):459–61.

71. Gresham C, Allen T. Investigational drug services: management implications. *Pharm Times*. 1993;59(Feb):3–12.

72. Hill DP, Browning DA. A perspective on investigational drug management. *Top Hosp Pharm Manage*. 1993;13(1):29–36.

73. Catania HF, Yee WP, Catania PN. Four years' experience with a clinical intervention program: cost avoidance and impact of a clinical coordinator. *Am J Hosp Pharm*. 1990;47:2701–5.

74. Mutnick AH, Streba KJ, Peroutka JA et al. Cost savings and avoidance from clinical interventions. *Am J Health-Syst Pharm*. 1997; 54:392-6.

75. Thomas P, Ross RN, Farrar JR. A retrospective assessment of cost avoidance associated with the use of nedocromil sodium metered dose inhaler in the treatment of patients with asthma. *Clin Ther.* 1996;18:939–52.

76. Seay RE, Edgren BE, Schilling GC. Cost avoidance using syringe pumps to administer fat emulsion in a neonatal intensive care unit. *Am J Hosp Pharm.* 1991; 48:1972–4.

77. Wermeling DP. Value of investigational drugs. *Am J Hosp Pharm.* 1993;50:1576. Letter.

78. Stolar MH, Gabriel T. Grant KL, et al. Pharmacy-coordinated investigational drug services. *Am J Hosp Pharm.* 1982;39:432–6.

79. http://www.hhs.gov/ohrp/policy/index.html#irbs.

80. http://ctep.cancer.gov/handbook/hndbk_16.html.

Chapter 31

The Literature of Pharmacy

William A. Zellmer, C. Richard Talley

Introduction

The literature of institutional pharmacy is the body of written work produced and used by practitioners, educators, and researchers in this field. That literature includes this handbook, for example, as well as any other information that institutional pharmacists use in their practices. The literature could be defined to include unpublished manuscripts and documents and everything on the Internet pertaining to the practice of pharmacy in hospitals and health systems. However, such informal publications are beyond the scope of this chapter, which is limited to the literature that is readily accessible by virtue of its formal publication.

Just as *institutional pharmacy* is a component of the broader profession of *pharmacy*, so the *literature of institutional pharmacy* is a component of the *pharmacy literature*. The pharmacy literature, in turn, is a component of the biomedical literature, which is a subcategory of the scientific literature. Some literature used in institutional practice is quite specific to this area of the profession (e.g., an article on inpatient drug distribution). However, a large part of the literature that is applied in institutional practice is the same as that used in other parts of the profession (e.g., a reference book on drug interactions) and in health care in general (e.g., reputable drug information and diverse publications in the biomedical literature focused on rational drug therapy).

The balance of this chapter discusses the link between the literature and the profession, uses of the literature, categories of literature, periodicals used in institutional pharmacy, use of periodicals for current awareness, computer-based literature retrieval services, books used in institutional pharmacy, contributing to the literature, the journal peer-review process, and controversies related to the literature. This chapter looks at the literature largely from the vantage point of general practitioners and managers in institutional pharmacy. Other perspectives might well produce a substantially different picture. For example, if the interests of the drug information specialist had been the focus, this chapter would have dealt more heavily with sources of clinical information, methods of literature retrieval, and techniques for evaluating published research. Likewise, if the interests of pharmacists directly involved in patient medication therapy management had been the focus, this chapter would have focused on methods of finding the latest information on rational drug therapy in all biomedical publications.

The Link between the Literature and the Profession

Many pharmacists take the literature of pharmacy for granted and do not appreciate the vital role that it has played, and continues to play, in shaping the profession. The earliest known form of pharmacy literature is a 4,000-year-old pharmacopoeia written on a clay tablet that documents the preparation of pharmaceutical dosage forms in Sumerian civilization.[1] The vast literature on drug therapy that was generated in Arabian culture between the 9th and 13th centuries is believed to have helped form the basis for pharmacy as an independent profession.[1] A profession, by definition, cannot exist without its own unique, scientifically-based literature. As Starr has indicated, professionals derive their authority from three distinctive claims[2]:

1. That a professional's knowledge and competence have been validated by a community of his or her peers

2. That this validated knowledge and competence rest on rational, scientific grounds

3. That the professional's judgment and advice are oriented toward a set of substantive values, such as health

The "rational, scientific grounds" for pharmacy are expressed through its literature. Further, the values of pharmacy—the things that it stands for as a health profession—are expressed and clarified through its literature. A career commitment to institutional pharmacy practice implies keeping up with the latest knowledge and thinking in the field (i.e., keeping up with the literature).

One of the ways of defining pharmacy is as a *knowledge system*:

> "[Pharmacy] is a system which generates or integrates knowledge about man in sickness and in health, takes knowledge from other sciences and arts, criticizes and organizes that knowledge, translates knowledge into technology, uses some knowledge to create products, devices, and instruments, transmits the knowledge through the education of practitioners and dissemination to others, to the end that an individual known as a patient may benefit from the particular knowledge system and its consequent skills. The thread which holds research, education and practice together in a rational system is *knowledge*."[3]

The obvious should be added: this knowledge is expressed through the pharmacy literature, in print and online.

Uses of the Literature

The literature may be used in three general ways: current awareness, research, and education. Most practitioners review professional journals primarily for current awareness. One of the thrills of pharmacy practice comes from reading an idea that sparks creative thinking about a problem that the reader is experiencing firsthand. Sometimes a pharmacist will first become aware of an important practice problem through an article in the pharmacy literature. Reading about the problems that other practitioners are facing can give institutional pharmacists a greater sense of community and help establish cohesiveness and *esprit de corps* within the discipline. Many pharmacists take pride in being conversant on contemporary pharmacy issues, and they attain their comfort with the issues of the day by reading the literature.

Whenever a practitioner consults the literature to find out what has been said about a particular subject, the research value of the literature comes to the fore. Use of the literature for research purposes may range from the informal to the formal. For example, one may consult a reference book to determine what package sizes a particular product comes in, or one may look up a journal article that relates to a practice problem. At the other extreme, one may do a comprehensive literature search on a well-defined subject area to prepare for a formal research project or to write a pharmacy and therapeutics (P&T) committee monograph on a new medication.

The literature is used extensively in both the education of pharmacy students and in the continuing education of pharmacists. Continuing education may be planned by a continuing education provider (e.g., a college of pharmacy, a professional society, or a pharmaceutical company) or may be self-directed by the practitioner. In either case, the content of the educational program will have a basis in the literature, the formal repository of the knowledge of the discipline. Many professional journals contain review articles and other content that is written especially for continuing education purposes. Often, those articles may be used to earn credit in those states that require continuing education to maintain a practice license.

Categories of Literature

The scientific literature is generally divided into three broad categories. The *primary literature* consists of the original reports of research and innovations in the field, original reports of research and innovations themselves. The *secondary literature* is made up of abstracting and indexing services. The *tertiary literature* includes review articles, reference books, and textbooks, and reflects experts' syntheses or overviews of subjects based on the primary literature.

This categorization is not entirely satisfactory for the literature of institutional pharmacy, especially with respect to news reports about developments in the profession. A news report in a pharmacy tabloid such as *Pharmacy Practice News* may be the first occasion for certain information to appear in print. However, such reports are hardly "original reports of research and innovations" in the sense of complete and carefully written articles by the individuals who performed research or developed an innovation. Hence, news would not seem to fit the definition of primary literature. Although news writing is often a synthesis based on observations of many events, the ephemeral nature of most news articles hardly permits them to be placed in the category of secondary literature. Nevertheless, news reports have some of the characteristics of the secondary literature in that they may be useful in leading one to more complete information about a subject (such as by identifying a person who was interviewed for a story). Perhaps the best solution is to create a separate category for news, such as *current affairs literature*.

The literature may also be classified according to the form in which it is produced. In this chapter, only the main forms are discussed, namely, *print periodicals, Internet-accessible versions of periodicals, printed books, and Internet- and PDA-accessible books.* Although not an exhaustive list, the following forms might also be considered by some to be a part of the literature of institutional pharmacy: package inserts; pamphlets and booklets; advertising and other promotional materials; the scripts for films, videotapes, and audiotapes; and Internet sites germane to pharmacy.

Another form of communication in institutional pharmacy is Internet-based discussions. The American Society of Health-System Pharmacists (ASHP) facilitates several such issue discussion groups (http://www.ashp.org/membership/idg/index.cfm?cfid=4208898&CFToken=54015177). The messages on these services are basically electronic forms of correspondence; no permanent record is kept of them, and they are not retrievable after they become old (typically within several months), at which point they are removed from the discussion thread. Because the information on Internet-based bulletin-board services has a short retrievable life, it is not considered a part of the literature of institutional pharmacy.

Periodicals Used in Institutional Pharmacy

The types of periodicals in institutional pharmacy include peer-reviewed journals, abstracting and indexing services, current affairs publications, newsletters, and company-sponsored publications. Many periodicals are not purely of one type. For example, although the *American Journal of Health-System Pharmacy* is primarily a peer-reviewed journal, it also carries news and occasionally publishes supplementary issues that are, to some extent, company-sponsored publications. It is common for a current affairs magazine such as *Drug Topics* to publish review articles that may be used for continuing education. Some company-sponsored publications consist largely of abstracts of articles from the primary literature.

Institutional pharmacists use journals from their own discipline as well as from pharmacy at large, the pharmaceutical sciences, medicine, and health care management. The most important periodicals to institutional pharmacists are listed in the Appendix 31-1. Most of these periodicals have archival value. (This means that major libraries either keep printed back volumes or have electronic subscriptions that include content from several years of back issues, or both.) In addition to these periodicals from the United States,

a number of English-language foreign journals are reviewed regularly by some institutional pharmacists. The most notable among these journals, listed in Appendix 31-1, are well-established periodicals that are supported through subscription revenue or advertising, or both, and that are available from bona fide publishers. There has been a proliferation of *throwaway* publications in pharmacy—publications that look like regular journals or newsletters but are funded by a single sponsor and that are often produced by an advertising agency and distributed free to pharmacists. The sponsor supports the publication for marketing purposes and generally will not make a long-term commitment to its existence. Although many of these periodicals contain information that pharmacists find interesting and useful, their quality varies greatly and they are not considered to be of archival value. Even the most comprehensive health sciences library does not maintain collections of throwaway periodicals. There are also numerous Internet sites that deal with matters of interest to pharmacists practicing in hospitals or health systems. The Internet sites of reputable, professional organizations and publishers are of great value in that they often have links to relevant background and can be substantially more current than printed materials. Unfortunately, there are countless Internet sites containing inaccurate and misleading information.

Use of Periodicals for Current Awareness

Many pharmacists spend a substantial portion of their time in keeping up with the current literature. It would not be unusual for an ambitious institutional pharmacist to regularly scan all of the periodicals listed in Appendix 31-1 (and often additional ones as well). Such scans are facilitated by subscribing to email-based distributions of the table of contents of many periodicals. Subscribers to some publications that have Internet sites in addition to print products can view the full text of published material, sometimes in advance of the mail distribution of printed journals. Internet-accessible journals also have powerful search engines that allow the reader to quickly find articles by full-text search for subjects or author. The most sophisticated of the electronic biomedical publications provide direct links to references cited in their content. These links allow the reader to see abstracts or, in some cases, full text of the cited papers. In addition, such publications often offer a host of services that assist the reader:

- View abstracts of earlier-published articles
- View full text of at least some of the articles archived
- See full text of many references cited in articles
- Search other biomedical publications within the entire PubMed file
- Order full text copies of any article ever published
- Receive email alerts of new publications by user-selected authors
- Receive email alerts of new articles published on user-selected topics
- Send articles to colleagues and friends by email
- For nonsubscribers, gain access to subscriber-only protected content through a variety of pay-per-view options

Table 31-1 compares the attributes of the online versions of several pharmacy periodicals.

Pharmacists who specialize in a particular area of practice may concentrate their attention on the literature in that area. Some pharmacy departments assign pharmacists to monitor specific journals and to bring to the attention of the whole staff articles that are especially relevant to the department's activities. Some departments conduct a journal club that meets regularly (e.g., monthly) to hear oral summaries by staff members of important articles from the current literature.

Internet- and Database-Assisted Literature Retrieval

Publishers, corporations, and even individuals devote substantial resources to provide and enhance Internet access to their information, and the advent of powerful Internet search engines (e.g., Google [www.google.com]) has made the Internet a major method of searching for information of all sorts. For example, a Google search of the subject, "computerized prescriber order entry," done on March 1, 2005, found more that 1,330 results in a fraction of a second. Scanning the descriptors of the results reveals the diversity of the information found: pharmacy association websites, other professional associations' sites, pharmacy journals, patient safety sites, individual hospital websites, various newsletters, and product vendors. Much of the information found in this fashion is germane to the issue but of unknown quality, focus, and bias. Further, it is quite time-consuming to explore all the informa-

tion found with the search. The same search in PubMed (www.ncbi.nlm.nih.gov) produced 17 results (articles published in medical, pharmacy, and nursing journals), and an Internet-based search of AJHP (www.ajhp.org) produced 19 results.

Structured search can be done efficiently through one of the numerous, reputable online database vendors. *International Pharmaceutical Abstracts (IPA)*, pharmacy's only abstracting and indexing journal, has special utility for current awareness. It covers more than 750 journals, and offers abstracts of articles that are of interest to pharmacy practitioners, educators, students, and researchers. *IPA* also includes abstracts of most presentations made at the ASHP Summer Meeting and Midyear Clinical Meeting. *IPA's* abstracts are grouped in 25 subject areas (such as pharmacy practice; legislation, laws, and regulations; adverse drug reactions; drug evaluations; and pharmaceutical education), which facilitates scanning issues for current awareness. Through its controlled index, *IPA* also offers subscribers a tool for searching for papers on a particular subject.

Appendix 31-1 lists contact information for several database vendors in the United States of interest to pharmacists. After users first register with a vendor, they receive complete instructions on how to access specific databases. Database producers and database vendors offer training seminars on online computer literature searching. In the "pay as you use" plans, users have an incentive to learn to be efficient in their searches because most vendors base their charges in part on the length of time of the user's connection with a database. Databases available on subscription basis do not have comparable connect-time considerations.

Some reference books and textbooks are also available through Internet-based subscriptions. Some of these can be accessed through personal digital assistants (PDAs). Books that may be searched by this method include *AHFS Drug Information, Handbook on Injectable Drugs, Martindale: The Extra Pharmacopoeia,* and *Medication Teaching Manual.*

Another method of information-retrieval is CD-ROM (compact disk, read-only memory) technology. Numerous pharmacy-related information sources (e.g., books, drug information compendia) have been produced in this format. Users of such CD products can search the database in much the same way as with an online service. The CD information product usually entails annual subscription purchase rather than per-use charges. The major shortcoming of this technology

Table 31-1

Comparative Attributes of Internet Site of Several Pharmacy Journals[a]

Journal Internet Address	Frequency (issues/yr)	Searchable (since)?	Abstracts (since)?	Full Text	References Linked
American Journal of Health-System Pharmacy www.ajhp.com	24	Yes 1965	Yes 1975	Yes 1997	Yes 2005
Annals of Pharmacotherapy www.theannals.com	12	Yes 1975	Yes 1978	Yes 1998	Yes 2003
Formulary www.formularyjournal.com	12	No	No	Yes 2001	No
Hospital Pharmacy www.hospitalpharmacyjournal.com	12	Yes 1999	No	Yes 1999	No
Journal of Pharmacy Practice www.jpp.sagepub.com	12	Yes 2001	Yes 2001	Yes 2001	Yes 2001
Pharmacotherapy www.extenza-eps .com	12	No 1999	Yes 1999	Yes 1999	No
The Consultant Pharmacist www.ascp.com/public/ pubs/tcp/archive.shtml	12	Yes 1996	No	Yes 1996	No
U.S. Pharmacist www.uspharmacist.com	12	Yes 1996	Yes 1996	Yes 1996	No

[a] As of 3/1/05.

is its static nature. CD-ROM products share with text-books the general limitation that their obsolescence begins upon their creation. A list of some vendors of CD-ROM products of interest to pharmacy is included in Appendix 31-1.

Books Used in Institutional Pharmacy

It is beyond the scope of this chapter to discuss thoroughly the books of institutional pharmacy. Hundreds of books are available that might be of some use in practice, and scores of new ones are published every year. Hence, one has to be selective about new acquisitions. A good way to learn about new books is to read the book review sections of periodicals such as the *American Journal of Health-System Pharmacy* and the *American Journal of Pharmaceutical Education*.

There would probably be strong agreement among institutional pharmacists with respect to a short list of books that should be available in every institutional pharmacy department. Many practitioners would want to own personal copies of some of the books on such a list. Included on the list would probably be a current medical dictionary, such as *Stedman's Medical Dictionary* or *Dorland's Illustrated Medical Dictionary*. This handbook, edited by Thomas R. Brown, would be on the list. Also present would be the current editions of ASHP's *Best Practices for Hospital & Health-System Pharmacy, AHFS Drug Information, Drug Facts and Comparisons, Martindale: The Extra Pharmacopeia, Physician's Desk Reference, Remington's Pharmaceutical Sciences, U.S. Pharmacopeia-National Formulary, USP DI, USP Dictionary of USAN and International Drug Names, American Drug Index,* and a general medical text such as Harrison's *Principles of Internal Medicine*. Further, Trissel's *Handbook on Injectable Drugs* has become a standard institutional pharmacy department reference book. Beyond this short list of basic books, many others will be found in pharmacy departments to aid them with specific needs related to their scope of services.

Contributing to the Literature*

It is well within the ability of every institutional pharmacist to write for publication in the pharmacy literature. Further, every practitioner has ideas and makes observations and innovations that are likely to have merit for publication.

There are two categories of reasons why pharmacists should want to contribute to the literature. The first stems from altruistic motives related to a desire to share what one has learned for the benefit of others and to help advance the profession of pharmacy. In the second category are more self-serving reasons relating to personal satisfaction, career development, and recognition. Although there can be some negative aspects associated with the latter reasons, such as submitting the least publishable unit (see section entitled Controversies Related to the Literature), vigilant journal editors can control most of them.

Notwithstanding these reasons for writing for publication, the vast majority of pharmacists never contribute to the literature. In part this is true because of some common myths about the publication process. One such myth is that frontline practitioners do not stand much chance of getting anything accepted for publication. If the following are substituted in the preceding sentence, one has a list of other common myths about journal publication: (1) pharmacists from small hospitals, (2) pharmacists from nonteaching hospitals, (3) pharmacists who do not belong to ASHP, (4) young pharmacists, and (5) old pharmacists.

There is no objective evidence that such biases exist among the peer-reviewed journals in pharmacy. The primary distinction between papers that are accepted for publication and those that are rejected relates to the quality of writing, including the quality of the ideas

expressed. There are very few naturally gifted writers in pharmacy; most authors have to work hard to produce clear, concise copy that holds the reader's interest and conveys a message worthy of the reader's time. In fact, the hard work required to produce a published paper is probably the main reason that most pharmacists do not write for publication in a professional journal.

It would not be unreasonable for a young pharmacist to develop a strategy for becoming a published author. This strategy could be an important component of a plan for building a fulfilling career, which in itself might be a component of an even larger plan for living a balanced, satisfying life. We all require creative outlets for personal growth, and publishing in a professional journal can be an avenue for fulfilling this need.

An early step for a pharmacist in a strategy for becoming a published author should be to build confidence in his or her ability to write. This can be done by taking on writing assignments in the pharmacy department (e.g., preparing meeting minutes, developing policies and procedures) and seeking feedback on performance. Pharmacists who lack academic preparation for good writing might consider taking courses part-time at a local college. Many reference books are available on writing, which may be obtained readily at a good public library or a full-service bookstore. The following two are worth adding to a personal library: *The Elements of Style*, 4th ed. and *Why Not Say It Clearly—A Guide to Scientific Writing*.[4,5]

Two useful books specifically about writing and publishing papers in the professional literature are *How to Write and Publish a Scientific Paper*, 3rd ed. and *How to Write and Publish Papers in the Medical Sciences*, 2nd ed.[6,7]

Before beginning to write a piece for publication, be sure that you have something important to say. A high proportion of papers rejected for publication are redundant with material already in the literature or deal with subjects that are deemed of insufficient importance to take up space in a journal.

Your first publication does not necessarily have to be a long article. Many journals like to receive short letters or reports on practical solutions to everyday

---

*A portion of this section is based on an editorial published previously by one of the authors (WAZ) in *Am J Hosp Pharm.* 1991;48:687. These comments relate to writing descriptive (not evaluative) reports and other general interest contributions for publication. For advice on writing research reports, see *Am J Hosp Pharm.* 1981;38:545–50. Advice on preparing review articles may be found in *Am J Hosp Pharm.* 1987;44:2264.

problems in pharmacy. These short communications are easier to write than full articles and are good confidence builders for the fledgling author. Also, keep in mind that college and residency projects often can be adapted for publication.

After selecting a topic to write about, study the journals that might be interested in your work. Peruse the material in recent issues and look for pieces similar to the one you plan to write. This will give you a model for your own writing and help you select the journal to which you want to submit your work. Keep in mind that some journals solicit nearly all of their papers. Unless your topic happens to coincide with a theme issue on the drawing board, such journals are unlikely to accept your paper. (To *solicit* a paper means that the journal staff identifies the topic of a prospective manuscript and recruits an author to write it. *Unsolicited* papers are submitted to journals by the authors without any explicit prompting by the publications.) If you are uncertain about whether a particular journal would be interested in reviewing a paper on your subject, email or call the editor to inquire.

After you have selected the journal, study its requirements for manuscripts carefully, looking at both the general instructions to authors and any special advice for the type of paper you will write. It pays to follow a journal's instructions diligently to avoid delays in its review of your work.

Before beginning to write your manuscript, check to learn if similar papers have already been published, especially within the past 5 years. One of the computerized literature retrieval services discussed earlier will aid this checking process. Cite relevant literature in your paper, but take extreme care not to plagiarize any of the articles you have reviewed.

You are now ready to begin writing. Strive to do an excellent job of organizing your thoughts and expressing them succinctly and clearly. Never submit a first draft to a journal. Even highly experienced authors will prepare three or more drafts before sending a paper to the editor. Have others whose writing ability you respect read and critique your paper when you think it is finished. Evaluate their comments with an open mind and do further revision if indicated. It is a good idea to set aside the finished paper for a few days and then give it one final reading with fresh eyes; this more detached scrutiny will often suggest additional polishing you will want to do. If you submit the paper to a journal through traditional mail, be sure to keep a copy for your files.

Most journals have Internet-based processes, which authors are encouraged to use in submitting their work. Most all publishers acknowledge receipt of a manuscript immediately. Several weeks later (the amount of time will depend on the paper's length and complexity), you will receive comments back from the journal's editorial staff. It is not unusual for the editors, based on their own analysis and the advice of outside reviewers, to ask for clarifications and to make suggestions for revision. Keep in mind that the editors' comments are based on their assessment of the needs of the journal's readers.

If the editors encourage you to resubmit your work, by all means do so, and do it promptly. There is a human tendency to avoid dealing with any type of negative feedback, which sometimes leads a novice author to set aside a returned paper and never get back to it. Recognize that tendency and work hard to overcome it. Although it may seem difficult to believe when you face a blunt list of things wrong with your paper, most editors have an honest desire to help you communicate your ideas in the most effective way. It will almost always be in your best interest to cooperate with the editors toward that end.

You may find that most of the editors' comments or suggestions make sense, and you will want to comply with them. Others may seem to be of borderline wisdom, and you must decide whether to follow them or defend your position. Still other criticisms may be clearly ill-founded, in which case you should hold your ground and tell the editors why. After you revise your paper, resubmit it with a cover letter that discusses in detail how you have handled all of the questions, comments, and suggestions.

If a journal rejects your paper, you have the option of submitting it to another publication. If you decide to do so, consider first revising it to take into account any criticisms passed on to you by the first editors. If your paper is not explicitly rejected but you wish to submit it elsewhere anyway (because, for example, it will not be possible for you to accommodate the requests for revision), you must first withdraw the paper from the journal to which you have already submitted it. One of the principles of author ethics is that a paper must not be sent to more than one journal at a time. If you do not respond to a journal's request for revision, the journal will still consider your paper a pending manuscript. If that paper later appears in print elsewhere without having been withdrawn from the first journal, your reputation will be sullied among that journal's editors.

The publication of your first paper in the professional literature will be a thrilling experience. Your family, friends, and boss will be impressed, and colleagues will bestow upon you all manner of flattery, both deserved and undeserved. Before the glow of that experience fades, begin planning your next paper.

The Journal Peer-Review Process

The steps that journals go through to ensure the quality of what they publish is called the *journal peer-review process*. It entails seeking the advice of experts with respect to the paper's merit for publication but also includes the review efforts of the editors themselves. The overall goal of the review process is to evaluate the quality of a manuscript in terms of its organizational structure, clarity of expression, and, fundamentally, contribution to the literature. This last factor means the extent to which a paper adds to the body of knowledge in a field.[8] Papers that are judged to make major contributions in this regard are given high priority for publication. The least meritorious papers are rejected. Most papers fall at various points on the scale between these two extremes.

Reviewers are asked to focus on the heart of a paper's content (writing style and organizational structure are scrutinized carefully by the editorial staff). It is not always possible to find reviewers who are fully knowledgeable in all of the key aspects of a paper. If a manuscript reports a study of the clinical pharmacokinetics of theophylline, for example, it might be necessary to select one or two reviewers who are clinical pharmacokinetics experts and another reviewer who is familiar with the nuances of theophylline therapy. Further, if none of these reviewers has expertise in study design and data analysis, another individual may be asked to analyze those aspects of the paper.

Specialized expertise is required to review the methods of data analysis in research reports. That is why many biomedical journals retain a statistical consultant who may be outside the immediate discipline represented by the journal.

Typically, journal editors will select two outside reviewers for a manuscript. Certain straightforward, brief communications (including letters to the editor) may be reviewed only by the journal's staff. Journals maintain lists of reviewers coded by areas of expertise. They also generally maintain a record of experience with each reviewer that covers, for example, promptness and helpfulness of reviews, to aid the staff in deciding which experts to use in the future. Most editors welcome volunteers for the review process. Reviewers contribute their time without remuneration as a service to the profession. Statistical consultants, however, are usually paid.

As an example of the magnitude of the review process for a large journal office, consider the operations of the American Society of Health-System Pharmacists, which publishes *American Journal of Health-System Pharmacy (AJHP)*. *AJHP* receives about 600 manuscripts per year. About 50% of these papers are eventually published in *AJHP*, most of them with substantial revision. Some of the papers published by ASHP are solicited, including many review articles. The manuscript review process is handled by five pharmacist editors who are full-time employees of ASHP. (These individuals apply their own expertise—in drug information, pharmacy education, and pharmacy practice as well as editing—in the peer review process, as a complement to the advice of outside reviewers). A reviewer file of more than 1,000 names is maintained.

The entire process of tracking manuscripts and reviewers at ASHP is achieved through Internet-based tools and email correspondence. This includes original receipt of submitted manuscripts, correspondence with authors and reviewers, searching for appropriate reviewers on a specific topic, maintaining records on reviewers, tracking a manuscript's progress through the review and editing steps, generating routine correspondence to authors and reviewers, and producing routine reports.

In the case of *AJHP*, the average lag time between submission of a paper and its publication is 6 months. About half of this time is consumed by the review by peers and editors. The other half is time required by authors to revise their submissions, editors to evaluate the authors' revisions, and production steps for page composition. Table 31-2 summarizes these steps.

There is substantial variability among journals in how they handle some of the specific steps in peer review. For example, whereas some pharmacy journals, including *AJHP*, mask the reviewers to the identity of the authors, other journals do not, in part because their editors believe that most reviewers would be able to discern the authors' identities or at least their institutional affiliations. Those who mask author identity believe that doing so reduces bias in the review process and is worth the effort for that reason.

Table 31-2

Steps in the Review and Publication of Manuscripts Submitted to *AJHP*

Step	Time Required for Completion
1. Receive manuscript electronically	
2. Assign corresponding editor	
3. Select reviewers	
4. Send manuscript to reviewers electronically	Steps 1–4 total less than one week
5. Receive reviewers' comments electronically	4–6 weeks
6. Independent critique by corresponding editors	2 weeks
7. Staff discussion and decision (pursue or release)	1 day
8. Request revision by author	within 2 weeks
9. Receive, evaluate, accept revision	4–6 weeks
10. Edit manuscript for clarity, conformance with journal style	2 weeks
11. Author review of copyediting	1 week
12. Page composition, issue collation, proofreading, electronic transmission to printer, prepress and press time by printer	4 weeks
13. Publish (print and electronic)	
Total	**22–24 weeks**

Table 31-2 shows typical elapsed time between steps as well as for the total cycle. *Corresponding editor* refers to a pharmacist-editor employed on the staff of ASHP. *Reviewers* are outside experts who are called upon to analyze papers and advise on their merit for publication. At step 7, the entire staff of pharmacists-editors meets to arrive at a consensus on how papers that have gone through the review process should be handled. At step 9, a paper may be rejected if the revision is highly unsatisfactory. At step 11, the author is sent a galley proof electronically for checking, which is the author's opportunity to review and approve editorial changes that have been made.

Most journals mask authors to the identity of the reviewers. However, reviewers occasionally ask that their identities be revealed in case the author wishes to contact them for clarification of their critique.

Some journals, including *AJHP*, exchange critiques among reviewers. By showing each reviewer what the other has said, individual reviewers have a basis for assessing the quality of their work, and they may learn about additional points to cover in future critiques.

Most editors consider the comments of reviewers advisory, not binding. The editors may well pursue a revision of a paper even though all of the outside reviewers are recommending rejection. Conversely, based on their perspective, the editors may reject a paper in the face of unanimous advice to accept. Factors that editors weigh in these decisions, which may not necessarily be points that reviewers considered, include the recent acceptance of other similar papers, the backlog of papers awaiting publication, and an assessment of author or reviewer bias or motive that is inconsistent with the objectives of journal publication. It is not unusual for the editors to be more familiar than outside reviewers with the literature in a particular area and for this to weigh heavily in the final decision. Further, if a paper has extraordinary problems in structure and writing style, the editors may decide that they cannot afford to devote the resources necessary for making it acceptable for publication, even though there may be some germ of merit buried within its pages. Although it is widely believed that the journal peer-review process improves the quality of the literature, it is not a guarantee of infallibility.[9]

Controversies Related to the Literature

Those who read and contribute to the literature should be aware of the major controversies associated with journal publishing. The debate on these issues has been going on for quite some time and is not likely to be resolved soon.

Perhaps the biggest concern about the literature is its proliferation. The "information explosion" is a ubiquitous reality. Further, the ease with which information can be posted to the Internet blurs the distinction between vetted material and that which is merely personal opinion or intentionally misleading.

The development of computerized literature searching services has been in direct response to the expansion of the primary literature and the overwhelming difficulty that individuals have in keeping up with all of the information published in their fields. The problem is compounded by the publication of information relevant to a particular discipline in the journals of other specialized fields.

This growth in the literature is related largely to genuine expansion of knowledge and the need to disseminate that knowledge. However, there are also abuses of the publishing enterprise that contribute to the growth of the literature. Because of the limited resources available for publishing, steps are being taken to curb those abuses.

The most prominent abuse stems from pressure on individuals, particularly those in academia, to publish more in order to advance their careers—the *publish or perish* phenomenon. Sometimes researchers will divide a project into several small aspects and attempt to publish a paper on each facet. Or they may take the ethically repugnant course of publishing the same work in more than one journal. The practice of writing up the least publishable unit has been referred to disparagingly as *salami slicing*. Sometimes individuals may be listed as coauthors, even though they had virtually nothing to do with writing the paper, solely because of the power they hold over the primary author.

Some academic institutions have made an important reform in their promotion and tenure systems in an effort to counter the pressure to publish many papers. Rather than weigh the number of publications of someone up for promotion, those institutions evaluate the quality of just a few publications selected by the candidate.

The journal peer-review process has been criticized on many fronts.[10] The objects of this criticism include the biases of reviewers, failure of the system to keep marginal papers from being published, and failure to detect errors and improprieties that wind up in print. There is a concerted effort underway by editors of biomedical journals to better understand issues such as these through educational conferences and research.

The research literature, including that of institutional pharmacy, has been criticized often for use of faulty statistical methods. As stated earlier, some journals have instituted expert statistical review of manuscripts to deal with this problem. A fundamental resolution of this issue would come from an upgrading of the statistical knowledge of researchers.

Another controversy in publishing in the biomedical literature is the concept of *open access publishing*.[11] This concept, championed by the former director of the National Institutes of Health, directs publishers of NIH research to make that content openly available to everyone. There is growing interest among some in expanding this concept to the content of all biomedical research. So far, there has been no credible business model imagined that would allow publishers to generate income adequate to fund this concept. The NIH proponents have suggested that this could be funded by fees paid by authors to their publishers, but the argument is specious. The process currently being used by the *New England Journal of Medicine*, in which all *NEJM* content older than 6 months is freely available, is an interesting experiment in open access publishing.

Summary

The strength and vibrancy of institutional pharmacy is explained by many factors, not the least of which is the literature of institutional pharmacy. This sector of the profession has been guided by a distinct literature separate from that of the rest of pharmacy for 60 years or more. This has helped create a strong identity for institutional pharmacy and has been an instrument for leadership and development of the discipline.

Use of the literature is a primary skill for practitioners of institutional pharmacy. In addition, many practitioners will want to plan to contribute to the literature as an aspect of their career development self-fulfillment.

Acknowledgments

Appreciation is expressed to the following individuals for their assistance in developing this chapter: Maryam R. Mohassel, Guy R. Hasegawa, Lori Justice, Edward

Millikan, Peter Cantor, Cheryl A. Thompson, Jill A. Sellers, Catherine Nichols Klein, Jane L. Miller, Dwight R. Tousignaut, and Michaelene W. Morgan.

References

1. Sonnedecker G. *Kremers and Urdang's History of Pharmacy.* 4th ed. Philadelphia: Lippincott; 1976:3–36.

2. Starr P. *The Social Transformation of American Medicine.* New York: Basic Books; 1982:15.

3. *Pharmacists for the Future: The Report of the Study Commission on Pharmacy.* Ann Arbor, MI: Health Administration Press; 1975:13.

4. Strunk W Jr, White EB, Angel R. *The Elements of Style.* 4th ed. Needham Heights, MA: Allyn & Bacon; 2000.

5. Matthews JR, Bowen JM, Matthews RW. *Successful Scientific Writing: A Step-By-Step Guide for Biomedical Scientists.* 2nd ed. Cambridge University Press; 2001.

6. Day RA. *How to Write and Publish a Scientific Paper.* 5th ed. Phoenix, AZ: Oryx Press; 2000.

7. Taylor RB. *Clinician's Guide to Medical Writing.* Springer; 2004.

8. Talley CR. Perspective in journal publishing. *Am J Hosp Pharm.* 1993;50:451.

9. Jefferson T, Wagner E, Davidoff F. Measuring the quality of editorial peer review. *J Am Med Assoc.* 2002;287:286–90.

10. Godlee F, Jefferson T. *Peer Review in Health Sciences.* 2nd ed. London: BMJ Publishing Group; 2003.

11. Open access publishing. http://www.pubmedcentral.nih.gov/about/openaccess.html.

Appendix 31-1
Periodicals Important to Institutional Pharmacists

The publisher's name and address are given below each journal's name. Each publication's emphasis, from the perspective of practicing pharmacists, is categorized according to this schema:

A—frontline pharmacy practice
B—pharmacy practice management
C—professional issues
D—pharmaceutical sciences
E—pharmaceutical education
F—drug therapy
G—current affairs
H—abstracting/indexing service

Institutional Pharmacy Journals

American Journal of Health-System Pharmacy (A,B,C,D,E,F,G)
American Society of Hospital Pharmacists
7272 Wisconsin Avenue
Bethesda, MD 20814
www.ajhp.org

Annals of Pharmacotherapy (A,C,F)
Harvey Whitney Books Company
P.O. Box 42696
Cincinnati, OH 45242
www.theannals.com

Formulary (B,F)
Advanstar Communications
131 West First Street
Duluth, MN 55802-7008
www.formularyjournal.com

Hospital Pharmacy (A,B,C,F)
Wolters Kluer Health, Inc.
111/West Port Plaza, Suite 300
St. Louis, MO 63146
www.hospitalpharmacyjournal.com

Pharmacotherapy (F)
Pharmacotherapy Publications, Inc.
11 Nassau Street
Boston, MA 02111
www.accp.com

The Consultant Pharmacist (A,B,C)
American Society of Consultant Pharmacists
2300 Ninth Street, South, Suite 515
Arlington, VA 22204
www.ascp.com

U.S. Pharmacist (A,F)
Jobson Publishing Corporation
1515 Broad Street
Bloomfield, NJ 07003
www.uspharmacist.com

General Pharmacy Periodicals

Journal of the American Pharmacists Association (A,B,C,G)
American Pharmacists Association
2215 Constitution Avenue, NW
Washington, DC 20037
www.aphanet.org

Pharmacy Times (A,B,C)
Medical World Communications
241 Forsgate
Jamesburg, NJ 08831
www.pharmacytimes.com

Pharmaceutical Sciences Journals

Journal of Pharmaceutical Sciences (D)
American Pharmaceutical Association
2215 Constitution Avenue, NW
Washington, DC 20037
www.aphanet.org

Pharmaceutical Research (D)
Springer-Science+Business Media B. V.
P.O. Box 14302
14197 Berlin
Germany
www.aapspharmaceutica.com

Pharmaceutical Education Journals

American Journal of Pharmaceutical Education (E)
(Web-only publication)
American Association of Colleges of Pharmacy
1426 Prince Street
Alexandria, VA 22314-2841
www.ajpe.org

Journal of Pharmacy Teaching (E)
The Haworth Press, Inc.
10 Alice Street
Binghamton, NY 13904-1580
www.haworthpressinc.com

Appendix 31-1, continued

Current Affairs Periodicals

Drug Topics (G)
Advanstar Communications
131 West First Street
Duluth, MN 55802-7008
www.drugtopics.com

F-D-C Reports (The Pink Sheet) (G)
F-D-C Reports
5550 Friendship Boulevard, Suite I
Chevy Chase, MD 20815
www.fdcreports.com

Medical Periodicals

Annals of Internal Medicine (F)
American College of Physicians
Independence Mall West, Sixth Street at Race
Philadelphia, PA 19106-1572
www.annals.org

Journal of the American Medical Association (JAMA) (F)
American Medical Association
P.O. Box 10946
Chicago, IL 60610-7827
jama.ama-assn.org

The Medical Letter on Drugs and Therapeutics (F)
The Medical Letter, Inc.
1000 Main Street
New Rochelle, NY 10801
www.themedicalletter.com

New England Journal of Medicine (F)
Massachusetts Medical Society
10 Shattuck Street
Boston, MA 02115
content.nejm.org

Health Care Management Periodicals

Hospitals & Health Networks (B,G)
Health Forum, Inc
1 North Franklin Street
Chicago, IL 60606
www.hhnmag.com

Modern Healthcare (B,G)
Modern Healthcare Magazine
360 N. Michigan Avenue, 5th Floor
Chicago, IL 60601
www.modernhealthcare.com

English-Language Foreign Journals

Canadian Journal of Hospital Pharmacy
Canadian Society of Hospital Pharmacists
Société canadienne des pharmaciens d'hôspitaux
Ottawa, Ontario KZE 7V7
Canada
www.cshp.ca

The Pharmaceutical Journal
Royal Pharmaceutical Society of Great Britain
1 Lambeth High Street
London, SE1 7JN
England
www.pharmj.com

Drugs
ADIS Press Limited
41 Centorian Drive, Private Bag
Mairangi Bay, Auckland 10
New Zealand
www.adisonline.info

The Lancet
Elsevier
360 Park Avenue South
New York, NY 10010-1710
www.thelancet.com

Major Online Sources for Searching Biomedical Publications

www.pubmed.gov/ (PubMed)

www.medlineplus.gov/ (Medline)

www.ovid.com (IPA)

www.uiowa.edu/nidis (IDIS)

www.ebsco.com (Academic Search Elite)

www.thomsonisi.com (Web of Science)

http://highwire.stanford.edu (Highwire Press)

www.biosis.org/products/ba (Biological Abstracts)

www.isinet.com/products/cap/ccc (Current Contents)

Appendix 31-1, continued

Email Addresses on Major Vendors of Biomedical CD-ROM Resources

http://www.ashp.org/ahfs/product_info.com (AHFS-DI drug
  information resources)

http://www.uiowa.edu/~idis (Iowa drug information products)

http://www.skyscape.com (PDA products for medicine, nursing, and pharmacy)

http://www.rxfactstat.com (free medical and pharmaceutical information)

http://www.medmatrix.org/reg/login.asp (clinical medicine resources)

http://www.micromedex.com/products (drug and disease information)

http://www.pdamd.com (hand-held information devices)

http://www.hannsonsoftware.com (pharmacy and medication-related software)

http://www.firstdatabank.com (drug knowledge integration)

http://library.dialog.com/bluesheets/html/bl0074.html (International
  Pharmaceutical Abstracts)

Chapter 32

Poison Control Centers

Daniel J. Cobaugh

Introduction

Poisoning is a significant international public health problem. In 2004, the Institute of Medicine estimated that 4 million poisonings occur in the United States annually.[1] The American Association of Poison Control Centers (AAPCC) reported over 2.3 million calls to poison centers regarding potential human poisonings in 2003.[2] Of these, over 1.3 million involved medications and 14.1% of the calls were received from health care facilities. Poison control centers have played an invaluable public health role for over 50 years.[3] The majority of U.S. poison centers are located in hospitals and many of these centers have historical roots in departments of pharmacy. Although poison centers were initially developed to address prevention and treatment of pediatric poisoning, their scope of services has expanded to include management of toxicities related to suicide, adverse drug events, substance abuse, and occupational and environmental exposures. In a post-September 11 environment, poison centers have become increasingly involved in community and regional preparedness efforts related to biological and chemical terrorism.[4–8] This chapter will provide an overview of contemporary poison center services, their role in the management of the wide variety of toxicities that are seen in hospitals, and the relationship between poison centers and departments of pharmacy.

Poison Center History

In 1953, Gdalman and Press established the first U.S. poison center in Chicago following recognition by the American Academy of Pediatrics Accident Prevention Committee that poisoning represented 49% of accidents treated by pediatricians.[3] The number of centers grew to 17 by 1957, and by 1978 there were 661 centers operating in the U.S. Many of these centers delegated case management responsibilities to staff in hospital pharmacies and emergency departments that were also responsible for other patient care activities. Absence of designated poison center staff in those settings led to inconsistencies in their overall scope of

activities and the quality of information provided.

In the early 1980s, the AAPCC initiated a movement toward regionalization of poison centers and certification of poison center staff. These quality-related activities, along with economic factors at the state and local level, dramatically changed the landscape for provision of poison control services in the U.S. The AAPCC established regional poison center certification criteria that focused on level of service, staff requirements, documentation, data collection, prevention programs, health professional education, and quality improvement activities.[9] Consolidation of poison centers ensued as state governments and the poison centers' host organizations, primarily hospitals, struggled with the increasing cost of poison control services. As of early 2005, there were 61 poison centers in the U.S. A 2002 survey by the AAPCC found that all U.S. poison centers currently receive some federal funding and 87% received state funds outside of Medicaid and block grants.[10] Almost 52% indicated that they continue to receive support from their host institution and less than 5% receive financial support from health insurers. In the 2002 AAPCC survey, 24 % of poison centers indicated that they receive funds through some other business relationship. In many cases, these centers are generating additional revenue through contractual arrangements with pharmaceutical and chemical manufacturers.[11] Along with responding to consumer inquiries about the health effects of the manufacturer's product, these poison centers play a role in collecting postmarketing surveillance information.[11] In order to maximize upon economies of scale in providing services to states with smaller populations, some large poison centers provide services to multiple states.

The Poison Center Enhancement and Awareness Act was originally signed into law in 2000 and reauthorized in 2004. This law authorizes federal grant support to poison centers and funding for the nationwide toll-free poison center number, enhancement of poisoning data collection, and establishment of a nationwide prevention program. One of the landmark results of this legislation was establishment of a single, nationwide toll-free telephone number that provides access to poison centers in all 50 states, the District of Columbia, and Puerto Rico. A single access number has enabled nationwide promotion of poison center services. One goal of establishment of this number was increased poison center awareness and utilization. Krenzelok and Mrvos described an 11.2% increase in poison center call volume following implementation of the nationwide toll-free number.[12]

In 2004, the Institute of Medicine completed a comprehensive review of poison center services in the U.S entitled *Forging a Poison Prevention and Control System*.[1] This report addressed several aspects of poison center services including system development, certification of centers and staff, and data collection and surveillance. Table 32-1 provides the 12 recommendations put forth by the IOM panel.

The AAPCC Toxic Exposure Surveillance System

The AAPCC Toxic Exposure Surveillance System. (TESS), developed in 1983, captures call data from all U.S. poison centers.[13] The TESS data set includes demographic, substance, and clinical data. Examples of clinical data collected include signs and symptoms of toxicity, treatments provided, and medical outcomes. Data collection occurs with the initial poison center call, during follow-up calls, and when bedside consultation occurs. The data collection software is integrated with the center's electronic medical record.

A TESS Annual Report that provides a comprehensive summary of the data collected through the system is published each year by the AAPCC.[2,14–32] Table 32-2 lists selected TESS data elements from these annual reports which can be accessed at http://www.aapcc.org/annual.htm. This site contains annual reports dating back to the system's origination in 1983.

TESS defines a therapeutic error as an unintentional deviation from a proper therapeutic regimen that results in the wrong dose, incorrect route of administration, administration to the wrong person, or administration of the wrong substance.[13] An adverse reaction is defined as an event that occurred with normal, prescribed, labeled, or recommended use of the product. In 2000, TESS began to collect additional information on therapeutic errors reported to poison centers.[33] The 2003 TESS data indicate that the top three scenarios for a therapeutic error were administration of an additional dose, a dosing error involving more than one

additional dose, and administration of the wrong medication.[2]

TESS data have been used for a variety of purposes including postmarketing surveillance, regulatory review, toxicology research, development of poison prevention campaigns and, most recently, real-time toxicosurveillance.[13] Pharmaceutical manufacturers have used TESS data in submissions to the U.S. Food and Drug Administration when prescription to over-the-counter switches are considered and when other types of regulatory reviews are conducted. In 1992, Litovitz and Manoguerra used a hazard factor analysis of TESS data to demonstrate a high pediatric mortality associated with iron-containing medications.[34] These data were used by the U.S. Food and Drug Administration in a regulatory review that preceded a mandated packaging of over-the-counter iron supplements in unit dose packages. Other investigators have used similar methodologies to characterize poisoning hazards in older adults.[35,36] Analysis of over 180,000 cases, reported over a 10-year period, revealed that major morbidity and death most frequently occurred from therapeutic errors involving heparin, colchicine, aminophylline/theophylline, lithium, and aspirin.[36] Analysis of adverse reactions found that biguanide hypoglycemics, cardiac glycosides, warfarin, antineoplastics, and heparin were most often associated with significant morbidity and mortality.

In response to potential acts of terrorism involving chemicals, the AAPCC has worked with the Centers for Disease Control and Prevention to develop systems for real-time toxicosurveillance using the TESS database. Data are uploaded from the poison center site to a central repository every 15 minutes. Toxicosurveillance systems have been developed to identify syndromic and product-specific trends in specific geographic locations. This toxicosurveillance technology could also be used for early recognition of emerging safety-related threats involving medications.

Scope of Poison Center Services

Poison centers' historic roots in the field of pediatric injury sometimes causes confusion among the public and health professionals regarding their contemporary role. It is sometimes assumed that poison center services are limited to the management of pediatric poisoning and poison prevention programs. Poison centers provide information regarding a wide spectrum of toxicologic emergencies that affect all age groups. Table 32-3 provides detailed information on the age

Table 32-1

IOM Recommendations for Forging a Poison Control and Prevention System[1]

1. All poison control centers should perform a defined set of core activities supported by federal funding that is tied to the provision of these activities.

2. Poison control centers should collaborate with state and local health departments to develop, disseminate, and evaluate public and professional education activities.

3. The U.S. Department of Health and Human Services (DHHS) and the states should establish a Poison Prevention and Control System that integrates poison control centers with public health agencies, establishes performance measures, and holds all parties accountable for protecting the public.

4. The Centers for Disease Control and Prevention (CDC), working with HRSA and the states, should continue to build an effective infrastructure for all-hazards emergency preparedness, including bioterrorism and chemical terrorism.

5. HRSA should commission a systematic management review focusing on organizational determinants of cost, quality, and staffing of poison control centers as the foundation for the future funding of this program.

6. Congress should amend the current Poison Control Center Enhancement and Awareness Act to provide sufficient funding to support the proposed Poison Prevention and Control System with its national network of regional poison control centers.

7. Congress should amend existing public health legislation to fund a state and local infrastructure to support an integrated Poison Prevention and Control System.

8. A fully external, independent body should be responsible for certification of poison control centers and specialists in poison information.

9. The Secretary of Health and Human Services should instruct key agencies to convene an expert panel to develop a definition of poisoning that can be used in surveillance activities (including the Toxic Exposure Surveillance System) and ongoing data collection studies.

10. DHHS should undertake a targeted education effort to improve health provider awareness of poisoning data collection as it relates to the Health Insurance Portability and Accountability Act (HIPAA) and state privacy regulations to mitigate their unintended chilling effect on poison control center consultation, including follow-up.

11. The Director of the Centers for Disease Control and Prevention should ensure that exposure surveillance data generated by the poison control centers and currently reported in the Toxic Exposure Surveillance System are available to all appropriate local, state, and federal public health units and to the poison control centers on a *real-time* basis at no additional cost to these users.

12. Federally funded research should be provided for (1) studies on the epidemiology of poisoning, (2) the prevention and treatment of poisoning and drug overdose, (3) health services access and delivery, (4) strategies to improve regulations and facilitate researchers' input into regulatory procedures, and (5) the cost efficiency of the new Poison Prevention and Control System on population-based outcomes for general and specific poisonings.

Table 32-2
Selected TESS Annual Report Tables

Age and Gender Distribution of Cases

Age and Gender Distribution of Fatalities

Chemical Substances Implicated in Human Exposure

Fatality Table

Exposure Site

Management Site

Medical Outcome by Age

Narrative Abstracts of Selected Fatalities

Pharmaceutical Substances Implicated in Human Exposure

Reason for Exposure

Route of Exposure

Substance Categories with the Greatest Number of Deaths

Substances Most Frequently Implicated in Human Exposures

Substances Most Frequently Implicated in Pediatric Exposures

Therapies Provided

distribution of poison center cases from 1999 through 2003. These toxicities may manifest as a result of accidental pediatric poisonings, suicide attempts involving medications and chemicals, adverse drug events, substance abuse as well as occupational and environmental exposure to toxic substances. In 2002, U.S. poison centers managed over 813,000 potential exposures involving patients 20 years of age or older.[2] Table 32-3 provides exposure reason data for a 5-year period from 1999 through 2003 as reported by the AAPCC.

As described in Table 32-4, poison center consultations can generally be characterized as involving either an accidental or intentional exposure. Examples of accidental exposures include pediatric poisonings, therapeutic medication errors, occupational exposures to lead, and environmental exposures such as carbon monoxide poisoning. Although they are accidental in nature, TESS classifies adverse reactions to medications and foods in a separate category.

Both the public and health professionals contact poison centers for toxicology information. Physicians or nurses in the emergency department and the intensive care unit represent the group of health professionals that most frequently seek poison center consultation. In 2003, 14.1% of poison center calls originated in a

health care facility.[2] As described in Table 32-4, poison centers were involved with the management of over 215,000 therapeutic errors and over 41,000 adverse drug reactions in 2003. The capability of poison centers to manage the toxicities that ensue subsequent to an adverse drug event or a therapeutic error, as well as their ability to collect extensive data regarding these cases, provides an opportunity for professional collaboration with hospital pharmacy departments.

Public and professional education is another component of a poison control center's scope of services. Poison prevention efforts have been a cornerstone of poison center activities since their inception.[3,9,37-44] Many centers employ one or more health educators who use a variety of prevention strategies to increase poison center awareness and decrease the frequency of poisonings. While these efforts have focused primarily on childhood poisoning, medication-related adverse event prevention in older people is also becoming a focus of prevention activities for some centers. The implementation of a nationwide toll-free poison center number has enabled development of nationwide awareness and prevention programs. Involvement in poison prevention activities provides an avenue for health-system pharmacists to carry out their valuable public health role.

Training of health professional students has also been a core poison center activity for decades.[45,46] These include pharmacy students, medical students, pharmacy residents, emergency medicine residents, pediatric residents, and a wide variety of other trainees. These educational programs have been validated through pretest and posttest assessment.[47] Poison centers also provide continuing education for a wide variety of health professionals who practice in the health care facilities in the center's geographic region.

Poison Center Operations

Poison centers are available 24 hours per day, 7 days per week to provide toxicology consultation. Use of the nationwide toll-free poison center number, 1-800-222-1222 (Figure 32-1), connects the public and health professionals to the poison center designated to serve the caller's geographic location.

Several types of health professionals provide the clinical toxicology expertise offered by poison centers. Calls to poison centers are initially managed by Specialists in Poison Information (SPIs) who are either pharmacists or nurses with specialized toxicology train-

Table 32-3
Calls to Poison Centers by Age, 1999–2003[2]

Year	≤ 5 Years	6–12 Years	13–19 Years	≥ 20 Years
1999	1,154,799	154,606	157,993	722,243
2000	1,142,796	151,221	160,505	696,171
2001	1,169,478	156,612	165,657	759,401
2002	1,227,381	159,487	171,731	803,520
2003	1,245,584	158,318	171,823	690,297
5 Year Total	5,940,038	780,244	827,709	3,671,632

ing.[48] The AAPCC offers a certification examination for SPIs who have worked for at least 2,000 hours in a poison center and have managed at least 2,000 human exposure cases. Poison Information Providers (PIPs) are also used in some centers. The PIP, who is supervised at all times by a SPI, is often a pharmacy student or paramedic.

Clinical and medical toxicologists provide 24-hour on-call support to the frontline poison center staff. Clinical toxicologists are most often pharmacists who have completed fellowship training in clinical toxicology and who have become board-certified by the American Board of Applied Toxicology.[49] All poison centers employ at least one physician who serves as the medical director and who is ultimately responsible for all clinical supervision within the center. Following completion of residency training in a primary medical specialty (e.g., emergency medicine, pediatrics, or internal medicine), these physicians complete 2-year medical toxicology fellowships and then become certified through the American Board of Medical Specialties subspecialty board in medical toxicology.[50]

Poison centers maintain extensive information regarding their service regions. The centers regularly survey the health care facilities in their region to collect information on the organization's capabilities. This includes the facilities ability to care for critically ill patients, the types and quantity of antidotes stocked, and their ability to emergently provide extracorporeal elimination procedures. The centers also establish consultative relationships with experts who have knowledge regarding local toxic risks such as hazardous materials, toxic plants, and poisonous snakes.

Poison Center Case Management

A comprehensive case management process results following each new call to a poison center. Initially, the SPI or PIP conducts a thorough assessment of the history of the exposure and determines the potential for development of toxicity. If there is potential risk for development of toxicity, the SPI first makes a decision regarding the most appropriate location for continued care of the patient. In 2003, 74.5% of poison centers cases were managed at the site of exposure, most often in the home, and did not require referral to a health care facility.[2]

Following the determination of the most appropriate treatment site, additional recommendations for patient management are provided. In some cases, the poison center recommends a use of a decontamination procedure in the home. For example, in over 1.1 million cases in 2002 and 2003 poison centers recommended some type of oral dilution of an ingested substance or irrigation, either ocular or dermal, following an exposure by one of these routes.[2,32] Historically, ipecac syrup was often recommended for gastric decontamination. However, the use of ipecac syrup to induce emesis has decreased dramatically over the last two decades and some poison centers have abandoned its use entirely. In 2005, the AAPCC published an ipecac treatment guideline that recommends its use in rare circumstances in which health care facility transport will be delayed significantly.[51] In some cases, observation is the only intervention that is required when a patient is not transported to a health care facility. In cases where observation and/or a decontamination procedure is recommended, the poison center will complete routine follow-up to monitor the patient's status.[52] If the ex-

Table 32-4
Reasons for Potential Poisoning Exposures, 1999–2003[2,30–33]

REASON	1999 NO.	%	2000 NO.	%	2001 NO.	%	2002 NO.	%	2003 NO.	%
Unintentional										
Bite/Sting	78,697	3.6	83,366	3.8	85,713	3.8	90,896	3.8	86,829	3.6
Environmental	51,751	2.4	50,370	2.3	57,209	2.5	64,330	2.7	60,493	2.5
Food Poisoning	46,054	2.1	41,110	1.9	41,319	1.8	42,690	1.8	36,556	1.5
General	1,460,073	66.3	1,418,573	65.4	1,455,602	64.2	1,498,801	63.0	1,502,401	62.7
Misuse	72,083	3.3	72,233	3.3	82,867	3.7	90,637	3.8	89,620	3.7
Occupational	42,088	1.9	36,975	1.7	35,472	1.6	35,882	1.5	32,952	1.4
Therapeutic Error	154,422	7.0	152,101	7.0	167,014	7.4	193,194	8.1	215,052	9.0
Unknown	2,897	0.1	7,937	0.4	6,645	0.3	4,167	0.2	3,991	0.2
Subtotal	1,908,065	86.7	1,862,665	85.9	1,931,841	85.2	2,020,597	84.9	2,027,894	84.7
Intentional										
Abuse	31,157	1.4	35,848	1.7	38,640	1.7	42,617	1.8	42,303	1.8
Misuse	35,261	1.6	35,811	1.7	37,078	1.6	41,246	1.7	40,989	1.7
Suspected suicide	154,355	7.0	162,473	7.5	176,221	7.8	181,894	7.6	186,024	7.8
Unknown	9,147	0.4	10,795	0.5	10,764	0.5	12,840	0.5	14,529	0.6
Subtotal	229,920	10.4	244,927	11.3	262,703	11.6	278,597	11.7	283,845	11.9
Other										
Contamination/tampering	5,010	0.2	4,675	0.2	5,537	0.2	5,336	0.2	4,777	0.2
Malicious	7,046	0.3	7,038	0.3	10,709	0.5	8,801	0.4	8,641	0.4
Withdrawal	Unavailable		Unavailable		5	0.0	420	0.0	776	0.0
Subtotal	12,056	0.5	11,713	0.5	16,251	0.7	14,557	0.6	14,194	0.6
Adverse Reaction										
Drug	32,742	1.5	31,245	1.4	35,646	1.6	41,215	1.7	41,335	1.7
Food	4,328	0.2	3,195	0.1	4,033	0.2	4,694	0.2	5,006	0.2
Other	8,139	0.4	7,913	0.4	9,519	0.4	11,224	0.5	12,461	0.5
Subtotal	45,209	2.1	42,353	2.0	49,198	2.2	57,133	2.4	58,802	2.5
Unknown	5,906	0.3	6,590	0.3	7,986	0.4	9,144	0.4	10,847	0.5
Total	2,201,156	100.0	2,168,248	100.0	2,267,979	100.0	2,380,028	100.0	2,395,582	100.0

pected response to home treatment does not occur or if a patient begins to display signs or symptoms of toxicity, transport to an emergency department (ED) is recommended. Poison centers are equipped to interface with the 911 system to arrange patient transport and to provide recommendations for out-of-hospital care to paramedics and emergency medical technicians. When transport to the ED is required, the poison center routinely apprises the ED staff of the patient's status and provides initial recommendations for care.

Over 525, 000 (21.9%) of cases reported to poison centers in 2003 were managed in health care facilities.[2] The poison center may have advised transport to a health care facility upon receipt of the call or they may have received a request for consultation from the facility as occurs in cases of iatrogenic toxicity. In these cases, clinical/medical toxicology consultation—either at the bedside or via the telephone—is often integrated

Figure 32-1
Toll-Free Poison Center Number

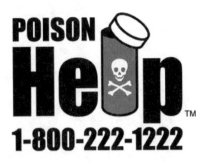

into the patient's care. These consultations address multiple aspects of the patient's care including key aspects of the physical examination and ongoing patient assessment, laboratory monitoring, gastrointestinal decontamination, antidote administration, the use of extracorporeal elimination measures (e.g., hemodialysis), and/or employing other poison-specific treatment strategies.

Given the potential for toxicologic ramifications from many medication-related errors and adverse events, the clinical/medical toxicologist is a critical member of the health care team that provides care to these patients. If the patient is hospitalized within the poison center's host institution, bedside consultation is often available. If the hospitalization involves another health care facility in the poison center's region, this consultation and the subsequent follow-up occur by telephone. Inclusion of the poison center and the clinical toxicologist in the team should result in enhanced patient care.

The decision to use a specific antidote (e.g., digoxin immune Fab) or an extracorporeal elimination procedure such as hemodialysis can be very complex. The clinical/medical toxicologist can also contribute to decisions about the need to monitor the patient in a critical care setting versus a medical/surgical floor. While timely use of interventions can be key to assuring good patient outcomes, decisions about their use must be judicious and based on a thorough understanding of the toxicologic characteristics of the implicated substance. The clinical/medical toxicologist is well positioned to provide guidance on the use of different toxicologic interventions

All poison centers interventions are documented and stored in an electronic medical record to document and maintain patient information. As mentioned previously, these medical records are integrated with the software used to collect data for submission to TESS.

Economic Impact

Since their inception, poison centers have struggled with maintaining secure and stable funding mechanisms. As mentioned previously, the majority of financial support has been provided by state governments and host institutions.[10] After the Poison Center Enhancement and Awareness Act was signed into law, a limited amount of federal funding was made available to fund the centers. In its report, the IOM recommended that "Congress should amend the current Poison Control Center Enhancement and Awareness Act to provide sufficient funding to support the proposed Poison Prevention and Control System with its national network of regional poison control centers."[1]

A key argument in the efforts to enhance poison center funding relates to the costs savings that result from poison center utilization. Miller found that the average public call to a poison control center for aid prevented $175 in other medical spending.[53] This was determined through analysis of incidence, medical spending, and payment sources data for poisoning. These authors found that in 1992 poison centers decreased the number of patients who received medical treatment but were not hospitalized for poisoning by approximately 24%. The number of hospitalizations was reduced by 12%.

References

1. *The Future of Poison Prevention and Control Services.* Washington: Institute of Medicine; 2004.

2. Watson WA, Litovitz TL, Klein-Schwartz W, et al. 2003 annual report of the American Association of Poison Control Centers Toxic Exposure Surveillance System. *Am J Emerg Med.* Sep 2004;22:335–404.

3. Burda AM, Burda NM. The nation's first poison control center: taking a stand against accidental childhood poisoning in Chicago. *Vet Hum Toxicol.* Apr 1997;39:115–9.

4. Krenzelok EP, Allswede MP, Mrvos R. The poison center role in biological and chemical terrorism. *Vet Hum Toxicol.* Oct 2000;42:297–300.

5. Crouch BI. Role of poison control centers in disaster response planning. *Am J Health-Syst Pharm.* Jun 15 2002;59:1159–63.

6. Forrester MB, Stanley SK. Calls about anthrax to the Texas Poison Center Network in relation to the anthrax bioterrorism attack in 2001. *Vet Hum Toxicol.* Oct 2003; 45:247–8.

7. Krenzelok EP. The critical role of the Poison Center in the recognition, mitigation and management of biological and chemical terrorism. *Przegl Lek.* 2001;58: 177–81.

8. LoVecchio F, Katz K, Watts D, Pitera A. Media influence on Poison Center call volume after 11 September 2001. *Prehospital Disaster Med.* Apr–Jun 2004;19:185.

9. Lovejoy FH, Jr., Robertson WO, Woolf AD. Poison centers, poison prevention, and the pediatrician. *Pediatrics.* Aug 1994;94:220–4.

10. 2002 Poison Center Survey. Available at: http://www.aapcc.org/2002_poison_center_survey_results.htm. Accessed March 30, 2005.

11. Krenzelok EP, Dean BS. A program of poison center services to business and industry. *Vet Hum Toxicol.* Apr 1987;29:172–3.

12. Krenzelok EP, Mrvos R. Initial impact of toll-free access on poison center call volume. *Vet Hum Toxicol.* Dec 2003;45:325–7.

13. Litovitz T. The TESS database. Use in product safety assessment. *Drug Saf.* Jan 1998;18:9–19.

14. Veltri JC, Litovitz TL. 1983 annual report of the American Association of Poison Control Centers National Data Collection System. *Am J Emerg Med.* Sep 1984;2: 420–43.

15. Litovitz T, Veltri JC. 1984 annual report of the American Association of Poison Control Centers National Data Collection System. *Am J Emerg Med.* Sep 1985;3: 423–50.

16. Litovitz TL, Normann SA, Veltri JC. 1985 Annual Report of the American Association of Poison Control Centers National Data Collection System. *Am J Emerg Med.* Sep 1986;4:427–58.

17. Litovitz TL, Martin TG, Schmitz B. 1986 annual report of the American Association of Poison Control Centers National Data Collection System. *Am J Emerg Med.* Sep 1987;5:405–45.

18. Litovitz TL, Schmitz BF, Matyunas N, Martin TG. 1987 annual report of the American Association of Poison Control Centers National Data Collection System. *Am J Emerg Med.* Sep 1988;6:479–515.

19. Litovitz TL, Schmitz BF, Holm KC. 1988 annual report of the American Association of Poison Control Centers National Data Collection System. *Am J Emerg Med.* Sep 1989;7:495–545.

20. Litovitz TL, Schmitz BF, Bailey KM. 1989 annual report of the American Association of Poison Control Centers National Data Collection System. *Am J Emerg Med.* Sep 1990;8:394–442.

21. Litovitz TL, Bailey KM, Schmitz BF, et al. 1990 annual report of the American Association of Poison Control Centers National Data Collection System. *Am J Emerg Med.* Sep 1991;9:461–509.

22. Litovitz TL, Holm KC, Bailey KM, et al. 1991 annual report of the American Association of Poison Control Centers National Data Collection System. *Am J Emerg Med.* Sep 1992;10:452–505.

23. Litovitz TL, Holm KC, Clancy C, et al. 1992 annual report of the American Association of Poison Control Centers Toxic Exposure Surveillance System. *Am J Emerg Med.* Sep 1993;11:494–555.

24. Litovitz TL, Clark LR, Soloway RA. 1993 annual report of the American Association of Poison Control Centers Toxic Exposure Surveillance System. *Am J Emerg Med.* Sep 1994;12:546–84.

25. Litovitz TL, Felberg L, Soloway RA, et al. 1994 annual report of the American Association of Poison Control Centers Toxic Exposure Surveillance System. *Am J Emerg Med.* Sep 1995;13:551–97.

26. Litovitz TL, Felberg L, White S, et al. 1995 annual report of the American Association of Poison Control Centers Toxic Exposure Surveillance System. *Am J Emerg Med.* Sep 1996;14:487–537.

27. Litovitz TL, Smilkstein M, Felberg L, et al. 1996 annual report of the American Association of Poison Control Centers Toxic Exposure Surveillance System. *Am J Emerg Med.* Sep 1997;15:447–500.

28. Litovitz TL, Klein-Schwartz W, Dyer KS, et al. 1997 annual report of the American Association of Poison Control Centers Toxic Exposure Surveillance System. *Am J Emerg Med.* Sep 1998;16:443–97.

29. Litovitz TL, Klein-Schwartz W, Caravati EM, et al. 1998 annual report of the American Association of Poison Control Centers Toxic Exposure Surveillance System. *Am J Emerg Med.* Sep 1999;17:435–87.

30. Litovitz TL, Klein-Schwartz W, White S, et al. 1999 annual report of the American Association of Poison Control Centers Toxic Exposure Surveillance System. *Am J Emerg Med.* Sep 2000;18:517–74.

31. Litovitz TL, Klein-Schwartz W, Rodgers GC, Jr., et al. 2001 Annual report of the American Association of Poison Control Centers Toxic Exposure Surveillance System. *Am J Emerg Med.* Sep 2002;20:391–452.

32. Watson WA, Litovitz TL, Rodgers GC, Jr., et al. 2002 annual report of the American Association of Poison Control Centers Toxic Exposure Surveillance System. *Am J Emerg Med.* Sep 2003;21:353–421.

33. Litovitz TL, Klein-Schwartz W, White S, et al. 2000 Annual report of the American Association of Poison Control Centers Toxic Exposure Surveillance System. *Am J Emerg Med.* Sep 2001;19:337–95.

34. Litovitz T, Manoguerra A. Comparison of pediatric poisoning hazards: an analysis of 3.8 million exposure incidents. A report from the American Association of Poison Control Centers. *Pediatrics.* Jun 1992;89: 999–1006.

35. Crouch BI, Caravati EM, Mitchell A, et al. Poisoning in older adults: a 5-year experience of US poison control centers. *Ann Pharmacother.* Dec 2004;38:2005–11.

36. Cobaugh DJ, Krenzelok EP. Geriatric poisoning severity: an analysis of poison center cases. *J Toxicol Clin Toxicol.* 2004;42:772.

37. Temple AR. Poison prevention education. *Pediatrics.* Nov 1984;74:964–9.

38. Oderda GM, Klein-Schwartz W. Public awareness survey: the Maryland Poison Center and Mr. Yuk, 1981 and 1975. *Public Health Rep.* May–Jun 1985;100:278–82.

39. McKaba J. Pharmacist involvement in poison prevention activities. *Am J Hosp Pharm.* Jul 1988;45:1496.

40. Baraff LJ, Guterman JJ, Bayer MJ. The relationship of poison center contact and injury in children 2 to 6 years old. *Ann Emerg Med.* Feb 1992;21:153–7.

41. Krenzelok EP. The use of poison prevention and education strategies to enhance the awareness of the poison information center and to prevent accidental pediatric poisonings. *J Toxicol Clin Toxicol.* 1995;33:663–7.

42. Schwartz L, Howland MA, Mercurio-Zappala M, et al. The use of focus groups to plan poison prevention education programs for low-income populations. *Health Promot Pract.* Jul 2003;4:340–6.

43. Spiller HA, Mowry JB. Evaluation of the effect of a public educator on calls and poisonings reported to a regional poison center. *Vet Hum Toxicol.* Aug 2004;46: 206–8.

44. Krenzelok EP, Mrvos R. Is mass-mailing an effective form of passive poison center awareness enhancement? *Vet Hum Toxicol.* Jun 2004;46:155–6.

45. Jordan JK, Dean BS, Krenzelok EP. Poison center rotation for health science students. *Vet Hum Toxicol.* Apr 1987;29:174–5.

46. Davis CO, Cobaugh DJ, Leahey NF, et al. Toxicology training of paramedic students in the United States. *Am J Emerg Med.* Mar 1999;17:138–40.

47. Cobaugh DJ, Goetz CM, Lopez GP, et al. Assessment of learning by emergency medicine residents and pharmacy students participating in a poison center clerkship. *Vet Hum Toxicol.* Jun 1997;39:173–5.

48. Mrvos R, Dean BS, Krenzelok EP, et al. A demographic profile of the Specialist in Poison Information. *Vet Hum Toxicol.* Aug 1994;36:330–1.

49. http://www.clintox.org/Abat/Index.html. Accessed April 1, 2005.

50. Wax PM, Donovan JW. Fellowship training in medical toxicology: characteristics, perceptions, and career impact. *J Toxicol Clin Toxicol.* 2000;38:637–42, discussion 643–4.

51. Manoguerra AS, Cobaugh DJ. Guideline on the use of ipecac syrup in the out-of-hospital management of ingested poisons. *Clin Toxicol (Phila).* 2005;43:1–10.

52. Litovitz TL, Elshami JE. Poison center operations: the necessity of follow-up. *Ann Emerg Med.* Jul 1982;11: 348–52.

53. Miller TR, Lestina DC. Costs of poisoning in the United States and savings from poison control centers: a benefit-cost analysis. *Ann Emerg Med.* Feb 1997;29: 239–45.

Chapter 33

Controlled Substances Management

George J. Dydek, David J. Tomich

Introduction

This chapter is directed at the pharmacy manager with the primary responsibility and oversight within a health-system pharmacy practice. This chapter is not intended to give a detailed description of applicable federal or state laws and regulations regarding the management of control substance medications (subsequently referred to as controlled substances), but rather this chapter will take a medication-use systems approach in examining the management of controlled substances in the health-system environment. Strategies and resources for the manager are offered. The approach taken in this chapter to the management of controlled substances is a medication systems approach, similar to the new Joint Commission on Accreditation of Healthcare Organizations (JCAHO) medication management standards instituted in 2004.[1] It allows for the systematic examination of controlled substances within an organization from selection and procurement through storage, inventory management, dispensing, administration, surveillance, and system evaluation.

There are several factors that influence the need or contribute to the necessity for the health-system pharmacy manager to emphasize the management of controlled substances and approach this oversight from a broad, medications systems perspective. The management of controlled substances is influenced first, by federal and state laws and regulations; secondly, by the concerns for patient safety as controlled substances are associated with medication errors resulting in adverse patient outcomes; and thirdly, by controlled substances that require astute management due to the ever increasing complexity of pharmacotherapy in the practice of pharmacy.

Federal and State Laws and Regulations

The overriding influence on the management of controlled substances in the health care environment are federal and state laws and regulations. The principal

federal law regulating controlled substances is the Controlled Substance Act (CSA), also referred to as Title II of the Federal Comprehensive Drug Abuse Prevention and Control Act of 1970, under Title 21 United States Code, starting at Section 801.[2] The Drug Enforcement Administration (DEA) is the federal entity charged with enforcing and implementing the CSA. The main mission of the DEA is working in concert with state agencies and other federal agencies (e.g., Food and Drug Administration) to prevent the diversion of controlled substances for illicit reasons. The DEA is able to carry out its mission through regulations contained in the Code of Federal Regulations (CFR), Title 21, starting at Part 1300. The health-system pharmacy manager must be familiar and have ready access to CFR Title 21. A good source for these regulations is the Food and Drug Administration website http://www.fda.gov/cdrh/devadvice/365.html or specifically relate to Part 1300 at.[3] The DEA provides an informative manual targeted for pharmacists that can be readily downloaded from their website.[4] Bookmarking the direct web link to the CFR Title 21 and maintaining either a hard copy or digital version of the DEA manual for pharmacists is highly recommended for any health-system pharmacy manager. Additionally, the DEA website (www.dea.gov) provides information related to CSA, with hyperlinks directly to government documents related to controlled substances. Controlled substances are classified according to their potential for abuse, accepted medical use, and potential for physical or psychological dependence which places them into different Schedules (I-V). A list of these classified medications can be viewed through a hyperlink from the DEA website.[5] State laws and regulations regarding controlled substances for the most part mirror the CSA and may have more stringent requirements, but not less than the federal law required in the CSA. Due to the variation in state law regarding controlled substances, it is beyond the scope of this chapter to detail

---

The opinions or assertions contained herein are the private views of the authors and are not to be construed as official or reflecting the views of the U.S. Department of Army or the Department of Defense.

every state law regarding these medications. Over the past two decades many states have adopted regulations granting prescribing privileges for mid-level practitioners. The health-system pharmacy manager needs to have a good understanding of State laws and regulations with regard to the prescribing authority of mid-level practitioners. The category of mid-level practitioners is comprised of a wide variety of health care disciplines. This may include nurse practitioners, nurse midwives, nurse anesthetists, physician assistants, optometrists, ambulances services, and pharmacists. Some state laws and regulations may not recognize some of these practitioners. The health-system pharmacy manager will need to actively seek out the state regulatory agency in the state where they practice for specific guidance. A source of information regarding some state and national activities involving controlled substances can be found at a website maintained by the National Association of Controlled Substance Authorities (NASCSA).[6] The primary purpose of the NASCSA is to act as a center for state and federal agencies as well as others to work together in preventing and controlling drug abuse. The website offers a variety of links and downloadable documents related to current issues regarding controlled substances.

Patient Safety

The national emphasis on patient medication safety issues has prompted greater vigilance and awareness on controlled substances management. This is evident by measures adopted by both The Institute of Safe Medication Practices (ISMP) and JCAHO. The ISMP has designated controlled substances, specifically opiates, both intravenous and oral preparations as *High Alert* medications.[7] Medication errors involving controlled substances have a greater risk of causing negative outcomes for patients. This designation for opiates has resulted from national reported medication errors through the United States Pharmacopoeia (USP)-ISMP Medication Errors Reporting Program. Data obtained from nationally reported medication errors collected through the USP-MEDMARX program revealed that medication errors involving controlled substances were among the most frequently reported. Morphine was second only to insulin as being associated with medication errors that cause patient morbidity.[8] The ISMP Medication Safety Alert program for acute care environments recently described problem errors relating to the use of patient-controlled analgesia. This problem specifically involved morphine toxicity due to inappropriate dosing.[9] A multitude of medications on the mar-

ket has contributed to medication errors due to names of the medications sounding or looking similar. The USP has identified controlled substances among the *Look-Alike/Sound-Alike* medications that may contribute to medication errors.[10] As part of JCAHO's 2005 National Patient Safety Goals (Goal: Improving the safety of using medications) they also identified some controlled substances as Look Alike/Sound Alike medications.[11]

Complexity of Pharmacotherapy

The complexity of pharmacotherapy continues to increase as new agents are introduced on the market and into the practice of pharmacy. An increasing number of patients are on multiple medications. Although the introduction of controlled substances on the market is not at the level of noncontrolled substances, many new formulations of older agents, such as morphine are now approved and available in a variety of different delivery forms and systems. This issue of medication complexity coupled with different delivery systems is highlighted in a case resulting in a death.[12] The case involved a controlled substance used in patient-controlled analgesia and underscores the importance of viewing the management of controlled substances from a broad medication system approach.

The health-systems pharmacy manager needs to gain the appreciation that the endpoint in the controlled substance management system must not only maintain compliance with legal requirements but enhance the medication-use management system and, thereby, have a positive impact on patient safety and patient outcomes. The pharmacy manager is further directed to the American Society of Health-System Pharmacists' *Best Practices for Hospitals & Health-System Pharmacy* to augment the proceeding sections of this chapter.

Selection of Controlled Substances

Formulary

In most health systems the selection of all medications to include controlled substance medications is jointly performed by a multidisciplinary, health care committee or team (e.g., the Pharmacy and Therapeutics Committee). As part of any formulary management process when any medication is considered for inclusion onto a formulary, an evaluation of the medication is done. Data on the safety, efficacy, toxicity, potential for adverse events and abuse, and the pharmacoeconomics related to the population served by the health system are reviewed. The same systematic formulary evaluation should be conducted for controlled substances. The pharmacy manager should consider the following:

- Location within the health system, other than the pharmacy, that the controlled substance will be stored

- Storage requirements for the controlled substances based on manufacturer requirements, such as refrigeration. As controlled substance inventory increases due to increased utilization and/or increase in formulary additions, the pharmacy manager needs to consider immediate needs and project ahead for appropriate space.

- Physical security requirements at the location to ensure federal or state standards are met

- Appropriate stocking levels both within pharmacy and outside in patient care areas

- Authorized access to the medication by health care staff

- Requirement for any prescribing restrictions based on providers' scope of practice

- Incorporation of the controlled substances into to any prescribing or clinical guidelines (i.e., pain guidelines)

- Specific requirements for medication ordering by prescribers (i.e., stop order requirements or taper order requirements)

- Health care staff and patient education requirements on the use of the controlled substances prior to release into the institution

- Any new polices and procedures that need to be addressed with the addition of the controlled substances

Risk Assessment

Use of a Failure Mode and Effects Analysis (FMEA) or similar process is useful when evaluating the controlled substances for formulary addition and prior to procurement and distribution within a health system.[13] The advantage of a FMEA type analysis for controlled substances creates an opportunity to allow the pharmacy manager to apply critical analysis to the medication-use system for controlled substances. The pharmacy manager can identify and examine potential deficiencies in federal and state legal requirements associated with physical security, accountability, documentation, and audit trail. A critical analysis of the processes involved

in the medication-use system for controlled substances can identify risk reduction strategies to enhance patient safety.

Procurement of Controlled Substances

Federal Registration Requirements

Procurement of controlled substances requires that the health-systems pharmacy be registered with the Drug Enforcement Agency (DEA) by submitting DEA Form 224, Application for New Registrant.[14] The registration is required to be renewed every 3 years with both the initial and renewal involving fees. The procurement of Schedule II's requires the use of DEA Form 222. The pharmacy manager needs to acquire a complete understanding of federal requirements for procurement and processes within the medication-use system to ensure integrity in accountability and documentation of controlled substances.

Inventory and Storage Management of Controlled Substances

Inventory and Record Requirements

Once the controlled substance has been procured, it is at this point, that a well-designed system to assure compliance with regulations pertaining to strict accountability and documentation is in place within the health-system pharmacy. The inventory system must allow for an audit trail of complete and accurate documentation of the controlled substance through the medication-use system from the point of procurement and receipt in the pharmacy, through storage and distribution points within the institution to administration to a patient. Accountability and documentation requires certain records in the management of controlled substances whether in paper or electronic format to be readily retrievable and maintained for 2 years. Records for Schedule II substances are segregated from all other records, whereas records for Schedules III–V substances are to be separated from other records or in a readily retrievable form. Under the definition of *readily retrievable* it is permissible to have the electronic storage of controlled substance records as long as they can be separated in a timely manner. Federal law and regulations require the following records to be maintained:

- Official order forms such as the official record of receipt and sale for Schedule II controlled substances, DEA Form 222

- Power of attorney authorizations to sign for DEA order forms

- Receipts and invoices for Schedule III–V controlled substances

- Initial inventory taken when a new DEA registration is required. The CFR requires the date and time of the initial inventory be documented; the name of the drug, strength, and dosage form; the number of units or volume and total quantity of the controlled substance.

- Biennial inventory is conducted following the initial inventory, with the same required information as in the initial inventory. An actual count is required for all Schedule II controlled substances. The inventory for Schedule III–V controlled substances allows for an estimated count, unless the container holds more than 1,000 dosage units and has been opened.

- Records of controlled substance distribution and dispensing records (i.e., prescriptions)

- Records, if required, relating to theft or loss (DEA Form-106)

- Inventory of controlled substances surrendered for disposal (DEA Form-41)

- Records of any transfers of controlled substances between pharmacies

- DEA registration certificate

All of the above records must contain the drug name, drug strength, dosage form, number of units or volume, and total quantity of the controlled substances.

Physical Security and Storage

Federal requirements for physical security for controlled substances require that the medications be in a "securely locked, substantially constructed cabinet" to deter theft and diversion. Pharmacies are allowed to place the controlled substances among the noncontrolled medications as long as there are barriers to theft of the controlled substances.[2,4] This requirement provides a lot of latitude in where the controlled substances can be stored. The pharmacy manager needs to evaluate the storage location of all controlled substances within their health system to consider the level and type of physical security warranted. In some cases a locked cabinet, with minimal stock levels, and limited access to health care staff may be sufficient security. In other cases the requirement for a safe with intrusion detection devices and alarm systems may be warranted.

Some suggested factors that a pharmacy manager should consider in making a determination of the level of security required, adapted from Title 21 CFR[15]:

- Location of the storage site (pharmacy, inpatient wards, surgical suites, ambulatory clinics)

- Level of activity of the storage site for controlled substances (bulk storage in the pharmacy, hospital ward, or clinic stock)

- Quantity of controlled substances expected to be stored at the site

- Dosage form of controlled substances handled at the storage site

- Level of physical security that the container provides that will be utilized for storage of the controlled substances (safe, fixed cabinet, movable cabinet, automated storage and dispensing device)

- Policies and procedures for restricting access to the storage site (authorized personnel, access code management, key control, and safe combination procedures)

- Adequacy of electronic detection and alarm systems

- Amount of unsupervised access, or potential for unsupervised access and procedures for handling patients and visitors

- Amount of oversight of health care staff, whether they have immediate access to the controlled substances or not

- Audit capability and inventory management of controlled substance at storage site

- Review of applicable state laws and regulations and institutional policies and procedures

Controlled substance medications come in different dosage forms and have different storage requirements as with any other medications. JCAHO addresses the requirements for storage of all medications and addresses controlled substances under their Medication Management (MM), standard MM 2.20. As with all MM standards, Standard MM 2.20 has several Elements of Performances (EP) that are accessed to determine compliance with the standard.[16] Under Standard MM 2.20, EP number 3, there is a requirement that all medications are to be "secured in accordance with the hospital's policy and law and regulation" to prevent unauthorized access.[1] JCAHO notes within that standard that the Centers for Medicare and Medicaid Services consider medications "secured" when they "are in locked containers in a room or are under constant surveillance."[1] EP 4, under that same standard (MM.2.20), addresses controlled substances to be "stored to prevent diversion according to state and federal laws and regulations."[1] Although the standard addresses the storage of controlled substances in the context of federal and state law, the health-system pharmacy manager would apply all the other EPs within MM 2.20 to controlled substances.

Automated Storage and Distribution Devices

The advent of automated storage and distribution devices has greatly enhanced the medication distribution system within health systems. The devices have provided for an enhancement in the management of controlled substances in both patient safety and in inventory control. The devices provide better inventory control over medications stored in patient care areas and when coupled with electronic data capture there is an enhancement in inventory control. The enhanced inventory control is provided through user identifiable access to the storage devices and a readable audit trail versus reliance on a paper inventory system to account for controlled system dispensing and administration. The system will truly be enhanced as more health systems adopt bar code technology applications at the point-of-administration. The American Society of Health-System Pharmacists provides an excellent overview of considerations for requirements in automated storage and distribution devices.[17]

Disposal of Controlled Substance Medications

Controlled substances that are required to be disposed of due to expiration, damage, or for other quality control reasons, need to be segregated. This requirement is expected with any noncontrolled substances and is specifically addressed in JCAHO Standards. The segregated controlled substances need to be inventoried separately from other (not designated for disposal) inventoried controlled substances, basically a separate set of books need to clearly indicate the medications for disposal. The CFR requires that the inventory for these medications include the inventory date, drug name, strength, and dosage form, total quantity or total number of units or volume, the reason for the substance being maintained in the disposal inventory, and whether the substance is capable of being used in the manufacturing of other controlled substances. A company that disposes of expired medications (a reverse distributor) may be used for controlled substances, as long as that distributor is registered with the DEA. The pharmacy manager can contact the local DEA Diversion Field Office to determine which reverse distributor is registered with the DEA. Complete inventory documentation of any transfer of controlled substances need to be retained as with other required records.

Ordering and Dispensing of Controlled Substances

Medication Orders

The ordering of medications is covered under Title 21 CFR, Section 1300. This section of Title 21 CFR defines a *prescription* as a means of ordering medication intended to be dispensed for a patient who is the ultimate user. The regulation goes on to clearly state that a *prescription* does not cover medication orders that are written for the purpose of being dispensed for immediate administration to a patient in a hospital setting. Pharmacists dispensing a prescription for controlled substances for patients in an ambulatory (outpatient) setting have strict requirements for container labeling. The same requirements for Schedule III-V controlled substances are not required for hospital dispensing from a Federal CSA perspective and is covered in Title 21 CFR.[18] The pharmacy manager should be aware that specific requirements for controlled substances dispensed in institutions may be covered within State law or regulations. The pharmacy manager that applies JCAHO requirements for medication orders and labeling of dispensed medications of controlled substances within a hospital will more than adequately cover any federal requirements.

Prescribers

Individual practitioners (physicians, mid-level practitioners) employed at an institution or hospital may conduct medications related activities such as administering, dispensing, or prescribing controlled substances under the hospital's DEA registration. These activities are allowed as long as the practitioner is engaged in the usual course of professional practice while in the employment of the hospital and allowed by state law and regulations. A detailed description of criteria for prescribing from the federal perspective can be found in the DEA-Pharmacist's Manual.[4] Pharmacy managers are advised to seek out state law and regulations regarding mid-level practitioners' prescription authority. Additionally, within health systems there may be established formulary prescribing restrictions placed on controlled substances based on clinical practice guidelines or through the hospital's credentialing process of restricting certain medication activities to individual practitioners.

Electronic Prescribing

There is continued movement across the nation to migrate most, if not all, of health care transactions currently being conducted on paper to an electronic format. There is a governmental initiative to migrate health care records to an electronic medical record. Certainly from a patient safety perspective, the migration of medication ordering has been identified as major tool to prevent medication related errors. Facsimile of Schedule II substances prescriptions has been authorized by the DEA since 1994. This authorization is allowed if an original prescription is presented at the time of actual dispensing of the controlled substances. Exceptions to this requirement for an original prescription are for medication orders related to home intravenous infusions for pain therapy, patients in long-term care facilities, and patients in hospice care. Facsimile prescriptions for Schedule III-V substances are authorized without the requirement for an original prescription to be presented at the time of dispensing. With the advent of physician computer order-entry and the strong movement within health systems across the nation to adopt this technology, both federal and state laws and regulations will need to address the electronic transmission of medication orders in the absence of paper. Both the DEA and state agencies are currently engaged in pilot projects to examine this technology to ensure appropriate security requirements in the electronic transmission of controlled substances prescriptions.

Administration of Controlled Substances

As has been highlighted previously, the three primary factors requiring increased scrutiny of controlled substances are attributable to federal and state laws and regulations, patient safety, and the complexity of pharmacotherapy. The pharmacy manager must take an active role in working primarily with the nursing staff to reduce the risk of controlled substances diversion and enhancing patient safety at the point of administration. The complexity of pharmacotherapy is certainly contributory to the environment of increasing the potential for medication errors, with multiple medications and dosage forms, medications with look-alike and sound-alike names, and the increased utilization

of infusion devices. Risk reduction strategies for reducing medication errors prior to administration on patient care units involve limiting the access to the controlled substances; limiting the availability of different products, especially look-alike and sound-alike identified controlled substances; requiring redundancies involving double check system; educating the health care staff and patient; and monitoring patients.[19]

Evaluation of Controlled Substances

Medication Utilization Evaluation (MUE) Program

A MUE Program can provide the pharmacy manager with a mechanism for examining the utilization of controlled substances within the health system. The MUE can be a tool to study the use of controlled substances throughout the medication-use system or to focus on one particular process of the system. If employed as part of a multidisciplinary program, it can be used to enhance patient safety and patient outcomes.

Controlled Substances Surveillance Program

Controlled substances by definition are medications that have various potential for abuse and diversion within the medication system. In concert with a MUE program is a controlled substances surveillance program. Controlled substances surveillance is a required program that every pharmacy manager must be actively engaged in. The deployment of automated storage and distribution devices previously noted has enhanced inventory control management of controlled substances. These devices not only serve as excellent inventory management tools for controlled substances but can serve as tools in any surveillance program. There are several commercial vendors on the market that offer storage devices with computer software enhancements, data capture, and report capabilities to allow the pharmacy manager in any health system monitor controlled substances. Wellman et al. describe an efficient computer assisted surveillance program utilizing data capture from automated storage and dispensing devices.[20] Any surveillance system built to monitor controlled substances will invariably have deficiencies. An article by O'Neal describes the inherent flaws in current automated surveillance systems and presents diversion scenarios with some recommendations for resolutions.[21] One recommendation is to ensure that controlled substances surveillance program information is readily available for pharmacy and nursing managers. Any controlled substances surveillance program will not only need to exploit automated data collection and analyses tools but also fully engage staff members within pharmacy and key departments or services outside the pharmacy. Further information related to the science of drug abuse and addiction can be found on the National Institute of Drug Abuse website at http://www.nida.nih.gov/.

Clinical Practice Guidelines

The pharmacy manager should not lose sight of the tremendous therapeutic potential that controlled substances offer when used appropriately. The use of clinical practice guidelines provides the opportunity to improve the quality of patient care through appropriate use of controlled substances. This is especially evident in the area of pain management, where there has been a tendency within the health care environment to allow controlled substances strict oversight and fear of abuse and diversion to hinder appropriate patient care. Clinical practice guidelines are part of any MUE program that strives to ensure appropriate utilization of medication and can be used as a tool in a controlled substances surveillance program. Further information on clinical practice guidelines can be explored on the National Guideline Clearinghouse website at http://www.guideline.gov/.

Policies and Procedures for Controlled Substances

As with any process within the medication-use system, it is imperative that policies and procedures for controlled substances management be developed and instituted within the organization (refer to the Chapter 22, The Policy and Procedure Manual). Policies and procedures are vital in the management of controlled substances and need to address the entire medication management system, from selection, procurement and storage, ordering, distribution and preparation, through administration and monitoring. The following are some subject areas under controlled substances management that need to be address in policies and procedures:

- Personnel authorized to procure controlled substances and required delegation of authority to order

- Normal procurement and emergency procurement procedures

- Receiving of controlled substances, to include staff responsibilities, storage location, and procedures for handling a discrepancy

- Inventory management and accountability in the pharmacy

- Inventory management and accountability in patient care areas

- Distribution procedures within the health system from the pharmacy to patient care areas, to include staff responsibilities and security of controlled substances during transfer

- Intravenous compounding of controlled substances to include disposal, distribution to patient care areas, and accountability

- Personnel authorized access to storage sites

- Disposal of controlled substances by pharmacy

- Handling of controlled substances returned from patient care areas

- Accountability of patient's own medications is a controlled substance

- Management of controlled substances in surgical and anesthesia services areas

- Management of controlled substances in automated storage and dispensing devices, to include staff responsibilities in stocking, quality control, discrepancies, problem solving with users, control of access codes, archiving of data, and surveillance report generation

- Handling of significant discrepancies anywhere in the health system, to include trigger points of when to engage outside agencies (DEA, state agencies, law enforcement)

- New employee orientation and ongoing competency assessment for the staff in dealing with controlled substances

Summary

Controlled substances medications are an integral and important component of many pharmacotherapy plans for patients. These medications have increased potential for abuse and misuse, Federal and State laws require increased oversight by the health-system pharmacy manager. This increased oversight by pharmacy requires compliance with legal aspects of medication management. All staff must be knowledgeable, competent, and vigilant. Their vigilance in the medication management system will enhance patient outcomes.

Controlled substances management will continue to present many challenges for the health-system pharmacy manager, who will continue to be counted on to provide leadership, by both health care organizations and societies, to devise effective and efficient methods for the management of controlled substances.

References

1. Rich DS. New JCAHO medication management standards for 2004. *Am J Health-Syst Pharm.* 2004;61:1349–58.

2. Fink JL, Vivuan JC, Reid KK, eds. *Pharmacy Law Digest.* 37th ed. St Louis: Facts and Comparisons; 2003: 125–67.

3. Code of Federal Regulations, Title 21, Food and Drugs, Parts 1300 to 1499. Available at: http://www.accessdata. fda.gov/scripts/cdrh/cfdocs/cfcfr/CFRSearch.cfm?CFRP artFrom=1300&CFRPartTo=1499. Accessed November 4, 2004.

4. Drug Enforcement Administration. Pharmacist's manual: an information outline of the Controlled Substances Act of 1970. April 2004. Drug Enforcement Administration's Office of Diversion Control. Available at: www.dea.gov. Accessed November 8, 2004.

5. Drug Enforcement Administration. Drug scheduling. Available at: http://www.dea.gov/pubs/scheduling.html. Accessed November 4, 2004.

6. National Association of Controlled Substance Authorities. Available at: www.nascsa.org. Accessed November 8, 2004.

7. Institute of Safe Medication Practice. Available at: http://ismp.org/MSAarticles/highalert.htm. Accessed November 4, 2004.

8. Hicks RW, Cousins DD, Williams RL. Selected medication-error data from USP's MEDMARX program for 2002. *Am J Health-Syst Pharm.* 2004;61:993–1000.

9. Institute of Safe Medication Practice. ISMP safety medication alert. May 29, 2002. Available at: http://www.ismp.org/msaarticles/pcaprint.htm. Accessed November 4, 2004.

10. United States Pharmacopoeia. USP quality review, 2004; 79:1–22. Available at: http://www.usp.org/patientSafety/briefsArticlesReports/qualityReview/qr792004-04-01. html. Accessed November 4, 2004.

11. Joint Commission on Accreditation of Healthcare Organizations. 2005 hospitals' national patient safety goals. Available at: http://jcaho.org/accredited+organizations/patient+safety/05+npsg/05_npsg_hap.htm. Accessed November 4, 2004.

12. Institute of Safe Medication Practice. ISMP safety medication alert. July 29, 2004. Available at: http://www.ismp.org/msaarticles/pca1.htm. Accessed November 4, 2004.

13. Cohen MR, Senders J, Davis NM. Failure mode and effects analysis: a novel approach to avoiding dangerous medication errors and accidents. *Hosp Pharm.* 1994;29:319–24, 326–8, 330.

14. Drug Enforcement Administration. Available at: www.DEAdiversion.usdoj.gov. Accessed November 4, 2004.

15. Title 21, Code of Federal Regulations, Chapter II, Subchapter L, Part 1301-Section 1301.71. Available at: http://www.accessdata.fda.gov/scripts/cdrh/cfdocs/cfcfr/CFRSearch.cfm?fr=1301.71. Accessed November 4, 2004.

16. Katzfey RP. JCAHO Shared visions—new pathways: the new hospital survey and accreditation process for 2004. *Am J Health-Syst Pharm.* 2004;61:1358–64.

17. Deffenbaugh JH, ed. ASHP guidelines on the safe use of automated medication storage and distribution devices. In: Hawkins B, ed. *Best Practices for Health-System Pharmacy. 2003–2004 Edition.* Bethesda, MD: American Society of Health-System Pharmacists; 2003.

18. Title 21, Code of Federal Regulations, Chapter II, Subchapter L, Section 306.24. Available at: http://www.accessdata.fda.gov/scripts/cdrh/cfdocs/cfcfr/CFRSearch.cfm?fr=1306.24. Accessed November 4, 2004.

19. Cohen MR. ISMP medication error report analysis, risk of morphine-hydromorphone mix-ups. *Hosp Pharm.* 2004;39:818–20.

20. Wellman GS, Hammond RL, Talmage R. Computerized controlled-substance surveillance: application involving automated storage and distribution cabinets. *Am J Health-Syst Pharm.* 2001;58:1830–5.

21. O'Neal BC. Controlled substance diversion detection: go the extra mile. *Hosp Pharm.* 2004;39:868–70.

Chapter 34

Legal Aspects of Institutional Pharmacy Practice

Francis B. Palumbo

Introduction

The laws and regulations governing the practice of pharmacy are both voluminous and detailed. Most apply to any type of pharmacy practice, but some are specific to certain types of practices such as institutional pharmacy.

Pharmacy is one of the most highly regulated professions. If one examines laws and regulations governing health professions, the others, such as medicine and nursing, are much less detailed. The reason for the comparatively pervasive regulation in pharmacy is that in regulating the profession, the states and federal government are also regulating the control and distribution of drug products. These include noncontrolled prescription drugs, controlled dangerous substances, and over-the-counter drugs. Some states include devices in their definition of the practice of pharmacy. Consider the fact that a state, rather than the federal government, grants pharmacists licenses or permits making them the custodian of hundreds of thousands of dollars worth of drug products, many of which are controlled dangerous substances with large street values, and one can begin to understand the societal need for so much regulation vis a vis other health professions. It is also important to note that when entering a regulated profession, one is expected to assume the burdens of being subjected to the regulation as the price for the rewards that accrue to membership in that profession.

Pharmacists' activities, whether in the institutional environment or in another setting such as the community, are governed by both federal and state law. Federal law (e.g., the Federal Food Drug and Cosmetic Act that will be discussed elsewhere in this chapter) applies primarily to the products that a pharmacist dispenses. Federal law also controls to some extent the practice of pharmacy. Examples include the Controlled Substances Act and its requirements for pharmacists and pharmacies and the Federal Food Drug and Cosmetic Act and its requirements for labeling, pharmacist manufacturing and compounding. The states, however, control primarily the practice of pharmacy via their police powers as granted by the United States Constitution. While states may have laws and regulations mirroring many of the federal laws, states retain the sole authority to grant licenses to pharmacists and to suspend those licenses for cause. States fiercely guard their control over the licensure of health professions and the facilities in which they practice such as pharmacies, hospitals, clinics, and nursing homes.

Sources of Legal Information

This chapter is written specifically for pharmacists and not for members of the legal profession. The pharmacist, nevertheless, is responsible for adhering to all applicable federal and state laws and regulations. This is reinforced by the fact that, in order to obtain a license to practice, the pharmacist must pass a pharmacy law examination. In practice, the pharmacist may often have need for information and there are a number of sources available to the pharmacist.

Statutes

A statute is a law that was passed by the Congress of the United States and signed into law by the President, or passed by the legislature of a state and signed into law by the Governor. Statutes are codified and may be found in law libraries, Internet sources, and legal search services such as Lexis-Nexis or Westlaw (the latter two generally require a subscription). The Federal Food Drug and Cosmetic Act is codified in Volume 21 of the United States Code.

Regulations

These are promulgated by the Executive Branch of the federal or state government (i.e., federal or state administrative agencies). In the federal system, an agency, such as the FDA, will publish a proposed rule in the Federal Register. After a period during which the public can comment on the proposed rule, the agency will generally publish a final rule in the Federal Register. This final rule (or regulation) now has the force of law. As a proposed rule, it did not. Regulations governing foods, drugs, cosmetics and medical devices can be found in Part 21 of the Code of Federal Regulations (CFR). States use a similar system of rule promulgation. Rules and regulations are published separately from statutes, so a search for information must include all of these sources.

Policies

While they do not have the force of law, federal and state agencies often publish policies or compliance policy guides (CPG) where they address an area of the law and inform the public about its enforcement mechanisms. CPGs are fairly common with the FDA and the industry knows that FDA is not likely to interfere if CPGs are followed. However, a party may deviate from a CPG for a variety of reasons. In the event that the agency pursues its enforcement mechanisms, the defending party has access to the courts to plead its case.

Other Sources

Newsletters, journals, textbooks, websites, and symposia are only a few of the other sources pharmacists may find useful in maintaining familiarity with current laws and regulations governing practice and products. State boards of pharmacy generally publish monthly or bimonthly newsletters that contain very useful information. In addition, state board personnel are often available to answer questions.

Food Drug and Cosmetic Act (FDCA)

As noted earlier, while state laws primarily govern the practice of pharmacy, the FDCA primarily governs products. The FDCA is the basic statute governing federal oversight of virtually all food, drugs, cosmetics and medical devices. The inventory of an institutional pharmacy is there largely because, under the FDCA, the FDA has determined that it may be marketed.

In 1906, Congress passed the Pure Food and Drug Act, providing that products were misbranded if their labeling was false or misleading. Unfortunately, that law did not provide for a determination of safety prior to marketing, and in 1937 over 100 patients died as a result of ingesting elixir of sulfanilamide. The vehicle used in manufacturing the elixir was diethylene glycol, a powerful toxin. This event prompted Congress to repeal the 1906 statute and pass the 1938 Food Drug and Cosmetic Act, one that continues to be in force although it has been amended many times since its passage. The 1938 FDCA provided that all drugs must be proven safe prior to marketing. If this law had been in force in 1937, the sulfanilamide tragedy could surely have been prevented. In 1961, another seminal event—the thalidomide tragedy—occurred. Thalidomide had been widely used in Europe, and its application for approval was pending at the FDA when reports of birth defects began to appear of children whose mothers had taken thalidomide for morning sickness. The FDA denied approval at that time. In fact, the 1938 law worked well, but the thalidomide tragedy provided the impetus Congress needed to make broader changes in the FDCA. Note that recently, FDA-approved thalidomide for use in Hansen's Disease (Leprosy), reflecting a more contemporary approach to benefit versus risk in the informed patient. In 1962, Congress amended the FDCA to require that all drugs be proven both safe and effective prior to marketing, including those approved between 1938 and 1962. The FDCA did not require proof of efficacy for drugs marketed before 1938. The 1962 amendments also provided for investigational drugs and the IND process. The institutional pharmacist is more affected by these particular provisions than community pharmacists because most of the clinical research is conducted in an institutional setting. The institutional pharmacist is often directly involved in these activities, serving as the repository of the key containing the identities of patients according to active or control status. In addition, the pharmacist may actually dispense the substances to the research subjects and may serve as part of the investigational group conducting and later publishing the results.

Under the FDCA, no new drug may be introduced into interstate commerce unless it has been proven safe and effective to the FDA's satisfaction. When a new drug is being studied in clinical trials, a legal mechanism known as the IND (Notice of Claimed Exemption for an Investigational New Drug) allows its shipment to investigators without violating the law.[1] The institutional pharmacist must be familiar with all stages of the IND (i.e., Phases I, II and III). Basically, Phase I involves a small number of healthy volunteers and is designed to examine the drug's safety. Phases II and III include volunteers who have the disease being studied. Phase II may include 200 patients while Phase III generally includes several thousand. All members of the investigation team must be very familiar with the requirements for protection of human subjects and the research design must include adequate protections. The study or studies must be approved by an institutional review board before they can proceed. In addition, the IND regulations address the qualifications of investigators, especially the lead investigator, who may conduct the research.[2] Pharmacists now often serve as investigators. At the conclusion of the IND process, the sponsor, generally the manufacturer, will submit a new drug application (NDA) to the FDA. The NDA includes all aspects of the new drug including but not limited to chemistry, pharmacology, kinetics, clinical studies, manufacturing, and labeling. An NDA is submitted for a single indication and when approved, the manufacturer may market the drug only for that indication. This restriction includes virtually every marketing function such as detailing and all advertising.

While the manufacturer is generally restricted to marketing the drug for approved uses only, physicians and other authorized prescribers may prescribe the drug for unapproved uses without violating the FDCA. Under the Food and Drug Administration Modernization Act of 1997 (FDAMA) manufacturers may, however, disseminate reprints and reference publications that include information on unapproved uses, subject to certain restrictions.[3] For instance, reprints of articles mentioning unapproved uses must be in peer-reviewed journals and must indicate on the face of the article that it contains unapproved use information. The manufacturer is also required to provide other information such as a bibliography. With regard to reference publications, the manufacturer may include such sources as textbooks as long as certain requirements are met. For instance, the manufacturer must not have any involvement in the production of the book. One major court case, *Washington Legal Foundation v. Friedman* has had a significant impact in this area. The Federal District Court had ruled the provisions of FDAMA relating to dissemination of off-label use information unconstitutional on First Amendment grounds.[4] The Court of Appeals subsequently vacated the District Court decision after FDA agreed to consider the FDAMA provisions as a safe harbor.[5] While manufacturers are uncertain about how to approach the issues of unapproved uses, following the letter of FDAMA is deemed to be a safe harbor.

The Pharmacy and Therapeutics (P&T) Committee

In the institutional setting, manufacturers are very interested in obtaining formulary status for their drugs. In its most basic form, a formulary is merely a list of drugs. Formularies can be unrestricted (i.e., any approved drug can be prescribed) or restricted in that there are only certain drugs that can be prescribed in the institution absent some special need and permission. Restricted formularies are the norm and are also widely used in managed care and other outpatient prescription reimbursement programs as they enable an institution or plan to take advantage of market leverage thereby obtaining more favorable discounts or prices. Manufacturers have an additional incentive in the institution in that they expect to enjoy spillover prescribing from the institution to the community thus increasing their market in both places.

Institutions, through their formularies, practice what is generally know as therapeutic substitution where the pharmacist substitutes the formulary product for that which was prescribed. Generally, this would require that the drugs be in the same class with the same general use and side effect profile. This is not legal practice outside the institution where the pharmacist may only substitute a *therapeutically equivalent* product (to be discussed). However, in the institutional setting, the formulary and prescribing restrictions are governed by the Pharmacy and Therapeutics (P&T) Committee. This is actually a committee of the medical staff, and a physician who admits patients to the hospital must agree to abide by the policies of the P&T Committee. Under present state laws, such arrangements can only work in closed settings, such as a hospital or HMO, where there is a closed medical staff that oversees a P&T Committee and where the pharmacies are part of the closed system. A community pharmacy that has a contract with a hospital or HMO to dispense prescriptions for its patients would not qualify as part of the closed system. The pharmacist generally serves as Secretary of the P&T Committee and has a great deal of influence over the process. Thus, in the institutional setting, the pharmacist is considered by the manufacturers to be an influential person and significant marketing efforts are directed toward the pharmacist. On the other hand, generally, a community pharmacist only has discretion over generics and is not the subject of such promotional activity by the manufacturers of brand name products.

Generic Substitution

Generic substitution is not an issue that is restricted to institutional pharmacy; it cuts across all areas of pharmacy practice and reimbursement for drug products. In a preceding section, the concept of therapeutic substitution in a closed system was addressed. Generic substitution presents different legal issues. Until the 1970s, states had laws forbidding the pharmacist from substituting a generic drug for the brand name without first obtaining the prescriber's authorization. These laws were collectively referred to as antisubstitution laws, and they placed the brand name companies at an advantage since prescribers were quite loyal to the brand companies and were reluctant to prescribe generics or switch from branded products. In retrospect, antisubstitution laws may have been consumer-friendly given that generic drugs of the time did not have to meet today's requirements and may not have elicited bioavailability profiles similar to the branded product. The generic industry was in a somewhat nascent stage and the requirements for approval were confusing.

During the 1970s, states, one after another, repealed their antisubstitution laws, allowing pharmacists the freedom to substitute a generic for a brand name prescription without obtaining prescriber approval. After Congress passed the Drug Price Competition and Patent Term Restoration Act of 1984 (Hatch-Waxman), a manufacturer must show that its generic product is bioequivalent to the innovator's patented product to obtain approval for marketing.[6] An abbreviated new drug application (ANDA) for a generic drug needs to include at least two bioavailability studies. FDA publishes the *Orange Book* where each innovator product, whose patent has expired, is listed along with the generic drugs that are deemed to be "therapeutically equivalent,"" (i.e., are bioequivalent and are "A" rated). In most states, a pharmacist may only substitute an "A" rated generic for the brand. Some states, however, grant the pharmacist the professional discretion to determine if a generic product is substitutable, regardless of whether it is "A" rated or otherwise accepted as a substitute in the state formulary. The discretion is typically directed toward whether the pharmacist believes the substitute is "therapeutically equivalent" as defined in a provision of the state substitution laws. For instance, Colorado's law permits equivalent drug product substitution if, *in the pharmacist's professional judgment,* the substitute drug product is therapeutically equivalent (i.e., contains "chemical ingredients of identical strength, quantity, and dosage form and of the same generic type, which will provide the same therapeutic effect") and interchangeable with the prescribed drug.[7] The institutional pharmacist needs to be aware that state law governs the substitution of a generic drug for the brand name. Nevertheless, if a prescriber specifies that the pharmacist is to dispense the brand name only, the pharmacist is bound by that instruction, despite any policies of, for example, an insurance company or state Medicaid program that will only pay for generics if they are available.

The substitution issue becomes further complicated when one considers drugs that were approved before Congress passed the 1938 FDCA. These are referred to as old drugs and may not be found in the *Orange Book.* In this case, there is no reference listed drug in the *Orange Book* and, generally, a generic for an old drug cannot be substituted for the brand. A few states, however, permit pharmacists to substitute drugs that are not contained in the *Orange Book* because the NDA or ANDA requirements did not apply to those drugs (e.g., pre-1938 drugs), or they are substitutable in the pharmacist's professional judgment. For instance, Maine's regulations permit substitution with a drug not listed in the orange book if based on the *pharmacists' professional judgment,* it meets the criteria of the definition for generic and therapeutically equivalent drug.[8] In fact, it is not unusual for old drugs to have their own brands even if they are the same generic drug.

Prescription Drug Marketing Act

Congress passed the Prescription Drug Marketing Act (PDMA) in 1987 to address a number of abuses in the marketing or diversion of prescription drugs.[9] The PDMA addresses four primary areas:

1. Bans the reimportation of American-made prescription human drugs from foreign countries
   a. except when reimported by the manufacturer, or
   b. for emergency medical care with permission of the Secretary of the Department of Health and Human Services

2. Regulates the distribution of prescription *drug samples*
   a. by banning the sale, purchase of, or trade (including the offer to sell, purchase or trade) in drug samples,
   b. by mandating storage, handling, and record keeping requirements for drug samples

3. Prohibits, with certain exceptions, the resale of prescription drugs purchased by hospitals, health care entities, and charitable institutions, and

4. Regulates prescription drug wholesale distributors
   a. by requiring the state to license them in the state where a wholesale distribution facility is located
   b. by requiring secondary wholesale prescription drug distributors (wholesale distributors who

are not authorized distributors of record [i.e., who do not have an ongoing business relationship with a manufacturer], to distribute that manufacturer's drugs) to provide a statement of origin or drug "pedigree" as part of certain sales of drugs.[10]

Distribution of samples is prohibited unless the prescriber has requested them and signs for them. In considering passage of the law, Congress considered a number of issues around the subject of samples. In some cases, samples were being diverted into the retail sector for sale as if they had been purchased through normal channels of distribution. Samples were designed for use by prescribers to give patients a starter dose of medication. The PDMA did not dispose of the practice of sampling. However, now manufacturer representatives must account for all of the samples sent to them or risk prosecution for violating federal law. Prescribers must sign for them and the manufacturer must have the signatures on file. Under the PDMA, the mere presence of a sample in a community pharmacy is evidence of violation of the law. In institutional pharmacies, however, the pharmacist may serve as custodian of the samples sent into the hospital and can assume responsibility for distributing them to the requesting prescribers. Clearly, this places a burden on the hospital pharmacist to account for all of the samples.

Under the PDMA, hospitals may not sell drugs to retail pharmacies or the retail sections of the hospital (e.g., an outpatient pharmacy) when those drugs were purchased at discount by virtue of their status as a hospital, particularly as a nonprofit. In fact, in 1938 Congress passed the Nonprofit Institutions Act providing that manufacturers could offer deep discounts to charitable entities without violating the Robinson-Patman Act (an antitrust law).[11] The matter was brought to a head in the case of *Abbott Laboratories v. Portland Retail Druggists Assn.* where the Supreme Court held that a hospital could only use discounted prescription drugs for its "own use," which was defined specifically as the following[12]:

(a) To the inpatient for use in his treatment at the hospital; to the patient admitted to the hospital's emergency facility for use in his treatment there; or to the outpatient for personal use on the hospital premises.

(b) To the inpatient, or the emergency facility patient, upon his discharge, and to the outpatient, all for off-premises personal use, provided these take-home dispensations are for a limited

and reasonable time, as a continuation of, or supplement to, hospital treatment.

(c) To the hospital employee or student for personal use, or for the use of his dependent.

(d) To the physician staff member for his personal use or the use of his dependent.

As a result of this case, hospitals must be very careful to track their inventory and, if they have a retail operation, to segregate the inventory purchased through traditional channels for sale from those purchased for the hospital's own use.

At the moment, the reimportation provisions have captured the attention of the public, lawmakers, policymakers and health professionals. The issues are complex and include not only reimportation but also another provision of the PDMA requiring state registration of wholesale distributors. As noted above, the PDMA provides that only the original manufacturer can reimport back into the United States. Of course, this law was never intended to prohibit the importation of prescription drugs from legitimate manufacturers in other countries. Prompted principally by rising prescription drug costs in the U.S., Congress passed the Medicine Equity and Drug Safety Act in 2000.[13] This law was intended to allow reimportation by pharmacists and patients (in addition to manufacturer). The law was never implemented, however, because the HHS Secretaries in office since the passing of the act could not certify that it would pose no additional risk to the public's health and safety and save money to the American consumer.

Congress continues to grapple with the Federal Food Drug and Cosmetic Act. Most of the recent interest with regard to drug access has been focused on obtaining prescriptions from Canadian sources. Some states and municipalities have even been encouraging or facilitating this activity despite its prohibition by law. The issue of whether patients are placed at risk of purchasing counterfeit or substandard drugs is critical in considering programs that bypass our current regulatory schemes. The Prescription Drug Marketing Act was amended in 1992 to require all prescription drug wholesale distributors to be registered in the state(s).[14] This federal law places the burden of registration on the states and has resulted in the registration of an estimated 6,000 wholesale distributors across the U.S.

Wholesale distributors are considered *authorized* if the manufacturer recognizes them as a legitimate supplier of the manufacturer's products. Three major authorized wholesale distributors are responsible for about 90% of the prescription medication distribution in the U.S. These major wholesale distributors indicate that they are able to obtain about 97% of their products directly from manufacturers and must rely on the secondary market (i.e., other wholesale distributors) for the remaining 3%. Not all prescription drugs dispensed to patients are obtained from these three sources. Pharmacies routinely purchase from these major wholesale distributors as well as from manufacturers and secondary wholesale distributors, many of whom wrongfully claim an authorized status (i.e., having a direct business relationship with the original manufacturer). Potential buyers are often unaware of the history or pedigree of the products they are buying. FDA has been quite concerned about this issue and has suggested that almost all counterfeit products may enter the stream of commerce through this unauthorized secondary wholesale distributor avenue.

The impact of such activities on pharmacy practice, including institutional pharmacy, can be substantial. With all of the questionable or illegal activity in the prescription drug supply, institutional pharmacists must now be more aware than ever of their sources of supply. If dealing through purchasing cooperatives, it is vitally important that the pharmacist has a high degree of confidence that the products are obtained from manufacturers or legitimate authorized distributors. Just like the drugs, pedigrees can be counterfeited so the importance of knowing your sources of supply cannot be overstated.

Pharmacist Compounding

One of the historical mainstays of pharmacy practice has been the ability of the pharmacist to compound prescriptions. Prior to the development of the pharmaceutical industry and preformulated dosage units, pharmacists compounded virtually all prescriptions. Later, when compounding became a small percentage of pharmacy practice, pharmacists continued to compound and schools continued to include compounding in their curricula. One tends to think of compounding as activity involving the traditional mortar and pestle. In the institutional setting, however, the mere act of adding a substance to an IV can be interpreted as compounding. From a regulatory perspective, compounding has been allowed as the FDCA was not intended to interfere with the practice of medicine, and physicians are able to prescribe substances that may not have been approved by the FDA. Whenever possible, a pharmacist would desire to engage in com-

pounding rather than manufacturing because, if the pharmacist were manufacturing, he or she would be required to register with FDA as a manufacturer and be subject to FDA regulations governing manufacturing. In some cases exposure to manufacturing regulations might be unavoidable. One major example is packaging and labeling unit dose forms from bulk drugs using machinery.

In 1992, in response to a number of problems in the compounding arena, FDA issued a Compliance Policy Guide (CPG) on pharmacist compounding. A CPG does not have the force of law, but it does put persons on notice as to how FDA views the law and how it may enforce the law. The CPG listed a number of factors that FDA said it would take into consideration when deciding whether a pharmacist was compounding or manufacturing. Later, in 1997, Congress included these factors in the FDCA, thereby giving them the force of law.[15] Pursuant to a recent 2002 Supreme Court case, however, the FDAMA provisions on compounding became essentially invalid.[16] As a result, FDA has now issued a new policy.[17] In cases where FDA believes a pharmacist is indeed manufacturing, FDA will consider certain factors when determining whether to take action. More specifically, FDA will consider whether the pharmacist engaged in any of the following activities:

- Compounding of drugs in anticipation of receiving prescriptions, except in very limited quantities in relation to the amounts of drugs compounded after receiving valid prescriptions

- Compounding drugs that were withdrawn or removed from the market for safety reasons

- Compounding finished drugs from bulk active ingredients that are not components of FDA approved drugs without an FDA sanctioned investigational new drug application

- Receiving, storing, or using drug substances without first obtaining written assurance from the supplier that each lot of the drug substances has been made in an FDA-registered facility

- Receiving, storing, or using drug components not guaranteed or otherwise determined to meet official compendia requirements

- Using commercial scale manufacturing or testing equipment for compounding drug products

- Compounding drugs to third parties who resell to individual patients or offering compounded drug products at wholesale to other state licensed persons or commercial entities for resale

- Compounding drug products that are commercially available in the marketplace or that are essentially copies of commercially available FDA approved drug products. In certain circumstances, it may be appropriate for a pharmacist to compound a small quantity of a drug that is only slightly different than an FDA-approved drug that is commercially available. In these cases, FDA will look to whether there is documented medical need.

- Failing to operate in conformance with applicable state laws regarding the practice of pharmacy

Taken alone, none of the above will necessarily move a pharmacist from compounding to manufacturing (although it could, depending on the circumstances of the case). Rather, the FDA will look at the total picture. The fate of this new CPG is still unknown since it was just recently issued.

Controlled Dangerous Substances

In 1970, Congress passed the Comprehensive Drug Abuse and Prevention Act, creating an entirely new framework for the regulation of controlled dangerous substances (CDS).[18] For example, this law provides for the schedules into which CDS currently reside. Schedules range from I through V. Schedule I drugs have no accepted medical use and have a high potential for abuse and thus cannot be prescribed or dispensed. The other schedules have acceptable medical uses and the abuse potential becomes lower as they progress from II to V.

Schedule II substances can only be prescribed if signed by the prescriber. There are certain exceptions for long-term care where a faxed order may suffice, depending on state law. Schedule II drugs require a new, signed prescription to be refilled. Many states have provisions for prescribers to telephone an emergency Schedule II provided that a written prescription is issued for the record within a specified period of time. For instance, in Maryland, this is 7 days. Schedule III through V prescriptions may be telephoned to the pharmacy and the prescriber may specify up to 5 refills within a 6-month period. Under federal law, Schedule V drugs are over the counter, but most states require a prescription.

The prescriber may only prescribe a CDS for a legitimate medical purpose, and the pharmacist has a cor-

responding responsibility to only dispense a CDS that he or she determines is for a legitimate medical purpose. This places a burden on the pharmacist to take steps to assure, to the best extent possible, that the prescription is indeed legitimate. The DEA publishes a guide for pharmacists which includes a number of helpful suggestions for verifying the legitimacy of CDS prescriptions.[19] Currently, the most controversial area is the management of pain with prescribing and dispensing of large amounts of CDS prescriptions.

Physicians and other prescribers register with the DEA in order to prescribe or dispense. Many states also require registration with the state. A prescribing physician must possess his or her own DEA registration number. One exception is for physicians in training in hospitals (interns or residents) who may prescribe under a single collective registration number with a unique suffix identifying the individual. However, this prescription is only valid inside the hospital. If a physician also practices outside the institution, he or she would need their own registration number for the outside activity. With regard to dispensers, pharmacies, rather than individual pharmacists, must register.

The institution must also account for all of its controlled substance. An inventory of all CDS must be taken every 2 years and sent to the DEA. During an inspection, whether routine or pursuant to an investigation, invoices and prescriptions will be examined to determine whether there are any deviations. The institution should control access to CDS very carefully. To that end, state regulations may, for example, provide that in a hospital all CDS on the floor must be counted at the change of each shift.

Poison Prevention Packaging Act

The Poison Prevention Packaging Act covers a wide variety of consumer products, including both prescription and over-the-counter drug products. As the name implies, its primary purpose is to protect vulnerable populations such as children from ingesting harmful substances. Over-the-counter drugs must be packaged in child-resistant containers. One product of a line may be exempted to account for the fact that many adults are physically incapable of opening a child resistant container. For example, if product X were available in 30s, 100s and 250s, the 30s may be contained in non-child-resistant packaging. With regard to prescription drugs, the Poison Prevention Packaging Act applies at the point of dispensing. Unit dose containers that are widely used in the inpatient setting need not be child resistant. The patient or the patient's physician may request that a particular prescription be dispensed in non-child-resistant packaging. A pharmacy may not honor a prescriber's letter indicating that all prescriptions written by him or her for all patients be dispensed in non-child-resistant packaging. Such requests must be handled on a patient by patient basis.

Health Insurance Portability and Accountability Act (HIPAA)

The states have laws governing patient confidentiality and, recently, the Federal Health Insurance Portability and Accountability Act (HIPAA) dealt with this issue at the federal level.[20] Where individual state laws on patient privacy are more stringent than HIPAA, the state laws generally control. Patient confidentiality has always been a sensitive issue where pharmacy is concerned. Pharmacy has one of the most efficient distribution systems in existence, yet there is a great need to assure the confidentiality of medical (including prescription) records. Many years ago, it was not uncommon for pharmaceutical representatives to be allowed to look through prescriptions to obtain a sense of how their company's sales were faring, and pharmacists sometimes allowed marketing companies to collect information directly from prescriptions. More recently, pharmacists and third parties such as PBMs market prescription data to interested parties. These data must be free of any patient or prescriber identifiers or any information that may enable one to decipher someone's identity. In practice, pharmacists and technicians must consider everything that occurs within the pharmacy to be confidential. Pharmacists must take care to counsel patients only in an environment where privacy is protected and must be careful to provide information only to those who are entitled to it.

While it is beyond the scope of this section to address every aspect of HIPAA as well as the laws of various states, there are some general precepts to bear in mind. Under HIPAA, the pharmacy is considered a *covered entity* and the patient's information in a pharmacy is considered *Protected Health Information (PHI)*. Disclosure of PHI without patient authorization is permitted only in certain instances, including, but not limited to, disclosure for treatment, payment, public health, and other limited matters. Disclosure to business associates (e.g., a software vendor that manages pharmacy information) may be allowed as long as the pharmacy maintains contracts with the business

associates providing that PHI will be adequately safeguarded. A pharmacist or technician may also provide information to the patient's insurance company for purposes of filing a claim for payment and to another pharmacist or prescriber for purposes of providing pharmaceutical care to the patient. Under HIPAA, pharmacies are required to have a private area where patients can discuss their health matters with the pharmacist and where other customers are not able to view or overhear protected health information. Many uses of PHI may require written patient authorization. Pharmacies must post notices to patients about HIPAA and their rights under HIPAA. There are many seemingly innocuous instances where the pharmacist or technician must be careful. For example, in general, a pharmacist or technician may not divulge prescription information to a spouse without the patient's authorization. This obviously poses some practical problems; for instance, a spouse will often pick up the other spouse's prescription. At the very least, any specific information should not be visible. The pharmacist must take every reasonable effort to assure confidentiality. If a prescription is delivered, the patient's name should be clearly marked on the outside without other prescription information. If a prescription is mailed, only the patient's name and mailing address should be on the mailing label. Clearly, an institutional pharmacist must consider relevant state law and HIPAA provisions in everyday practice.

Negligence

By virtue of being a licensed health professional, the pharmacist must live up to the public's and the profession's expectations. This involves practicing according to the standards of the profession. Sometimes, the standard of practice is breached and the patient may be injured because of a pharmacist's negligence. In order for the injured party (plaintiff) to prevail in a negligence suit, he or she must prove a number of elements: duty, breach of duty, causation, and damages. There are basically two types of negligence—ordinary negligence and negligence on the part of a professional. Ordinary negligence applies to everyone, not only professionals, and could involve occurrences in our daily activities. In an ordinary negligence case, duty is defined as what the reasonable person would expect (reasonable person standard). The reasonable person is represented by a judge or jury. For example, a reasonable person would expect a driver to stop at a stop sign.

Professional negligence is handled differently. Duty is generally defined by standards of practice, which are often substantiated by expert witness testimony. With an issue such as placing the wrong medication in a bottle, there may be only one expert since the issue is rather clear. However, cases involving more complex issues may require expert testimony on both sides of a case. For instance, if the issue were whether an interaction is clinically significant, there may indeed be differences of opinion among the experts and this will need to be determined by the court. Experts will give opinions about the correct standard of care and whether the pharmacist's actions violated such standard(s) (breach of duty). The plaintiff must also demonstrate that the breach of duty was the proximate cause of the damages he/she suffered. Finally, the plaintiff must also have suffered actual damages and must be able to document them.

The plaintiff's recovery may be limited or perhaps completely foreclosed if the injury resulted from his/her own negligence. For example, suppose a plaintiff who had been taking a blue tablet for five years receives and ingests a red tablet that causes his injury. While it is not necessarily an open and shut issue, the judge or jury may find that the plaintiff should have at least contacted the pharmacy about the apparent change, and by not inquiring, he or she has also been negligent. Such failure to heed reasonable steps can affect the injured person's recovery. Most states employ the doctrine of comparative negligence where the court determines the percentage of negligence attributable to both the defendant and the injured-plaintiff and allocates awards accordingly. For example, if the court finds that defendant-pharmacist was 80% negligent and the plaintiff was 20% negligent, a jury award of $100,000 would require the defendant-pharmacist's insurance company to pay $80,000. Several states employ the doctrine of contributory negligence where the least bit of negligence on the plaintiff's part would preclude any recovery at all.

It is important for the pharmacist to maintain adequate malpractice (negligence) insurance coverage. The institution generally maintains that coverage for its employees. It is incumbent upon each pharmacist to make sure that he or she is named in the insurance policy. The institution has a strong incentive to maintain coverage since it would undoubtedly be named in any lawsuit and may be found liable under the doctrine of corporate liability. This doctrine essentially places with the institution the responsibility to ensure that its patients receive care that meets standards of the profession. Institutional pharmacists who also work outside of the institution (for example, moonlighting at a local pharmacy) will not be covered by the institution's policy for outside activities and should purchase their own policies to be fully protected. Fortunately, and unlike some other health professions, pharmacist malpractice insurance is quite inexpensive.

Summary

The practice of pharmacy (institutional, community or outpatient) is a highly regulated profession and business. The voluminous laws and regulations concerning pharmacy practice are written for the protection of the public and not necessarily the health professional. It is the pharmacist's responsibility to maintain current knowledge of the laws, including any changes.

Acknowledgments

The author wishes to gratefully acknowledge the assistance of Ravi Upadhyay, a graduate of the University of Maryland School of Law.

References

1. 21 C.F.R. § 312 et seq.
2. 21 C.F.R. § 312.53.
3. Food and Drug Administration Modernization Act of 1997 § 401, 21 U.S.C. § 360aaa et seq.
4. *Washington Legal Foundation v. Friedman*, 13 F.Supp. 2d 51 (D.D.C. 1998).
5. *Washington Legal Foundation v. Henney*, 202 F.3d 331 (D.C. Cir. 2000).
6. Drug Price Competition and Patent Term Restoration Act of 1984, 21 U.S.C. § 355.
7. Colo. Rev. Stat. Ann. §§ 12-22-102 – 12-22-124 (West 2004).
8. Code Me. R. 02-392 CH. 11 § 6 (2004).
9. Prescription Drug Marketing Act of 1987, Pub. L. No. 100-293, 102 Stat. 95 (codified as amended in scattered sections of 21 U.S.C.).
10. Angarola RT, Beach JE. The prescription drug marketing act: a solution in search of a problem? *Food Drug Law J.* 1996;51(1):21–55.
11. Nonprofit Institutions Act, 15 U.S.C. § 13c .
12. *Abbott Laboratories. v. Portland Retail Druggists Assn., Inc.*, 425 U.S. 1, 9 (1976).
13. Medicine Equity and Drug Safety Act of 2000, Pub. L. No. 106-387, 114 Stat. 1549 (codified as amended in 21 U.S.C. § 384).

14. Prescription Drug Amendments of 1992, Pub. L. No. 102-353, 106 Stat. 941 (codified as amended in scattered sections of 21 U.S.C.).

15. FDAMA § 127, 21 U.S.C. § 353a (held unconstitutional).

16. *Western States Medical Center v. Thompson,* 535 U.S. 357 (2002).

17. FDA Center for Drug Evaluation and Research. Compliance policy guide, § 460.200 pharmacy compounding. Available at: http://www.fda.gov/ora/compliance_ref/cpg/cpgdrg/cpg460-200.html. Accessed February 14, 2005.

18. Comprehensive Drug Abuse and Prevention Act, 21 U.S.C. § 801 et seq.

19. Drug Enforcement Agency, Dept. of Justice. A pharmacist's guide to prescription fraud. Available at: http://www.deadiversion.usdoj.gov/pubs/brochures/pharmguide.htm#char. Accessed February 15, 2005.

20. Health Insurance Portability and Accountability Act of 1996, Pub. L. No. 104-191, 110 Stat. 1936 (codified as amended in scattered sections of 18, 26, 29 and 42 U.S.C.).

Chapter 35

Specialization in Pharmacy

Cindy C. Selzer

Introduction

In recent years, there has been a heightened awareness in the pharmacy profession on issues related to specialization in pharmacy practice. Multiple factors have contributed to this specialization and the topic has evoked intellectual, political, and emotional statements from individual practitioners, pharmacy educators, and organizational representatives. This chapter outlines some of the concepts that are integral to professional specialization, reviews the background of specialization in pharmacy, and discusses the current process for specialty recognition and certification in pharmacy.

Basic Concepts and Terminology

To understand the concept of pharmacy specialization, one must be able to distinguish between differentiation in pharmacy practice and pharmacy specialization. The following discussion attempts to clarify the meaning of these terms and to elaborate on these concepts.

Differentiation

Pharmacy practice has evolved from an era of drug distribution to an era of drug information and clinical pharmacy with an emphasis on pharmaceutical care. The expansion and evolution of pharmacy practice has led to the differentiation or diversification of practice opportunities for pharmacists. Differentiation occurs when a practitioner concentrates on a specific aspect of practice. Pharmacy practice differentiation can be attributed to several factors and includes the following: the rapid development of new drugs and drug delivery systems; changes in the health care delivery system; an increase in the acuity of illness of institutionalized patients; increased emphasis on patient outcomes and quality of health care; and the rapid proliferation of drug information.

Pharmacy practice today is a highly differentiated system in which pharmacists perform specific roles. These roles are defined by a number of factors.

- *Place of Practice*—Examples include, but are not limited to, community pharmacists, hospital pharmacists, managed care pharmacists, home health pharmacists, consultant pharmacists, and pharmacists in the pharmaceutical industry.

- *Primary Function*—Primary functions of the pharmacist may include patient care, drug information, management, research, and/or drug development.

- *Level of Patient Care*—Emergency care, critical care, long-term care, ambulatory care, acute care, and home health care are patient care areas in which pharmacists are involved.

In addition to practice differentiation, there has been a differentiation in pharmacy education and postgraduate education. With the adoption of the entry level Doctor of Pharmacy degree, the pharmacy work force has experienced a shift in its educational statistics. Currently, there are 89 colleges and schools that offer the Doctor of Pharmacy, also known as Pharm.D., as the first professional degree. In addition, the Pharm.D. degree is also available as a post BS degree, which is offered by 31 colleges and schools. Doctor of Pharmacy degrees were awarded to 6,649 students as their first professional degree in 2002–2003. Doctor of Pharmacy degrees were awarded to 895 post-BS students in 2002–2003.

The evolution of postgraduate pharmacy education has paralleled changes in pharmacy practice differentiation. Pharmacists have various opportunities to receive advanced postgraduate education and training. Both pharmacy residencies and fellowships are available and offer different areas of focus.

A pharmacy residency is an organized, directed, postgraduate training program in a defined area of pharmacy practice.[1] The general purpose of a pharmacy residency is to prepare pharmacists for the practice of pharmacy; therefore, direct patient care and practice management are the areas of emphasis. Residency training has many advantages: a wide variety of patient care experiences, competitive advantages in the job market, networking opportunities, career advice and planning, and professional vision. Residencies may be accredited or nonaccredited programs. The American

Society of Health-System Pharmacists (ASHP) grants accreditation to practice sites with pharmacy residencies upon fulfillment of requirements. ASHP accreditation may also occur in partnership with other pharmacy organizations, such as the American College of Clinical Pharmacy (ACCP), American Pharmaceutical Association (APhA), Academy of Managed Care Pharmacy (AMCP), American Society of Consultant Pharmacists (ASCP), and others. Currently, the three types of accredited residency programs are managed care pharmacy practice residencies, pharmacy practice residencies, and specialized residencies. Specific career goals dictate the type of residency, in addition to, the practice setting. Practice settings vary with each residency program; additionally, residency programs may have multiple practice settings. Community, ambulatory care, home infusion, long-term care, inpatient care, and managed care are a few examples of residency program practice settings.

Pharmacy practice residencies are designed "to develop competence, skills, and application of drug therapy knowledge in providing the broad scope of pharmaceutical services needed in a practice setting."[2] Pharmacy practice residencies may provide a general experience or offer a specific emphasis, such as community care, managed care, and home care. For more information on pharmacy practice residencies, please see Chapter 13, Residency Training for Practice.

Specialized pharmacy residencies have developed in conjunction with differentiation of pharmacy practice. As pharmacy services expanded into discrete patient care areas, there was an accompanying need to train pharmacists with a more focused knowledge base in complex drug therapy management. Specialty residencies are designed to build upon the acquired skills of a pharmacy practice residency. Completion of a pharmacy practice residency or equivalent experience in pharmacy practice is a prerequisite for an accredited specialty residency. Although completion of a pharmacy practice residency or equivalent experience in pharmacy practice is preferred, it is not always required for a nonaccredited specialty residency program.

Specialized residencies do not participate in the Residency Match Program so the specific programs must be contacted directly. One should contact the programs in the fall for the specific application requirements and prerequisites, application process, job description, and benefits. For example, the salary of a specialty resident is generally higher than that of a pharmacy practice resident. Attendance at the ASHP Midyear Clinical Meeting (MCM) and participation in the Personnel Placement Service (PPS) is especially important for those interested in completing a specialized residency program. Both the MCM and PPS are excellent forums to meet people from the various programs and begin the interviewing process.

Fifteen ASHP accredited specialized residencies are available. These specialty areas are listed as follows: clinical pharmacokinetics, critical care, drug information, geriatrics, infectious diseases, internal medicine, managed care pharmacy systems, nuclear pharmacy, nutrition support, oncology, pediatrics, pharmacotherapy, pharmacy practice management, primary care, and psychiatric pharmacy. Other available specialized residency programs, in areas such as cardiology, nephrology, and emergency medicine, are numerous but are not currently accredited. A directory of accredited and nonaccredited specialized residencies is available at the ASHP website (www.ashp.org) and the ACCP website (www.accp.com). Those interested in pursuing a specialized residency are also encouraged to discuss program options with their faculty, clinical preceptors, and other pharmacy contacts.

"A pharmacy fellowship is a directed, highly individualized, postgraduate program designed to prepare the participant to become an independent researcher."[1] Fellowships provide experience in the scientific research process under the close direction and instruction of a qualified researcher. Fellowship programs are available in a wide variety of areas such as cardiology, infectious diseases, pediatric transplantation, and critical care. Pharmacy fellows possess pharmacy practice skills in the area of study; however, they will only spend a small portion, if any, of their time in patient care activities. Fellowships are not currently accredited; however, ACCP offers Peer Review of Fellowships. This review process is not intended to standardize fellowship programs but to assure quality and assist preceptors in improving their fellowship program. Eighty fellowship programs are listed in the current ACCP directory with 20 programs having the distinction of a Peer Reviewed Fellowship.

The interest in postgraduate education has increased, especially in recent years. Residency applications, the number of participating programs, and available pharmacy residency positions set records in 2004.[3] The desire for specialized training; recognition of new and challenging roles; and increased knowledge and experience are the most frequently cited reasons for residency training. In addition, the involvement of preceptors, residents, and fellows in didactic pharmacy education and clerkship training may also contribute to student interest in residency and fellowship training.[4] The availability and advancement of postgraduate training has played an important role in the development and recognition of pharmacy specialties.

Specialization

Differentiation and specialization are not equivalent. Differentiation, as described above, results from a distinction in place or practice, function, or level of patient care. True specialization in pharmacy is based on a unique core of scientific knowledge and practice skills. Specialization is an indicator of professional maturity and growth.

In pharmacy, the specialty recognition process is intended to assure the public that the pharmacy specialist has attained a high level of competence and skill. Another purpose of specialty recognition is to inform other professional colleagues of the pharmacy specialist's educational and training accomplishments, thereby assuring that a patient referred to the specialist will be completely served. Among other aims of specialty recognition are the stimulation of research, enhancement of training programs, and overall advancement of the pharmacy specialty. Pharmacy specialization and specialty recognition are not self-serving efforts to legitimize pharmacy as a clinical profession; rather, they constitute another phase in the evolution of the profession.

Specialized practice areas in pharmacy have developed as a result of practice differentiation. Practitioners with a specific expertise or focus in some differentiated practice areas are sometimes referred to as *specialists*. The use of the term *specialist* is often used to indicate a specific expertise or focus of practice rather than an individual's credential. It is becoming increasingly common to see the term *specialist* used in position descriptions for clinical practice positions regardless of the existence of that practice area as a formally recognized pharmacy specialty. For example, a position listing may seek a *drug information specialist* even though there is no formally recognized specialty in this practice area. This imprecise terminology can be quite confusing and possibly misleading to other health professionals and the public.

Practice differentiation leads to recognition of specialized practice needs. As differentiated practice areas develop a unique knowledge base and skill, postgraduate training experiences have developed to foster the growth of a specialized practice area. As practitioners in these specialized practice areas conduct research and scholarly activities, they contribute to further maturation of the specialized practice area. At this point, the specialized practitioners have made significant progress in the development of a specialty and may wish to petition for recognition of the specialized practice area as a formal pharmacy specialty. This process is discussed in detail later in this chapter.

Credentialing in Pharmacy

Various professions have developed specific procedures to grant credentials to individuals or programs in the profession. Credentialing is a process that entitles an individual or program to hold a position or exercise authority. The Council on Credentialing in Pharmacy recognizes three fundamental types of credentials: college or university degrees; licensure and relicensure; and certificates, awards or postgraduate work.[5]

Licensure/Relicensure

A pharmacy license is granted to an individual by a governmental agency to guarantee the public a minimal level of professional competence. For pharmacists, this governing body is the State Board of Pharmacy. In order to obtain licensure, a pharmacist must graduate from an accredited pharmacy program with the necessary documentation of intern/extern hours. The North American Pharmacist Licensure (NAPLEX®) exam must be successfully completed in addition to the respective state's law exam, usually the Multistate Pharmacist Jurisprudence Examination (MPJE®). Some states also require the completion of courses or proof of recent coursework in specified areas, such as medication errors, to obtain a pharmacist license.[6]

Most states require a specified number of continuing education (CE) credits per year in order to maintain licensure. Specific details on number of CE credits required are easily found on the website for the respective state's Board of Pharmacy. A pharmacist may obtain CE credits by attending presentations or completing self-study programs. The American Council on Pharmaceutical Education (ACPE) or an equivalent accrediting body should approve continuing education for pharmacists. In addition, the Board of Pharmacy may mandate the type of CE required, specific areas of CE required, and the type of CE accreditation required.[7]

Accreditation

Accreditation is a process used to review and evaluate

educational or training programs rather than individuals. The process is controlled by the profession and assures the public, as well as the profession, that the program has met established standards for producing a high-quality learning experience.

Examples in pharmacy include the accreditation of pharmacy degree programs and continuing education programs by the American Council on Pharmaceutical Education (ACPE). As discussed previously in this chapter, ASHP accredits pharmacy residency programs, in addition to, technician training programs.

Certificate Programs

Certificate programs are a type of continuing education program. A pharmacy certificate program provides an in-depth program on a specific topic commonly encountered in pharmacy practice. Examples of certificate programs include asthma, diabetes management, hyperlipidemia, and anticoagulation. These programs typically follow a planned curriculum, have a didactic and experiential component, develop new practice skills, enable new practice competencies, and qualify for CE or academic credit. Upon completion, the pharmacist receives a certificate of completion for that specific area of pharmacy practice. Although the pharmacist will gain experience and education to develop clinical skills, certificate programs do not assess competency or expertise in that area.

Certification

Certification is the process of credentialing an individual in a recognized practice area or pharmacy specialty. Certification is recognition that a pharmacist has met eligibility requirements, successfully passed an examination, and is competent to practice in the specified area. The profession usually controls certification; however, multidisciplinary certifications are available. Examples of this type of credential are the Certified Anticoagulation Care Provider (CACP) and Certified Diabetes Educator (CDE). These certifications are available to several disciplines including nurses, pharmacists, and physicians.

Three groups offer certification specifically for pharmacists. These are as follows: the Board of Pharmaceutical Specialties (BPS), the Commission for Certification in Geriatric Pharmacy (CCGP), and the National Institute for Standards in Pharmacist Credentialing (NISPC). Pharmacy certificate programs are often confused with certification. However, the certification process encompasses a greater scope and depth of knowledge and practice than offered in a certificate program. Of the three available pharmacist certifications, the BPS certification is the oldest and its certification process is detailed later in this chapter. Further information on the CCGP and NISPC certification can be found elsewhere.[5]

Importance of Credentialing in Pharmacy

Pharmacists are finally gaining recognition for their contribution to patient care. The benefits of pharmacist involvement on patient care teams have been clearly demonstrated.[8–11] In addition, pharmacists have gained recognition as health care providers from agencies such as Medicaid.[5] Therefore, it may become necessary in the future to establish procedures beyond licensing to ensure pharmacist's competence to provide specific patient care services.[12] These procedures may include the use of existing credentialing procedures or the development of new competencies.

Board of Pharmaceutical Specialties Recognition and Certification

A formal process to recognize pharmacy specialties and certify pharmacy specialists has existed since 1976. At that time, the BPS was created to serve as the certification agency for the pharmacy profession. The BPS was born as a result of recommendations made by the APhA Task Force on Specialties in Pharmacy. In 1973, APhA created this task force in order to respond to the changes occurring in health care and in pharmacy practice. In its final report, the task force's conclusions were as follows: (1) pharmacy specialties may exist in the future; (2) an official board with independent decision-making authority should be established; and (3) this board should be empowered to certify individuals as specialists.[13]

The task force emphatically stated its belief that a specialty certification process should exist for the benefit of society, not only for the mere benefit of the pharmacy profession. To ensure this belief, the task force drafted a set of criteria that should be met by any group seeking the recognition of a specific practice area as a pharmacy specialty. These criteria are discussed in a later section. In addition, the task force outlined an organizational structure and certification process that are nearly identical to those of the BPS today.

The BPS is an independent organization that is governed and financed by the APhA. The Mission of the BPS is "to improve health through recognition and promotion of specialized training, knowledge, and skills in pharmacy, and board certification of pharmacists."[14] The primary responsibilities of the BPS as outlined in its bylaws are as follows: (1) grant recognition of pharmacy specialties; (2) establish standards for certification and recertification of pharmacy specialists; (3) objectively evaluate pharmacists seeking specialty certification and recertification; and (4) serve as a source of information and coordinating agency for pharmacy specialties and specialists.[15] The BPS is comprised of nine members: six pharmacist members, two other health care professionals, and one public member. The BPS Executive Director and each chair of the Specialty Councils serve as nonvoting members of the Board.

Current Specialties

Currently, there are five recognized specialty practice areas by BPS. These practice areas include nuclear pharmacy (1978), nutrition support pharmacy (1988), pharmacotherapy (1988), psychiatric pharmacy (1992), and oncology pharmacy (1996). To receive certification in one of these specialty areas, candidates must meet eligibility requirements to sit for the certification exam, in addition to successfully passing the examination. The specialty of nuclear pharmacy currently has 463 Board Certified Nuclear Pharmacists (BCNP). Nutrition support pharmacy has 330 current Board Certified Nutrition Support Pharmacists (BCNSP). There are 473 Board Certified Oncology Pharmacists (BCOP). Psychiatric pharmacy has 493 Board Certified Psychiatric Pharmacists (BCPP). The largest group of the specialty areas is pharmacotherapy with 2,637 Board Certified Pharmacotherapy Specialists (BCPS). Presently, there are 4,526 pharmacist specialists certified by BPS. In addition, specialty certification examinations have been administered to worldwide sites, including Hong Kong, Madrid, and Singapore.[16]

Specialty Petition Development

An individual or group may petition the BPS to recognize a specific area of pharmacy practice as a specialty. Specific instructions for petitioners must be followed and are available at www.bpsweb.org. BPS has seven criteria with corresponding guidelines that must be met within the petition. The intention is to give the petitioner an opportunity to clearly state that the proposed area of specialty practice meets the criteria and merits specialty recognition. These criteria were initially adopted by the APhA House of Delegates in April 1975 and later amended in 1997. The criteria that must be met in the submitted petition are as follows.[17]

1. *Need*—The need for the proposed specialty is established by examining the public health or patient care needs that are best met by pharmacists in the proposed specialty area. In addition, there must be documentation that public health and welfare may be at risk if the services of the proposed specialists are not provided.

2. *Demand*—Statements by members of the public and nonpharmacy leaders characterize the demand for the proposed specialty. The petition must include estimates of filled and unfilled positions in the proposed specialty area.

3. *Number and Time*—There must be a reasonable number of individuals who devote a significant amount of time in their practice to the proposed specialty area.

4. *Specialized Knowledge*—Documentation is provided to demonstrate that the proposed specialty area has a unique body of knowledge that is based in the biological, physical, pharmaceutical, and behavioral sciences. Administrative and managerial services within pharmacy are not applicable to this criterion.

5. *Specialized Functions*—Evidence of the specialized functions and skills required by a practitioner in the proposed specialty area should be provided.

6. *Education and Training*—Comprehensively describe the type of education and training programs necessary to produce practitioners in the proposed specialty area.

7. *Transmission of Knowledge*—Demonstrate a transmission of knowledge in the proposed specialty area through professional scientific literature, workshops and/or meetings.

After preliminary review by BPS, the petition is released to solicit comments from pharmacists, other health care professionals, and the public to determine the merit of each petition. After careful consideration, the BPS either approves or rejects the petition to recognize a pharmacy specialty.

Certification of a Specialty

Once a specialty is recognized, the BPS appoints a Specialty Council of content experts. Each Council is comprised of six pharmacists practicing in the recognized specialty and three other pharmacists. The Specialty Council develops an effective certification process in conjunction with a professional testing firm that has been contracted by the BPS. The charges of the Specialty Council are as follows: (1) to recommend standards and requirements for certification and recertification of pharmacists in the specialty, (2) to develop and administer specialty certification examinations, and (3) to recommend qualified individuals to the BPS for certification or recertification as specialists.

Two of the major tasks of the Specialty Council include using the discrete knowledge areas and practice behaviors identified for the specific pharmacy specialist and establishing the eligibility requirements for individuals interested in taking the certification examination.

Development of the certification process is comprehensive, rigorous, and time-consuming. It is reasonable to expect a 2- or 3-year delay between recognition of a specialty and administration of the first specialty examination in that area.

Added Qualifications

The growing complexity of health care systems, patients, and the profession of pharmacy has lead to increased differentiation within previously recognized specialties. In order to accommodate this differentiation, BPS implemented the process of *added qualifications* for pharmacist specialists already certified. "The term 'Added Qualifications' is used by BPS to denote the demonstration of an enhanced level of training and experience within one segment of a specialty practice area recognized by the Board."[18] Cardiology and infectious diseases are the currently approved areas of added qualifications within the pharmacotherapy specialty. Applicants requesting review for the added qualifications must be current Board Certified Pharmacotherapy Specialists and submit the required application, fees, and portfolio by the yearly deadline. Applicant's portfolios are then reviewed and if approved, the added qualification is conferred upon the applicant. The applicant must reconfirm the added qualification every seven years by resubmitting their application, fees, and updated portfolio. Complete details on the application process for added qualifications are available at www.bpsweb.org.

Advantages of Certification

Pharmacists receive numerous rewards for obtaining specialty certification. Personal rewards include advanced knowledge in a specialty area; enhanced self-worth; and improved marketability. Recognition and acknowledgment from employers and colleagues are evidenced by increased acceptance by health care professionals, public recognition, monetary rewards, job promotions, and increases in job responsibilities.[19] Examples of employers and specific benefits awarded to specialty certified pharmacists are as follows: (1) United States Department of Defense—specialists may receive bonus pay; (2) United States Public Health Service—specialists may receive bonus pay; and (3) North Carolina State Board of Pharmacy—specialists may apply for specific prescribing privileges.[20]

Specialty certification improves the pharmacist's ability to provide comprehensive patient care. Improved pharmaceutical care benefits the patient, other health care professionals, the health care system, and the payers of health care and pharmacy services.[8–11,21] Examples of these improvements include substantial reductions in adverse drug reactions; fewer complications with medication therapies; reduction in unnecessary medications; improved laboratory monitoring of medications; and shorter hospital stays.[20] However, the public and payers have not yet realized the value of specialty certification in pharmacy.[19]

Summary

Specialization in pharmacy has stemmed from the differentiation of practice and postgraduate training experiences. It is a natural step in the maturation of a profession. Practice differentiation and specialization presents pharmacists with a challenging opportunity to serve as a force in society for the safe, appropriate, and cost-conscious use of medications. Several segments of the pharmacy profession—practitioners, educators, associations, accrediting bodies, and regulatory agencies—must be aware that the role of the pharmacist in providing high-quality, contemporary pharmaceutical care is expanding, and as it does, the profession is developing and recognizing pharmacy specialties.

Suggested Readings

American Society of Health-System Pharmacists (ASHP). Best practices for health-system pharmacy. Available at: http://www.ashp.org/bestpractices/index.cfm.

American Society of Health-System Pharmacists (ASHP). Draft ASHP accreditation standards for specialized pharmacy practice residencies. Available at: http://www.ashp.org/rtp/pdf/May2002DraftStdSpec Res.pdf.

Bucci KK, Knapp KK, Ohri LK, et al. Factors motivating pharmacy students to pursue residency and fellowship training. *Am J Hosp Pharm.* 1995;52:2696–701.

The Council on Credentialing in Pharmacy. Credentialing in pharmacy. *Am J Health-Syst Pharm.* 2001;58:69–76.

Professional development: the 2001 ASHP blue book. Available at: http://www.ashp.org/student/BlueBook 2001.pdf.

Shane-McWhorter L, Fermo JD, Bultemeier NC, et al. National survey of pharmacist certified diabetes educators. *Pharmacotherapy.* 2002;22(12):1579–93.

References

1. American Society of Health-Systems Pharmacists (ASHP). Definition of pharmacy residencies and fellowships. *Am J Hosp Pharm.* 1987;44:1142–4.

2. American Society of Health-Systems Pharmacists (ASHP). Pharmacy residencies. Available at: www.ashp.org. Accessed May 2005.

3. Accreditation Services Division of the ASHP. *The Communiqué.* 2004;7:1–3.

4. Bucci KK, Knapp KK, Ohri LK, et al. Factors motivating pharmacy students to pursue residency and fellowship training. *Am J Hosp Pharm.* 1995;52:2696–701.

5. The Council on Credentialing in Pharmacy. Credentialing in pharmacy. *Am J Health-Syst Pharm.* 2001;58:69–76.

6. Florida Department of Health. Florida pharmacist examination application and information. Available at: http://www.doh.state.fl.us/mqa/pharmacy/ph_home.html. Accessed May 2005.

7. Indiana State Board of Pharmacy. Continuing education requirements. Available at: www.in.gov/hpb/boards/isbp. Accessed May 2005.

8. Kucukarslan SN, Peters M, Mlynarek M, et al. Pharmacists on rounding teams reduce preventable adverse drug events in hospital general medicine units. *Arch Intern Med.* 2003;163:2014–8.

9. Leape LL, Cullen DF, Clapp MD, et al. Pharmacist participation on physician rounds and adverse drug events in the intensive care unit. *JAMA.* 1999;282:267–70.

10. Boyko WL Jr, Yurkowski PJ, Evey MF, et al. Pharmacist influence on economic and morbidity outcomes in a tertiary care teaching hospital. *Am J Health-Syst Pharm.* 1997;54:1591–5.

11. Cupit GC. The role of the clinical pharmacist in the institutional setting. *J Clin Pharmacol.* 1981;21:251–2.

12. Galt KA. Credentialing and privileging for pharmacists. *Am J Health-Syst Pharm.* 2004;61:661–70.

13. Cohelan J, Edwards WJ, Fenninger LD, et al. Final report: APhA task force on specialties in pharmacy. *J Am Pharm Asso.* 1974;NS14:618–22.

14. Board of Pharmaceutical Specialties. Mission statement. Available at: www.bpsweb.org. Accessed May 2005.

15. Board of Pharmaceutical Specialties. The pharmacy specialty certification program: over 20 years of service to the public and the pharmacy profession. Available at: www.bpsweb.org. Accessed May 2005.

16. Board of Pharmaceutical Specialties. News release—results of BPS examinations announced, November 30, 2004. Available at: www.bpsweb.org. Accessed May 2005.

17. Board of Pharmaceutical Specialties. Petitioner's guide for recognition of a pharmacy practice specialty. Available at: www.bpsweb.org. Accessed May 2005.

18. Board of Pharmaceutical Specialties. Guide to added qualifications. Available at: www.bpsweb.org. Accessed May 2005.

19. Pradel FG, Palumbo FB, Flowers L, et al. White paper: value of specialty certification in pharmacy. *J Am Pharm Assoc.* 2004;44(5):612–20.

20. Board of Pharmaceutical Specialties. 2004 recertification guide. Available at: www.bpsweb.org. Accessed May 2005.

21. Gourley DR, Fitzgerald WL Jr, Davis RL. Competency, board certification, credentialing, and specialization; who benefits? *Am J Manag Care.* 1997;3(5):795–801.

Chapter 36

Evidence-Based Medicine

Suellyn J. Sorensen

The institutional pharmacist is continually involved in therapeutic decision making. These therapeutic decisions are made in several different settings: inpatient rounds, ambulatory clinics, development of order sets, guidelines, clinical pathways, computer-assisted decision support tools, and when formulary decisions are made at the Pharmacy and Therapeutics (P&T) committee level. In all of these settings it is important for the institutional pharmacist to use an evidence-based approach to clinical decision making. The remainder of this chapter is dedicated to the evidence-based approach to pharmacotherapeutic decisions.

Evidence-Based Medicine Overview

Evidence-based medicine is the practice of using the best scientific evidence from the literature to make medical decisions.[1,2] This evidence may range from published case reports to randomized controlled clinical trials. The topic of evidence-based medicine emerged from suggestions in the 1980s that only 10–20% of physician's interventions were supported by objective data.[3,4] An evidence-based medicine working group published a manuscript in the *Journal of the American Medical Association (JAMA)* in 1992 that laid the foundation for a shift in practice paradigms. They described a past and present state of medical decision making. The past relied largely on clinical intuition by seasoned practitioners, and the future state should be one that incorporates the medical literature into every clinical decision that is made.[1] This shift is possible due to the large number of clinical trials that are available today and computer software that allows us relatively easy access and searching capabilities. Technology has allowed for a world of booming medical information systems.

This evidence-based approach to practicing medicine was not initially received by the medical community with open arms. There was much skepticism and debate regarding this approach.[5–7] However, over time the medical community has learned to understand the concept more accurately through subsequent publications and dialog on the topic.[8] With increased use of evidence-based medicine, more publication on the topic, and increased discussions, the definition has evolved over time. Evidence-based experts recognize that decisions should not be based solely on scientific evidence.[9] Empirical observations by the clinician constitute potential evidence that needs to be factored into the analysis of scientific evidence. Patient circumstances, values and preferences also play a role in clinical decisions. Therefore, the contemporary definition of evidence-based medicine is more appropriately defined as integrating current best evidence with clinical expertise, pathophysiological knowledge, and patient values and preferences in making decisions about the care of individual patients.[10,11] The challenge today is not convincing health care providers that evidence-based medicine should be practiced but giving practitioners the tools needed to navigate through the medical literature and efficiently and effectively analyze this information.

A series of publications in *JAMA* have been published by the evidence-based medicine working group to assist the busy physician in translating the results of medical research into clinical practice.[12] These user guides began in 1993 and have continued through 2000.[9,12] They assist the clinician with navigating through and analyzing the medical literature. Each guide focuses on a specific type of article (e.g., therapy, diagnosis, practice guidelines, economic analysis) and organizes each set into three basic questions: Are the results of the study valid? What are the results? Will the results help me in caring for my patients? Many of the principles outlined in this series are applicable to pharmacotherapeutics.

Evidence-based therapeutics is essentially a component of evidence-based medicine. Etminan et al. defined evidence-based pharmacotherapy as an approach to decision making whereby the clinician appraises the scientific evidence and its strength in support of his therapeutic decision.[13] As mentioned previously, this article will focus on the application of evidence-based therapeutics by pharmacists. Today pharmacy students complete coursework in drug information and biostatistics through their doctor of pharmacy (Pharm.D.) education. Many of the principles learned in these courses are applicable to evidence-based therapeutics in the practice of pharmacy. Therefore, it is not an extreme change in practice for pharmacists and has been widely accepted by pharmacists for many years. The most difficult part for pharmacists is the component that physicians have been practicing for decades: clinical intuition and experience and judgments related to patient values and preferences. These are the pieces that historically have not been a large component of pharmacy practice. With the evolution of Pharm.D. curriculums and clinical pharmacists, pharmacists are gaining comfort and experience in this area and, hence, are more qualified and better able to incorporate these pieces into evidence-based therapeutic decisions. As Guyatt et al. pointed out, evidence of treatment does not always mean that treatment should automatically be given.[9] The decision requires a judgment about the balance between benefits and risks. Values and preferences can differ; therefore, the best course of action will vary between patients and clinicians. Understanding and applying this concept can often be difficult for the pharmacist that does not have a great deal of contact with patients and their family members. The challenge for the pharmacist is to incorporate patient values and preferences into evidence extracted from the literature in making sound therapeutic decisions and when understanding decisions made by physicians.

Importance of Using Evidence in Clinical Decision Making

Uncovering the *Truth*

Applying concepts of evidence-based therapeutics to clinical decision making is important for several reasons. The breadth and depth of information in the literature can be overwhelming. A systematic approach to sorting through all of this information is essential. Decisions made based on data and scientific evidence helps to eliminate bias.[13] Bias can not be completely eliminated and the quality of published studies can vary widely; therefore, it is important for the pharmacist to learn how to critically appraise clinical trials and other forms of evidence in the literature. Randomized controlled clinical trails (RCCT) are the best study design to determine the most accurate estimate of efficacy and safety. RCCT have confirmed the value of many pharmacotherapeutic options today and disproved or clarified the usefulness of others.[2] Perhaps the best example is hor-

mone replacement therapy for postmenopausal women. The Nurses Health Study, a large cohort observational study designed to determine the risk of hormone replacement therapy in postmenopausal women reported that estrogen replacement therapy may actually be cardioprotective.[14,15] These results were incorporated into clinical practice guidelines and for many years patients were prescribed long-term hormone replacement therapy to prevent cardiovascular events. However, a follow-up randomized controlled clinical trial (Women's Health Initiative) found no reduction in overall risk of nonfatal myocardial infarction or coronary death with estrogen replacement therapy.[16] The study also found that the risk may actually increase for recurrent coronary heart disease.[17] Clinical intuition and results of a cohort study failed to uncover the lack of benefit and potential harm with estrogen replacement therapy. For a detailed analysis on the discrepancy between these observational studies and randomized trials, the pharmacist is referred to Nananda and Pauker's perspective.[18]

Increasing Accountability

Payers are holding institutions accountable for safe, quality, cost-effective health care and are embracing the practice of evidence-based medicine. Many payers are requesting, and, in some cases, mandating the use of order sets, practice guidelines, clinical pathways, and computer-assisted decision support tools that are evidence-based in order to receive reimbursement. Accreditation and safety groups are also requesting the use of these tools to decrease errors in health care.

The Leapfrog Group is providing quality incentive and reward programs aimed at improving health care in both inpatient and outpatient settings. The Leapfrog incentive and reward program is designed to raise awareness among purchasers, health plans, and health care providers about innovative schemes that are already in place to improve the quality and affordability of health care. The Leapfrog Group was founded in 2000 by the Business Roundtable and includes more than 150 Fortune 500 corporations and other large private and public sector health benefits, representing more than 34 million enrollees.[19] The quality component of many of their performance measures utilizes evidence-based medicine to determine best practice.

The Centers for Medicare and Medicaid Services (CMS) administers a comprehensive quality improvement program designed to monitor and improve utilization and quality of care for Medicare beneficiaries.[20] CMS supports quality initiatives in the following practice areas: home health, hospital, nursing home, and physician. Under the hospital initiative, beginning October 1, 2004, hospitals failing to voluntarily report data on the 10 starter set measures will see a reduction of 0.4% to their Medicare payments. A few examples of these initiatives include: aspirin on arrival in patients with an acute myocardial infarction, antibiotic timing in community-acquired pneumonia, and angiotensin-converting enzymes (ACE) inhibitors in heart failure patients with left ventricular systolic dysfunction. A complete listing of these initiatives may be found at http://www.cms.hhs.gov. These initiatives were developed based on supportive evidence in the literature.

The Agency for Healthcare Research and Quality (AHRQ) has set quality indicators based on readily available hospital inpatient administrative data.[21] They were developed to assess the effects of health care programs and policy choices, guide future policy making, and accurately measure outcomes. AHRQ has also launched the National Quality Measures Clearinghouse (NQMC). NQMC is an open, searchable database of quality measures from various governmental non-governmental and professional sources. All measures are supported by evidence.

The Institute for Clinical Systems Improvement (ICSI) also focuses on quality through supportive evidence. ICSI is a collaboration of health care organizations and is sponsored by six Minnesota health plans. Their objective is to help members identify and accelerate the implementation of best clinical practices for their patients. ICSI is involved in practice guideline development and formalizing the process for developing and reviewing hospital order sets.[22]

The Leapfrog Group, CMS, AHRQ, and ICSI are examples of payers and organizations that are actively involved in quality initiatives that are based on evidence and best practice. Therefore, to receive certain levels of reimbursement, incentives, and quality grades hospital administrators are forming committees to develop evidence-based best practice guidelines, programs, order sets, and decision tools. Pharmacists are an essential component to these teams. Almost all patients in the hospital receive medications, many of which are complex and expensive. Pharmacists must know or learn how to apply evidence-based medicine skills to these initiatives. Pharmacists have and will need to become proficient at retrieving, critically analyzing, and applying evidence to patient care.

Is There Evidence for Evidence-Based Medicine?

One would assume that there would be an enormous amount of evidence to support the practice of evidence-based medicine. In reality, there is very little published in the literature on the effectiveness of evidence-based practice in terms of outcomes. The evaluation thus far has been in the area of teaching medical residents and students. These studies demonstrated that the skills can be taught, and that when taught these skills, the trainee is more knowledgeable about therapeutic guidelines than his or her counterparts.[1,11] Clearly, there is a need for more research to support the widely accepted practice of evidence-based medicine.

Evidence-Based Medicine Resources

Time constraints are usually sited as the biggest reason clinicians do not practice evidence-based medicine. Searching for relevant publications and then extracting the important and applicable information can be a daunting task. There are several readily available resources to most clinicians to assist with this process. The Internet and/or your hospital/institution library may serve as a vehicle to access this information.

Databases

Cochrane Collaboration

The Cochrane Collaboration was founded in 1993 and named after the British epidemiologist, Archie Cochrane. It is an international not-for-profit organization that produces and disseminates systematic reviews of health care interventions and promotes searching for evidence in the form of clinical trials and other intervention studies.[23]

Cochrane Library

The Cochrane Library consists of an updated collection of evidence-based medicine databases, including the Cochrane Database of Systematic Reviews.[23] The Cochrane Library is designed to provide high-quality evidence to people providing and receiving care, researchers, teachers, payers, and administrators. You can browse and search abstracts on their website or subscribe to the CD-ROM or the Wiley InterScience website to receive access to the full review. Many hospital, medical, and pharmacy libraries subscribe to this database.

Cochrane Database of Systematic Reviews

The Cochrane Database of Systematic Reviews is published quarterly as part of the Cochrane Library.[23] The systematic reviews are a rapidly growing collection of frequently updated, systematic reviews of the effects of health care. The reviews are prepared by health care professionals who volunteer to work in one of the many Collaborative Review Groups. Editors oversee the preparation and maintenance of the reviews. Systematic reviews are mainly of randomized controlled clinical trials. Trials are included or excluded on the basis of rigorous quality criteria to minimize bias. Data are often combined statistically, with meta-analysis, to increase the power of the findings of numerous smaller studies that would not produce reliable results on their own. New reviews are added with each issue of The Cochrane Library. Protocols for reviews currently being prepared are also available that include the background, objectives, and methods of reviews in preparation.

The Database of Abstracts of Reviews of Effectiveness

The Database of Abstracts of Reviews of Effectiveness (DARE) Database is likely to be a very useful Cochrane Database for clinical pharmacists and medicine physicians.[23] DARE contains critical assessments of systematic reviews from various medical journals. It is in the form of abstracts of systematic reviews from all over the world. These abstracts cover topics such as diagnosis, prevention, rehabilitation, screening, and treatment.

Other Cochrane Databases

The Cochrane Central Register of Controlled Trials (CCTR) is a collaboration with the National Library of Medicine and Reed Elsevier to produce a bibliographic database of definitive controlled trials.[23] This collaboration was an effort to produce an unbiased source of data that can identify all relevant studies. Other Cochrane Databases include the Cochrane Methodology Register, the NHS Economic Evaluation Database, Health Technology Assessment Database, and the Cochrane Database of Methodology Reviews (CDMR).

Zynx

Zynx Health was founded in 1996 and is a subsidiary of the Hearst Corporation. It is a commercial provider of evidence-based clinical content to health care organizations.[24] Zynx Health identifies best practice, facilitates the creation and use of evidence-based clinical guidelines, pathways, order sets, and protocols based on their critical appraisal and synopsis of the medical literature. The Zynx Knowledge management tool assists subscribers with meeting regulatory and accreditation requirements.

Clineguide

Clineguide is similar to Zynx Health in that it is a commercial provider of a clinical knowledge system.[25] It focuses more on point of care decision support and relies on the clinical content from other vendors. It is a resource for disease, drug, laboratory, and best practice information. It is designed to be integrated with electronic medical records, or can be used stand alone.

Evidence-Based Medicine Reviews (EBMR)

Evidence-Based Medicine Reviews is an Ovid Database that combines articles into a searchable database from the Cochrane Collaboration's Cochrane Database of Systematic Reviews, Best Evidence, and the National Health Services Centre for Reviews and Dissemination.[26,27] The database contains links to Medline and full text journals. Using Ovid's Medline you can enter a term and select the EBMR limit and a small number of high-quality articles will appear.

Best Evidence

Best Evidence is produced by the American College of Physicians (ACP).[26,27] It is the electronic version of two journals, ACP Journal Club and Evidence-Based Medicine. It is a database of summaries of articles from major medical journals and includes expert commentaries.

Journals

ACP Journal Club and Evidence-Based Medicine contain structured abstracts of and expert commentary on high-quality, clinically important studies from many medical journals.[26,27] The ACP Journal Club is a publication of the American College of Physicians and Evidence-Based Medicine is a joint publication of the British Medical Journal Group. ACP Journal Club focuses on articles that are methodologically sound and clinically relevant in internal medicine. Whereas, Evidence-Based Medicine focuses on articles that are methodologically sound and clinically relevant in internal medicine, family practice, surgery, psychiatry, pediatrics, and obstetrics and gynecology.

Websites

Netting the Evidence

Netting the Evidence is an Internet resource for evidence-based medicine.[27] The site includes a library of key publications on evidence-based practice. It contains links to other evidence-based medicine websites, and it contains a listing of evidence-based journals and databases.

Centre for Evidence-Based Pharmacotherapy

The Centre for Evidence-Based Pharmacotherapy was established in 1995 by pharmacy professor Alain Li Wan Po to undertake research in the methodology of medicines assessment, epidemiology, and pharmacoeconomics.[27,28] The research completed at the Centre is funded by the Department of Health and pharmaceutical companies. The Centre also undertakes meta-analyses and systematic reviews.

Clinical Practice Guidelines

There are several clinical practice guidelines available on the Internet. Primary Care Clinical Practice Guidelines (http://medicine.ucsf.edu/resources/guidelines) and the National Guideline Clearing House (NGC) (www.guideline.gov) would be of great interest to pharmacists.[27] Each site contains practice guidelines that are evidence-based and critically appraised with a standard methodology. Table 36-1 lists websites for Evidence-Based Medicine Resources.

Process for Using Evidence-Based Pharmacotherapy

You are working late one evening in the central pharmacy of a large teaching hospital. You receive medication orders for a 100-mg dose of gentamicin with subsequent orders for pharmacy to dose and monitor serum concentrations. If you were to apply evidence-based pharmacotherapy to this clinical scenario, you would need to use a stepwise approach as outlined below.

Identify/Formulate the Question

It is important to identify the specific question that you are trying to answer before retrieving the evidence. If your question is well-formulated, it will save you an enormous amount of time searching for evidence. The question should be focused and include the following elements: the patient being addressed, the intervention being considered, the comparison intervention, and the outcomes of interest.[2] In order for a question to be formulated with these elements, the pharmacist needs to retrieve more information about the patient. The pharmacist needs to find out why gentamicin is being used and if the physician has identified target serum concentrations. After this information is gathered, the following sentence would be an example of a well-formulated question. How should gentamicin be dosed (extended interval or traditional) in this 65-year-old patient with methicillin-resistant staphylococcus aureus (MRSA) prosthetic valve endocarditis to achieve gram positive synergy with vancomycin, and what serum concentrations should be achieved?

Searching for the Evidence

The next step is for the pharmacist to search for scientific evidence to support the answer to the question. One may ask another colleague or expert in the area, review practice guidelines or textbooks, search an electronic database of systematic reviews, or conduct a

Table 36-1
Websites for Evidence-Based Medicine Resources

The Cochrane Collaboration	http://www.cochrane.org
The Cochrane Library	http://www.thecochranelibrary.com
Zynx Health	http://www.Zynx.com
Clineguide	http://www.clineguide.com
Evidence-Based Medicine Reviews	http://www.ovid.com/site/catalog/DataBase/904.jsp
ACP Journal Club	http://www.acpjc.org/
Evidence-Based Medicine	http://ebm.bmjjournals.com/
Netting the Evidence	http://www.//shef.ac.uk/scharr/ir/netting/
Centre for Evidence-Based Pharmacotherapy	http://www.aston.ac.uk/lhs/teaching/pharmacy/cebp/
Primary Care Clinical Practice Guidelines	http://medicine.ucsf.edu/resources/guidelines
National Guideline Clearing House	http://www.guideline.gov

MEDLINE search of the primary literature.[12,28] In most situations, the correct answer is likely to be discovered in practice guidelines, systematic reviews, or the primary literature. Colleagues' answers are often biased and based on their past experiences, and colleagues often share what they were taught and not what they learned from reviewing the most current scientific literature. This does not mean that a pharmacist should not consult others when answering a question. Colleagues' opinions are pieces of the puzzle and should be factored into the decision-making process after the scientific evidence is reviewed. Textbooks are often helpful for general information on a topic but not for answering specific questions. Textbooks also have the disadvantage of not being updated on a regular basis.

To answer the question above it would be most effective and efficient to start with reviewing practice guidelines. If further information is needed, a search for systematic reviews would be necessary. The primary literature would be the last step in answering the question. Reviewing and critically appraising practice guidelines for the treatment of endocarditis would assist in answering the question. Searching MEDLINE or PubMed by entering a search term and selecting the EBMR limit would quickly identify systematic reviews on gentamicin dosing and the treatment of prosthetic valve endocarditis. If systematic reviews are not available or the quality is lacking, then the primary literature will be the best source for answering the question.

Evaluate the Evidence

Every piece of literature is subject to human error and bias. Therefore, it is important to complete your own critical appraisal of the available evidence. Each type of evidence carries its own set of advantages and disadvantages. There are limitations on the conclusions that can be drawn from certain study designs. Statistical methods can be manipulated based on desired outcomes by authors, or the statistics applied may not reflect the best statistical test, given the study design.

Implementation

The final step in the process of using evidence-based pharmacotherapy is to implement the best evidence into clinical practice or decisions for individual patients or groups of patients. In the gentamicin dosing scenario, the pharmacist would want to dose gentamicin for this individual patient based on the best evidence that was discovered and reviewed. Subsequently, the pharmacist may want to work with a pharmacy or hospital committee to develop standard gentamicin

dosing guidelines based on best evidence. These guidelines would need to be updated periodically to ensure that new evidence is factored into dosing decisions.

Types of Evidence

Case Reports

Case reports describe single-case experiences with resulting outcomes. More than one case may be reported in a single publication. This is often referred to as a case series. Case reports are written to inform the medical community of possible benefit or harm from a particular treatment.[13,29] In general, case reports should not be used to make clinical decisions, because they lack a hypothesis and are not scientific studies. However, there are times when case reports will be the only evidence available in the literature. In this situation a decision may have to be made based on published clinical experience in case reports.

Cohort Studies

A cohort is a group of patients or study subjects. Cohort studies are observational studies that are usually conducted with large groups of patients to identify a particular benefit or harm from a given treatment.[13,29] Cohort studies identify two groups of patients (cohorts), one which receives active treatment (treatment group) and one which does not receive treatment (control group). The two groups are studied over time to see which group develops the outcome of interest. An example of a cohort study is the Nurses Health Study described previously, in which two groups of women were followed over time to determine the benefits verses risks of hormone replacement therapy. The biggest drawback to this type of study is the lack of control over confounding factors. The biggest advantage to this type of study is the large number of patients that can be enrolled and it is relatively inexpensive to conduct compared to randomized controlled clinical trials.

Case-Controlled Studies

A case controlled study is a retrospective study that identifies patients that have experienced a particular outcome (cases) and those that have not experienced a particular outcome (controls). The study looks back in time to identify characteristics that may be linked to the outcome of interest in case patients. Case-controlled studies are most useful in evaluating rare outcomes that take years to develop; however, they are subject to patient selection bias.

Retrospective Studies

Retrospective studies look back in time to evaluate events that occurred in the past.[13,29] A case-controlled study is one example of a retrospective study. Other types of retrospective studies report results from a particular treatment or intervention but case patients are not always matched with control patients. These studies are also subject to bias because patients are not randomized to treatment, investigators and patients are not blinded to treatment, and the setting is not controlled. Retrospective studies are less expensive and time consuming to conduct than randomized controlled clinical trials. An advantage to retrospective studies is that they reflect actual practice and how treatment is being used in real clinical practice.

RCCT

In RCCT, patients are randomly assigned into treatment or control groups and then followed over time for the variables/outcomes of interest.[13,29] The randomization process ensures that patient have an equal chance of being placed in the treatment or control group. This allows for equal chance that a patient may have a particular characteristic that may affect the study outcome. RCCT are the best study design used to discover the truth about the effects of treatment or an intervention. RCCT have confirmed the value of many pharmacotherapeutic options today and disproved or clarified the usefulness of others. The main disadvantage of RCCT is that they are time consuming and costly to complete.

Systematic Reviews and Meta-Analyses

There are several different types of review articles. Systematic reviews are an excellent tool for the clinical pharmacist to use when trying to answer a specific therapeutic question or dilemma. An example of a specific therapeutic question that may be answered effectively and efficiently using a systematic review would be: When is the optimal time to initiate antiretroviral therapy in patients infected with the human immunodeficiency virus (HIV) to prevent HIV complications and delay death? What evidence supports this recommendation? Systematic reviews will synethize the results of multiple primary studies by using explicit reproducible criteria in the selection of articles for review in an attempt to eliminate bias and random error.[30] Systematic reviews are different from other types of reviews in that they are scientific investigations themselves with preplanned methods. This differs from general review articles (narrative reviews) in that they are not designed

to answer a specific question and they do not use preplanned methods for primary literature selection. General reviews offer a broad overview of a topic with a summary of select primary literature studies. General reviews would be most useful to the clinician when trying to gain general knowledge on a particular topic rather than when trying to answer specific questions.

There are two different types of systematic reviews, qualitative and quantitative reviews.[30] A quantitative systematic review uses statistical methods to combine the results of two or more studies. A quantitative review is often referred to as a meta-analysis. A qualitative review summarizes the results of primary studies using predetermined methods but does not use statistical methods to combine the results of studies. Many of the evidence-based medicine resources described previously are excellent sources for retrieving systematic reviews. Several of them conduct their own systematic reviews with varying degrees of rigor. Perhaps the most rigorous and well know is the Cochrane Library and Database for Systematic Reviews.[23] Zynx Health, Clineguide, and the Centre for Evidence-Based Pharmacotherapy are examples of other resources that also conduct their own systematic reviews.[24,25,28] Each site provides a description of how they conduct their reviews. The most efficient and effective way to find a systematic review for the specific question at hand is to tap into your electronic databases that are available to you.[31] MEDLINE is the largest and most readily available database for retrieving literature. Pharmacists are extensively educated on the use of MEDLINE in their Drug Information course during pharmacy school. However, unless the pharmacist recently graduated, they may not be familiar with the updated and added features of MEDLINE. Ovid's MEDLINE allows the user to enter a search term and then to limit that search to Ovid's Evidence-Based Medicines Reviews (EBMR) Collection. As described previously, EBMR combine multiple reviews into a searchable database.

Clinical Practice Guidelines

Clinical practice guidelines have been defined as "systematically developed statements to assist practitioner and patient decisions about appropriate health care for specified clinical circumstances."[39] Clinical practice guidelines are developed by a group of experts in the defined clinical area. These experts review the literature to provide support for their recommendations. The recommendations are often graded based on the strength of the evidence. In the past, practice guidelines have not followed a true evidence-based approach, in that they did not follow the steps outlined above. These steps require the formation of a question that contains the four key elements described previously, the search for evidence, the evaluation of the evidence, and determining how to incorporate the evidence into practice. Newer guidelines that are developed today are incorporating these evidence-based steps into their approach. Take, for example, the Seventh ACCP Conference on Antithrombotic and Thrombolytic Therapy Evidence-Based Guidelines.[32] The name of this guideline was changed to reflect the evidence-based approach that was incorporated into this seventh update. This included the explicit definition of questions, eligibility criteria for including studies, and the specification of values and preferences underlying recommendations where they were particularly relevant.

Practice guidelines usually grade the strength of their recommendation based on the strength of the recommendation and the quality of evidence for the recommendations. A series of publications in *JAMA* outlined a method for grading health care recommendations using a hierarchy from overviews of observational studies with inconsistent results to overviews of randomized controlled trails with consistent results.[33–35] Guidelines do not all follow the same rating system; however, they are all based on the same core principles.[32,34,36] Guidelines should clearly define upfront how they rated their recommendations.

Analyzing the Evidence

Primary Studies

When evaluating and analyzing the primary literature, the pharmacist must critically appraise the study to validate the accuracy of the results and conclusions. Readers cannot and should not take the recommendations and conclusions as truth and apply this to clinical practice if they have not completed a critical appraisal of the study. Critical appraisal involves the detailed assessment of design, procedures, analysis, and interpretation of a trial.[13] As mentioned previously, even RCCT are subject to bias, and as pharmacists we need to uncover this bias if it is apparent. Etminan et al. composed the following questions to help identify factors that affect the strength of the primary evidence: Were the inclusion and exclusion criteria clearly stated? Was the study randomized? Was there adequate concealment of blinding of both study participants and investigators? Was compliance with the medication measured? Was the sample size adequate to detect the

outcome? Were all patients accounted for in reporting the results? What were the endpoints measured? Was the selection of cases and controls appropriate? Is the temporal relationship correct? Is there a dose response relationship?[13] It is important to ask these questions when evaluating and analyzing the primary literature.

Evaluating the Results

Several papers provide an excellent explanation for evaluating the results of a clinical trial.[2,13,37] The pharmacist is encouraged to consult these references for more detailed explanations or case examples. Askew suggests making a list of efficacy endpoints of the trial by listing the percentage of patients with a particular outcome in the treatment group and the percentage of those in the control group.[37] These percentages can then be used to calculate the size of the effect. The relative risk reduction (RRR) and absolute risk reduction (ARR) are parameters used to determine the magnitude of the drug effect.[37] The relative risk (RR) is the ratio of the incidence of an event in the treatment group to the incidence in the control group.[13] The RRR estimates the comparative risk reduction between treatment and control groups. The ARR is the difference in event rate between treatment and control groups. If you divide 100 by the ARR, you get another parameter, the number needed to treat (NNT). The NNT is the number of patients needed to treat with a specified therapy in order for one patient to benefit from treatment.[29] This parameter is useful because it puts the magnitude of the effect into context. They are all calculated as follows:

ARR = event rate in the control group – event rate in the treatment group

NNT = 100/ARR

RR = event rate in the treatment group/event rate in the control group

RRR = ARR/event rate in the control group or 1 – RR

The ARR determines the actual differences in outcome between the two groups. For example, if 10% of patients died in the control group and 5% died in the treatment group, the ARR for death would be 5%. The RRR also determines the difference in outcome between the two groups but takes into account the frequency of the event in a controlled population. For example, if 10% of the control group and 5% of the treatment group died, the RRR for death would be 50% with the treatment. In this example, the NNT is

20 in order for one patient to benefit from treatment. Only looking at the RRR can be misleading. In the above example, if we halved the percentage of patients in each group who died, the ARR would be 2.5% but the RRR would still be 50% and the new NNT is 40 in order for one patient to benefit from treatment. Hence, RRR overemphasizes the potential benefits of treatment and does not take into account the baseline risks of subjects in the trial.[13] As RR stays constant, absolute risk may change along with an individual patient's baseline risk.[13] The NNT also has its drawbacks in that it is based on the average baseline risk of all the patients in the study.[13] This means that you have to treat a larger number of patients to prevent one death than you would need to treat in a less-healthy population. Pharmacologic interventions can therefore be tailored to the specific patient risk to obtain the optimal therapeutic benefit for the patient and society.[2,13] These same equations and parameters can be applied to adverse effects.

Determining Statistical Significance

To determine the statistical significance of the RR, RRR, and ARR one must understand statistical indicators of significance. The p value and the confidence interval are used to determine statistical significance of studies. Usually a p value of less than 0.05 represents statistical significance.[13] The lower the p value, the lower the probability that the observed result occurred by chance. The p value does not provide the possible range of the true difference. The confidence interval (CI) is an estimate of the range within which the true treatment effect lies. The 95% confidence interval is the range of values within which we are 95% certain the true value lies. If the CI of ARR includes 0 or the CI of RRR includes 1, the difference between the treatment and control groups is not significant.[37] A wide confidence interval is a reason for a clinician to be cautious about recommending therapy based on the results of the study.[13]

Integrative Studies

Assessing the Quality of a Systematic Review

All types of research evidence, including systematic reviews require critical appraisal to assess their validity and to determine if and how they will be useful in the clinical situation at hand. Several publications have focused on how to determine or assess the quality of a systematic review.[31,38] These eight questions may assist the pharmacist when evaluating the quality of a review: (1) Did the review article address a focused question? (2) Is it likely that important, relevant studies were missed? (3) Were the inclusion criteria used to select articles appropriate? (4) Was the validity of the included studies assessed? (5) Were the assessments of studies reproducible? (6) Were the results similar from study to study? (7) What are the overall results and how precise are they? (8) Will the results help in caring for patients?

Assessing the Quality of Clinical Practice Guidelines

Hayward et al. provide a users' guide for practice guidelines.[39] They use the same basic questions as the users' guides for original research articles, overviews, and decision analyses. Are the recommendations valid? If they are, what are the recommendations and will they be helpful in patient care? Guidelines need to clearly specify their methods for selecting the evidence, grading the evidence, and making recommendations. They also need to provide information about how they chose options and outcomes, decided on values, and the relative values of different outcomes. If these are not defined, the user should question the usefulness and validity of the recommendations. Two additional questions are important in determining validity: Is the guideline likely to account for important recent developments?, and Has the guideline been subject to peer review and testing? One also needs to determine how strong are the recommendations, what is the impact of uncertainty associated with the evidence and values used, and if the recommendations are practical and clinically important.

Summary

Applying the principles of evidence-based medicine is important for the institutional pharmacist when selecting and evaluating pharmacotherapeutic regimens. The application of evidence-based medicine assists the clinician in uncovering the *truth* regarding treatment benefit and risk. Pharmacists need to make a concerted effort to develop the skills needed to practice true evidence-based medicine. Practicing evidence-based medicine is more than just conducting a literature search on a topic. It involves identifying and formulating a good question, searching for the evidence, critically analyzing and evaluating the evidence, and implementing the best evidence into clinical practice after considering patient circumstances, values, and preferences and your clinical expertise and pathophysiological knowledge. A big challenge for pharmacists can be incorporating clinical expertise, patient circumstances, values, and preferences into evidence extracted from the literature in making sound therapeutic decisions and when understanding decisions made by physicians. This is a challenge because not all pharmacists have adequate contact with patients and their family members. With the role of the institutional pharmacist evolving into a patient focused clinician, pharmacists are better able to incorporate these pieces into evidence-based decision making. Practicing evidence-based medicine strengthens confidence in therapeutic decisions that may be conveyed to physicians, patients, and payers.

References

1. Guyatt G, Cairns J, Churchill D, et al. Evidence-based medicine. A new approach to teaching the practice of medicine. *JAMA*. 1992;268:2420–5.

2. Chiquette E, Posey LM. Evidence-based medicine. In: DiPiro JT, Talbert RL, Yee GC, et al., eds. *Pharmacotherapy A Pathophysiologic Approach*. 5th ed. New York: McGraw-Hill; 2002:19–29.

3. Reidenberg MM. Clinical pharmacology: the scientific basis of therapeutics. *Clin Pharmacol Ther*. 1999;66: 2–8.

4. Ellis J, Mulligan I, Rowe J, et al. Inpatient general medicine is evidence-based. A-Team, Nuffield Department of Clinical Medicine. *Lancet*. 1995;346:407–10.

5. Sackett D. Evidence-based medicine. *Lancet*. 1995;346: 1171. Letter.

6. Fowler PBS. Evidence-based medicine. *Lancet*. 1995; 346:838. Letter.

7. Grahame-Smith D. Evidence-based medicine: socratic dissent. *BMJ*. 1995;310:1126–7.

8. Marwick C. Proponents gather to discuss practicing evidence-based medicine. *JAMA*. 1997;278:531–2.

9. Guyatt GH, Haynes RB, Jaeschke RZ, et al. Users' guides to the medical literature: XXV. evidence-based medicine: principles for applying the users' guides to patient care. *JAMA*. 2000;284:1290–6.

10. Ellrodt G, Cook DJ, Lee J, et al. Evidence-based disease management. *JAMA*. 1997;278:1687–92.

11. Sackett DL, Rosenberg WMC, Gray JAM, et al. Evidence-based medicine: what it is and what it isn't. *BMJ*. 1996;312:71–2. Editorial.

12. Oxman AD, Sackett DL, Guyatt GH. Users' guides to the medical literature: I. how to get started. *JAMA*. 1993;270:2093–5.

13. Etminan M, Wright JM, Carleton BC. Evidence-based pharmacotherapy: review of basic concepts and applications in clinical practice. *Ann Pharmacother*. 1998;32: 1193–200.

14. Stampfer MJ, Colditz GA, Willett WC, et al. Postmenopausal estrogen therapy and cardiovascular disease. ten year follow-up from the nurses' health study. *N Engl J Med*. 1991;325:756–2.

15. Grodstein F, Stampfer MJ, Manson JE, et al. Postmenopausal estrogen and progestin use and the risk of cardiovascular disease. *N Engl J Med*. 1996;335:453–61.

16. Rossouw JE, Anderson GL, Prentice RL, et al. Risks and benefits of estrogen plus progestin in healthy postmenopausal women: principal results from the Women's Health Initiative randomized controlled trial. *JAMA*. 2002;288:321–33.

17. Hulley S, Grady D, Bush T, et al. Randomized trial of estrogen plus progestin for secondary prevention of coronary heart disease in post-menopausal women. Heart and Estrogen/progestin Replacement Study (HERS) Research Group. *JAMA*. 1998;280:605–13.

18. Nananda FC, Pauker SG. The discrepancy between observational studies and randomized trials of menopausal hormone therapy: did expectations shape experience? *Ann Intern Med*. 2003;139:923–9.

19. The Leapfrog Group for Patient Safety Rewarding Higher Standards. Available at: http://www.leapfrog group.org/rewards_compendium. Accessed November 13, 2004.

20. Centers for Medicaid and Medicare services (CMS) quality indicators. Available at: http://www.cms.hhs.gov/ quality/hospital. Accessed November 13, 2004.

21. Agency for Healthcare Research and Quality (AHRQ) quality indicators. Available at: http://qualityindicators. ahrq.gov. Accessed November 13, 2004.

22. The Institute for Clinical Systems Improvement (ICSI) health care guidelines. Available at: http://www.icsi.org. Accessed November 13, 2004.

23. What is the Cochrane Collaboration? Available at: http://www.cochrane.org Accessed November 13, 2004.

24. Zynx Health. Available at: http://www.zynx.com. Accessed November 13, 2004.

25. Clineguide. Available at: http://www.clineguide.com. Accessed November 13, 2004.

26. Ovid Technologies Field Guide. Available at: http:// gateway.ut.ovid.com. Accessed November 13, 2004.

27. Netting the Evidence. Available at: http://www.shef.ac. uk/scharr/ir/netting/first.html. Accessed November 13, 2004.

28. Centre for Evidence-Based Pharmacotherapy. Available at: http://www.aston.ac.uk/lhs/teaching/pharmacy/cebp/ cebpmain.html. Accessed November 13, 2004.

29. Allen J. Applying study results to patient care: glossary of study design and statistical terms. *Pharmacist's Letter*. 2004;20:1–14.

30. Cook DJ, Mulrow CD, Haynes RB. Systematic reviews synthesis of best evidence for clinical decisions. *Ann Intern Med*. 1997;126:376–80.

31. Hunt D, L, McKibbon KA. Locating and appraising systematic reviews. *Ann Intern Med*. 1997;126:532–8.

32. Hirsch J, Guyatt G, Albers GW, et al. The seventh ACCP conference on antithrombotic and thrombolytic therapy: evidence-based guidelines. *Chest.* 2004;126: 172S–173S.

33. Guyatt GH, Sinclair J, Cook DJ, et al. Users' guides to the medical literature: XVI. how to use a treatment recommendation. *JAMA.* 1999;281:1836–43.

34. Wilson MC, Hayward RS, Tunis SR, et al. Users' guides to the medical literature: VIII. how to use clinical practice guidelines: B. what are the recommendations and will they help you in caring for your patients? *JAMA.* 1995;274:1630–2.

35. Guyatt GH, Sackett DL, Sinclair JC, et al. Users' guides to the medical literature: IX. a method for grading health care recommendations. *JAMA.* 1995;274:1800–4.

36. Guidelines for the use of antiretroviral agents in HIV-1-infected adults and adolescents, October 29, 2004. Developed by the panel on Clinical Practices for Treatment of HIV Infection convened by the Department of Health and Human Services (DHHS). Available at: http://AIDSinfo.nih.gov. Accessed November 13, 2004.

37. Askew JP. Journal club 101 for the new practitioner: evaluation of a clinical trial. *Am J Health-Syst Pharm.* 2004;61:1885–7.

38. Oxman AD, Cook DJ, Guyatt GH. Users' guides to the medical literature. VI. how to use an overview. Evidence-Based Medicine Working Group. *JAMA.* 1994;272: 1367–71.

39. Hayward RS, Wilson MC, Tunis SR, et al. Users' guides to the medical literature: VIII. how to use clinical practice guidelines: A. are the recommendations valid? *JAMA.* 1995;274:570–4.

Chapter 37

Ethics for Pharmacists

Robert A. Buerki, Louis D. Vottero

I pay thy poverty, and not thy will.
—*William Shakespeare*

About 400 hundred years ago, William Shakespeare penned *Romeo and Juliet.* In the apothecary scene, Romeo, seeking a poison, is cautioned by the apothecary, "Mantua's law is death to any he that utters them." Persisting, Romeo plays on the poor living and practice conditions evident in the pharmacist and his surroundings: "Thy world is not thy friend, nor the world's law: The world affords no law to make you rich; Then be not poor, but break it and take this." As Romeo offers 40 ducats for a dram of poison, the apothecary hesitates, "My poverty, but not my will, consents." Insists Romeo, "I pay thy poverty, and not thy will," and thus introduces the world to "pharmaceutically assisted suicide." (*Romeo and Juliet,* Act V, Scene I)

Introduction

In the practice of pharmacy, core activities such as dispensing and counseling reflect the varied and significant professional responsibilities pharmacists encounter in today's multilayered health care system. More specialized tasks, such as therapeutic interchange, add deeper and more complex obligations, while fully implemented pharmaceutical care imbues professional pharmacy practice with renewed requirements for virtuous behavior. In addition, recent advances in medical care, such as drug-releasing implants and pharmacogenomics, reflect the high level of technology common in 21st-century medical and pharmacy practice, many of them presenting unique ethical and moral dilemmas. Other shared practice responsibilities, such as evidence-based prescribing, clinical protocols, institutional review boards, drug budgets, and drug availability, clearly demonstrate how decisions about medicine and pharmacy practice are connected with public life and the social system of modern democracies.[1] In many situations, intense moral dilemmas formerly not encountered are emerging as pharmacists, physicians, and others are confronted with decisions or interventions correlative to the complicated and complex aspects of emerging procedures such as pharmaceutically assisted death, off-label drug use, clinical trial code-breaking, and more assertive patient advocacy. Such *modern* dilemmas appeal for solutions that are rational, based on defensible ideas, understandable, and accepted by society as a whole.

Pharmacists provide vital services to mankind, in various domestic and foreign cultures, and are confronted, concerned, and confounded by practice situations that they find deeply disturbing. Some of these situations, which are often unrelated to clinical procedures or medical intervention, may involve such basic human rights as the right to privacy and dignity or even the right to be told the truth. In recent years, pharmaceutical educators have embraced the practice philosophy of pharmaceutical care with its "emotional commitment to the welfare of the patients as individuals who require and deserve pharmacists' compassion, concern, and trust."[2] This listing of professional practice values, especially trust and compassion, is considered to be fundamental to the patient-pharmacist relationship and anticipates a set of ethical values that may be the essential guide to the moral decision-making that will define professional pharmacy practice for many decades.

Throughout the 19th and 20th centuries, American pharmacists sought to maintain ethical standards as an integral part of their emerging professional character. Expanded patient contacts resulted in improved patient care, more rational drug therapy, and higher rates of compliance; however, these intensely personal, even intimate, contacts have increased pharmacists' exposure to ethical and moral dilemmas. Resolving these ethical conflicts remains a constant challenge to even the most experienced pharmacists; however, resolution of these conflicts through reflective ethical reasoning can lead pharmacy practitioners not only to a greater sense of personal worthiness, but may also represent the most laudable aspect of professional behavior within their practice. The apothecary serving Romeo knew it was against the laws of Mantua to deliver a dram of poison: Was it also unethical or, perhaps, immoral?

Pharmacy as a Moral Community

In the early part of the 20th century, a respected pharmacy educator wrote that "ethics is the science of human duty," a terse statement, yet one that defines the breadth of ethics in today's world.[3] More recently, two renowned medical ethicists examined the fundamentals of the professional-client relationship and declared that any actions involving humans are value-laden and consequently are "moral in nature."[4] Like all professionals, members of the pharmacy profession are "bound together by a common course of education, traditional values, and communal aspirations, all of which lead to an agreed upon professional purpose"; moreover, like other professionals, pharmacists are viewed as a moral community.[5] Pharmacy educators have underscored the moral nature of professional pharmacy for decades, asserting in 1927 that "the character and personality of pharmacists are of primary importance" and concluding in 1950 that "the outstanding factor determining the future of the profession of pharmacy is fundamentally moral in nature."[6,7] Thus, ethics and responsibility encompass the moral dimension of the pharmacy profession; this realization—that the intrinsic nature of the profession of pharmacy rests on moral values—helps to shape the relationship between the profession as a group, its members, and the individuals who receive professional pharmacy services.

The Importance of a Professional Ethic

Professionals are given certain legal prerogatives by society, such as a license to practice and a quasimonopoly to operate in a certain professional arena. In return for these prerogatives, a profession accepts responsibility to maintain a standard of conduct beyond conformity to law or technical skill. This standard of conduct, this common concern for collective self-discipline, this control of a profession from within, is known as *professional ethics*.

Deciding what is right or wrong, good or bad, virtue and vice, rights and responsibilities, and taking the moral point of view is the essence of ethics and ethical issues. Ethics is an action concept; doing something, taking an action, making a decision about what is the correct pathway for behavior when confronted with a moral dilemma. *Professional pharmacy ethics*, that is, moral behavioral standards applied to professional pharmacy practice dilemmas, controls only members of the pharmacy profession, not society at large. Ethics is closely related to two other systems designed to control society, law and morals. *Law* refers to regulations established by a government applicable to a certain political subdivision. Law controls all people within a certain political subdivision, not a particular group in society. By contrast, *morals* are generally accepted customs of right living and conduct, and an individual's practice in relation to these customs. Noncompliance by an individual to any one of these three systems may result in certain sanctions. Breaking a rule of law may incur not only fines, but imprisonment; nonconformance to a moral tenet may bring a feeling of shame; nonobservance of a professional ethic criterion could lead to disciplinary measures, even expulsion, from the group controlled by the ethic. Table 37-1 summarizes the differing characteristics of law, morals, and ethics.

Foundations of Ethical Decision Making

All persons, pharmacists included, draw upon a wide range of experiences and influences that converge to form their personal value systems. The influences of our parents, friends, teachers, religious leaders, and others all combine to forge a basic value system that continues to expand during our years of professional pharmacy education and practical experience and into our professional practice. Our professional decisions flow from this unique, highly complex set of values we have acquired. All pharmacists, whether they are aware

Table 37-1
Comparison of Systems of Societal Control

System	Applies to	Control from	Form
Ethics	Specific group	Within the group	Codes of ethics
Law	Specific area	Outside the group	Legislation
Morals	Individuals	Conscience, religious beliefs	Religious writings

of it or not, are constantly making ethical choices, deciding what is the right course of action given a specific moral dilemma, taking a course of action that is the best of any alternative; it is the action that one *ought* to do.

What are the agreed-upon personal values or ethical practice standards of the 21st-century American pharmacist? Is it possible to identify time-honored moral principles, ethical theories, or virtues so associated with the practice of pharmacy that they are embodied in every "ethical" pharmacy practitioner? Are the ethical norms reflected in our Code of Ethics for Pharmacists defined by a national body representing pharmacists, or is ethical conduct merely what most pharmacists informally agree is right or proper?

Framers of the earliest standards of professional medical and pharmacy practice presumed that their rules (codes) would reflect their patients' best interests. Primarily based upon the ancient Hippocratic principle of doing good (*beneficence*) and avoiding evil (*non-maleficence*), these codes essentially reflected paternalistic attitudes that posed challenges to patient autonomy and often opened professional veracity to question. For example, the basic principle that underlies the Hippocratic Oath enjoins physicians to work for the benefit of the sick according to their "ability and judgment" without necessarily including their patients in the decision-making process surrounding their treatment program, thus ignoring "freedom of choice" as an essential human value. More recently, additional moral principles such as *justice*—strategies or acts that ensure the fair allocation of goods and services; *respect for autonomy*—strategies or acts that respect the self-determination of other persons; and *fidelity*—strategies or acts that stress faithfulness and promise keeping—have been included as important action guides. Various aspects of medical and pharmaceutical practice, such as medical confidentiality, respect for life, patients' rights, patient advocacy, health politics, and the nature of the patient-pharmacist relationship, emphasize the need for a fundamental grounding for any concept of ethics.

For centuries, gifted individuals have attempted to encapsulate rules for ethical behavior into fundamental theories. These ancient and modern ethical theories may be considered under a broad classification scheme that distinguishes two basic types of ethical theory: *Consequentialism*, an ethical theory concerned only with the outcomes or consequences of actions, and *nonconsequentialism*, an ethical theory based upon the

actions themselves without particular regard to their consequences. A particular action becomes right or wrong in the first case by evaluating the benefit or harm the patient—and all others concerned—might derive from the given action. For example, lying to a patient may be permissible to the consequentialist if it results in some benefit to the patient or others. The nonconsequentialist, on the other hand, would reason that lying to a patient is wrong by definition, whether or not the lie might ultimately provide some benefit to all parties.

Another conceptual basis for ethical practice in pharmacy involves studying the underlying values and virtues of its practitioners and the traits of character most associated with these values and virtues. *Virtue* is often defined in terms of traits of character that are valued as a human quality; that is, by looking at the virtues of individuals, we are able to gauge their character, and can better understand the attitudes with which they approach moral decisions. *Values* are standards that are considered important or that have worth or merit; values are expressed by behaviors or standards that a person endorses or tries to maintain. Some writers believe that the actions of present-day pharmacists are best characterized by the virtues of *honesty, dedication, carefulness,* and *dependability*.[8] The American public, through the Gallup Polls, tell us that pharmacists are one of the most respected of all American professionals in terms of honesty and ethical standards.[9] A listing of values and behaviors for professional pharmacists is presented in Table 37-2. This wide range of values with their attendant behaviors is often apparent in professional pharmacy practice as the public observes reoccurring instances of fair dealing and equity, patient-centered services, and faithfulness.

Yet another approach for grounding ethical pharmacy practice is a consideration of human rights and professional duties and the inherent tension that can exist between these concepts. In recent decades, the importance of human rights, reflected in the tenets of liberal individualism, has emerged as a driving force in American society. In response to this societal mandate, nearly every institution and professional association in the health care field has embraced the notion of patient rights to some extent. *Rights* may be defined as justified claims that individuals or groups can make on others or upon society, and may emanate from two distinct sources: *natural rights*—such as the right to life and the right to die—which are inherent to the human condition, and *bestowed rights*—such as the right to

Table 37-2
Values and Behaviors for Professional Pharmacists

Values	Attitudes	Professional Behavior
Altruism (concern for the welfare of others)	Commitment Compassion Generosity	Gives full attention to patients Assists other health care personnel Sensitive to social issues
Equality (having the same rights, privileges, or status)	Fairness Self-esteem Tolerance	Provides services based on needs Relates to others without discriminating Provides leadership in improving access to health care
Esthetics (qualities of objects, events, and persons that provide satisfaction)	Appreciation Creativity Sensitivity	Creates supportive patient care
Freedom (capacity to exercise choice)	Openness Self-direction Self-discipline	Respects each individual's autonomy
Human Dignity (inherent worth and uniqueness of an individual)	Empathy Kindness Trust	Respects the right of privacy Maintains confidentiality
Justice (upholding moral and legal principles)	Integrity Morality	Acts as a health care advocate Allocates resources fairly Reports incompetent, unethical, and illegal practices
Truth (faithfulness to fact or reality)	Accountability Honesty Rationality	Documents actions accurately Protects the public from misinformation about pharmacy

Source: Adopted from *Essentials of College and University Education for Professional Nursing: Final Report.* Washington, DC: American Association of Colleges of Nursing; 1986:6–7.

privacy and the right to health care—which must be granted by others, such as a government, an institution, or individuals. Other types of rights include *legal rights* and *moral rights.*

Rights not only form a significantly symbolic underpinning to our society, but also exert a powerful force in the development of our system of health care. Increasingly, Americans have claimed the right to a wide gamut of governmentally assured health care services, including the right to receive prescription drugs through such programs as Medicare and Medicaid. Recently, federal legislation extended patients' privacy rights with respect to their "individually identifiable health information."[10] Every right carries with it a correlative *duty,* that is, an obligation on someone

else to behave in a certain manner; for example, the bestowed right of health care assistance to the medically indigent through Medicaid implies an obligation on all health care practitioners to provide that assistance in an equitable manner. Similarly, the right of patients to be fully informed about their therapy obliges pharmacists to provide such information to patients and to warn them about possible serious side effects and adverse reactions.

The Code of Ethics for Pharmacists

Society expects a profession, through its collective members, to generate its own statement of acceptable and unacceptable behavior, usually in the form of a *code of ethics,* a detailed, explicit operational blueprint of norms of professional conduct, a recital of desirable and undesirable actions having an impact on the character of a profession and its functional reliability. The behavioral pattern established in a code of ethics is generally enforced through a peer-review mechanism associated with a professional academy or association.

The Code of Ethics for Pharmacists, adopted by the American Society of Health-System Pharmacists in 1996, is strikingly different from all code statements previously adopted by pharmacists. Earlier codes were very practice-specific, and often narrowly focused merely on practice events encountered by pharmacists with patients, physicians, other health care professionals, or fellow pharmacists. The Code of Ethics for Pharmacists (Table 37-3), with its preamble and eight principles, avoids this detailed approach and instead uses general recommendations and general norms as its framework.

The preamble to the Code is a straightforward expression of purpose that provides a simple, clear declaration of the role that pharmacists play in medication use, namely to "assist individuals in making the best use of medications." This obviously refers not just to the patient, but to all individuals who are linked to the medication-use system, including physicians, nurses, administrators, pharmaceutical manufacturers, insurance executives, hospital administrators, government officials, and all others who formulate drug use policy. Such a sweeping statement of role responsibilities positions pharmacists as critical to all drug therapy situations. The preamble concludes by declaring that the principles embodied in the code are "based on moral obligations and virtues." This declaration of a moral foundation for a professional code of ethics is unique among American health professions and sets the aspirational tone that is carried forward throughout the Code.

Principle I of the Code sets the stage for the rest of the Code by defining the relationship that exists between patients and pharmacists. By establishing the patient-pharmacist relationship as a "covenant," the Code serves notice that pharmacists respond to this relationship by observing certain moral obligations, assuring that pharmacy practice is not merely transactional. The concept of a covenant relies upon giving and receiving; pharmacists are offered the "gift of trust" from their patients; in return, pharmacists promise to help individuals achieve optimum benefit from their medications, to be committed to their welfare, and to maintain their trust. Indeed, trust and confidence may well be the central values of any relationship between health care professionals and their patients. Since the nature of the patient-pharmacist relationship forms the bedrock of professional practice, its nature and the resulting moral obligations deserve sincere reflection upon the part of every pharmacist.

A number of the Code principles encompass values and virtues that sustain professional pharmacy practice: care, compassion, autonomy, dignity, honesty, and integrity. Such values and virtues recognize that the well-being of patients is a primary practice imperative of pharmacy; to achieve this outcome, pharmacists must consider both needs defined by science and those needs expressed by their patients.

Other Code principles outline duties of pharmacists toward professional competence and respect for other health care professionals. In the presence of patients who need pharmaceutical services, pharmacists make an implicit public "profession" that they have special skills and knowledge that will contribute to their patients' best interest. This declaration of a special competence and its use in the interest of others is the central act of a profession, carrying with it all the obligations that make the declaration authentic. Thus, pharmacists have a duty to posses and maintain competent knowledge and abilities, especially as new medications, devices, and technologies become available. At the same time, the Code alerts pharmacists to willingly accept the limits of their knowledge and practice competencies and to ask for the consultation of colleagues and other health professionals or refer the patient to the most appropriate service.

Finally, the Code affirms that pharmaceutical services provided by pharmacists to individuals, communities, or to society have both private and public aspects. Private aspects include the personal well-being of individuals in their social environment, while the public character derives from the fact that health care today is considered to one of the primary benefits of our society, at the same level as the right to work, the right to a clean environment, and political rights. In all of this, the Code anticipates that pharmacists will be fair and equitable when health resources are allocated, balancing the needs of patients and society.

Table 37-3
Code of Ethics for Pharmacists[a]

Pharmacists are health professionals who assist individuals in making the best use of medications. This Code, prepared and supported by pharmacists, is intended to state publicly the principles that form the fundamental basis of the roles and responsibilities of pharmacists. These principles, based on moral obligations and virtues, are established to guide pharmacists in relationships with patients, health professionals, and society.

I. A **pharmacist** respects the covenantal relationship between the patient and pharmacist.

Considering the patient-pharmacist relationship as a covenant means that a pharmacist has moral obligations in response to the gift of trust received from society. In return for this gift, a pharmacist promises to help individuals achieve optimum benefit from their medications, to be committed to their welfare, and to maintain their trust.

II. A **pharmacist** promotes the good of every patient in a caring, compassionate, and confidential manner.

A pharmacist places concern for the well-being of the patient at the center of professional practice. In doing so, a pharmacist considers needs stated by the patient as well as those defined by heath science. A pharmacist is dedicated to protecting the dignity of the patient. With a caring attitude and a compassionate spirit, a pharmacist focuses on serving the patient in a private and confidential manner.

III. A **pharmacist** respects the autonomy and dignity of each patient.

A pharmacist promotes the right of self-determination and recognizes individual self-worth by encouraging patients to participate in decisions about their health. A pharmacist communicates with patients in terms that are understandable. In all cases, a pharmacist respects personal and cultural differences among patients.

IV. A **pharmacist** acts with honesty and integrity in professional relationships.

A pharmacist has a duty to tell the truth and to act with conviction of conscience. A pharmacist avoids discriminatory practices, behavior or work conditions that impair professional judgment, and actions that compromise dedication to the best interests of patients.

V. A **pharmacist** maintains professional competence.

A pharmacist has a duty to maintain knowledge and abilities as new medications, devices, and technologies become available and as health information advances.

VI. A **pharmacist** respects the values and abilities of colleagues and other health professionals.

When appropriate, a pharmacist asks for the consultation of colleagues or other health professionals or refers the patient. A pharmacist acknowledges that colleagues and other health professionals may differ in the beliefs and values they apply to the care of the patient.

VII. A **pharmacist** serves individual, community, and societal needs.

The primary obligation of a pharmacist is to individual patients. However, the obligations of a pharmacist may at times extend beyond the individual to the community and society. In these situations, a pharmacist recognizes the responsibilities that accompany these obligations and acts accordingly.

VIII. A **pharmacist** seeks justice in the distribution of health resources.

When health resources are allocated, a pharmacist is fair and equitable, balancing the needs of patients and society.

[a] This code was approved by the membership of the American Pharmaceutical Association on October 27, 1994.

Ethical Decision Making in Pharmacy Practice

Given some understanding of the available systems that can be used as a foundation for ethical decision making, it is useful to develop a framework for the process of making these decisions. Regardless of whether the choice of behavioral standards is ethical theory, principles, virtues, rights, or codes, the resolution of ethical dilemmas in pharmacy practice needs to be based on objectivity and critical thinking. Several models are available that view ethical decision-making as a generalized problem-solving process that can be easily learned. The following four-step process encourages pharmacists to not only make professional decisions based on reflection and reason but also ensures that the resulting choice is defensible and validated in ethical terms. The four steps are (1) *identifying the problem,* (2) *developing alternative courses of action,* (3) *selecting one alternative course of action,* and (4) *considering objections to the alternative selected.*

1. *Identifying the Problem*—Given a true moral dilemma, it may appear deceptively simple to define or identify the problem; nevertheless, the clear identification of an ethical problem sets the stage for systematic problem analysis. At this step, it is essential to identify all parties who may be affected by any course of action taken, whether they are individuals, institutions, or organizations. A possible road map for use in problem identification includes the following self-explanatory steps: identify all technical facts, identify moral parameters, identify legal constraints, and identify relevant human values.

2. *Developing Alternative Courses of Action*—The development of alternative courses of action is often extraordinarily difficult because in many cases only one alternative leaps to the mind, while other alternatives are discarded as not meriting serious consideration. However, this step in the problem-solving process is of great importance as it is a plea for thoroughness in deciding which of several equally satisfying actions should be taken. This step must be completed with diligence; each alternative will contain relevant ethical principles that will have to be identified as well as any ethical assumption associated with it. Other ethical issues may emerge as an indirect result of this exhaustive process and will expand the field of ethical inquiry.

3. *Selecting One Alternative Course of Action*—The third step in this proposed problem-solving process involves selecting the one course of action that best fits your personal and professional value system. In selecting your course of action, it is imperative that you be able to identify the specific foundation upon which you made your selection and the process of reasoning which led you to your conclusion. Be able to defend your selection on ethical grounds keep-

ing in mind that more than one action may be acceptable in a given situation.

4. *Considering Objections to Alternative Selected*—Finally, it is important in the resolution of ethical problems to anticipate the objection that might arise as the result of your decision. These objections usually arise from three sources: factual errors, faulty reasoning, and conflicting values. With practice, pharmacists should be able to minimize or even eliminate factual errors in any ethical analysis. Eliminating faulty reasoning in ethical analysis is somewhat more challenging, requiring justification of the selected alternative on the criteria of both relevancy and sufficiency. For example, if the alternative selected is "to tell the truth," it must be supported with defensible reasons, such as community standards, religious beliefs, or statements from a code of ethics. To justify your choice with a personal standard—"I always tell the truth"—may be relevant but not sufficient.

Applying Ethical Decision Making in Pharmacy Practice

With some knowledge of the foundations that can assist the ethical decision-making process—ethical theories and principles, virtues, rights and duties, and professional codes—and a general understanding of a process model for reaching these decisions, we may now turn our attention to ethical decision making in pharmacy practice. In doing so, we need to realize that the real-world settings of professional pharmacy practice often exert external influences that may affect our ethical decision making, influences such as professional authority, technical competence, practice setting rules and policies, or economic forces. These external influences are integral to the dilemma and need to be factored into the decision-making process. The following case is structured to demonstrate the effect of such external influences; it also provides an example of how one might use the ethical analysis model described above.[11]

The Pharmacist as a Patient Advocate

Mrs. McGuire is 70 years old and hospitalized due to severe and debilitating back pain. She has a history of degenerative disk disease that resulted in having two cervical disks fused and a metal rod placed in her neck. She has no relatives and is a past employee of an urban tertiary teaching hospital, where she is now a patient; she therefore knows many of the employees. Because of her previous relationship with the head of the pharmacy department, she placed an urgent call to William Johnson, Pharm.D., the head of the pharmacy department, because, as she said, she needed someone to "serve as her advocate" while she was in the hospital. Bill Johnson remembered Mrs. McGuire as a pleasant person but somewhat dogmatic and demanding. He assured her he would confer with the clinical pharmacist in charge of her therapeutic regimen and "look out for her." Within 24 hours, Bill had met with both Mrs. McGuire and the charge pharmacist. Mrs. McGuire was outraged because she was being denied the kind of pain medication that she was accustomed to taking. "This new stuff doesn't work and I won't take any more of it," she complained. When Bill investigated the matter further, he discovered that the charge pharmacist had refused to dispense opioids for Mrs. McGuire, which prompted the prescribing physician to make the regimen modification that resulted in the unwanted drug. "As my advocate, Dr. Johnson, I want you to set this straight," Mrs. McGuire pursued. The charge pharmacist, an experienced and capable Pharm.D., quietly defended his position to Bill by claiming it was his duty to protect Mrs. McGuire from the potential harm that is inherent in opioid use. Does Bill Johnson face an irresolvable moral dilemma? Where is the harm, if any, resulting from the pharmacist's refusal to dispense the requested opioid?

Step One: Problem Identification

Bill Johnson is confronted with a complex dilemma that has engaged pharmacists in their professional practice for decades, the right to exercise personal judgment in withholding a prescribed medication from a patient.[12] This issue raises important questions about individual rights and public health. Who prevails when the needs of patients conflict with the personal held morals of the health care provider? This case not only involves the pharmacist who withheld the opioid drug, but also the chief pharmacist who is not serving as a therapy specialist, but rather as a patient's advocate, a role that is part of the guiding ethical principles of the American Society of Health-System Pharmacists.[13]

This is an ethical dilemma with many conflicting viewpoints. As head of the pharmacy department, Bill Johnson had assumed the authority of a "triple agent": As department head he represents the administrative policies and values of the hospital and the immediate

health care structure; as a pharmacist and the head of pharmacy services for the hospital, he affirms the values and virtues of professional pharmacy practice; finally, as a patient advocate for Mrs. McGuire, he needs to protect Mrs. McGuire's patient rights and interests. The charge pharmacist also needs to consider the influences of his ethical decision-making as an employee of the institution.

The right to refuse to participate in acts that conflict with personal ethical, moral, or religious convictions is accepted as an integral and essential element of a democratic society. Pharmacists have refused to honor prescriptions (mainly for emergency abortive medication) for many years, a practice that is likely to continue. American courts have held that pharmacists, like all health care professionals, owe their patients a duty of care; many states offer some level of protection for those health care professionals who refuse to provide certain services. More recently, several dozen states have taken the idea of "conscientious objection" and applied it legislatively to pharmacy practice, attempting to screen objecting pharmacists from sanctions such as civil lawsuits, criminal liability, or professional and employment repercussions. Unlike conscientious objectors to a military draft for whom choice is limited by definition, pharmacists choose to enter a profession that is bound by fiduciary duties, and willingly enter the profession of pharmacy and adopt its corresponding ethical and legal obligations. In addition to authenticating the existence of true conscientious objection, Bill must examine the action of the charge pharmacist more closely to ensure himself that the action has not moved beyond the duty to care for the patient and become invasive.

The core premise of this situation is that by denying Mrs. McGuire access to an opioid drug, the charge pharmacist has acted on his assumed obligation to protect her from possible harm (the principle of nonmaleficence). At the same time, he may have deprived Mrs. McGuire of her right of self-determination (respect for autonomy), since she was not consulted about the switching to a nonopioid, pain-relieving medication. The pharmacist may claim his own "right to self-determination," however; professional autonomy has its limits: it can be argued that when a pharmacist's objection directly and detrimentally affects a patient's health, the patient's interest should come first. Perhaps as compelling for meeting the patient's needs in this case are statements embedded in the Code of Ethics for Pharmacists: "A pharmacist promotes the good of every patient in a caring, compassionate, and confidential manner," and "a pharmacist seeks justice in the distribution of health resources." Such guiding principles seem to have a chilling effect on a pharmacist's claim to conscientious objection as a basis for professional practice decision making.

Step Two: Develop Alternative Courses of Action

Bill Johnson has several courses of action available to him. He could sanction the action taken by the charge pharmacist and try to convince Mrs. McGuire of the merits of the new therapy, perhaps emphasizing the risks involved with using an opioid medication. This is an attractive action-course for Bill; it satisfies his administrative responsibilities and it demonstrates strong support of the pharmacy department staff. Mrs. McGuire may be miffed, but with some careful counseling she could be persuaded of the merits of the modified therapy plan. The charge pharmacist should be pleased; the chief pharmacist has supported and endorsed his personally held moral value—the right to conscientious objection.

Bill also has the option to intervene directly and request the charge pharmacist to return to the therapy plan and accommodate the wishes of Mrs. McGuire, who is a long-time friend and a former employee. This approach would satisfy any concerns that the hospital administration might have and would meet Mrs. McGuire's needs. The charge pharmacist would probably be disappointed, but would at least continue to be involved in managing Mrs. McGuire's therapy.

Assuming that the prescribing physician is comfortable with a therapy plan recommended by the charge pharmacist, Dr. Johnson could move toward finding a reasonable and respectful balance between the needs of Mrs. McGuire and the moral stance of the charge pharmacist. This third alternative course of action is more inclusive than the first two suggested but is also more difficult to conclude, and it may make Bill appear to be indecisive to his administrative superiors who would anticipate rapid, clear solutions to any perceived treatment problems.

Finally, the chief pharmacist could look at other strategies that are beyond the realm of moral reasoning. For example, he could simply remove the "offending pharmacist" from Mrs. McGuire's therapy team and replace him with someone who has more liberal view concerning opioid therapy. This is an expedient action, and would appear decisive to the administrative staff, but obviously such behavior simply ignores the moral issues involved.

Step Three: Select One Alternative Course of Action

The heart of this dilemma is the notion of the right of the charge pharmacist to refuse to fill a prescription for an opioid drug because of a perceived potential harm to the patient. Three options may be considered: (1) the charge pharmacist has an absolute right to object to opioid therapy for Mrs. McGuire; (2) he has no right to object; or (3) he has a limited right to object. The first two options are extreme and contain some severe constraints that are ethically indefensible. To allow the charge pharmacist an absolute right to conscientious objection respects his claim of professional autonomy but lessens or even ignores Mrs. McGuire's right to self-determination. Furthermore, one of the unexpected effects of this action is a possible untoward affect on the health of the patient, since she now refuses therapy. Another potential problem with this approach, not discussed earlier, may be drawn from consideration of the *principle of double effect*, which simply states that an action with both good and bad effects is ethically permissible: If filling an opioid prescription is morally permissible, only the good effect (relieving pain) is intended, even if the bad effect (abusing opioids) is foreseen, and there is proportionality between the good and bad. In applying this principle to the case of Mrs. McGuire, only the proportionality aspect applies, and any challenge to proportionality would fail since the obligation to prevent serious evil or harm arises only when an action seriously interferes with one's life plans or style, and withholding opioids from Mrs. McGuire does interfere with her routine.

The second suggested alternative requires the complete denial of the charge pharmacist's right to refuse to fill the opioid prescription, an action that forces the pharmacist to completely abandon his moral standards. This seems heavy-handed. Society expects health care professionals to discard personal moral and religious standards in life-and-death situations. Mrs. McGuire's medical care at this point is not at this stage; therefore, this alternative is more than problematic and should be ignored.

The third alternative—finding a reasonable and respectful balance between the needs of Mrs. McGuire and the moral stance of the charge pharmacist—remains the action of choice. By recognizing and respecting the right of self-determination for both the patient and the pharmacist, this alternative calls for a compassionate duty of care. The charge pharmacist must be prepared to limit the reach of his personal objection; as a health care professional pledged to serve the public, it would be unreasonable for him to expect Mrs. McGuire to acquiesce to his personal convictions.

Step Four: Consider Objections to the Alternative Selected

Bill Johnson realizes there may be objections to reworking the therapy plan and including the Mrs. McGuire in the discussion. Hospital administration may be concerned about delays and an appearance of indecisiveness; the prescribing physician may have qualms about rehashing a therapy scheme for a third time. Nevertheless, the case facts show that the moral principle of respect for autonomy was slighted in denying the patient an opioid drug; there is an ethical imperative for correction. In addition, there is a strong possibility that a consideration of social justice and its obligation to promote the fair and equitable distribution of medical care (in this case an opioid medication) would result in the physician and pharmacist returning to the patient's bedside and beginning anew.

Summary

Nearly 50 years ago, George F. Archambault, a leader in American pharmacy, issued a call to America's hospital pharmacists to define and codify their professional practice mores.[14] The recently adopted Code of Ethics for Pharmacists satisfies this call and demonstrates in positive and certain terms the moral foundation of America's pharmacists. As we have seen, pharmacists practicing in the American health care system increasingly encounter ethical dilemmas that are profound in scope. Nevertheless, those pharmacists who embrace a professional practice that builds upon moral principles and virtues will find expanded opportunities for ethical decision making as they strive to meet the challenges of providing pharmaceutical care in the 21st century.

References

1. Dressing RP, Flameling J. Ethics in pharmacy: a new definition of responsibility. *Pharm World Sci.* 2003;25(1):3–10.

2. Penna RP, ed. The *Papers of the Commission to Implement Change in Pharmaceutical Education: Background Paper II: Entry Level, Curricular Outcomes, Curricular Content and Educational Process.* Alexandria, VA: American Association of Colleges of Pharmacy; 1994:10.

3. LaWall CH. Pharmaceutical ethics: a historical review of the subject with examples of codes adopted or suggested at different periods, together with a suggested code for adoption by present-day associations. *J Am Pharm Assn.* 1921;10(11):895.

4. Pellegrino ED, Thomasma DC. *A Philosophical Basis of Medical Practice: Toward a Philosophy and Ethic of the Healing Professions.* New York and Oxford: Oxford University Press; 1981:178.

5. Buerki RA, Vottero LD. Ethics and pharmaceutical care. In: Knowlton CH, Penna RP, eds. *Pharmaceutical Care.* 2nd ed., Bethesda, MD: American Society of Health-System Pharmacists; 2003:301.

6. Charters WW, Lemon AB, Monell LM. *Basic Material for a Pharmaceutical Curriculum.* New York: McGraw-Hill Book Company, Inc.; 1927:3.

7. Elliott EC. *The General Report of the Pharmaceutical Survey, 1946–49.* Washington, DC: American Council on Education; 1950:4.

8. Baldwin HJ, Alberts KT. Detailed cases and commentary: introduction. In: Smith M, Strauss S, Baldwin HJ, et al., eds. *Pharmacy Ethics.* New York and London: Pharmaceutical Products Press; 1991:452.

9. Carlson DK. Nurses remain at top on honest and ethics poll. *Gallup Poll Monthly.* 2000;422(Nov):45–8.

10. Health Insurance Portability and Accountability Act of 1996, Public Law 104-191, 104th Congress, August 21, 1996, 42 USC 1320d-2.

11. The foundation for this case is taken from: Nelson K. Ethics in practice: the case of Ms. M. *JONA's Healthcare Law, Ethics, and Regulation.* 2003;5(4):2003.

12. For a current review of this issue, see: Cantor JC, Baum K. The limits of conscientious objection—may pharmacists refuse to fill prescriptions for emergency contraception? *N Eng J Med.* 2004;351:2008–12.

13. ASHP Statement on Pharmacist's Decision-Making on Assisted Suicide (9915); reaffirmed by the Council on Legal and Public Affairs and by the Board of Directors in 2001.

14. Archambault GF. Ethical standards: Professional conduct and responsibilities. *Bull Am Soc Hosp Pharm.* 1956;13(5):445.

Chapter 38

Facility Planning and Design

Kenneth N. Barker, Elizabeth A. Flynn, David A. Kvancz

Introduction

This chapter describes the facility planning process, along with the role of the pharmacist in this process. The purpose is to prepare the reader for participation in a facilities planning program, so that he or she can then apply this process to the enormous amount of detail involved, whether for a new facility or remodeling.

This chapter does not offer *standard plans*, because experience has shown that such plans do not recognize the significant variation in hospitals due to the differences in their marketing strategies and local needs. The use of standard plans is a poor and misleading substitute for pharmacy planning founded on a thorough in-house study of future needs, functions, and operations that would yield a true picture of the facilities needed.

Topics to be addressed include the factors affecting facility needs, the hospital facility development process, current pharmacy planning and use of space, functional programming, the architectural design process, the process of designing for efficiency and flexibility, human factors in pharmacy, specialty work areas (e.g., sterile preparation and satellite pharmacies), and implementation.

Significance

Consider this. If a major mistake is made in planning the pharmacy, all pharmacy staff members will have to get up and face it, and work in it, every day of their professional lives.

At this time, the United States is facing one of the largest hospital building booms in U.S. history. As the result of the need to replace aging 1970's hospitals, the graying of the baby-boom generation, and the introduction of new technologies, the United States is predicted to spend more than $16 billion for hospital construction in 2004, rising to $20 billion per year by the end of the decade.[1] This once-in-a-lifetime construction program offers an opportunity to rethink hospital design, and especially to consider how improved design can help increase effectiveness in delivering care,

improve patient safety, and reduce staff stress and fatigue.[2]

One precept of architecture is that *form follows function*. The wisdom of this is seen most clearly in its violation (i.e., when obsolete buildings and fixtures limit the efficiency and effectiveness with which functions can be performed). With a greater need for efficiency in operations than ever before, capital investments in buildings or remodelings that offer the prospect of lower operating costs in the short run are in demand. Special attention is now being given to *evidence-based design*, reflecting the growth of a body of rigorous research, linking the physical environment of hospitals to staff performance and patient outcomes, and overall health care quality.[2]

This is good news for the pharmacy that is inefficient now and whose administrative pharmacists understand the planning process and can draw upon such pharmacy-related research to effectively justify the changes needed.

Factors Affecting Facility Needs

External Factors

The factors affecting the facility of an institution are many and varied. Those external to the individual departments include the following:

- Changes in government or third-party reimbursement systems may directly affect planning priorities and resources

- The adoption of new information technologies hospital-wide, such as computerized physician order entry and bar code-medication administration systems, may alter the work systems or even some functions of the pharmacy staff

- Changes in laws, regulations, codes, and standards are important. For example, the requirements for the preparation of sterile preparations are subject to new guidelines.

- Changes in the hospital's patient mix due to aging and degree of illness are of great importance

- Competition for patients via a demonstrated emphasis on the quality and personalization of care manifested in layout and design of patient areas is receiving increasing attention. Offering new services demanded by patients must be considered. Bed capacity and projected occupancy rates are vital to know. Hospital programs and services may need to be added or expanded (e.g., ambulatory and home health care services, sleep labs, and specialty hospitals).

- Automation of the medication system outside the pharmacy (e.g., bar code-based nursing procedures) can drastically change the work systems of the pharmacy department

- Increased patterns of prescription drug use are resulting in an increase in drug orders, thereby increasing pharmacy workload and storage needs. The rise or decline in alternative therapies may affect drug use, as when drugs replace surgical procedures. The development of new dosage systems (e.g., implanted devices) may create a need for pharmacy space dedicated to the storage of the many new high-tech medical devices involved in drug administration. One study has found that 67% of the doses nurses administer must first be prepared for administration, a task delegated to the pharmacy in unit dose systems.[3] Trends in other departments can have an important effect on many aspects of drug storage and distribution.

- Any change in hospital mechanical service systems, such as the decision to add (or shut down) a pneumatic tube system, can affect pharmacy greatly

- Concern for drug-related crime may warrant special security concerns

- Anticipation of terrorist activities may require special drug storage areas

- Confidentiality concerns, heightened as a result of the HIPAA regulations, may affect how prescriptions are labeled, records maintained, and where patient counseling must be performed

- The pharmacy manpower shortage is prompting the use of pharmacists who perform order entry and editing from their home (a telepharmacy application)

Internal Factors

Factors internal to the pharmacy department that influ-ence facility needs include decisions about the functions to be performed, such as whether the pharmacy will provide not only drug distribution and pharmaceutical care to inpatients but highly specialized clinical services as well. Larger hospitals may require specialized pharmacy services for trauma patients, and clean rooms for the preparation of sterile preparations and chemotherapy.[4]

In a smaller hospital, a decision to expand to 24-hour service may necessitate a pharmacy design capable of being operated by a single pharmacist working alone on the night shift, with attendant concerns for the safety of the pharmacist and the security of areas away from view. Outpatient service functions have grown and may include not only on-site outpatient pharmacies serving discharge patients and hospital personnel, but also off-site prescription pharmacies in physician office buildings and home infusion services.[5] Changes in work systems, such as the decision to recentralize the distribution process, may result in the need to close satellite pharmacies on the patient care units and expand the central pharmacy area. Assembly line picking will require a different layout than will modular picking stations.[6,7] Automation as in automated dispensing and intravenous (IV) compounding machines obviously will have considerable impact in terms of the rearrangement of workflow and consequent changes in facilities (e.g., automation service areas). Robotic distribution systems may require a prepackaging operation, which may be located internally or off-site (or outsourced). Changes in the use of personnel such as the redeployment of pharmacists for clinical tasks may result in the substitution of auxiliaries for professionals in some cases, necessitating new checking procedures and the need for new *checking stations*. Office space for clinical pharmacists may be sought in the patient care areas, or (grouped) near the central pharmacy, weighing the advantages of access and availability of a *bedside* location against the advantages of face-to-face consultation with colleagues, and central pharmacy support and supervision. Personnel additions obviously must be accommodated in terms of additional work stations, chairs, air-conditioning capacity, etc. Increased emphasis on continuing education and on-the-job training may necessitate special teaching and training areas, which may be shared. A change in hospital policy to return to warehousing can drastically change the reserve storage needed. And, finally, new equipment such as required for gene therapy, will place new demands on utilities and air handling systems.

All of the above demonstrate the considerable interaction between what is happening in or to the hospital, and the physical facility in which it happens.

Hospital Facility Development Process

The cash flow difficulties experienced by many hospitals today have turned the master planning process around, such that financial concerns have become paramount. Master planning today is conducted with financial consultants, who review the fiscal viability of both present and proposed services, preparing pro formas for comparison. A high priority goes to those health care services likely to generate cash flow the quickest, in many cases.

Because most hospitals are reimbursed at a flat rate for any given disease state, there is great incentive to redesign inpatient areas for maximal efficiency and for hospitals to specialize in the areas in which they are most efficient (e.g., cardiac care) while dropping other inpatient services entirely. At the same time, the competition for patients has also placed heavy emphasis on making *profitable* patient facilities inviting and attractive to patients. Because of financial incentives for minimizing a patient's inpatient stay without losing them from the health care system, great economic pressure is exerted on hospitals to substitute outpatient care for inpatient care wherever possible. The result, at the departmental level, is that many department heads face instructions to cut back on plans (reduce space) related to some inpatient services while developing plans for the expansion of those which offer better reimbursement or for outpatient services (e.g., outpatient dispensing, home health care services).

A separate issue is the availability of capital. Many hospitals face the need to renovate or build anew for efficiency in a new strategic focus, but they have great difficulty in raising capital (e.g., for a pharmacy *clean room*). In summary, it is a difficult time to build or renovate a hospital, but the need for changes is compelling hospitals into such construction projects.

The hospital facility development process of today may be outlined as follows:

1. Marketing plan developed, beginning with a review of the entire array of services offered in the context of utilization, market share, staffing (physician and other), financial performance, technology, and *fit* within the strategy of a parent health care system. Physician availability must be assessed when considering present and pro-

posed services. Ambulatory care services may need to be unbundled for delivery in multiple locations to enhance patient convenience. Public input via patient satisfaction surveys may be sought. Joint ventures with local medical group practices may be considered.[8]

2. Competition examined, from both other hospitals and alternative modes of treatment, such as freestanding ambulatory care centers

3. Existing facility resources evaluated, a process that may heavily influence whether to renovate or build anew

4. Financial capability evaluated, focusing primarily on the question of raising capital, a problem made more complex by a history of the industry's difficulties in controlling operating costs

5. Environmental constraints evaluated, including growth zones limited by regulations, legal codes, and local politics

6. Impact of information technology developments that can effect design and include the hospital-wide computer system, medication dispensing, patient and product-tracking systems, medical records of all kinds, and security

7. *Framework for planning* statement developed, to include hospital mission statement, activity projections, priorities, organization plan, schedule, and monitoring and evaluation procedures

All of these concerns are considered as the hospital periodically reformulates its framework for planning statement, which is the cornerstone of any specific facility planning project.

The planning of the pharmacy must proceed as part of the process for designing the rest of the facility because of the relationships described above. It is essential for the director of pharmacy to understand the facility development process if he or she is to have any influence on it, and see that the needs of the pharmacy department are given their proper due, in the proper place, and at the proper time.

The steps or stages of the facility planning process, which typically consumes 2–3 years and sometimes longer, are shown below.

Steps in Facility Planning Process

1. Strategic master facilities plan developed, which sets forth the implications of the hospital strategic plan in terms of the facilities needed to

accommodate all planned activities, along with a timeline to show when facility needs will occur. The pharmacy department should have its own master facilities plan, keyed to its strategic plan, and congruent with that for the hospital.

2. Analysis of existing facility resources compiled, including *as-built* plans, space inventory room by room, equipment list showing age and replacement value, site surveys, assessment of structural, mechanical, and electrical systems, code conformity, and traffic patterns

3. Functional program compiled, including block diagrams that show department components, flow and traffic relationships, phases in development, new versus renovated space, gross cost estimate, and a statement of assumptions and priorities

4. Architectural schematic plans drawn, including alternatives, showing layout and design of departments and relationships plus workflow of staff, materials, and patients (includes a brief description of fixtures, mechanical and electrical systems, and a cost estimate)

5. Architectural design developed, adding all other architectural details, including the last review by the users

6. Construction contract documents drawn up, including final drawings for regulatory approval and bidding plus the final cost estimate

7. Construction begun, including demolition, construction, equipment ordering, and inspection

8. Occupancy implemented, including installation of equipment, orientation of staff, moving, post-occupancy evaluation, and follow-up

As the major processes described above move along, it is not difficult to see why a department traditionally thought of as *small* (8% of the typical hospital operating budget) may find that it exerts little control or influence over its own destiny. This need not happen if pharmacists understand the process and the opportunities it affords them for influence. For example, the pharmacist can begin by taking every opportunity to assert that, from the facilities planning standpoint, the *pharmacy function* includes control of all medications and related information in the hospital and extends far beyond the walls of the pharmacy to include nursing unit design, decisions about hospital communication, transportation, and security systems, etc.

Current Pharmacy Planning and Space Utilization

Facilities Surveys

The 1989 edition of the *Lilly Hospital Pharmacy Survey,* sent to directors of hospital pharmacies and yielding a response rate of about 37% (2,048 pharmacies), found that the average hospital had a slightly smaller central pharmacy area than in the previous year, down from 7.5 square feet per bed to 7.1 square feet.[9]

A national survey based on a stratified random sample of hospitals (response rate 45.6%) showed that the pharmacies in the most common types of hospitals (general medical surgical, nonprofit, short-term) occupied about 7 square feet per bed. Pharmacies in government hospitals of all kinds had the most space; whereas pharmacies in for-profit hospitals had only a little more than half the space of the not-for-profit hospitals. For every hospital type, little correlation between bed size and total pharmacy space was noted.[10] This finding was not as surprising as it may sound, because as hospitals grow in size, new functions are added, while the original functions may not require additional space as a result of economies of scale.

It is impossible to evaluate the adequacy of current space allocations in hospital pharmacies without knowing the services they are attempting to provide and the work systems and personnel to be accommodated.

The recommended approach to determining pharmacy space needs is the functional planning approach (see below), based on an in-house evaluation of individual hospital needs, rather than the method of relying on comparisons with other pharmacies and other hospitals.

Planning Process

Too often the pharmacist's input in the planning process is minimal. The administrator may inform the pharmacist at the last minute about the location and the space that have already been determined for the pharmacy. The pharmacist is then shown a proposed plan, which already has been drawn up by the architect. Another undesirable approach is to contact commercial vendors of pharmacy fixtures and ask them to submit the design for the pharmacy. Such firms can be very helpful after needs have been defined (i.e., *after* the functional program has been written). Otherwise, the designs proposed may feature unneeded quantities of the particular line of fixtures the vendor sells.

The planning approach recommended is called *functional planning*. This is an organized and systematic approach based on the architectural principle that states *form follows function*. The implication is that a hospital, along with each department, should be planning from the inside-out—with its functional requirements dictating the arrangement, the characteristics, and even the appearance of its final structure.

The planning team should include the hospital administrator, the architect, and consultants, plus the department heads. The administrator's role is to define the hospital's goals and to allocate resources. The pharmacist's role is to identify the functions the pharmacy must perform, the work systems to be used, the physical environment needed, and serve as the ultimate authority for overseeing compliance with professional and legal standards. The architect's role is to translate all of this into architectural plans.

The functional planning process typically involves the following three phases:

1. Strategic master facilities plan

2. Functional programming

3. Architectural design

The specific responsibilities of the pharmacist on the planning team are to (1) develop a strategic master facilities plan for the pharmacy, (2) prepare the functional program for the department, and (3) work with the pharmacy design specialist or architect as they design schematic plans to meet the functional program specifications.

The strategic master facilities plan (SMFP) reviews the long-range plans of the hospital to identify future demands upon the pharmacy department. The current and long-range goals of the pharmacy are reviewed for congruence. A statement of the functions the pharmacy must plan to perform, now or in the foreseeable future, is developed along with a timeline for anticipating the need.

The functional program (FP) is a volume of detailed performance specifications for the facility needed. These specifications provide the pharmacy design specialist or architect with details which include all major operations, work flows, and workloads. An exhaustive catalogue of general and specific work areas is created. Each work area is then analyzed with regard to such requirements as personnel to be accommodated, fixtures and equipment, storage needs, transportation and communications, services, utilities environmental controls, security considerations, etc. The arrangement of work areas is analyzed and a configuration and location are recommended. Finally, space needs are calculated by work area, and provision for flexibility and growth are considered, working with the designer or architect.

The schematic plans are drawn in response to the performance specifications set forth in the functional program. This design process involves the synthesis of physical environments which satisfy the FP requirements, which are then reconciled with the practical limitations of hospital-wide planning (e.g., location, financial). In addition to meeting functional requirements, the design process adds the expression of organizational values, comfort, way-finding and attractiveness (esthetics).

The planning process described above has been found to be an important key to achieving new levels of productivity and quality in pharmacy operations.

The specific steps in planning a pharmacy facility using the functional planning process are shown in Table 38-1. Functional programming encompasses steps A through H. Architectural design overlaps functional programming and includes steps G through J.

The purpose of the functional program is to describe individual pharmacy operations and the demands (i.e., performance requirements) of each on the facility, in the form of a written report. It may include diagrammatic plans (e.g., bubble diagrams) but does not get into the drawing of schematic plans, which comes after the functional program has been completed.

During the next phase—architectural design—the architect will translate these needs into physical space, equipment, and furnishings.

Functional Programming

The functional program usually begins with a formal statement of the purpose, goals, and specific objectives of the pharmacy service for the future and then lists the specific functions to be performed. Long-range goals, including those for future growth and expansion plus a timetable for their implementation over the next 5–10 years, should be included. (This information should be already available in the separate strategic master facilities plan document for the department, prepared during Phase I.)

Functions

A function is defined as "a system of one or more tasks to serve a stated purpose." Some typical pharmacy functions include reviewing and editing orders; dis-

Table 38-1
Functional Planning

Steps	Primary Responsibility
A. Identify hospital purpose and goals	Administrator
B. Derive pharmacy goals and objectives	Pharmacist
C. Identify functions	Pharmacist
D. Determine workflow	Pharmacist
E. Identify work areas	Pharmacist
F. Specify requirements for each work area re:	Pharmacist
1. Workload	
2. Equipment and fixtures	
3. Storage	
4. Personnel	
5. Materials handling	
6. Communications	
7. Services	
8. Security	
9. Utilities	
10. Environment	
G. Find optimal arrangement for work areas	Pharmacist and Architect
H. Find optimal location	Pharmacist and Architect
I. Develop trial schematics, calculate space	Pharmacist and Pharmacy Design Specialist/Architect
J. Develop architectural design	Architect

pensing unit doses to inpatients; compounding of IV admixtures; purchasing; storage; and administration (the terminology used may differ from one pharmacy to another).

The key point is that an effort should be made to identify every specific function to be performed in the new facility, along with the methods and the systems to be used. For example, the type of drug distribution system to be used and whether or not satellites will be built should be known. If such decisions have not been made, then little further progress is possible until they are. (A systems analysis may be advisable, to take advantage of the opportunity to design a new system and the new facilities together for optimum efficiency of performance. Designing a new facility for an inefficient system may have the undesirable long-term effect of *designed-in inefficiency*.) Facilities can and should

be designed to be flexible (and how to do this is addressed later), but good predictions about future work systems are essential to contain costs.

Workflow Analysis to Identify Work Area

Workflow analysis is performed to examine what the workflow will be in order to identify all of the tasks along the way. In the new plan, each and every task must have a place where it can be performed, and that place must be properly equipped and have the proper environment. Such places are designated work areas (general and specific). This is a systematic approach to ensure that the plans provide a work area for each and every task.

Workflow analysis for the purpose of facilities design is significantly different from that for systems analysis, for example, in that the focus is limited to only those items having implications for facilities.

The analysis is begun by examining each function to be performed and the workflow involved. Workflow is defined as "the sequence of activities in response to a work order," such as a physician's medication order. The way to begin is to identify each different work order (i.e., anything that causes work to begin), such as a requisition received for filing, or even a printout indicating that inventory is low and that a purchase order should be initiated.

The way this approach generates a basic list of work areas is illustrated below. In this example, the procedure for the filing of an IV admixture order is listed on the left-hand side. Then, proceeding down the right side, the idea is to stop at each step and try to picture mentally the physical activity that will take place in that step and then give each workplace in that mental picture a generic name, such as *computer station* or *hood*. In this way, a list of all of the work areas needed is generated as in Table 38-2.

A work area is defined as "a place where work of a similar nature is performed." A work area may be only a desk, a counter, or one section of a long counter, the corner of a room, or the whole room itself. Some work areas typically found in a hospital pharmacy are presented below, where they are organized into general and specific work areas:

Dispensing to Outpatients

1. Waiting
2. Receiving and dispensing
3. Order entry
4. Prescription filling counter
5. Communications and references
6. Inspection
7. Compounding, nonsterile
8. Compounding, sterile
9. Counseling
10. Management

Once all of the work areas needed is identified, it is possible to proceed. The next step calls for the examination of each of these work areas to identify and specify for each the workload, personnel, inventory, and equipment to be accommodated, services and utilities needed, etc.

It will be advantageous to group the work areas to the degree possible. For example, the functional programming specifications for the several specific work areas contained in one small office can usually be combined and considered together under the general work area title for the entire office. This would not be the case in an IV admixture center, for example, where the laminar flow hood would have special utility requirements.

Workload Analysis

The most important determinants of the space requirements of a hospital pharmacy performing a given set of functions are (1) workload, (2) equipment and fixtures, (3) storage needs, and (4) personnel to be accommodated.

It is useful to differentiate between the extrinsic workload, which is the demand on the pharmacy from outside the department, and the intrinsic workload, which is that generated from within, as when a drug is prepackaged, creating a need for a label to be generated.

Table 38-2
Creating the Work List

Task	Work Area
1. Work order received	Pass-through window
2. Label prepared	Computer station
3. Solution, additives, and supplies obtained	Active storage solutions Active storage additives Active storage supplies
4. Assembled/checked in hood	Hood
5. Put in pass-through refrigerator	Refrigerator
6. Waste items discarded	Waste receptacle

To estimate the workload (whether extrinsic or intrinsic) for any work area, the work units must first be identified. Some typical work units in a hospital pharmacy include the number of physicians' medication orders received for processing, the number of drug information requests, and the number of batches of drugs to be prepackaged. Such workloads may be analyzed and reported according to the volume per day; the distribution by hour of the day; or the distribution across a sufficient number of days to include the normal cycles and fluctuations that have implications for facility design.

A convenient way to collect workload data is to arrange to have every form time-date stamped as it is processed, for tabulation later. Often such data are already being collected for departmental reports. Otherwise, direct observation may be needed to count and record work units during typical time periods.

When a new facility is planned where none previously existed, the best approach is to begin by examining data from an institution of similar size and with similar programs and services.

Current workload data must be adjusted to reflect changes expected in the future. Formulas for forecasting the extrinsic workload of the pharmacy, based on the past and present number of patient days, for example, are available. Adjustments should be made for important trends, asking questions such as these: Does the hospital plan to increase or decrease bed capacity? Will patient mix change? (This can *greatly* affect the pharmacy workload). Is the hospital planning to discontinue certain programs, such as obstetrics, or to add others, such as home health care? Will recent medical staff decisions change the number or types of medications ordered in the future?

The study of expected workload will reveal, for example, whether the IV admixture center will require one hood or two and how many printers will be needed. Without such information, the final plans might not include a place for these extra items of equipment.

Equipment and Fixtures

The cost of equipment may be the single most important cost associated with a new facility. It not only may constitute the greatest portion of the total initial expenditure but also will be a determining factor in the day-to-day operating expenses of the facility for the long run.

The selection of the equipment for the pharmacy department should be based on an analysis of the work that the equipment is needed to do. Questions relating to how the work will be done (e.g., the degree of computerization and automation) must be addressed. If some equipment will be built into purchased fixtures, this also must be known.

The solution is to study the nature of the work at each work area, the volume involved, and the methods to be used. Based on this information, an initial equipment list can be generated. Then, published lists can be consulted for items overlooked. The purchasing agent will be a source of information about standard items such as office equipment.

A high initial cost should not be a deterrent to the consideration of equipment that has a favorable net effect on operating costs for the long run. A method for determining the most cost-effective alternative is *life cycle costing*. The use of consultants is helpful and justified in the selection of expensive equipment for more complex operations, such as computer applications and unit dose packaging.

In composing the equipment list, it is important to distinguish between fixed and movable equipment. Fixed equipment is that which requires installation and becomes attached to the building. For example, fume hoods, autoclaves and walk-in refrigerators are fixed equipment. Movable equipment includes furniture, carts, and printers. A separate list is important, because fixed equipment often is included in the hospital construction contract, whereas movable equipment may be bid separately.

The physical environment needed to accommodate each piece of equipment must be considered. For example, there may be a need for extra space around the sides to give access for repairs and maintenance. Some equipment manufacturers will even supply a template to show the access space requirements for each equipment item. Space must be provided for the operator to stand or sit and for the storage of supplies and accessories. Temporary storage space for incoming materials and outgoing products is needed. Trash cans and areas for waste materials are sometimes overlooked.

General characteristics to be sought in all equipment are standardization throughout the pharmacy (and hospital), compatibility with existing equipment, modularity, and flexibility. Each of these points will be addressed later.

Remember, every item of equipment ordered is going to have to be put somewhere, and the best time to provide a place for it is at the time the facility is being planned.

Storage

Storage fixtures may or may not appear on the final equipment list, as they may be treated as part of construction. However, they should be treated as equipment in the functional program to ensure that they receive proper consideration.

To estimate the type and amount of storage space needed, it is best to actually measure the amount of space currently occupied by all inventory, supplies, etc. The space now occupied by current stock should be measured with a tape measure, shelf by shelf and drawer by drawer, so that the planner can form an accurate mental picture of the block of space needed to accommodate the contents. Then the average height, width, and depth needed for all of the stock on one shelf, for example, should be estimated. These data then should be broken down by class and summarized in terms of linear front feet, square feet, and cubic feet. Although such measurements will be approximate, this approach has the important advantage of avoiding the distortion that comes from the common approach of measuring the outside dimensions of existing shelving units, which too often are no longer optimal for the items stored there. When such data are collected by operating personnel, these persons can be instructed to adjust their estimates to reflect the latest developments, including departmental objectives regarding inventory levels.

The results obtained should be presented in the functional program in the form shown in Table 38-3.

Storage requirements may be organized and reported according to the classes of storage as listed below:

A. Frequency of Use
   1. Most used
   2. Less used
   3. Deep reserve

B. Environmental Requirements
   1. Air-conditioning
   2. Refrigeration
   3. Freezing
   4. Protected from light

C. Security Requirements
   1. Controlled drugs (by schedule)
   2. Alcoholic beverage

D. Special
   1. Disinfectant-proof
   2. Autoclave-proof

The compilation of these data in this way makes it possible to enlist the skills of the architects, consult-ants, fixture vendors, and other outside experts to suggest solutions beyond the storage fixtures traditionally seen in pharmacies. There has been a great need for improvements, and the recent economic pressures to reduce space use everywhere has resulted in many new and innovative approaches, all requiring a three-dimensional analysis of space requirements.

The active storage areas of the pharmacy may include one or more cart-filling station, arranged in U-shaped alcoves. In some centralized operations, carts may also be filled on an assembly-line basis, cafeteria style. Unit dose dispensing systems generally require about 25% more storage space than other systems.

The arrangement of stock should give first priority to placing all of the fast-moving stock together near the front to minimize personnel travel time. Traditionally, most pharmacies have organized their stock by dosage form (i.e., all oral solids together, all oral liquids, injections, etc.). Though this allows for economy of shelf space, the value of pharmacy labor wasted is likely to be much greater.

Shelving that is open and adjustable is often quite adequate, versatile, and inexpensive. Cabinets and drawers cost considerably more and are generally less efficient to use. Angled adjustable shelving provides gravity feed. These can be designed to be replenished from the rear to minimize drug stock deterioration.

Rotary storage carousels, both horizontal and vertical, can offer fingertip retrieval of the most used drugs. Such carousel storage units may be viewed as expensive but the cost of their use should be weighed against the value of the labor saved, and they may reduce dispensing errors. Some are efficient only when no more than two persons are involved in filling orders from the same carousel. Beyond that point, the one-at-a-time access feature of the type of storage reduces its efficiency.

For bulk storage, rail-mounted shelving is recommended for its space-saving features, because fewer aisle spaces are needed.

Regarding refrigeration, unit dose dispensing systems require a greater amount of refrigerated storage for injectables and liquids. The commercial reach-in type, such as that used in food stores, eliminates the time involved in opening and closing doors.

For reserve and bulk refrigerated storage, prefabricated cold rooms are available and can be made secure for controlled drugs.

Deep reserve storage items, such as IV solutions in cartons, often are kept on pallets or on *fork-lift service-*

Table 38-3
IV Reserve Storage

Class and type	Linear ft.	Shelf Space Needed for Current Stock Levels	
		Square ft.	Cubic ft.
IVs and administration sets	198	444	1,274
Floor space—pallets	12	42	108
Total	210	486	1,382

able steel shelving in a locked room that may be remote from the pharmacy.

A trend towards *just-in-time* purchasing can have a profound effect on the need for reserve storage; however, some hospitals are returning to warehousing, so this must be checked.

With respect to the storage of controlled drugs, the current emphasis is upon sophisticated electronic alarm systems, rather than sturdier vaults and safes. The regional agent of the Drug Enforcement Administration (DEA) should be contacted for an interpretation of the current regulations and requirements.

The problem of storing flammables is familiar to the architect, and the architect should be the one responsible for complying with all applicable codes and regulations, which vary from state to state. Many hospital pharmacies no longer have their own flammables room. Sealed containers of alcohol eliminate the need in some cases and, in other cases, the hospital may provide a flammables room for use by all. In the case of shared storage facilities, the means for adequate security over pharmacy-controlled items may need to be provided.

Personnel

The number of personnel to be accommodated in the pharmacy is another factor of major importance in the design of a new pharmacy. The trend towards redeployment of the pharmacists for practice in the patient care areas has prompted considerable debate about the location of offices for such clinical practitioners. Some pharmacies will need such office located in the separate patient care areas, while others may want offices clustered centrally near the main pharmacy with only clinical substations (e.g., desk plus computer) for their use on each floor.

The architect will need to have documented the number of persons who will be in each area during normal work times as well as peak work periods, to be able to provide adequate working space, the proper number of chairs, the necessary air-conditioning capacity, etc. The architect should be supplied the expected staffing pattern, as well as the hours of operation. The expected presence of individuals being *trained* should not be overlooked.

Communications

Communication systems needed by the pharmacy should be analyzed, with thought given not only to telephone systems but also to telecommunication needs, facsimile reproduction, bulletin boards, and access to all hospital-wide systems.

The pharmacy telephone systems should provide separate telephone numbers for business and professional calls, with calls related to patient care answered by a pharmacist directly. Dispensing areas should be designed so that the pharmacist can talk privately on the phone without being overheard. Telecommunication, facsimile, and computer terminals will have special requirements regarding location, space, and utilities that must be checked with the manufacturer. The use of wireless alternatives to the standard telephone system is already widespread: technology choices must be coordinated at the hospital-wide level.

Materials Handling

The hospital will likely provide central materials-handling systems such as service elevators, dumbwaiters, pneumatic tubes, or messenger service for use throughout the hospital for all departments. When planning this system, the architect should be reminded that the pharmacy will be a major user, for both drug products and documents, sending and receiving more units (in unit dose systems) than any other department. The architect should also be advised that pharmacy has some unique, special requirements such as a rapid response for stat orders and security for controlled drugs during transit. Documented for the architect should be the volume of this workload, its distribution by time of day, and size and weight of the largest and smallest units to be transported.

Before a costly and complicated automated transportation system is recommended, the advantages of the "ancient" manual cart delivery and messenger services should not be overlooked. These offer a relatively maintenance-free system, featuring carriers with built-in, highly versatile "computers" (the human brain) for observation, control, recording inventory, feedback, and on-the-spot problem solving. Also, the cost of expanding such systems is minimal.

Care should be taken that all carts will pass through all doors, including elevator doors and passageways, and that they will roll satisfactorily on the type of flooring anticipated. If automated delivery carts are used, be sure the grades they must climb are not excessive, and that they are secured from the hijacking of the cart and components.

Services from Other Departments

Services from other departments on which the pharmacy may depend must be identified so that the architect can locate them as close to the pharmacy as possible. Such services include centralized purchasing, centralized receiving, library, cashier and waiting areas for outpatients, and access to autoclaves.

Security

The hospital pharmacist must deal with security problems at a variety of levels, including the detailed requirements for the various cases of controlled drugs; the regulations for alcohol and alcoholic beverages; the regulations regarding prescription and nonprescription drugs; and concern for the confidentiality of patient information—all in addition to the normal security for the protection of the employees and property.

Security considerations may include limiting the number of doors and others means of access to storage areas, the reinforcements of door and wall materials (e.g., requiring that walls be built to extend vertically from slab to slab), the quality and types of door locks, electronic controls, and the control of keys (e.g., no master keys).

Visual surveillance of all doors and high-security areas may be needed if the pharmacy is to be staffed by one person at night. Automatic door locks, bullet-proof glass, and special alarm systems are being installed in an increasing number of pharmacies.

However, there is concern that such devices too often interfere with the pharmacist-patient interaction, which is important in providing optimal pharmacy services.

Utility and Environmental Controls

The functional program prepared by the pharmacist should give particular attention to the requirements of the special work areas unique to pharmacy. The typical architect can anticipate the requirements of a normal office, for example, but not for an IV admixture center. The architect should also be alerted to the need for emergency power for the refrigerators, freezers, laminar air flow hoods, and the security alarm systems.

Arrangement of Work Areas

Once all work areas are known and the individual requirements have been identified, the next step is to analyze and recommend how they should be arranged in relation to each other. Factors to be considered include the flow of products and information, points of input and output, access to fixed or shared equipment (e.g., dumbwaiter), joint use of personnel and equipment, need for visual supervision, and the desire to minimize travel and delay time between work areas.

Those general work areas that probably should not be physically separated are order review, distribution, and extemporaneous compounding and packaging. General work areas that may be separated when adequate communications and transportation can be provided are administration, batch compounding and packaging, and deep reserve storage.

The desired location of the work areas with respect to corridors and elevators should be recorded. For large complex facilities, there are systematic, quantitative methods for calculating the best arrangements of work areas.[11] Such a quantitative analysis involves the determination of personnel and material flows between the work areas. A From-To Chart (see Figure 38-1) can be used in estimating the flow, or travel frequencies, of personnel and material between each pair of work areas. The evaluation of travel frequencies can be based on either workflow analyses or observation. The results of the travel frequency analyses can be ranked and classified into five closeness ratings (see Figure 38-2).

A second code system that describes the reasons for each relationship is also used in the chart.

The qualitative analysis is used to account for factors other than the relationships of workflow. Such factors include managerial decisions (e.g., decisions made for security reasons).

In addition to the previous five closeness ratings, undesirable (symbol: X) may be used to indicate occasions when two work areas should be segregated. For example, it is undesirable to locate the controlled drug distribution area adjacent to the main entrance.

A work area relationship diagram can be used in facilitating the layout design (see Figure 38-3). The squares (work areas) are shifted around until a "neat" layout (fewer lines crossing) is obtained. The next step is to adjust the design by considering the physical constraints (i.e., location of entrance, physical shape) of the pharmacy and size of each work area. The result of this process is traditionally called a *bubble diagram* (see Figure 38-4). Computer software programs are available for the preparation of such analyses.

Rendering the Functional Program

The functional program is a written report, composed mostly of lists, tables and diagrams, summarizing the data collected. The architect's task is to interpret this material and translate it into visual concepts and physical forms. Therefore, every effort to help the architect through a concise presentation that pinpoints and summarizes the key information will be greatly appreciated.

The table of contents for a typical functional program may include the following:

1. Introduction: departmental purpose, design issues (e.g., regulatory), assumptions
2. Functions (now and in the future)
3. Work flows (for operations with implications for facility design)
4. List of general and specific work areas
5. Workload analysis (for key work areas)
6. Equipment and fixture list (dimensions, space required)
7. Storage requirements (type, space required)
8. Other work area requirements special to pharmacies (environment, controls, utilities)
9. Arrangement of work areas
10. Ergonomics (human factors design requirements)

Space considerations should begin with the categorization of all pharmacy space into five major types: primary activity, support, administrative, educational, and research. (Note: Some planners include educational and research under administration.)

The recommended approach is first to locate the primary activity spaces (e.g., dispensing) and then locate the appropriate support and administrative spaces. Support space would include all reserve drug storage areas, for example.

The next step should be to draft the bubble diagram as shown in Figure 38-4.

Figure 38-1

From-To Chart Showing Number of Trips per Day between Each Work Area

TO \ FROM	A	B	C	D	E	F	G	H	I	J
A		42	4	36			12			16
B	35			8	8		6	13	92	12
C	6								3	3
D	24	13			16	4	4		256	16
E		12						10	4	14
F				7			6	6		10
G	12	6		4		8		16		
H		13		4	10	6	16		30	
I		124	3	212	4			30		
J	16	12	3	16	14	10				

Legend: A. Entrance, Main
B. Central Drug Distribution
C. Controlled Drug Distribution
D. Central IV Admixture Compounding and Distribution
E. Preparations, Nonsterile
F. Preparations, Sterile
G. Receiving (into pharmacy)
H. Storeroom
I. Dispatching Center
J. Lockers and Lounge

Figure 38-2
Work Area Relationship Chart

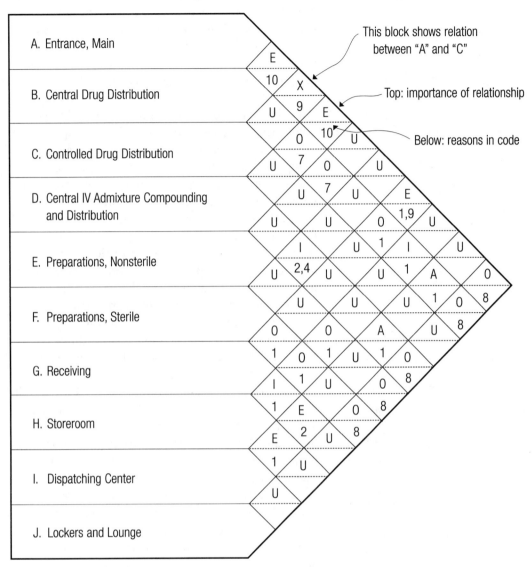

Code	Reason
1	Flow of materials
2	Common personnel
3	Common equipment
4	Supervision
5	Personal contact
6	Common records
7	Communication
8	Spec. management
9	Security
10	Interdept. trips

Rating	Definition
A	Absolutely necessary
E	Especially important
I	Important
O	Ordinary closeness OK
U	Unimportant
X	Undesirable

Figure 38-3
Work Area Relationship Diagram

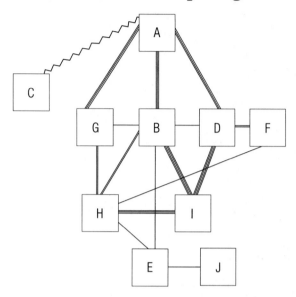

Legend:

A. Entrance, Main
B. Central Drug Distribution
C. Controlled Drug Distribution
D. Central IV Admixture
E. Preparations, Nonsterile
F. Preparations, Sterile
G. Receiving
H. Storeroom
I. Dispatching
J. Lockers and Lounge

Legend	
▬▬▬	A Rating
══	E Rating
──	I Rating
──	O Rating
	U Rating
∿∿	X Rating

Architectural Design Process

Role of the Architect

From the architect's viewpoint, the creative part of a facilities design project represents only about 20% of total effort, but it is "the fun part." This is important to know, because it suggests that the best time to capture the architect's personal (and creative) interest in a project is at the very beginning of the design process. If given the opportunity to truly understand the department, the architect can significantly improve the effectiveness of that department through designs unfamiliar to pharmacists.

The design of any facility, from the viewpoint of the architect, involves three major factors: utility, amenity, and expression. *Utility* simply means it is functional and efficient. A good functional program is the key to helping the architect address this factor. The term *amenity* refers to satisfying the human requirements for the people who will work there. Chief concerns are ease of access and movement, personal comfort, and safety and health protection. The term *expression* means the symbolic aspects or image the facility should project to others when they see it. For example, if the appearance of a dispensing window is to encourage patient counseling, its design should convey the message that an important pharmacist-patient communication occurs here, the privacy of which must be protected.

A collaborative approach between the architect and the pharmacist can produce designs that encourage the pharmacist to use the best professional practices and that discourage poor practice. For example, to promote personal contact between the pharmacist and patient, the normal positions of the pharmacist and of the ambulatory patient can be designed for their encounter to place them face-to-face in proximity (without a clerk between them, and without a place for a reluctant pharmacist to "hide").

The role of the pharmacy design specialist (consultant) has achieved special importance in recent years, as the role of the pharmacist has undergone many important changes with major implications for changes in the design of pharmacy facilities. Once essentially salespersons for a particular line of fixtures, today some architectural firms employ (or engage) such specialists for their recognized expertise in planning complex pharmacy facilities. It is recommended that a pharmacy design specialist be employed as an (independent) consultant to the design process.

Space

How much total space will the pharmacy need, and where should it be located? These will be among the first questions to which answers will be sought by the planning team. However, a good answer requires the comprehensive analysis of pharmacy needs described here, which are then modified and integrated with the needs of the other departments by the hospital architect.

To estimate the pharmacy space required, the architect studies the functional program and adds space for halls and internal passageways. Next, the architect proceeds to develop one or more alternative proposed schematic drawings for the pharmacy, seeking the

HANDBOOK OF INSTITUTIONAL PHARMACY PRACTICE

Figure 38-4
Bubble Diagram

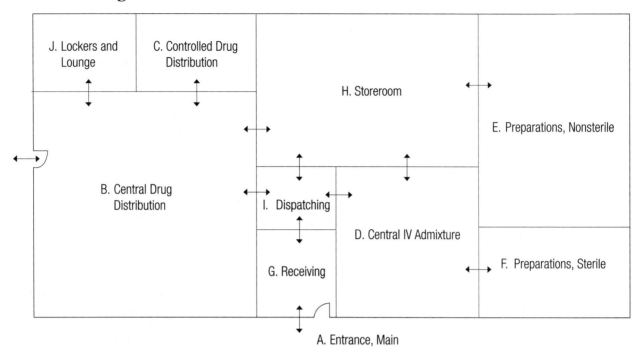

shape and location called for within the hospital plan. Architects can usually provide a computerized version of the schematic plan in a computer-aided design (CAD) format, which can be viewed in color by pharmacy staff using a viewer (e.g., Volo View by Autodesk) and marked with comments. Once the planning team agrees on one, then pharmacy space needs can be finally determined by measuring the space that plan occupies.

The above description of the process for determining space is the best approach and defies the use "standard" space allocation formulas without proper attention to the needs of a particular pharmacy function in a particular setting. Hospital pharmacy functions and services are changing dramatically as new roles emerge for the pharmacist; and these changes cannot be ignored. Some hospital systems have tried to standardize departmental space needs, unsuccessfully.

Location

The question of the location of the pharmacy should be brought to the attention of the architect and the planning team at the earliest time. This is because it is too common for the pharmacy to be thought of as a department that can be located almost anywhere, and

it is, therefore, given a low priority in the competition for prime locations.

The location of the inpatient pharmacy distribution areas must provide ready and full access to the hospital's materials-handling systems. When pharmacy satellites are involved, service to those satellites must be adequate and fast. Therefore, it is common to locate the inpatient pharmacy close to the central core of elevators and dumbwaiters, but access to a modern adequate pneumatic tube system, conveyors or automated carts may also meet the need.

If the inpatient pharmacy is to serve off-site locations such as home therapy centers, then access to a loading dock for speedy transfer of drug preparations (e.g., IV admixtures) is important.

If outpatients are to be served, the outpatient pharmacy dispensing area should be located somewhere along the normal patient traffic flow, perhaps sharing the same waiting room and cashier with the rest of the outpatient clinics. This consideration often necessitates separating the outpatient pharmacy from the inpatient pharmacy, which occurs more frequently as the number of hospital beds increases.

The location of a drug information center (or any area designed to encourage physician "drop-ins") will need to be located on a route heavily traveled by physicians, such as near the hospital library or a medical staff lounge.

The location of pharmacy satellites varies widely, depending on the specific functions they serve. The ideal location for a general satellite providing both distributive and clinical pharmacy services to a general medical or surgical service is adjacent to or directly opposite the nurses' station (most current satellites are located some distance away only because they were not part of the original plan). All satellites should be located to allow face-to-face communications with the users (nurses and physicians) and to ensure that this primary projected benefit of the use of satellites is obtained.

Satellites designed exclusively for clinical pharmacy services should be accessible from both the nurses' station and the physicians' work areas. Satellites designed to serve other pharmacy satellites, such as IV admixture preparation units located in two or three sites throughout a multilevel hospital, should be located to maximize access to the hospital materials-handling systems.

Offices for clinical pharmacy specialists may be required to be located in particular patient care areas to maximize the expertise that comes from specialization and total immersion in only one area. However, some pharmacy directors differ and wish all such offices to be adjacent or near the central pharmacy for better coordination, the sharing of expertise, and management.

Administrative offices may be separate from the inpatient and outpatient pharmacies. Bulk and reserve inventory can be maintained in remote locations provided the pharmacy controls all access to drug storage areas.

Designing for Efficiency

Work Systems

Designing a pharmacy for efficiency includes beginning with an efficient work system, which may require a systems analysis *before* trying to design a facility to accommodate the system. This is especially important if extensive automation has been implemented since the system in place was created, since automation can change efficiency in unexpected ways.

Efficiency is simply the ratio of output (e.g., unit doses dispensed) per resources input (e.g., labor, space). One of the most effective ways to achieve efficiency is to reexamine the work systems at the beginning of the

planning process and then design the facility for optimal performance of the new improved systems. Systems analyses typically begin with flow-charting to look for tasks that can be combined, eliminated, or automated.[12] Queuing theory and computer-simulation models of pharmacy operations can be used to identify mathematically the (theoretically) most efficient operation, although this can become quite complex.[13–15]

To illustrate the application of queuing theory, its use has shown that the assembly-line method of dispensing, used mostly by military pharmacies, where the task of dispensing is broken down in various elements performed by various personnel in different locations, is efficient only where strict scheduling is possible. The most efficient way to provide service for orders that arrive at random and that require varying periods of time to dispense is to have this done in one place by one person (like McDonald's).

A systems change that can have a great impact on efficiency and on facilities needs is the alteration of the use of personnel (e.g., as when the work of a professional is redesigned and part of it delegated to an auxiliary worker).[16,17] For this reason staffing studies, if planned, should always precede facilities design.

Systems changes that have been shown to improve the efficiency of the pharmacy given the proper facility for their performance include prepackaging, standardization of quantities issued, minimization of the variety of inventory items (as possible via a formulary system), mechanization, automation, and improved use of personnel.[18–20]

Task-Oriented Design

In the task-oriented design approach, a facility is viewed as a series of interrelated task centers, and the design of each general work area is based on the specific task to be performed there.

This approach contributes to efficiency through the reduction of the number of steps it takes to complete a task. Obviously, if the time consumed by such travel can be minimized, the work will be more efficient. Consider the distance traveled in an outpatient pharmacy in which the pharmacist must go to the door to receive the prescription, return to get a label typed, put the label on, travel to obtain an empty container, travel to obtain the drug, return the stock bottle, and then deliver the prescription to the door. The travel time involved can be evaluated mathematically by multiplying the number of trips times the distance per trip.

Perhaps the most obvious application of this approach is the separating of the most-used stock from the lesser used stock and the grouping of the former close at hand. The dispensing workplace should be designed to facilitate such a stock arrangement, instead of grouping drug stock by dosage forms. Modular boxes can be used for ampules and other small items.

Minimizing motion is another way to improve efficiency through the use of a task-oriented approach. This begins with the recognition of the geometry and mechanics of human movement and proceeds to design the workplace to "fit" the human.[21] The natural boundaries for human movement are circular (e.g., the hand rotating around a stationary wrist, the forearm rotating around a stationary elbow, and the extended arm and trunk rotating around the waist). Most equipment and building materials are rectangular, but rectangles do not fit the human body very efficiently, since some areas are harder to reach than other areas. The consequences are increased fatigue, lower productivity, and more mistakes. Task-oriented pharmacy fixtures are commercially available.[22]

Human Factors in Pharmacy

Human factors engineering (ergonomics) is a specialty within industrial engineering that focuses on the design of facilities, tasks, and work environments so that they match human capacities and limitations.[23] Recognizing that humans have limited reach distances and that the environment affects performance can lead to improvements in worker efficiency, accuracy, and job satisfaction.

Appropriate lighting levels for pharmacy work areas range from 50 to 150 foot-candles. Such levels are necessary for accurate and efficient visualization of written documents and working on video display terminals (VDTs).[24] Increasing the lighting level from 100 to 146 foot-candles was associated with a significantly lower dispensing error rate in a high-volume outpatient pharmacy.[25]

When sound levels rise above 70 decibels, which is the same level as a typical conversation, it becomes difficult to carry on a comprehensible conversation. Label printers, telephones, loudspeakers, and other sources of sound may exceed the 70-decibel level. Unpredictable, uncontrollable, or irregular noises can have an adverse impact on worker performance.[26,27] Therefore, the design of the facility should protect against excessive noise levels as well as annoying sounds.

Counters that are too low require workers to lean over, which may lead to back problems; counters that are too high require workers to hold their arms higher than their normal relaxed position, leading to muscle fatigue. Chair heights that are not adjustable can impair blood circulation to the lower leg, which results in discomfort. Inadequate leg room has resulted in significantly more complaints of sore shoulders, neck, and back pain.[28]

Research-based recommendations regarding the design of a computer terminal work station are available.[29] The following guidelines are offered:

- *Adjustability*—The heights of the keyboard (24–34 inches above floor), screen (35–50 inches from floor to top of screen), and chair (15–21 inches above floor) should all be adjustable within the ranges noted in order to accommodate the majority of workers.[28] A chair developed for VDT work stations has been described.[29] The screen should be placed so that it is 10–25 degrees below the horizontal plane (line drawn from eyes parallel to ground). This is considered the normal line of sight and will prevent neck strain. The angles of the chair's backrest and VDT should both be adjustable.[28,29]

- *Minimum Glare*—Place the VDT so that sunlight and light from other sources cannot be seen on the screen. Glare can be severe enough to prevent reading text accurately—and can also lead to worker discomfort. The surrounding walls and furniture should be a dark color.[29]

- *Lighting Levels*—For the work area surrounding the VDT, the lighting level should be at least 50 foot-candles.[29]

Three-Dimensional Space Planning

The 3-D approach to space planning is important for efficiency and use of space. Every wasted square foot of floor space is expensive to build and will cost many dollars per year to maintain.

Storage needs should be calculated and supplied to the architect and consultants in terms of three dimensions—linear front feet, square feet, and cubic feet—to provide the maximal flexibility to explore space-saving solutions.

An alternative to the use of additional floor space for storage is, for example, vertical space, such as storage on suspended balconies to use the otherwise unusable space near the ceilings in storage rooms. Rail-mounted shelving is efficient and easy to use. The efficiency comes from the elimination of aisles between the shelves. Aisles can then be "moved" wherever needed by simply pushing apart particular shelves, offering access to the item needed.

A third approach, particularly important in the pharmacy where many small items are stocked, is to make maximal use of the space at the back of each shelf and between the shelves. The area for picking of unit doses should be compressed, to minimize travel and motion. To accomplish this, the storage containers for unit dose packages should be designed take up a minimum of the front-of-the-shelf space; long, thin, modular boxes are ideal for this. The use of relatively shallow shelves that are easily adjustable is recommended so that shelves can be placed as close together as possible to conserve space.

Designing for Flexibility

The practice of hospital pharmacy is in a period of great change, with considerable uncertainty about the future. This places a high priority on designing to "build in" flexibility throughout. A recommended approach involves a growth plan, the core concept, and the use of flexible fixtures. Flexible fixtures are those that are modular, interchangeable, movable, and self-contained.

Growth Plan

There should be a growth plan for the pharmacy that provides zones of transition, or space buffers, between the pharmacy and the space external to it. For horizontal expansion, the zone of transition may be an easily movable storage room located in the expansion path. Vertical expansion to another floor is also possible via stairway and elevator, but that is usually more disruptive of workflow and internal control.

Such transition zones should be outlined in the comprehensive master facility plan for the hospital, and it behooves the pharmacist to achieve recognition of his or her needs in this regard.

The development of the pharmacy growth plan should begin by analyzing future needs at the individual work area level. This is because an increased workload does not affect work areas uniformly. For example, a second computer terminal may be needed before a second laminar floor hood, and both may be needed before a second refrigerator. The goal is a growth plan that is essentially unidirectional.

Core Concept

The core concept facilitates unidirectional growth by calling for all fixed items to be placed where they will not have to be moved. Examples of such items include plumbing, dumbwaiter, and pneumatic tube stations.

Flexible Fixtures

Truly flexible fixtures should be expandable as the workload increases and should be adaptable to changes in work methods. To achieve these goals, fixtures should be modular, to allow additional units to be ordered and inserted as the workload increases. Such units may be rearranged as work methods change and to allow the substation of new upgraded component sections to replace those that have become outmoded or obsolete.

Fixtures should not be difficult to finish and repair, and should be easily adjustable. For example, the storage of drugs in modular boxes on adjustable shelves is preferable to casework, cabinets, and drawers. Likewise, prefabricated expandable cool rooms give greater flexibility than large refrigerators.

Fixtures, including storage shelving, should be movable, although expensive castor and lift systems are not justified for one or two moves per year. Built-in fixtures and custom-built casework should be avoided.

Fixtures should be designed for grouping in self-contained task centers for the performance of a particular task in any location to which it may be moved. For example, an ambulatory care pharmacy with two outpatient dispensing task centers can be designed to be capable of being separated and each moved to a different outpatient clinic if needed as workload expands.

Pharmacy Satellites

Satellite pharmacy facilities have undergone pronounced changes in recent years, with a clear trend away from those designed to primarily accommodate distributive functions. It has been recommended that a satellite should serve no fewer than 85 beds of the same "medical type."[30,31] Fricker and Davis published information on satellite sizes with additional information about functions performed.[32]

The satellites needed today are usually for special purposes as follows:

1. Operating rooms

2. Oncology, for chemotherapy

3. Pediatrics

4. The emergency room

Replacing the distribution-oriented and staffed satellite of yesterday may be no more than a pharmacy substation (e.g., desk area) on the nursing unit, used for order entry by pharmacy personnel, and in clinical practice.

Cabinet-based drug vending machines may be located in the medication room of the nurses' station, which is a location superior to the open hallway from the viewpoint of safety and control. Such *pharmacy satellite* areas must be provided with adequate lighting and control of access. The design specifications for accommodating particular automated systems should be obtained from the manufacturer.

Functions

Functions typically found in satellite pharmacies include the following:

- First-dose distribution, orals, IVs
- Routine drug distribution (cart-filling)
- Compounding parenteral agents
- Drug therapy monitoring
- Order review, editing, and computer entry
- Provision of drug information to professionals
- Cardiopulmonary resuscitation (CPR) team participation
- Distribution, controlled substances
- Consultation with physicians, nurses (remote or in satellite)

After the workflow for each function is determined, a list of work areas can be generated. The major work areas required may include the following:

- Order receipt
- Order processing and preparation
- Compounding, parenteral agents
- Storage, active
- Storage, reserve
- Dispatching
- Clinical services area

Special design needs and problems for satellite facilities include the following:

- If a drug distribution is a function, fast and reliable transportation from the central pharmacy for drugs and supplies is essential, especially in smaller satellites with limited storage space. This is particularly true where slow response times led to the implementation of some satellites in the first place.[31]
- Space should be provided for visiting professionals, if increased interaction is desired. A conven-

ient, but quiet, area will promote this type of interaction.

- For a delivery mechanism between satellite and nursing unit, the advantages and disadvantages of pneumatic tube systems or some other method of transportation should be considered.

A unique, interprofessional image opportunity is created by the satellite pharmacy's design, since it is a highly visible pharmacy area. The image of the department should be reflected in every aspect of the design, from "looking efficient" to providing adequate storage (preventing clutter and disorganization), to selecting an interior design that emphasizes professionalism and welcomes interaction with other professionals

Compounding of Sterile Preparations

The sterile preparation work area in hospital pharmacy has likely been affected by professional, regulatory and accreditation organizations more than any other part of the pharmacy facility. Publication of USP Chapter 797, *Pharmaceutical Compounding—Sterile Preparations,* in The United States Pharmacopeia and The National Formulary (USP) is the latest set of standards to attempt to improve the quality of sterile preparations in hospitals. Kastango and Bradshaw published a primer on USP Chapter 797 that details the history of efforts to improve sterile preparation quality as well as covering the key parts of the new USP chapter.[33] Hospital pharmacists have been motivated to follow the information in USP 797 by the Joint Commission on Accreditation of Healthcare Organizations (JCAHO), who will be evaluating compliance during accreditation surveys.[34] Chapter 28, Sterile Preparations and Admixture Programs, in this handbook contains details about the impact of USP 797 on pharmacy facilities. Compliance with previous ASHP technical assistance bulletins on the quality of sterile preparations was found to be only 9.3% for risk level 2 and 3 agents in a 2003 publication, illustrating that extensive changes will be needed by many pharmacies to comply with either the ASHP guidelines or the USP Chapter 797.[35,36] Relative costs and quality impact of complying with USP 797 are described for each aspect of USP 797 by Kastango and Bradshaw.[33]

Reports are available describing the process of designing and building cleanrooms and sterile preparation areas.[37,38] These reports are helpful in learning the scope of such an undertaking but need to be updated with the new information from USP 797.

Several unique characteristics of the sterile preparation area that should be brought to the attention of the architect include special equipment (e.g., barrier isolators, autoclaves), product mix (premixed from manufacturers, outsourced items, workload for compounding from nonsterile ingredients), interaction with other pharmacy work areas (such as the order entry area for original orders), and environmental demands (additional air conditioning capacity due to laminar airflow clean bench heat generation and air filtration needs). Incorporation of barrier isolators into sterile preparation areas is favored by some for preparation of high risk agents and other functions, based on costs.[30–42]

Implementation

Preparation

The implementation of the next facilities planning project should begin the day after a facility is occupied! This statement is to make the point that facilities planning should be a continuous process. The ideal plan for the facility should be a constantly evolving concept that is periodically fixed and translated into architectural plans and physical structures whenever the opportunity arises. This viewpoint is essential if the pharmacist is to cope effectively with the short deadlines so often encountered. For example, as noted previously, the first thing asked of the pharmacist will be to recommend the space and location of the new pharmacy, which is not known until close to the very end of the functional planning process.

Recommended references include the out-of-print Department of Health and Human Services publication, *Planning for Hospital Pharmacies*, still available in many pharmacy school libraries; the workbook and CD-based reference *SpaceMed2004—A Space Planning Guide for Healthcare Facilities*, (available at http://www.space-med.com/Details-Overview.htm); and a pharmacy design bibliography.[43–45] Auburn University Harrison School of Pharmacy has a research program involving the design of pharmacy facilities.

Pharmacists should visit other hospital pharmacy departments but be selective. They should pick those less than 10 years old or those that have been remodeled recently, and those providing the kinds of services (or performing the kinds of functions) that they expect their own facility to provide. In particular, they should look for those where substantial planning was involved and the plan was carried out. Some bad examples (which will not be difficult to find) should be included; researchers have found they often learn more from failures than from successes.

Pharmacy Director's Role in Promoting the Project

The design of a contemporary pharmacy facility needs to effectively support the mission and vision of the health care organization and the department of pharmacy and can have a significant impact on operational efficiency and effectiveness. It also can affect the recruitment and retention of professional and technical staff. As such, adequate workspace and efficient workflows need to be planned for all current department operational, educational and research activities. Further, significant consideration needs to be given to the long-term strategic plans of the organization and department as these may reduce or increase future space needs. Typically, a director of pharmacy will have very few opportunities to plan for a significant renovation or the construction of a new pharmacy facility. Therefore, facility design is a critical strategic planning activity in the leadership of a department.

Despite this, many directors of pharmacy delegate the details of analyzing, planning and designing a pharmacy facility to in-house or external architects. These individuals can bring a wealth of experience to the project, especially from an aesthetic design, building code, and construction perspective. However, they are often unfamiliar with general pharmacy practice activities, workflow patterns, workload volume variation impact, functional area relationships and specific legislative, regulatory and accreditation requirements. If such expertise is not present, the director should strongly consider the engagement of consultants with experience in specific areas (e.g., workflow analysis, standards and guidelines for sterile preparations, security systems, automation, receiving and storeroom management, ambulatory pharmacy design).

Given most health care organizations' limited capital budgets, a newly renovated or constructed pharmacy facility will likely be utilized with only minor modifications for many years to come. In the past, pharmacy facilities were not thought to require significant capital dollars for either design or construction plus operating equipment. However, with the advent of central pharmacy automation equipment for drug preparation, packaging, storage, and dispensing, along with specially-constructed sterile preparations areas, a significant increase in both physical space and capital funding to incorporate these technologies is now essential for this new era.

As a result, the director of pharmacy will likely need to spend significant time and effort, perhaps over a prolonged time period, educating health-system administrators about the need for adequate space and workflow design, in order to minimize the potential for process and system induced medication errors and maximize personnel productivity. The development of an objective facility design justification document is essential to gaining administrative support for adequate space and capital funding. In addition, consensus building among key stakeholders outside of the pharmacy department who are the recipients of pharmacy services (nursing, medical staff, etc.) is key to appropriate review and approval.

The design of a new or renovated space for operations and services can be a critical factor in the overall success of a contemporary department of pharmacy, and thus it is essential for the director to make the most of the opportunity. In addition to any architects or consultants, key pharmacy department members should be involved with the development of ideas and design drafts early on. All pharmacy staff members should be kept informed as to the project objectives, issues, etc., and actively solicited for their contributions and viewpoints as the project progress through the design process. By so doing, the completed design will likely address in the best possible manner the primary issues of patient safety, personnel productivity, morale and retention for many years to come.

Timetable

Some 2–3 years may elapse between the initial planning and occupancy of the pharmacy. The timing of most of the major deadlines, as the project moves from one stage to the next, will be established by the planning committee. It is essential to know these dates, and to be on the mailing list for updates and changes.

Personnel Involvement

Whenever a new work area is being designed, the people who will be working in the area should be asked for suggestions and should be allowed to review the final design. They will be able to offer many practical suggestions to help design a more efficient workplace. This also helps to promote a more positive attitude toward the new facility.

A program for orientation of employees to the new facility should be undertaken. When major projects are involved, this may include not only printed materials, lectures, and review of the plans but actual simulation by "walking through" the new work systems planned for the new facility.

It seems to be human nature for personnel to expect new facilities to work perfectly and to solve all previous problems. They never do, of course, and it is typical for a negative reaction to surface right after the first few days of occupancy. The solution is to warn employees of this phenomenon in advance, to promote more realistic expectations. Then, provide a mechanism to note and acknowledge problems as they occur and make employees feel confident that these problems are being addressed. A simple device is a log book in which problems can be noted by the employees as they occur each day. At the end of the day, the supervisor should read and initial each entry, to signal to the employee that the problem has been noted. Some problems can be resolved by bringing them back to the group and challenging its members to find a way to "make the facility work better under the unexpected circumstances." Given a supportive environment, novel solutions to seemingly insurmountable problems often emerge.

Suggested Readings

Huntzinger PE. Pharmacy renovation: one pharmacist's experience. *Hospital Pharmacy.* 2003;38(10):935–41, 946.

King C. Planning facility expansion for pharmacy (letter). *Am J Hosp Pharm.* 1982;39:36–7.

Newton DW, Trissel LA. A primer on USP chapter <797>. *Infusion.* 2004;10(4):38–41.

Summerfield MR, Gurwitch KD, Scholz RL, et al. Establishing a pharmacy department for a large pediatric hospital: managerial problems, opportunities, and lessons. *Am J Hosp Pharm.* 1991;48(Jul):1463–6.

References

1. Babwin D. Building Boom. *Hospitals & Health Networks.* 2002;76(3):48–54.

2. Ulrich R, Zimring C, Quan X, et al. *The Role of the Physical Environment in the Hospital of the 21st Century: A Once-In-a-Lifetime Opportunity.* The Center for Health Design, Robert Wood Johnson Foundation; September 2004.

3. Pepper GA. Nursing workforce issues and implications. *ASHP Midyear Clinical Meeting.* 2004;39(DEC):PI-6.

4. Rapp CD, Mullin FW, Galvan E. Design of a comprehensive pharmacy facility within a level I trauma center. *ASHP Midyear Clinical Meeting.* 1992;27(Dec):P-445D.

5. Pelham LD. Facility design, construction, and implementation of home infusion satellite services. *ASHP Midyear Clinical Meeting*. 1993;28(Dec):P-296(D).

6. Bonner JE. Assembly line cartfill: alternative for a more efficiently operated and cost effective cartfill area. *ASHP Annual Meeting*. 1993;50(Jun):MCS-31.

7. Hammond JM, Buth JA. Modular pharmacies: Air Force design concept. *Journal of Pharmacy Practice*. 1990; 3(Dec):361–4.

8. Jackson W. Master planning: old vs. new. *Healthcare Design*. 2004;11(4):51.

9. Flohrs W, ed. *Lilly Hospital Pharmacy Survey, 1989*. Indianapolis, IN: Eli Lilly and Company; 1989.

10. Alexander VB, Barker KN. National survey of hospital pharmacy facilities: space allocations and functions. *Am J Hosp Pharm*. 1986;43(Feb):324–30.

11. Francis RL. *Facility layout and location: an analytical approach*. 2nd ed. Englewood Cliffs, NJ: Prentice Hall; 1992.

12. Barker KN, Harris JA, Webster DB, et al. Consultant evaluation of a hospital medication system: synthesis of a new system. *Am J Hosp Pharm*. 1984;41(Oct): 2016–21.

13. Johnson RE, Myers JE, Egan DM. Resource planning model for outpatient pharmacy operations. *Am J Hosp Pharm*. 1972;29(May):411–8.

14. Myers JE, Johnson RE, Egan DM. Computer simulation of outpatient pharmacy operations. *Inquiry*. 1972;9(Mar): 40–7.

15. Lin AC, Jang R, Sedani D, et al. Re-engineering a pharmacy work system and layout to facilitate patient counseling. *Am J Hosp Pharm*. 1996;53(Jul 1):1558–64.

16. Barker KN, Smith MC, Winter ER. Work of the pharmacist and the potential use of auxiliaries. *Am J Hosp Pharm*. 1972;29(Jan):34–53.

17. Dostal MM, Daniels CE, Roberts MJ, et al. Pharmacist activities under alternative staffing arrangements. *Am J Hosp Pharm*. 1982;39(Dec):2098–101.

18. Guerrero RM, Nickman NA, Bair JN. Work activities of pharmacy teams with drug distribution and clinical responsibilities. *Am J Hosp Pharm*. 1995;52(Mar 15): 614–20.

19. Guerrero RM, Nickman NA, Jorgenson JA. Work activities before and after implementation of an automated dispensing system. *Am J Health-Syst Pharm*. 1996; 53(Mar 1):548–54.

20. Pierce RA, Rogers EM, Sharp MH, et al. Outpatient pharmacy redesign to improve work flow, waiting time, and patient satisfaction. *Am J Hosp Pharm*. 1990; 47(Feb):351–6.

21. Hepler C. Work analysis and time study. In: Brown TR SM, ed. *Handbook of Institutional Pharmacy Practice*. 2nd ed. Baltimore, MD: Williams & Wilkins; 1987:77.

22. Swensson ES. Innovative design in hospital pharmacy facilities. *Am J Hosp Pharm*. 1971;28(Jun):440–6.

23. Chapanis A. *Man-Machine Engineering*. Monterey, CA: Brooks/Cole Publishing; 1965.

24. Niebel B. *Motion and Time Study*. 7th ed. Homewood, IL: Richard D. Irwin; 1982.

25. Buchanan TL, Barker KN, Gibson JT, et al. Illumination and errors in dispensing. *Am J Hosp Pharm*. 1991; 48(Oct):2137–45.

26. Flynn EA, Barker KN, Gibson JT, et al. Relationships between ambient sounds and the accuracy of pharmacists' prescription-filling performance. *Human Factors*. Dec 1996;38(4):614–22.

27. Holahan C. *Environmental Psychology*. New York: Random House; 1982.

28. Grandjean E. The design of workstations. *Fitting the Task to the Man: A Textbook of Occupational Ergonomics*. 4th ed. New York: Taylor & Francis; 1988:36–81.

29. Sanders MS. *Human Factors in Engineering and Design*. New York: McGraw-Hill Book Company; 1987:354–8.

30. Barker KN. *Planning for Hospital Pharmacy Facilities*. HEW Publication NO. FRA 74-4003. Rockville, MD: U.S. Department of Health, Education, and Welfare, Health Resources Administration, Health Care Facilities Service; 1974.

31. Barker KN. Medication distribution systems. In: Brown TR, ed. *Handbook of Institutional Pharmacy Practice*. 2nd ed. Baltimore, MD: Williams & Wilkins; 1987.

32. Fricker MP, Davis NM. Space requirements for pharmaceutical functions in selected nonuniversity hospitals. *Hospital Pharmacy*. 1983;18(Dec):645–7, 650–2, 655–9, 662–4.

33. Kastango ES, Bradshaw BD. USP chapter 797: establishing a practice standard for compounding sterile preparations in pharmacy. *Am J Health-Syst Pharm*. 2004 Sep 15;61(18):1928–38

34. Thompson CA. JCAHO gears up to survey sterile compounding practices. *Am J Health-Syst Pharm*. 2004; 61(10):980, 984, 986.

35. American Society of Health System Pharmacists (ASHP). ASHP guidelines on quality assurance for pharmacy-prepared sterile products. *Am J Health-Syst Pharm*. 2000;57(12):1150–69.

36. Morris AM, Schneider PJ, Pedersen CA, et al. National survey of quality assurance activities for pharmacy-compounded sterile preparations. *Am J Health-Syst Pharm*. 2003;60(24):2567–76.

37. Schumock GT, Kafka PS, Tormo VJ. Design, construction, implementation, and cost of a hospital pharmacy cleanroom. *Am J Health-Syst Pharm*. 1998;55(5):458–63.

38. Allan EL, Barker KN, Severson RW, et al. Design and evaluation of a sterile compounding facility. *Am J Health-Syst Pharm*. 1995;52(Jul 1):1421–7.

39. Karolchyk S. Barrier isolators: new, high tech option for the preparation of sterile admixtures. *Indian Journal of Natural Products*. 2001;5(6):422–3.

40. Pilong A, Moore M. Conversion to isolators in a sterile preparation area. *Am J Health-Syst Pharm*. 1999; 56(Oct 1):1978–80.

41. Sabra K, Wilson H, Gallelli JF. Use of isolators in centralized IV additive services in hospital pharmacies. *Hospital Pharmacy.* 1996;31(Oct):1257–63.

42. Rahe H. Sterile compounding with barrier isolation technology. *Int J Pharm Compound.* 2001;5(4):254–8.

43. Barker KN. Planning a hospital pharmacy facility. *Am J Hosp Pharm.* 1971;28(Jun):423–31.

44. Hayward C. *SpaceMed200—A Space Planning Guide for Healthcare Facilities.* Ann Arbor, MI: SpaceMed2004; 2004.

45. Barker K, Flynn E. Basic bibliography: facility design. *Hospital Pharmacy.* 1999;34(Feb):250.

46. King C. Planning facility expansion for pharmacy (letter). *Am J Hosp Pharm.* 1982;39:36–7.

Chapter 39

Marketing Pharmaceutical Services

Mickey C. Smith

Introduction

Every practicing pharmacist is involved in marketing. Just as one can't *not* communicate, anyone providing a service or product to others can't *not* market. Pharmacists who are unaware of the marketing function that they perform risk doing it poorly. Acknowledgement of the importance of marketing to the practice of pharmacy will not guarantee that one will do it well, but it is certainly an important step in the proper direction.

This chapter will concentrate more on the philosophy of marketing pharmaceutical services in institutions than on techniques. This choice is based on the judgment that marketing must be sold to pharmacists before it can be taught to them. We are way behind in this, because educators have eschewed instruction in marketing, favoring instruction in the clinical area. If we achieve nothing else here, we hope to show that, over the long-term, good pharmacy *practice* (our products and services) can be more effective through good pharmacy *marketing*.

Definitions

The definition of *marketing* from the American Marketing Association is as follows:

> Marketing is the process of planning and executing the conception, pricing, promotion, and distribution of ideas, goods, and services to create exchanges that satisfy individual and organizational objectives.[1]

A somewhat more practical definition is that of Hillestad and Berkowitz[2]:

> Marketing is the process of *understanding* customer wants and needs, *listening* to those wants and needs, and then, to whatever extent possible, *designing* appropriate programs and services to meet those wants and needs in a timely, cost-effective, competitive fashion. It is the process of molding the organization to the market, rather than convincing the market that the organization provides what they need.

Both of these definitions make it clear that in a successful marketing program, everyone benefits. Whether or not the pharmacy administrator recognizes it, he or she regularly engages in what may be called marketing activities. Marketing is a discipline that can be used not only to *attain* management objectives, but also to *identify* them. The central concepts underlying marketing are communication and the exchange of value for effort to increase and satisfy demand for existing products and services; rather, it seeks to identify and respond to the needs, differences, and perceptions of its clients and consumers.

Pathak has described the exchange process in marketing[3]:

> Although most definitions of exchange and marketing revolve around dyadic or restricted exchanges (two-party reciprocal relationships), exchange relationships in modern society are becoming more complicated because of specialization due to division of labor, the use of money as a medium of exchange, and the increasing number of participants. Complex exchanges (a system of mutual relationships between at least three parties) and interactive changes are more commonplace in today's society, especially in the pharmaceutical marketplace.
>
> Pharmaceutical marketing, as a subspecialty of marketing, can be defined as a process by which a market for pharmaceutical care is actualized. It encompasses all the activities carried out by various individual or organizations to actualize markets for pharmaceutical care.
>
> The emphasis in pharmaceutical marketing is on pharmaceutical care, and not just on drugs. Any article, service (see Table 39-1), or idea needed to anticipate and to remove gaps in pharmaceutical care should be included in the discussion of pharmaceutical marketing. The marketing of many clinical pharmaceutical services and programs is as much a part of pharmaceuti-

cal marketing as is the marketing of drug products. In other words, pharmaceutical marketing is not synonymous with, but is significantly broader than, the marketing of pharmaceuticals.

The emphasis in this definition is on pharmaceutical care, indicating that the justification for the existence of pharmaceutical marketing is the patient, and not the manufacturer or the pharmacist.

Any party interested in the exchange for pharmaceutical care may undertake pharmaceutical marketing activities. Hospital pharmacies, community pharmacies, third-party insurance companies, consulting pharmacies, and many other organizations and individuals, in addition to pharmaceutical manufacturers and drug wholesalers, are involved in pharmaceutical marketing.

Marketing Planning

Successful marketing requires careful planning. Many pharmacy directors have a reasonably good system for determining and controlling expenses and mistakenly believe that this is an annual planning or market planning process. Others confuse budgeting with planning. Although budgeting and forecasting are important in the development of market plans, they are not the sole ingredients for a market plan, which when completed will contain answers to such questions as those shown in Table 39-2.

A typical marketing planning sequence should include the following six steps:

1. Setting the mission

2. Conducting an internal and external analysis

3. Determining the strategy action match and marketing objectives

4. Developing action strategies and marketing mix

5. Integrating the plan and making revisions

Providing appropriate control procedures, feedback, and integration of all plans into a unified effort.

The Mission

Definition of pharmacy mission has an intimate, chicken-and-egg relationship to market boundary definition. On the one hand, mission must be defined, at least in part, in terms of market scope. On the other hand, the market cope should emerge from the mission. *Mission*

is a broad term that refers to the total perspectives or purpose of a pharmacy. Traditionally, the mission of a *business* corporation was framed around its product(s), and mottoes such as "Our business is textiles," "We manufacture cameras," and so on were the norm. In contrast, consider the mission statement in a Glaxo Laboratories annual report:

We are in the business of providing pharmaceutical products of the highest quality that alleviate pain and suffering and enhance human health and longevity.

To this end we commit all of our efforts to the discovery, development, production and marketing of medicines of the highest quality and efficacy.

The mission is neither a statement of current activities nor a random extension of current involvements. It signifies the scope and nature of the pharmacy service, not just as it is today, but as it could be in the future. The mission plays an important role in evaluating opportunities for diversification.

The mission deals with the questions: "What type of services do we want to offer at some future time? What do we want to become? At any given point in time, most of the resources are frozen or locked into their current uses, and the outputs in services and/or products are, for the most part, defined by current operations. Over an interval of a few years, however, environmental changes place demands on the business for new types of resources; pharmacy management has the option of choosing the environment in which the pharmacy department will operate and acquiring commensurate new resources rather than replacing the old ones in kind. This explains the importance of defining the mission. The mission should be so defined that it has a bearing on both strengths and weaknesses.

In order to arrive at a mission statement for a pharmacy department, it is valuable to have input from the various constituencies of hospital or clinic. A difficulty in developing market-based plans in health care is the *number of constituencies* whose opinions must be assessed.

Internal and External Analysis

The first consideration in the strategic process is to recognize the individuals and groups that have an interest in the fate and nature of the pharmacy department and the extent and nature of their expectations.

In order to apply the marketing approach to its

Table 39-1
Service Marketing

Special Considerations of Marketers of Service

1. Services cannot be stockpiled.
2. The entire service mix is usually not visible to the consumer.
3. The intangibility of services makes pricing difficult.
4. The intangibility of services makes promotion difficult.
5. The existence of a direct service organization-consumer relationship makes employee public relations skills important.
6. Services often have high costs and low reliability.
7. Peripheral services are frequently needed to supplement the basic service offering.

Basic Differences between Services and Products

Services	Products
1. Services are often intangible. Services are acts, deeds, performances, efforts. Most services cannot be physically possessed. The value of a service is based on an experience; there is no transfer of title.	1. Products are tangible. Products are objects, things, materials. The value of a product is based on ownership; transfer of title takes place.
2. Services are usually perishable. Unused capacity cannot be stored or shifted from one time to another.	2. Products can be stored; product surpluses in one period can be applied against product shortages in another period.
3. Services are frequently inseparable. One cannot separate the quality of many services from the service provider.	3. Products can be graded or built to specifications. The quality of a product can be differentiated from a distribution channel member's quality.
4. Services may vary in quality over time. It is difficult to standardize some services because of their labor intensiveness and the involvement of the service user in diagnosing his or her service needs.	4. Products can be standardized through mass production and quality control.

activities, the pharmacy must develop a marketing perspective: an awareness of and sensitivity to the exchange relationships it depends on for its very existence. This calls for first identifying the groups or markets with which the pharmacy director and pharmacy staff exchange values. Primary internal markets for pharmacy are the organization itself and the patient population. In a hospital, other internal markets are the medical staff, other departments' employees, volunteers, and trustees. External pharmacy markets include the community, families, visitors, suppliers, regulators, donors and supporters, professional associations, and colleagues employed elsewhere.

The exchanges between a pharmacy and its markets can be very complex and vary with each individual encounter. The values exchanged between a pharmacy staff member and the organization involve wages or salary, fringe benefits, security, social rewards, and

Table 39-2
Some Marketing Planning Questions

Where is the market?
  1. Needs and demands

Where are you now?
  2. As an institution
  3. As a department
  4. As an individual
  5. With respect to the environment and competition
  6. With respect to capabilities and opportunities

Where do you want to go?
  7. Assumptions and potentials
  8. Objectives and goals

How do you want to get there?
  9. Policies and procedures and levels of initiative
  10. Strategies and programs

When do you want to arrive?
  11. Priorities and schedules

Who is responsible?
  12. Organization and delegation

How much will it cost?
  13. Budgets and resource allocations

How will you know if you did it?
  14. Feedback and review sessions
  15. Continuous monitoring

feelings of accomplishment and responsibility in exchange for the pharmacist's time, effort, loyalty, and support of organizational objectives. Patients exchange money, approval, and gratitude for pharmacy care, relief of symptoms, pain, and anxiety, health teaching, primary preventive measures, and attentiveness.

Examination of the pharmacist-physician relationship from an exchange of values perspective is a complex exercise. Within the entire hospital organization, the physician exchanges patient referrals in return for a fully equipped workplace, service, prestige, and a number of conveniences. Pharmacy service is part of this exchange, but what the pharmacist receives of value is not as easy to define. In addition to being consumers of services, physicians have been called marketing intermediaries, the sales force of the hospital, and competitors. The attending physician is responsible for admitting the patient, providing medical care, and writing orders for medications, treatments, and patient activities that the pharmacist carries out. Therefore, the pharmacist does not have complete control of all of his or her exchange relationships with the patient and physician. In order to apply a marketing approach to pharmacy administration, internal and external markets with which the nursing division exchanges values must be identified, segmented, and analyzed. A marketing information and research program can be designed to systematically monitor the attitudes and desires of these markets so that strategies can be developed to satisfy them.

The attitudes, perceptions, needs, and wants of the market must be monitored in some systematic way so that strategies can be developed for satisfying them. This is done by means of various types of marketing research and feedback systems that collect, process, and analyze information. The motivation for new or continuing pharmacy services should not be emotional enthusiasm but marketing information that objectively identifies the potential markets, market needs, and financial feasibility of services.

The pharmacy director must consider present and future needs to forecast volume and frequency of demands for services, and the types of programs and services desired and required by patients, physicians, and staff. He or she must project the reimbursement demands, the numbers of pharmacy personnel, and the skills and knowledge personnel will need to meet at least some of the needs, preferences, and expectations of patients, physicians, and other markets. These demands are not created by market research, but their discovery can lead to a more efficient, effective, and appropriate exchange of values.

Qualitative Studies

Markets often have perceptions of their needs that differ from the pharmacy administrator's perceptions of their desires and expectations. In the qualitative phase, the market segments are given an opportunity to verify or challenge the administrator's assumptions. Feedback can be solicited from patients, families, visitors, nurses, physicians, personnel department, patient representatives, and others.

The director can use focus group discussions to identify general attitudes toward the services provided and those that are desired by patients or to identify pharmacy staff attitudes and needs. The in-depth individual interview may be used in lieu of focus group discussions or to clarify issues raised by a focus group.

Quantitative Studies

Questionnaires and brief personal or telephone interviews are the survey techniques most often used for quantitative market research. Existing internal and external sources should be tapped before new survey research instruments are developed so that market research studies complement existing marketing information rather than duplicate it. Because quantitative research can be very costly in time and money, it is essential that the pharmacy director seek expert assistance if he or she does not have the research skills necessary to plan and execute the studies. Even with careful design and sample selection, an internal market research study may be fraught with problems. Employees' biases may affect the way they ask questions of patients. The interviewed patient is subject to bias in some responses if he or she knows who is sponsoring the research. Confusing market research with promotion activities by attempting to educate or *sell* the target market under consideration is less likely to occur if market research experts are consulted. The bias of managers protecting their own turf must also be considered in evaluating market information and research. For example, a patient evaluation form designed with several levels of choice can provide ongoing data about patients' expectations and perceptions of pharmacy services.

Goals, Objectives, and Strategies

Goals and objectives flow from and must be consistent with the mission. There are differences of opinion about the definition of each. Goals are often described as long-term (5–15 years) accomplishments consistent with the mission. Objectives are often shorter term and should always be measurable. These terms are used interchangeably in practice, but within a department a commonly understood definition of both is essential.

Objectives form a specific expression of purpose, thus helping to remove any uncertainty about policy or about the intended purpose of any effort. Properly designed objectives permit measurement of progress and determination of whether adequate resources are being applied or whether these resources are being managed effectively. Finally, objectives facilitate the relationships between units, especially in a diversified department where the separate goals of different units (e.g., outpatient and home care) may not be consistent with some higher purpose.

Despite their overriding importance, defining objectives is far from easy. Defining goals as the future becomes the present is a time-consuming and continuous process. In practice, many pharmacy departments are run either without any commonly accepted objectives and goals or with conflicting objectives and goals. At times, the objectives may be defined in such general terms that their significance for the job is not understood.

Strategy in a pharmacy department is concerned with the basic goals and objectives of the business, the product-market matches chosen on which to compete, the major patterns of resource allocations, and the major operating policies used to relate the pharmacy to its institutional environment.

Each functional activity (e.g., marketing) makes its own unique contribution to strategy formulation at different levels. The marketing function represents the greatest degree of contact with the external environment, the environment least controllable.

In its strategic role, marketing consists of establishing a match between the department and its environment to seek solutions to problems of deciding how the chosen endeavor may be successfully run in a competitive environment by pursuing product, price, promotion, and distribution (see below) perspectives to serve target markets. Marketing provides the core element for future relationships between the department and its environment. It specifies inputs for defining objectives and helps in formulating plans to achieve them.

Strategy specifies the direction. Its intent is the evolution of the market to the advantage of the pharmacy and the parent institution. Thus, a strategy statement includes a description of the new competitive equilibrium to be created, the cause-and-effect relationships that will bring it about, and the logic to support the course of action. Planning articulates the means of implementing strategy. A strategic plan specifies the sequence and timing that will alter relationships.

Marketing Strategies

The fourth component of a marketing program is the management phase in which research information is translated into strategies and tactics that meet the markets' needs. In addition to the overall marketing strategy for the organization, subordinate strategies, or road maps, must be devised for each market segment if exchange relationships are to be managed to meet the pharmacy department's and consumers' long- and short-range objectives. Tactics are the programs used along the strategic path to accomplishing short-term objectives.

In a marketing approach to pharmacy, the target markets' needs and expectations, rather than those of the organization, guide nontechnical strategic decisions. When the actual service meets expectations, the consumer will be happy.

Marketing strategy involves decisions basic to the daily functioning of the nursing division: whom to serve, what services to offer; how to promote these services; where to serve; whom to hire; what to pay; and what to charge. Marketing strategy and tactics use combinations of the four elements known as *the four Ps* of the marketing mix: *product, promotion, place,* and *price*. These elements are the tools marketers use to satisfy markets.

The key to success in understanding and applying the marketing mix is having "the right product in the right place at the right time with the right promotion"—and for the right price. Marketing research and the management elements of planning, organizing, directing, and controlling are involved in developing the marketing objectives of the organization flow from these activities.

The definitions we use for the marketing mix components listed above are as follows:

- *Product*—The *benefits* or positive *results* that markets derive from using the services you offer in the way you offer them.

- *Promotion*—What markets are informed of the department's product, place, price and how.

- *Place*—The distribution channels and physical distribution practices through which markets use your services.

- *Price*—The total cost that markets must bear in order to use the services offered. (These are not necessarily monetary but may include time, inconvenience, etc.) Elaboration on these definitions follows.

Product

In marketing terms, a product is anything that fills a need or want and includes services, individuals, organizations, and ideas, in addition to physical objects. When the product is an idea, its exchange is called *social marketing*. Health care as a product has three components: services offered, physical characteristics of the institution, and personnel. It is the personnel who are most important to the patient markets.

There are four distinct characteristics of services that should be considered in planning service marketing strategies. Services are *intangible* commodities, requiring a measure of confidence in the provider's abilities. A service is *inseparable* from its provider and is consumed as it is produced. It is *perishable* and cannot be stored until it is needed. Finally, service quality is highly *variable* depending upon the abilities, and even the moods, of the provider.

The marketing strategy should include offering services that are desired by the marketplace, remembering that a consumer values a service in direct proportion to its perceived benefits. Services also should be distinguishable from those offered by competitors. If the pharmacy administrator does not believe that the services offered compare favorably with those of the competition, the services should be improved before being promoted.

Place

Place or distribution decisions are the second component of the marketing mix. As with the other elements of marketing strategy, place decisions are based on patient, physician, employee, and other target group preferences and not on what the pharmacy director wants to provide. The department must decide how to make its services accessible and available to the target markets. Place decisions involve what services will be offered in each location.

As part of place decisions, one should consider the concept of *atmospherics*: the intentional design of space to create feelings such as well-being, safety, and competence. Some of management's attitudes toward patients, visitors, employees, physicians, trustees, and the community will be perceived by these target groups through the facilities and conveniences provided for them.

Price

Price decisions include consideration of direct and indirect costs associated with a valued product or service. The price of a staff member to the organization involves wages, fringe benefits, recruitment and orientation costs, and some indirect costs such as managerial effort, waiting, and psychological costs. For patients, indirect costs may include discomfort, pain, anxiety, disruption of lifestyle, economic distress, costs of babysitters, and transportation. The director who can identify the total price of the exchange to both parties is more likely to achieve marketing success in the long run.

The director of pharmacy in many hospitals may be directly involved in setting fees and hospital rates, and it is very important that he or she understand how the prices for pharmacy services and pharmacy revenue centers are determined. There are three stages in setting prices. First, the price objective is determined: maximizing use or profits, cost recovery, fairness, and other goals. Second, pricing strategy must be planned based on competition, demand, or actual cost. The last stage considers whether price change is warranted and how such a change can be implemented. These stages also apply to wage and salary price decisions.

Often, the third-party payment system in the health care sector obscures the price of health services from users and providers. Third-party payers also limit the ability of health care providers to price services competitively, because penalties may be imposed when price reductions are implemented. Since physicians usually admit their patients to hospitals of the physician's choice, the voluntary exchange relationship of a free market is violated by both physicians and third-party payers.

Promotion

As the successful organization must do more than make attractive products and services available, promotional strategies are used to develop persuasive communication between the organization and its markets. The end result of this communication should meet the markets' needs as well as the organization's goals. Too often the promotion element of the marketing mix is thought of as *marketing* in and of itself.

An important caveat for the pharmacy administrator to remember is that "everything about the organization talks, but not all of it will promote the organization." Services, employees, facilities, actions, and attitudes communicate something about the pharmacy and the hospital organization. When these factors are recognized as sources of marketing promotion, their impact can be realistically assessed. Other forms of promotional efforts will not override the daily personal communication an organization has with its markets.

Evaluation

Evaluating the results of strategic and tactical programs is part of the management phase of marketing and may demonstrate a need for altering the marketing mix. Four levels of marketing outcomes can be assessed in the evaluation program: awareness, change of attitudes, conviction, and action or behavior. The director can measure marketing effectiveness by analyzing use of services and programs, revenues and expenses, patient compliance and satisfaction, turnover rates, number of unfilled positions, continuing education program attendance, and many more indicators. As program outputs are measured against marketing plans, new problems and challenges surface that need additional market research, different strategies and tactics, and further evaluation, all of which demonstrates the dynamic nature of marketing management.

Each pharmacy administrator should develop a marketing perspective and view marketing problems as a managerial responsibility. The organization has marketing problems when it fails to meet the desired exchange relationships with its markets. These problems exist when there is a gap between a target market's needs and what is offered by the pharmacy to patients, nursing staff, physicians, community, or regulating agencies. Unfortunately, pharmacy has not always viewed all of these groups as target markets. In the exchange with the patient, the fact that the patient is purchasing pharmacy service has been obscured by the way charges are billed as drug products.

The market planning model begins with an analysis of the needs, preferences, and perceptions of current and potential consumers as well as the capabilities of the organization. Marketing information and research are the basis for this analysis or audit. Specific strategies are determined for each market segment, following mission statements, goals, objectives, implementation of marketing plans, and evaluation.

A pharmacy director cannot undertake a marketing approach to pharmacy service without the support and commitment of the hospital administrator, board of trustees, staff, medical staff—the groups that are, in essence, the consumers as well as colleagues. To be committed and supportive, these groups must understand the rationale, purposes, goals, objectives, strategies, and tactics of marketing.

Internal Marketing

Sometimes, if not often, administrators are keenly aware of the need to market to their various external customers, but overlook the necessity of *internal* marketing (i.e., marketing within the pharmacy organization).

For most services, the server cannot be separated from the service. The accountant is a significant part of the accounting service, the physician a significant part of the medical service, and the pharmacist a vital part of the pharmacy service. In reality, customers "buy" the people when they buy a service. Service, after all, is a performance and the performance is often labor-intensive.

Thus, for labor-intensive service firms especially, the quality of employees influences the quality of service which, in turn, influences the effectiveness of services marketing. To practice services marketing successfully, pharmacy organizations must practice *internal marketing* successfully. They must market to their own employees and to employee prospects, competing as imaginatively and aggressively for internal customers as for external customers.

Internal marketing is attracting, developing, motivating, and retaining qualified employees through job-products that satisfy their needs. It is a *philosophy* of treating employees as customers and it is a *strategy* of shaping job-products to fit human needs.

The ultimate goal of internal marketing is to encourage effective marketing behavior; the ultimate goal is to build an organization of staff willing and able to create true customers for the firm. The ultimate strategy of internal marketing is to create true customers of employees. "A knowledgeable, satisfied employee is our best marketing agent."[4] Treat your employees the way you want them to treat your customers.

Thinking like a marketer cannot be restricted to external marketing. By satisfying the needs of its internal customers, an organization enhances its ability to satisfy the needs of its external customers. In this section, we present seven essentials in the practice of internal marketing.*

1. *Compete for Talent*—Hiring the best possible people to perform the service is a key factor in services marketing. Yet many pharmacy organizations act as though this were not the case. Many have ill-defined or too low standards for the personnel they hire.

   One of the principal causes of poor service quality is hiring the wrong people to perform the service. In one study conducted with customer-contact employees from five major commercial service firms, it was found that employees who felt their units were not meeting service standards also felt their company was not hiring people qualified to do their jobs.

Why do so many pharmacists permit the wrong people to carry the pharmacy flag in front of customers? Part of the answer is the failure to think and act like a marketer when it comes to human resource issues. The same organizations that compete intensively and imaginatively for customers often compete meekly and mundanely for employees.

Here are some recommendations: Aim high, use multiple methods, cast a wide net, and segment the market. It is tempting, given the intense competition for capable employees, to lower hiring standards. Smart marketers ignore this temptation and instead work harder than competitors to find the right people. Smart marketers aim high. They develop ideal candidate profiles for each type of position based on customer service expectations, and they use these profiles in recruiting candidates. They interview multiple candidates for one position, involve multiple employees in the interviewing process, and interview the more promising candidates on multiple occasions. They are tenacious in their pursuit of talent.

2. *Offer a Vision*—The attraction, development, motivation, and retention of quality employees require a clear vision worth pursuing. A paycheck may keep a person on the job physically, but it alone will not keep a person on the job emotionally. People delivering service need to know how their work fits in the broader scheme of operations, how their work contributes to the overall organization. They need to understand and believe in the goal to which they contribute; they need to have a cause because serving others is just too demanding and frustrating to be done well each day without one.

   Great internal marketing organizations stand for something worthwhile and they communicate this vision to employees with passion. *Passion* is a strange word to use in this context, but it is the word that best captures the fervent commitment to the goal-oriented values that distinguish the best internal marketing companies from others.

3. *Prepare People to Perform*—Preparing people to perform and market the service enhances every sub-goal of marketing: attracting, developing, motivating, and retaining superior employees.

---

* This section is based on the work of Berry LL, Parasuraman A. *Marketing Services*. New York: The Free Press; 1991.

Unfortunately, servers are often ill-prepared for the service role. They receive training, but it is too little, or too late, or not the kind of training they need. Or they may receive adequate technical skills training, but do not receive enough *knowledge*; they learn *how* but not *why*.

A common mistake is to view employee skills and knowledge development as events rather than an ongoing process. The inclination to put employees through a specific training program and then to consider them *trained* is both strong and wrong. Staff need to learn continuously as learning is a confidence builder, a motivating force, and a source of self-esteem. What managers perceive as unmotivated employee behavior is often *unconfident* employee behavior. Employees are unlikely to be motivated to perform services they do not feel competent and confident to perform.

4. *Stress Team Play*—Service work is demanding, frequently frustrating, and sometimes demoralizing. It is common for service providers to be so stressed by the service role that they become less caring, less sensitive, less eager to please. What customers perceive as impersonal or bureaucratic behavior is often the coping behavior of weary servers who have endured too many hurts in the real world of service delivery. In effect, the experience of serving becomes a negative.

One important dynamic in sustaining servers' motivation to serve is the presence of service *teammates*. An interactive community of coworkers who help each other, commiserate, and achieve together is a powerful antidote to service burnout. Team involvement can be rejuvenating, inspirational, and fun. It also raises the stakes for individual performance. Letting down the team may be worse than letting down the boss. Few motivators are more potent than the respect of teammates. Deep down, people want to identify with a group, to make a contribution, to express themselves and exercise their creativity. They want to strive together … to meet goals. They want to feel good about their jobs, because this translates into feeling good about themselves.

One way teamwork bolsters the will to serve is by enhancing the ability to serve. For servers to come through for their customers, others within the organization must come through for them. Teamwork enhances internal service.

The more people and functions involved in the chain of services leading to the end service, the greater the need for service teams. You have to ask, "How complex is the work?" The more complex, the more suited it is for teams.

5. *Leverage the Freedom Factor*—Human beings were not meant to be robots. Yet managers treat them this way when they use thick policy and procedure manuals to severely limit employees' freedom of action in delivering service. Rule book management undermines employees' confidence in managers, stifles employees' personal growth and creativity, and chases the most able employees out the door in search of more interesting work.

Rule book management usually does not benefit end-customers either. Un-empowered employees deliver regimented, "by-the-book" service when a creatively tailored "by-the-customer" service is really needed. While managers rein in servers, customers wish they could be served by "thinking servers."

Rules are needed, of course. We are not advocating the elimination of policies and procedures; what we are advocating is thinning the rule book to its bare essentials. Good internal marketing involves giving servers the opportunity to create for their customers and achieve for themselves.

Practicing the other facets of internal marketing encourages empowerment. A strong, well-defined vision guides employee behavior and fewer rules are needed. Skill and knowledge development gives employees the confidence to innovate for customers. The interdependencies and shared goals of team play stimulate individual initiative.

Empowering employees is not easy. Some employees would prefer everything spelled out so they would not have the additional pressure of creative problem-solving and the risk of making errors in judgment. It is, after all, less work and less risky to tell a customer that nothing can be done.

Pushing authority and responsibility downward into the organization, close to the customer, requires determination, patience, and conscious efforts to thin the rule book. Most service companies would benefit from task forces that review existing policies and procedures with the mandate to modify or discard those that unnecessarily restrict service freedom. Pharmacies would also benefit from training and education programs that teach front-line servers values, not just rules. And performance measurement and reward systems need to encourage creativity and initiative on behalf of customers.

6. *Measure and Reward*—The goals of internal marketing are thwarted if employee performance is not measured and rewarded. People at work need to know that they will be measured on how well they do and that it is worthwhile to do well. Job-products that offer the opportunity for achievement are most likely to fit the needs of human beings, yet achievement remains unidentified and uncelebrated without measurement and rewards.

Unfortunately, many service companies do a poor job of building an achievement culture. Performance measurement systems often focus exclusively on *output measures,* such as size or accuracy of transactions, and ignore *behavioral measures,* such as customer perception of the responsiveness or empathy of the service. Moreover, performance feedback to employees may be infrequent or not presented constructively. Sometimes measurement leads to no apparent consequence; the employees who perform well fare no better than others in compensation, advancement, or recognition.

Firms intent on rewarding the best performers often focus too narrowly on financial incentives and do not reap the benefits of multiple forms of recognition. The key to an effective reward system is an effective performance measurement system that identifies who deserves the rewards. An effective system measures performance that most contributes to the company's vision and strategy, and it does so in a clear, timely and fair manner. Convoluted or complicated systems fail to focus employee attention—one of the principal objectives of performance measurement. Infrequent feedback does not provide the regular reinforcement that the objectives of teaching and continual improvement require.

The feedback of service performance information to employees can be a powerful intervention strategy for behavioral management. In a surprisingly large number of cases, service employees have little idea of how they are doing. Regularly displayed feedback can keep employees aware of their performance and, as shown in the studies reviewed, lead them to increase desirable service behaviors.

Performance measurement and reward systems symbolize an organization's culture in a powerful way. Employees know that management measures and rewards are what are important. Thus, it is beneficial to disseminate performance measurement data to the appropriate senior executives. People in the trenches performing work that at least some of the time is intrinsically rewarding need to know that significant others in the organization will be aware of their performance.

Here are some reward-system guidelines:

- Link rewards to vision and strategy. Reward performance that moves the organization in the intended direction.

- Distinguish between competence pay (compensation for doing one's job) and performance pay (extra rewards for outstanding performance).

- Use multiple methods to reward outstanding performers, including financial rewards, non-financial recognition, and career advancement.

- Remember the power of a pat on the back. Rewards need not always be elaborate or expensive; the sincerity of the recognition is most important.

- Compete for the sustained commitment of employees. Develop enduring reward systems and use short-term programs such as sales contests sparingly or not at all.

- Stress the positive. Use reward systems to celebrate achievement rather than to punish.

- Give everyone a chance. Avoid the trap of rewarding people in some positions but not in other positions. Remember that *all* employees perform some kind of service for someone, their performance can be measured and they need the opportunity to excel and be recognized.

- Reward teams and not just individuals. Reinforce team play with team rewards, while also rewarding superior individual performers.

All but the smallest organizations have three groups of employees: those who, for whatever reason, are not performing well; those who are performing competently but not exceptionally;

and those who are outstanding. Effectively measuring and rewarding employee performance affects all three groups. Some members of the bottom group either leave or improve. Members of the middle group have reason to strive for improvement. And members of the top group are less likely to feel unappreciated and leave. Words alone won't work. What is measured and rewarded, recognized or promoted will work.

7. *Know Your Customers*—Marketing's oldest axiom is to know the customer. We spoke of this earlier in the section. Satisfying customers requires that decision-makers first understand their wants and needs. Employees are customers too, buying job-products from their employers. Designing job-products that attract, develop, motivate, and retain these internal customers demands sensitivity to their aspirations, attitudes, and concerns. Assumptions about what employees want and feel often are wrong, and practicing the art of marketing research is as important in internal marketing as in external marketing. Don't ask if you really don't want to hear. Don't ask if you only seek your preconceived answer. Value the input, value the participation, and explain why their ideas are being sought and how they will be used.

An organization can be only as good as its people. A service is a performance, and it is usually difficult to separate the performance from the people. If the people don't meet customers' expectations, then neither does the service. Investing in people quality in service business means investing in product quality.

To realize its potential in services marketing, a firm must realize its potential in internal marketing—the attraction, development, motivation, and retention of qualified employee-customers through need-meeting job-products. Internal marketing paves the way for external marketing services.

A Word about the Marketing of Pharmaceuticals

The reader is urged to consider the discussion of marketing concepts, provided early in the section, as they regard the activities of the pharmaceutical industry. The ultimate goal of *good* pharmaceutical marketing is to match patient needs with the best, most appropriate medication in an efficient and effective way. Not all pharmaceutical marketing practices and firms meet all of these criteria. Institutional pharmacists, noting inefficiencies and other inappropriate or ineffective practices have often established rules to control the marketing of pharmaceuticals in and to their institutions. The reader is urged only to work to assure that such rules, instituted for valid reasons, do not themselves interfere with the mutual achievement of the goal of the very best patient care.

Summary

Whether recognized or not, whether proactively practiced or not, marketing is a part of institutional pharmacy practice. Recognition of the need for marketing and effective implementation of a marketing program will result in better pharmacy services and better patient care.

References

1. American Marketing Association. AMA board approves new marketing definition. *Marketing News.* 1985; 21(5):1.

2. Hillestad SG, Berkowitz EN. *Health Care Marketing Plans: From Strategy to Action.* Homewood, IL: Dow Jones-Irwin; 1984.

3. Pathak, D. Introduction to pharmaceutical marketing. In: Smith, MC. *Principles of Pharmaceutical Marketing.* Philadelphia: Lea and Febiger; 1983.

4. Berry LL. Parasuraman A. *Marketing Services.* New York: The Free Press; 1991.

Chapter 40

Integrity of the U.S. Drug Supply

*Thomas J. McGinnis, Ilisa B.G. Bernstein**

Overview of the U.S. Drug Distribution System

The intricate web of federal and state laws has created a drug distribution network in the United States that instills high public confidence in the delivery of safe and effective drug products. This network is a *closed* system that involves several entities, including Food and Drug Administration (FDA) registered manufacturers and state licensed wholesalers and pharmacies. These entities move drug products from the point of manufacture to patients and provide the American public with multiple levels of protection against receiving unsafe, ineffective, or poor quality medications. This system evolved over the last century as a result of legislative requirements that drugs be treated as potentially dangerous consumer goods that require professional and regulatory oversight to protect the public health. The result has been a level of safety and quality assurance for drug products that is widely recognized as the world's "gold standard."

The current regulatory system for drug distribution offers several layers of protection and quality assurance of the drug products within the system. First, as required under the Food, Drug, and Cosmetic Act (FD&C Act), FDA maintains high standards for drug approval. Second, once the drug is approved, the manufacturer must continue to comply with current Good Manufacturing Practice (GMP) regulations to ensure that the quality of the product is consistent throughout the manufacturing process. Third, the specific registered facility where the product is manufactured remains subject to periodic inspection by FDA. Fourth, pharmacies and wholesalers who sell or distribute drug products in the U.S. must be licensed or authorized by the states in which they operate and are subject to inspection. Fifth, there are limited channels of entry into the American drug supply, thereby reducing the opportunity to place counterfeit or poor quality medications into the U.S. commercial distribution system. However, once a product leaves this closed system, FDA and the states' ability to assure that it is an authentic FDA-approved product or that it has been properly handled is significantly hampered.

Entities Involved in Drug Distribution

Manufacturers

Drug manufacturers may be small businesses or multinational giants with global operations and sales. Regardless of their size, drug manufacturers making medications for sale in the U.S. must register with FDA, list their drugs with FDA, and be subject to FDA inspection. They must also comply with rigorous good manufacturing practice regulations. Often, an FDA-approved product may be manufactured in a facility outside of the U.S. Even in these instances, the facility must be registered with and inspected by FDA. FDA periodically samples products in the distribution system to test them against standards for the product. Failure to meet the standards usually results in recall of the product from the drug distribution system by the manufacturer of the product.

Wholesalers

Currently, there are three large wholesalers who account for about 90% of the primary drug wholesale market. In addition, there are an estimated 7,000 regional and small wholesalers who may have full or partial product lines and sell nationally or regionally. Some of these wholesalers concentrate in the *secondary* wholesale market (i.e., they purchase drug products from wholesalers and resell to other wholesalers, including large wholesalers, as well as to hospitals and retail pharmacies). A wholesaler may purchase from another wholesaler for several reasons, for example: (1) to take advantage of price discounts available on certain legitimate drug products, (e.g., when a manufacturer or wholesaler has a temporary overstock or a wholesaler purchases excessive product on speculation that the manufacturer will raise prices); (2) for low

---

*The views and opinions expressed here do not represent those of the Food and Drug Administration.

volume transactions (e.g., involving drugs that are used only occasionally or in special populations); (3) when a quick turnaround is needed, (e.g., to meet a temporary or unexpected increase in demand for a drug); or (4) to sell to a remote area (e.g., a small rural community). Wholesalers are licensed and inspected by the state board of pharmacy or other state authority, such as a department of health. Wholesalers who repackage or relabel drugs must register with FDA and are subject to inspection.

Pharmacies

Pharmacies are at the end of the closed distribution chain. The pharmacist dispenses the drug to the patient upon receipt of a valid prescription written by a licensed practitioner authorized by the state to prescribe prescription drugs. At this point in the drug distribution chain the drug is still expected to conform to FDA-approved specifications so that pharmacists can assure their patients that the drug being dispensed meets strength, quality, and purity standards and is safe and effective. Unfortunately, over the years, pharmacists have been involved in compromising the integrity of the distribution system by buying prescription drugs from manufacturers or wholesalers who operate outside of the legitimate, closed U.S. distribution system.

Figure 40-1 depicts three models showing the movement of drugs through the U.S. drug distribution system (the dotted lines indicate potential illegal sales).

In the simplest situation, the manufacturer sells directly to a pharmacy. However, in many instances, there can be one or more wholesalers, or even a repackager, who handles the drug before it reaches the pharmacy. It is in these intermediate steps that the greatest opportunities for compromising the security of the U.S. distribution system exist. It is the "Achilles' Heel" of an otherwise closed distribution system.

Regulatory Framework for Drug Distribution in the U.S.

The movement of drugs through the supply chain is overseen and enforced by federal and state regulatory authorities. FDA has jurisdiction over the drug products themselves, including how and where they are manufactured, labeled, packaged, and held, and over the entities that handle the drug products in the supply chain. However, the states are primarily responsible for oversight of wholesalers, pharmacies, and pharmacists.

Federal

There have been a number of cases over the years regarding counterfeit and diverted prescription drugs. However, in 1985, two incidents alerted Congress to the need to take steps to ensure greater control over the drug distribution system in the U.S. First, over 2 million counterfeit tablets of a birth control pill entered the U.S. supply chain from Panama and were distributed throughout the U.S. That same year, a counterfeit version of Ceclor™, a widely used antibiotic, found its way into the U.S. drug distribution system from a foreign source.

As a result, in 1987 Congress enacted the Prescription Drug Marketing Act (PDMA). Among other things, the PDMA requires that wholesalers of prescription drugs be licensed by the state. The PDMA also requires wholesalers to provide a statement of origin, also known as a drug *pedigree*, which contains information about each prior sale, trade, or purchase of the prescription drug and accompanies that product to subsequent wholesalers who sell, trade, or purchase that drug and who add information to the pedigree. The pedigree information accompanies the drug product up to and including its sale to a retail pharmacy. Under the PDMA, manufacturers and certain *authorized* wholesale distributors are exempt from providing or transmitting a pedigree for a particular drug product on to the next entity that purchases the drug. Authorized distributors are wholesalers who have an ongoing relationship with the manufacturer for a particular drug product.

In 1999, FDA published final regulations that, among other things, clarified specific pedigree requirements. FDA subsequently stayed the provisions concerning the pedigree requirements (21 CFR §§203.3 (q), (u) and 203.50) because of concerns expressed by industry, trade associations, and Congress about problems related to passing a pedigree on between wholesalers. Such concerns included the high cost and logistical problems associated with maintaining and providing or transmitting a pedigree, and the potential for record-keeping failures and counterfeiting the paper pedigree document itself. However, the requirement for unauthorized wholesale distributors to transmit a pedigree to all wholesale customers is contained in the PDMA statute itself and remains in effect.

In 2004, FDA announced that it would continue to stay the implementation of these provisions of the regulations until December 2006 in order to give industry

Figure 40-1
Drug Distribution Models

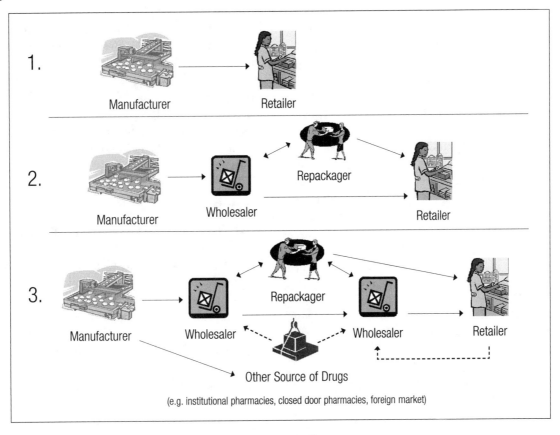

1. Manufacturer → Retailer

2. Manufacturer → Wholesaler → Repackager → Retailer

3. Manufacturer → Wholesaler → Repackager → Wholesaler → Retailer

Other Source of Drugs
(e.g. institutional pharmacies, closed door pharmacies, foreign market)

time to move toward implementing an electronic pedigree. FDA is monitoring the industry's progress toward development of an electronic system to track and trace a product through the supply chain from the point of manufacture to the end user of the drug product (see section Securing the Integrity of the Drug Supply Chain, below, for further discussion on electronic track and trace). In 2006, FDA will determine whether to further stay the pedigree regulations or take other appropriate action.

State Authority

Each state has its own laws and regulations governing the sale, distribution, storage, and handling of drug products. Each state also has its own licensing and registration system for pharmacists and wholesale distributors. The scope and coverage of these systems varies from state to state.

Many states have or are in the process of strengthening their state requirements governing the licensure

and oversight of wholesale drug distributors. The National Association of Boards of Pharmacy (NABP) recently updated their Model Rules for Licensure of Wholesale Distributors. These model rules serve as a template law for states to adopt and include stronger measures to ensure the legitimacy and integrity of wholesalers (e.g., disclosure requirements, background checks, due diligence before transacting business, posting of a bond), to reduce incentives for counterfeiting (e.g., increased penalties), and measures to ensure the integrity of the drug product (e.g., pedigree requirements, use of authentication technologies, and strengthened storage, handling, and record-keeping requirements).

Integrity/Concerns of the Prescription Drug Supply Chain

On its face, it appears that the distribution chain for drug products in the United States is fairly straightforward: manufacturers sell their products to whole-salers, who in turn sell the products to hospitals, other health care institutions, or retail pharmacies, who in turn dispense medicines to patients upon receipt of prescriptions. It is not until the system is studied in greater detail that one begins to appreciate the complexities and vulnerability of the distribution chain and the potential for exploitation or abuse.

Even though the U.S. drug distribution system is among the safest in the world, vulnerabilities in the system create opportunities for unscrupulous activity. In 2004, FDA released the Counterfeit Drug Task Force Report, which describes several of these vulnerabilities. Such activities include counterfeiting, diversion, incomplete or fraudulent pedigrees, inadequate or lack of authentication of the drug product, repackaging, tamper-evident packaging requirements for OTC drugs, and illegal importation.

Counterfeit Drugs

Counterfeiting of medications is a particularly devious practice. Drug counterfeiters not only defraud consumers, they also deny ill patients the therapies that can alleviate their suffering and save their lives. In some countries, counterfeiting is endemic, with some consumers having a better chance of getting a fake medicine than a real one. In the U.S., a relatively comprehensive system of laws, regulations, and enforcement by federal and state authorities has kept counterfeiting rare. In recent years, however, there have been growing efforts by well-organized counterfeiters who use sophisticated technologies and well-financed criminal operations to profit from drug counterfeiting at the expense of American consumers. Figure 40-2 illustrates that the number of counterfeit cases FDA has opened over the last 7 years has been rising steadily.

Diversion

Diversion is the sale of drugs outside of the distribution channels for which they were originally intended. Diverted drugs can originate domestically, when there is illegal redirection of drugs from otherwise legitimate sources. For example, free samples supplied to health care providers or lower-priced drugs intended for non-profit clinics, hospitals or Medicaid programs may be diverted and illegally sold into the U.S. distribution system. Diverted drugs can also originate from a foreign country. For example, diversion occurs when donated or lower-priced product that is intended for use in one country is, instead, shipped to and sold in another country where the market price is higher. Counterfeit drugs also are associated with the practice of diversion. Diversion facilitates the entry of counterfeit drugs into the U.S. distribution system. Those individuals or entities that sell or purchase diverted drugs are less able to verify the integrity of these drugs because they are purchased outside the normal distribution chain and without the usual regulatory safeguards. This allows unscrupulous peddlers to commingle authentic drugs with counterfeit, substandard, or otherwise adulterated or misbranded products in the U.S. distribution system.

Incomplete Pedigrees

A pedigree is a statement of origin that traces the drug from the point of manufacture and contains information about all transactions related to the distribution of the product until it reaches the end user. It is also referred to as *chain-of-custody* documentation. Not all wholesalers are required to provide pedigrees under federal law. However, when they are required, products with incomplete pedigrees, such as pedigrees that are missing one or more transactions along the chain of distribution, are more difficult to track and trace to establish authenticity than products that have complete pedigree information.

Inadequate or No Authentication

It is important for purchasers in the U.S. drug distribution chain to have confidence that the products they are purchasing are genuine. One method of determining whether a drug is genuine is by product authentication. Counterfeiters are using tools and processes to copy drug products and their labeling and packaging to such an exact degree that even the manufacturer of the authentic product has difficulty determining whether a product is real or fake. On the other hand, there are new and emerging technologies that can be used to identify counterfeits. Unfortunately, these authenticating technologies often are not incorporated into the drug product, labeling, or packaging.

Repackaging

Many drugs in the distribution system are also *repackaged*. In the U.S., wholesale drugs in bulk containers are often repackaged into smaller containers prior to sale to a pharmacy. Repackaging operations are per-

Figure 40-2
Counterfeit Drug Cases Opened by FDA per Year

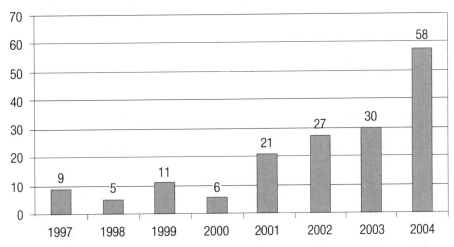

formed by independent entities, wholesale distributors, or by distribution centers owned by large pharmacies. In the current distribution system products are repackaged for several legitimate reasons, such as to improve efficiencies for automated systems or to make unit dose packages. In Europe, products are packaged by the original manufacturer in quantities that relate to a course of treatment (*unit of use*), usually obviating the need for repackaging. Repackaging may destroy the anticounterfeiting measures used in the original packaging and labeling of the drug. It may also provide a point of entry for expired, adulterated, or counterfeit drugs into the distribution system because they may be repackaged in a way that makes them appear to be legitimate products.

Tamper-Evident Packaging

Currently, prescription drug products are not required to utilize the tamper-evident features that are required for OTC drug packaging. Without tamper-evident features, the original packaging may be reused for counterfeit or diverted product and thereby be more easily passed off as legitimate product. The reuse of old prescription drug containers found in trash facilities or taken from hospitals and clinics is also a significant problem because no tamper-evident feature has to be replicated, thereby enabling easy reuse of the packaging to distribute counterfeit, adulterated, or unapproved drugs. While tamper-evident packaging is important, it is also worth noting that counterfeit drugs can be

repackaged into legitimate-appearing packaging (including features intended to mimic legitimate tamper-evident features), so that packaging alone cannot assure that drugs have not been counterfeited or are not otherwise unsuitable for human use.

Importation of Drugs through the Mail or Courier Services

When consumers purchase medications from outside the U.S. (e.g., Internet purchases, cross-border purchases), a portal of entry is created for counterfeit or substandard drugs to enter into the U.S. distribution system. For example, counterfeiters can take advantage of this entryway by combining many small purchases of drugs from foreign countries into one unit and selling the consolidated unit to U.S. wholesalers or other unsuspecting entities. Due to the extensive resources involved in preventing small quantities of drugs from entering the U.S., as the volume of unapproved drug imported through the mail or courier services increases, it is more difficult for FDA and Customs and Border Protection to use their existing resources to identify and stop unsafe importations. The FDA and the states do not have oversight or authority over the foreign marketplace. Under current law, the FDA only has authority over foreign manufacturers when they submit to FDA oversight as part of a new drug application (NDA; see 21 USC 355). In addition, under current law, FDA has no authority to inspect or assess the practices used in foreign drug distribution systems. Obtaining drugs from a foreign distribution system further exacerbates the existing vulnerabilities that facilitate domestic diversion. However, unlike entities engaged in domestic diversion, counterfeiters located in foreign countries generally remain outside the reach of U.S. law enforcement.

Securing the Integrity of the Drug Supply Chain

Counterfeiting of prescription drugs is a growing global concern. To respond to this emerging threat, FDA developed a comprehensive framework of ways to combat counterfeiting. Because no one measure will solve this problem, FDA's Counterfeit Drug Task Force Report calls for a multilayered strategy, with cooperation by all participants in the drug supply chain and consumers.

Counterfeiters are increasingly sophisticated in the methods they use to introduce finished dosage form counterfeits into the otherwise legitimate U.S. drug distribution system. Some criminal operations seek to introduce finished drug products that closely resemble legitimate drugs yet may contain only inactive ingredients, incorrect ingredients, improper dosages, subpotent or superpotent ingredients, or are contaminated. To counter these threats, the U.S. drug supply chain is moving toward greater use of anticounterfeiting measures to protect the product and the public health.

Anticounterfeiting Measures

Authentication Technologies

Authentication technologies are used to verify that a product is genuine and not a fake. Manufacturers are currently using a variety of authentication technologies on a product-by-product basis. Authentication technologies may be overt (easily visible to the eye, such as color shifting inks and holograms), covert (not visible to the eye, requiring special equipment to visualize, such as chemical markers, fluorescent inks, and invisible bar codes), or forensic (not visible to the eye, requiring sophisticated analytic equipment to identify, such as taggants and chemical markers). Figure 40-3 lists authentication technologies that are used or may be used in the future for drug products. Pharmacists and consumers could easily identify overt technologies. However, special equipment (e.g., readers) or forensic analysis would be needed to authenticate the product, packaging, or labeling on which covert technologies are used. An important consideration of manufacturers

incorporating authentication technologies into the product, packaging, or labeling is that it increases the cost of drug product. In addition, because enterprising counterfeiters can eventually defeat many anticounterfeiting technologies, these technologies must be changed at frequent intervals. Consequently, not all products will use authentication technologies and manufacturers may do a cost-benefit analysis to determine if the cost justifies the measures.

Manufacturers are just starting to incorporate overt and covert technologies in drugs likely to be counterfeited. However, an infrastructure for authenticating products with authentication technologies is not available yet in the U.S. To be most useful for the U.S. drug distribution system, all entities would have to have the ability to authenticate the product. This means that they would need appropriate devices to authenticate covert measures, know what the legitimate overt measures are on the genuine product and how to authenticate those measures, and an up-to-date system for communicating changes since manufacturers will need to change authentication measures frequently to stay ahead of counterfeiters.

Track and Trace Technologies

Track and trace technologies are used to follow and monitor the movement of a product as it travels through the distribution system. Typically, a unique number is assigned to packages, cases, or pallets of drugs. The unique number can be incorporated into radio frequency identification (RFID) electronic tag or into a bar code. The unique number is then read and associated with other product-specific information that is in a database, which can be used to verify that the

Figure 40-3
Types of Anticounterfeiting Technologies

Authentication Technologies	Tracking Technologies
■ Taggants ■ Substance ■ Watermark ■ Planchettes ■ Optical Pigments & Dyes ■ Inks ■ Holograms	■ Radio Frequency Identification Devices (RFID) ■ Bar codes

product is authentic and to list all of the transactions associated with the product, thereby creating an electronic pedigree. RFID involves the attachment of electromagnetic chips/tags that contain specific product information and a unique serial number, called a *license plate*. Figure 40-4 shows the flow of the RFID-enabled drug product through the drug supply chain. The RFID system includes the tags, antennae affixed to the tags, readers to receive data from the tags, and an information database that is used to manage the data. Figure 40-5 shows an example of an RFID tag and antenna. RFID may be the most promising way to accomplish product track and trace because it does not require line-of-sight reading and has numerous associated benefits, including inventory management, theft control, recall management, and reduced labor costs due to automation. Several efforts are underway to test the feasibility of RFID use in the drug supply chain. RFID technology is already in use on some highway toll booths to electronically collect tolls and, thus, speed traffic flow, with RFID tags placed on the automobile windshield and the tag readers placed in toll booths. Airports are also starting to RFID tag luggage to make sorting and tracking more efficient.

What Pharmacists Can Do to Protect against Counterfeit Medications

Pharmacists are in an important position to protect patients from receiving counterfeit drugs. They are the last stop, or gatekeepers, before a counterfeit drug reaches the patient. Pharmacists should take steps to minimize the risk of exposure to counterfeit drugs, be vigilant in their efforts to identify suspect counterfeit drugs, know how to counsel patients if a counterfeit drug is suspected or identified, and report suspect counterfeit drugs to FDA or the drug manufacturer.

Minimize the Risk

There are several steps that pharmacists can take to minimize the risk of drug diversion or the entry of counterfeit drugs into their drug supply. The American Society of Health-System Pharmacists suggests that hospital or other institutional pharmacy managers reevaluate their pharmacy security measures and consider the following:

- Monitoring access by cameras and ID readers
- Using automated supply stations where additional controls are needed

Figure 40-4
Flow of RFID Tagged Product through Supply Chain

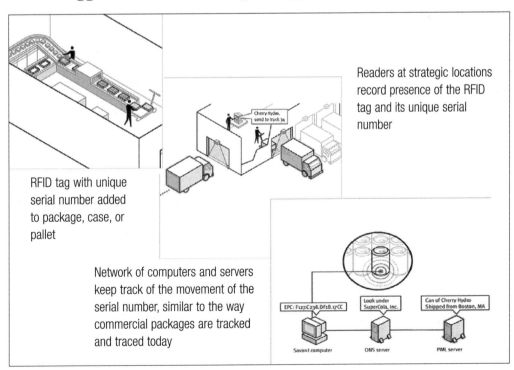

Readers at strategic locations record presence of the RFID tag and its unique serial number

RFID tag with unique serial number added to package, case, or pallet

Network of computers and servers keep track of the movement of the serial number, similar to the way commercial packages are tracked and traced today

Figure 40-5
Sample RFID Tags

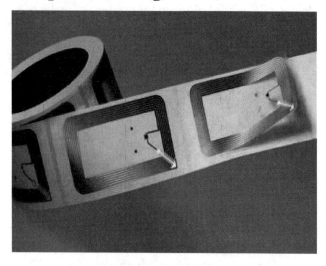

- Assuring delivery of drugs directly to the pharmacy, not to a loading dock
- Altering drug packages for products in inventory to make them less resellable (e.g., mark the box with the hospital name; tear off box tops)
- Completely destroying empty drug packages and vials so that they cannot be removed from the trash and refilled with counterfeit product
- Removing drugs considered at risk for diversion from floor stock
- Reconciling purchasing records with billing or administration records
- Assuring that staff placing drug orders are not *receiving* inventory
- Using sequential purchase order numbers to increase accountability
- Using invoice approval as an additional verification of appropriate purchasing
- Safeguarding drug product returns to help minimize unguarded access by counterfeiters

In addition, pharmacy purchasers must know with whom they are doing business. They must ensure that the wholesalers they buy from are state licensed and legitimate. Pharmacists should be suspicious of secondary wholesalers with whom no previous business relationship exists, especially when those wholesalers offer products that are in short supply or when their prices are suspiciously low. Pharmacists should also review policies for medication acquisition with the pharmacy and therapeutics committee at their institution to assure that necessary controls are in place.

Be Vigilant to Identify Suspect Counterfeits

Pharmacy staff should be educated about the problem of counterfeiting and how to identify situations in which they should suspect a counterfeit drug. Pharmacists should investigate whenever a patient has an atypical adverse event, unusual side effect(s), or unexplained treatment failure in order to determine if a counterfeit or defective drug may be the cause. They should be alert to changes in drug manufacturing or packaging and inform patients of these changes made by the manufacturer. It is important for pharmacists to take comments and complaints about products seriously, investigate them promptly, and report them when deemed necessary. Many counterfeit products have been discovered only after patients complained of a change in effectiveness, a change in the taste of their oral medication, or that an injection was stinging when it had never stung before. All of these complaints by patients have led to the discovery of counterfeit products in the drug distribution system. Pharmacists should be mindful that expensive drug products and drugs in short supply are more likely to be counterfeited or diverted than other medications. Box 40-1 lists some counseling points for patients.

Pharmacists should pay particular attention to products considered to be at high risk for counterfeiting. The NABP maintains a national list of drugs highly likely to be counterfeited. The list is shown in Box 40-2. This list is routinely updated as needed and can be found at www.nabp.net.

Box 40-1
Counseling Points for Pharmacists

Patients should be told to contact their pharmacist or health care provider if:

- They experience new or unusual side effects
- The drug looks, tastes, or smells abnormal
- They experience pain or redness that is out of the ordinary at the site of injection
- Their signs and symptoms persist or recur with continued treatment

Reporting

Suspect counterfeit drugs should be reported promptly to FDA's MedWatch program or the drug's manufacturer. MedWatch is an FDA program for voluntary reporting of adverse events and product problems related to drugs, devices, and dietary supplements. Reports can be made to MedWatch from FDA's website at www.fda.gov/medwatch or by calling 1-800-442-1088. FDA and the manufacturer typically work together to determine whether the product in question is counterfeit or genuine.

Summary

Patients must have confidence that the drugs they take are safe and effective. The U.S. drug distribution system is one of the safest, most highly regulated, and sophisticated systems in the world. In order to maintain its high degree of integrity, the drug distribution system and the entities involved, including manufacturers, wholesalers, and pharmacists, must continue to evolve as modern challenges threaten this integrity.

References

1. The prescription drug marketing act report to congress. Rockville, MD: FDA; June 2001. Available at: http://www.fda.gov/oc/pdma/report2001/.

2. *FDA Counterfeit Drug Task Force Interim Report.* Rockville, MD: FDA. October 2003.

3. *HHS Task Force on Drug Importation: Report on Prescription Drug Importation.* Washington, DC: Department of Health and Human Services; December 2004.

4. First interim report of the seventeenth statewide grand jury. In the Supreme Court of the State of Florida. Case No: SC02-2645. February 2003.

5. Second interim report of the seventeenth statewide grand jury: report on recipient fraud in Florida's Medicaid program. In the Supreme Court of the State of Florida. Case No: SC02-2645. December 2003.

6. *Model Rules for Licensure of Wholesale Distributors.* Mt. Prospect, IL: National Association of Boards of Pharmacy; February 20, 2004.

7. Combating counterfeit drugs: a report of the Food and Drug Administration, February 2004. Available at: http://fda.gov/oc/omotoatoves/counterfeit/report02_04.html.

8. Board of directors report on the council on professional affairs. ASHP House of Delegates session. 2004. Available at: http://www.ashp.org/aboutashp/PolicyGovernance/CouncilsComms/COPA.pdf.

Box 40-2
NABP National Specified List of Susceptible Products[a]

- Combivir® (lamivudine/zidovudine)
- Crixivan® (indinavir)
- Diflucan® (fluconazole)
- Epivir® (lamivudine)
- Epogen® (epoetin alfa)
- Gamimune® (globulin, immune)
- Gammagard® (globulin, immune)
- Immune globulin
- Lamisil® (terbinafine)
- Lipitor® (atorvastatin)
- Lupron® (leuprolide)
- Neupogen® (filgrastim)
- Nutropin AQ® (somatropin, E-coli derived)
- Panglobulin® (globulin, immune)
- Procrit® (epoetin alfa)
- Retrovir® (zidovudine)

- Risperdal® (risperidone)
- Rocephin® (ceftriaxone)
- Serostim® (somatropin, mannalian derived)
- Sustiva® (efavirenz)
- Trizivir® (abacavir/lamivudine/zidovudine)
- Venoglobulin® (globulin, immune)
- Viagra® (sildenafil)
- Videx® (didanosine)
- Viracept® (nelfinavir)
- Viramune® (nevirapine)
- Zerit® (stavudine)
- Ziagen® (abacavir)
- Zocor® (simvastatin)
- Zofran® (ondansetron)
- Zoladex® (goserelin)
- Zyprexa® (olanzapine)

[a] As of Jan. 2005. Go to www.nabp.net for most current list.

9. Board of directors report on the council on administrative affairs. ASHP House of Delegates session. 2004. Available at: http://www.ashp.org/aboutashp/ PolicyGovernance/CouncilsComms/COAA.pdf.

10. ASHP strategies to protect against drug counterfeiting. October 6, 2003. Available at: www.ashp.org/practice manager/ashp/anti-counterfeitingstrategies.pdf.

11. *Pharmaceutical Anticounterfeiting Insight Report.* Greenwood Village, CO: Lew Kontnik Associates; April 20, 2004.

12. Consent decree for condemnation and permanent injunction. In the United States District Court for the Northern District of Illinois Eastern Division. Case No 03 C 6495.

13. New FDA initiative to combat counterfeit drugs. Rockville, MD: FDA. Available at: http://www.fda.gov /oc/initiatives/counterfeit/backgrounder.html.

14. Young, D. FDA embraces RFID to protect drug supply. *Am J Health-Syst Pharm.* Dec 2004;61:2612.

15. NABP educates pharmaceutical industry on new VAWD program. News release. Mt. Prospect, IL: National Association of Boards of Pharmacy; November 11, 2004.

16. NABP and FDA Partner on combating counterfeit drugs. News release. Mt. Prospect, IL: National Association of Boards of Pharmacy; February 18, 2004.

17. Electronic safety net: NABP exploring the creation of a clearinghouse for pedigree data. News release. Mt. Prospect, IL: National Association on Boards of Pharmacy; November 16, 2004.

18. FDA. Prescription Drug Marketing Act of 1987: Final Rule. 64 Federal Register 67720. December 3, 1999.

19. FDA. Prescription Drug Marketing Act of 1987. Final Rule: Delay of Effective Date. 69 Federal Register 8105. February 23, 2004.

Index, continued

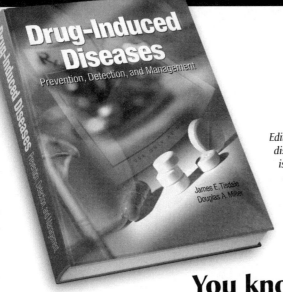
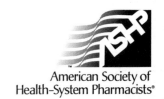